PSYCHIATRIC DISORDERS – TRENDS AND DEVELOPMENTS

Edited by **Toru Uehara**

Psychiatric Disorders – Trends and Developments
Edited by Toru Uehara

Published by InTech
Janeza Trdine 9, 51000 Rijeka, Croatia

Publishing Process Manager Ivana Zec

Technical Editor Teodora Smiljanic

Cover Designer InTech Design Team

Additional hard copies can be obtained from orders@intechopen.com

Psychiatric Disorders – Trends and Developments, Edited by Toru Uehara
p. cm.
ISBN 978-953-307-745-1

For EU product safety concerns:
IN TECH d.o.o., Prolaz Marije Krucifikse Kozulić 3, 51000 Rijeka, Croatia,
info@intechopen.com or visit our website at intechopen.com.

Meet the editor

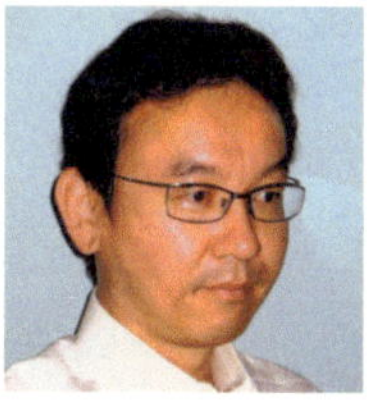

Dr. Toru Uehara is currently an Associate Professor of mental health at the General Health Support Centre, Gunma University, Japan. He has been working in the area of neuropsychiatry, psychosomatic medicine and clinical psychology for over 20 years and published over 60 papers in English peer-reviewed journals, over 80 in Japanese journals, as well as 35 invited chapters in books. He is a board member of several Japanese societies or associations in these fields. His research and clinical interests focus on child and adolescent psychiatry, eating disorders, expressed emotion, family psychoeducation, neuroimaging, diagnosis and evaluations, psychosocial factors and campus mental health.

Contents

Preface

Due to their prevalence, pervasiveness and burden inflicted on men and women of today, psychiatric disorders are considered as one of the most important, sever and painful illnesses. This impairment of cognitive, emotional, or behavioural functioning is in some cases tragic. Aside from knowing the physical organic factors, such as infections, endocrinal illnesses or head injuries, the aetiology of psychiatric disorders has remained a mystery. However, recent advances in psychiatry and neuroscience have been successful in discovering subsequent pathophysiology and reaching associated bio-psycho-social factors.

This book consists of recent trends and developments in psychiatry from all over the world, presented in the form of multifarious and comprehensive articles. The first two sections of the book are reserved for articles on schizophrenia and depression, two major illnesses present in this field. The third section of the book is reserved for addiction psychiatry, related not only to socio-cultural but also biological alterations. The last section of the book, titled "Biological Neuropsychiatry", consists of three topics - updated molecular biology, fundamental neuroscience and clinical neuropsychiatric conditions. Doubtlessly, this book will be fruitful for future developments and collaboration in "world psychiatry".

In the first section, "Schizophrenia", Dr. Somenarain describes how the prefrontal cortex (PFC) controls the activity of many subcortical structures via the excitatory axons of pyramidal neurons. Cognitive behaviour and motor planning are also investigated. The author presents novel findings about PFC and schizophrenia according to decreases of microtubule-associated proteins, loss of dendrites and spines, decreases in neurogranin and the role of antipsychotic drugs. Dr. Jutzeler et al. review the characteristics in schizophrenia of event-related potentials and current preclinical models of Electroencephalogram abnormalities. The authors discuss potential requirements of future model and methods to provide insight into pathophysiological mechanism and facilitate the development of new treatments. Dr. Carlino et al. perform a meta-analysis of studies measuring serum concentrations of Brain-derived neurotrophic factor to elucidate whether or not this neurotrophin is abnormally produced in patients with schizophrenia. Additionally, the authors identified factors that might contribute to different findings in literature. Dr. Krzystanek et al. describe their data on "Neurocognitive Expression of Hypofrontality in Long Term Schizophrenia", and suggest that creating the treatment strategy considered hypofunction of the N-methyl-D-aspartic acid receptor model can be a new research direction. Dr. Douma et al. discuss experimental data in chapter "Linking Stress and Schizophrenia: a Focus on Prepulse Inhibition". Professor Gregoric Kumperscak focuses on childhood and adolescent schizophrenia and other early-onset psychoses, and concludes that early-onset schizophrenia has worse prognosis than the adult-onset one; early diagnosis followed by treatment is essential. As the author indicates, to diagnose schizophrenia properly, a thorough knowledge of negative and positive symptoms, prodromal state symptom varieties, as well as full range of normal developmental changes is indispensable. Dr. Verhaegen et al. discuss "Verbal Behavior Analysis as a Diagnostic and Psychopharmacological Strategy for Differentiating Paranoid and Disorganized Schizophrenics" and describe potential relationship between these discontinuities, syndrome's specificities and how they relate to the question of incoherence. The authors emphasize pragmatic, cognitive, and formal methodology for dialogue analysis to specify and differentiate between the various schizophrenic syndromes.

In the second section, "Depression", Dr. Dedic et al. introduce some basic concepts with respect to the question what and how animal models are able to contribute to our understanding of mood disorders, and give an overview of the most popular behavioural tests and mouse models with a particular focus on major depression. Also, the authors review latest views on the importance of introducing gene/environment interactions into animal models of etiologic relevance. Dr. Benton and Dr. Whiltshire discuss several key molecular and neurochemical alterations that have been linked with depressive disorder, and present future directions for biological alterations in depression. Msc. Pereira et al. give us a comprehensive review of epidemiological and clinical aspects in developed and developing countries about depression during pregnancy. Dr. Guiard summarizes a new class of antidepressants in the treatment of psychiatric disorders, and describes serotonergic, noradrenergic and dopaminergic pathways in the brain, as well as specific symptoms of depression. The author addresses the possibility that triple reuptake inhibitors may exert part of their antidepressant activity by preventing/reversing algesia in depressed patients.

In the third section, "Addiction psychiatry", we can read powerful articles which cover many issues around substance abuse. Prof. Lurigio mentions that drug abuse and dependence disorders are chronic but treatable brain diseases, involving compulsive drug-seeking and drug-using behaviors that persist despite immediate or potentially harmful consequences for users and their families and communities. As the author suggests, in order to deal with this serious threat to public health and safety, resulting in healthcare expenditures, poor work productivity and academic or job losses, we should develop assessment, treatment matching, relapse prevention, the use of medications and adjunctive services. Dr. Maior et al. highlight the importance of neuropharmacological data, originated in non-human primate studies, towards our understanding of the mechanisms of cocaine addiction. Dr. Novak et al. present an overview of current state of knowledge about the nonmedical use of prescription medications in the U.S.A. The authors also provide us with a summary on pharmacological properties that are likely to confer selective use of particular drug class for nonmedical use. Dr. Aartsen alarms that the knowledge about causes, consequences and characteristics of older people who are addicted to alcohol, cannabis, cocaine and heroin is still very limited. The author emphasizes that the development of effective prevention of substance abuse in older adults, as well as effective therapies, is therefore strongly hampered. Since the anti-smoking trends have been observed in many countries, Prof. Muehlig's chapter on current state of knowledge on the phenomenon of tobacco addiction, and tobacco use related disorders, is very appropriate. Dr. Krzysztof et al. introduce "Comorbidity of a Serious Mental Illness with an Addiction to Psychoactive Substances" according to experiences at the Center for Mental Health and Addiction Treatment, and at the Center for Addiction Treatment, "Familia", in Poland, specializing dual diagnosis.

In the last section, "Biological Neuropsychiatry", we can find three types of articles related to molecular biology, neurochemistry and psychogenic movement disorders. Tohyama et al. describes available information on molecular cascades and their association with mental diseases, involving the susceptibility genes, DISC1, PACAP, TRAP1 and Dysbindin in major psychiatric disorders, such as schizophrenia, depression and bipolar disorder. Dr. Rex and Dr. Fink introduce integrated reviews on the relationship between neurotransmitter and behaviours, focusing on serotonin (5-hydroxytryptamine, 5-HT) and anxiety disorders. They investigated whether anxiolytics of different drug classes inhibit 5-HT release in, for example, herbal products. Abnormal movements and postures resulting from primary psychiatric disease are popular but difficult conditions because these may be mimicked by some neuro-psychogenic factors, including akinesia, hyperkinesia, tremor, myoclonus, and dystonia. Dr. Dallocchio reviews empirical evidence concerning clinical manifestations of psychogenic movement disorders (PMDs) and summarizes how PMDs are currently diagnosed, investigated and treated.

Doubtlessly, this book will be fruitful for future developments and collaborations in "world psychiatry".

I would like to thank all the authors and contributors in book project "Psychiatric Disorders – Trends and Developments". Special thanks are also due to Ms. Ivana Zec, editorial management and InTech – Open Access Publisher. Finally, the editor would like to express his gratitude to all readers.

Assoc. Prof. Dr. Toru Uehara
General Health Support Centre, Gunma University, Gunma,
Japan

Part 1

Schizophrenia

1

Neuropathology of the Prefrontal Cortex Neuropil in Schizophrenia

Latchman Somenarain
Bronx Community College, CUNY Bronx, New York
USA

1. Introduction

Schizophrenia is a brain disease with a multitude of symptoms and deficits in several areas of the brain. While the search for the neuropathological mechanisms of most diseases of the brain remain a forefront in the frontier of brain research, studies in schizophrenia has progressed significantly within the last three decades; however, the central etiological mechanisms of this devastating disease remains a mystery. A new impetus was gained with the landmark study by Johnstone et al., (1976) using computed tomographic (CT) scans, reported dilation of the lateral ventricles in a small group of chronic schizophrenic patients. Following this study, numerous more sophisticated neuroimaging studies using techniques such as magnetic resonance imaging (MRI) and positron emission tomography (PET) scans, consistently showed ventricular enlargement, sulcal widening and cortical atrophy in schizophrenia (Reveley et al., 1982; Andreasen et Al., 1988, 1990, 1994; Lawrie and Abukmeil 1998; Van Horn and McManus 1992). Lateral ventricle studies showed a 20-75% increase in the ventricular to brain ratio (Daniel et al., 1991; Van Horn and McManus 1992) and a median 40% increase in volume using MRI (Lawrie and Abukmeil, 1998). Additionally, some of these volumetric studies also showed an 8% decrease in the overall temporal lobe and 4-12 % decrease in volume of medial temporal structures, such as the hippocampus, parahippocampus and amygdala (Lawrie and Abukmeil 1998). Of significant importance are imaging studies of monozygotic twins discordant for schizophrenia. In all pairs studied the affected twin had the larger ventricles (Reveley et al., 1982; Suddath et al., 1990) and smaller cortical and hippocampal size (Noga et al., 1996). These studies were supported by data from family studies, which showed that the affected relatives had larger ventricles and smaller brain volume (Honer et al., 1994; Sharma et al., 1998; Silverman et al., 1998). Buchanan et al., (1998), in an effort to identify reductions in specific subregions of the frontal lobe, found a 13% decrease in the inferior prefrontal grey matter compared with an average 5% decrease in other frontal regions. MRI studies of subcortical structures showed small decreases in the thalamic volume of schizophrenics (Andreasen et al., 1994; Buchsbaum et al., 1996; Byne et al., 1997, 2001, 2002; Jones 1997, Popken et al., 2000; Young et al., 2000; Brickman et al., 2004). Structural imaging findings and macroscopic changes in the brain provided the impetus for more stereomorphometric and immunocytochemical investigations of the cytoarchitecture of cortical and subcortical structures of post-mortem brains. One particular area of major interest has been the prefrontal cortex (PFC).

The prefrontal cortex is located in the frontal lobe. It is rostral to premotor and primary motor areas. The PFC is the prominent cortical projection of the medial dorsal (MD) nucleus of the thalamus (Takagi 1980; Yarita et al., 1980; Price et al., 1981). It also receives reciprocal connections from areas of the diencephalon, mesencephalon and limbic system as well as cortical afferents of visual, auditory and somatic origin (Barbas et al., 1989: Barbas 1992). It is one of several association areas in the brain and is concerned with cognitive behavior and motor planning. The prefrontal cortex can be divided into several subregions; however, there are two main regions: the prefrontal association cortex proper, located on the dorsolateral surface of the frontal lobes, and the orbitofrontal cortex, located on the medial and ventral portions of the frontal lobe (Leonard 1972). In primates, the mid-dorsolateral PFC is targeted as a locus for working memory processes, and it encompasses the region within and above the principal sulcus (Broadmann's areas 46 and 9). In recent years, many studies have focused on the prefrontal cortex as a site of perturbation in schizophrenia (Benes et al., 1991; Shapiro, 1993; Davis and Lewis, 1995; Perone-Bizzozero et al., 1996; Beasley et al., 1997; Glantz and Lewis, 1997; Honer et al, 1997; Garey et al., 1998; Selemon and Goldman-Rakic, 1999; Kalus et al., 2000; Buxhoeveden et al., 2000; Lewis et al., 2001; Pierri et al., 2001, 2003; Broadbelt et al., 2002, 2006, 2008; Jones et al, 2002; Kindermann et al., 2004; Kolluri et al., 2005; Vostrikov et al., 2007; Subroto et al., 2009; Somenarain et al., 2010). Functionally, the prefrontal cortex is involved with attention, memory, orderly thinking and planning (Goldberg 1995), cognitive functions which have been shown to be impaired in schizophrenia and patients with damage to the prefrontal cortex (Weinberger et al., 1988), all of which are altered in schizophrenics.

Much evidence points specifically to the dorsolateral prefrontal cortex (DLPFC) as a site for dysfunction in schizophrenia (Weinberger et al., 1986; Buchsbaum et al., 1990; Benes 1991; Pakkenberg 1993; Goldman-Rakic and Selemon 1995, 1997; Lewis 1995, 1997; Harrison 1999; Andreasen 2000; Thune et al., 2001; Jones et al., 2002; Broadbelt et al., 2002, 2006; Miguel-Hidalgo et al., 2005; Kolluri et al., 2005; Somenarain et al., 2010). Schizophrenics perform poorly on tasks that require the use of working memory (Baddeley 1986). The intricate nature of working memory was first identified in studies of human cognition (Norman 1970, Baddeley 1986). Working memory allows one to simultaneously keep several pieces of information in mind for a few short seconds. For example, a newly read phone number is stored until it is dialed and after it is immediately forgotten. Morphological post-mortem studies in the DLPFC showed an increase in neuronal density (Benes et al., 1991; Selemon et al., 1995) without a change in the number of neurons (Pakkenberg 1993; Thune et al., 2001). Both Benes et al., (1991) and Selemon et al., (1995) hypothesized that increases in neuronal density without a change in the number of neurons would imply a change in the DLPFC neuropil, which includes the axon terminals, dendrites and dendritic spines that are the site for most cortical synapses. This was corroborated by several studies that showed a decrease in the synapse-associated protein synaptophysin (Karson et al., 1996; Perrone-Bizzozero et al. 1996; Glantz and Lewis 1997). A study by Buxhoeveden et al., (2000) reported reduced neuropil space in area 9 of schizophrenics. There are consistent findings of reduced spine density in layer III pyramidal neurons of the temporal cortex, BA 22 and 38, and frontal cortex, BA 10 and 46 (Garey et al., 1993, 1998; Glantz and Lewis 2000; Kolluri et al., 2005). Understanding the significance of these alterations requires an understanding of which elements of the DLPFC circuitry are disturbed. Functional maturation of the DLPFC circuitry in monkeys and humans seems to be uniquely protracted. It does not become functionally mature until after puberty (For a review see Lewis 1997). Human PET studies by Chugani et al., (1987) showed cerebral blood flow in the frontal cortex does not reach adult levels until 15 to 19 years of age. This seems to correspond with the appearance of clinical symptoms during late adolescence in schizophrenia. Additionally, adult levels of performance on some cognitive tasks, like delayed-response tasks, subserved by the DLPFC are not achieved until after puberty in both monkeys and humans (Fuster 1989).

Several studies have examined the morphology of pyramidal cells in the prefrontal cortex. Two studies showed a decrease in soma size and others decreased spine density (Garey et al., 1993, 1998; Glantz and Lewis 2000). Soma size is directly proportional to dendritic and axonal arborization (van Ooyan et al., 1995; van Pelt et al., 1996); therefore, a decrease in soma size, as seen in schizophrenics, might lead to decreases in dendritic arborization. The studies on spine density, Garey et al., (1998), examined the prefrontal cortex in general and not specific brain areas whereas, Glantz and Lewis (2000) examined areas 46 and 17.

2. Decreases in MAP2

More recently, studies by Jones and collaborators have investigated areas 9 and 32 of the prefrontal cortex (Jones et al., 2002, Broadbelt et al., 2002, 2006, 2008; Somenarain et al., 2010). These studies targeted the pyramidal cell and its ultrastructure: dendrites, spines and structural proteins. They first showed significant decreases in Microtubule Associated Protein (MAP2), a protein found in dendrites and cell bodies, in layers III and V of areas 9 and 32 of the prefrontal cortex Jones et al., (2002). Microtubule-associated proteins (MAP) are proteins that promote tubulin capacity to self-associate into microtubule polymers (Herzog and Weber 1978). Microtubule-associated proteins can also interact with actin filaments and with components of the intermediate filament proteins thus, pointing to their functional role in the regulation of the functional organization of the cytoskeletal network of neurons (For review see Maccioni and Cambiazo 1995). The family of neuronal MAPs includes high-molecular-mass components, namely MAP-1A, MAP-1B, MAP-1C, MAP-2A, and MAP-2B; the neuronal MAP-3; MAP-4 is found in both neuronal and nonneuronal cells; and intermediate-size polypeptides such as tau; and the small 70-kDa MAP-2C. MAPs have been found to be compartmentalized in neurons, with MAP1 being widely distributed, while MAP2 is essentially a dendritic protein and tau an axonal component. The majority of MAPs have a rather widespread distribution among different cell types and even tissues, but certain MAPs have been found localized in specific cells and not in others (For review see Maccioni and Cambiazo 1995).

MAP2 was first described by Murphy and Boresy (1975). It is an abundant protein in brain tissues which copolymerizes with brain microtubules in vitro and promotes the polymerization of tubulin. High levels of MAP2 can be found in the somatic and dendritic compartments, but not axons (Matus and Bernhardt 1986). In dendrites MAP2 is associated with microtubules and has an active role in the development and maintenance of dendritic processes by promoting polymerization of tubulin to form microtubules (Hirokawa et al., 1988). Because of its role in microtubule assembly and its selective association with dendrites, MAP2 has been implicated as playing a major role in the molecular mechanisms regulating dendritic growth and stabilization (Matus and Bernhardt 1986). Therefore, assembly and stability of microtubules are regulated by MAP2. MAP2 is a sensitive cross-linker and adjustable spacer in dendritic architecture. The phosphorylation state of MAP2 modulates its interaction with microtubules. In low-phosphorylation states MAP2 binds to microtubules and increase microtubule assembly and/or stability. Increased phosphorylation decreases these effects (Audesirk et al., 1997). Hely et al., (2001) proposed a model which suggests that dephosphorylated MAP2 favors elongation by promoting microtubule polymerization and bundling; whereas, MAP2 phosphorylation which increases microtubule spacing could cause dendritic branching. This is through the action of CAMKII being activated by elevated calcium concentrations, which is regulated upstream by calmodulin and neurogranin. Dendritic branching is due to changes in the cytoskeleton through the interaction of microtubules and actin filaments. Any factor that can alter microtubule dynamics will affect the dendritic architecture. The MAP family of proteins is known to regulate many factors of microtubule dynamics such as, deploymerization, bundling, spacing, and interaction with actin filaments (for review see Maccioni and Cambiazo 1995).

3. Loss of dendrites and spines

The loss of MAP2 immunostaining in their first study (Jones et al., 2002) suggests a loss of dendritic material on the pyramidal cells. The second study from their lab reported decreases in the primary and secondary basilar dendrites in area 32 of the prefrontal cortex (Broadbelt et al., 2002). There are mainly two types of neurons in the cortex, pyramidal and non-pyramidal neurons. The pyramidal neurons constitute about 70% of the cortical neurons and the non-pyramidal neurons about 25% (Powell 1981). The pyramidal neurons have a pyramidal shape cell body with an apical dendrite extending towards the pial layer and several basal dendrites on the base of the cell body. These neurons are the primary cortical projection neurons and are of major interest in this regard. Their axon collaterals extend for considerable distances horizontally through the gray matter and give rise to clusters of axon terminals in the superficial layers, which are organized as a series of stripes 2 μm wide and 1.8 mm long (Levitt et al 1993). There are reciprocal connections among these stripes and over 90% of the synapses furnished by these collaterals target the dendritic spines of other pyramidal cells (Metchitzky et al., 1995). It was suggested that these connections could provide the substrate for reverberating cortical circuit that coordinates and maintains the activity of spatially segregated, but functionally-related populations of DLPFC pyramidal neurons during the delay phase of the delayed-response task (Lewis and Anderson 1995).

The dendrites have tiny projections called spines which are the sites for synaptic inputs to the neuron. Spines are protrusions of the neuronal membrane consisting of a head connected to the neuron by a thin spine neck. They can be found on the dendrites, the soma and on the axon hillock (Mates and Lund 1983). Spines are the site of synaptic transmission and about 90% of the synapses on spines are excitatory (Mates and Lund 1983). There are three types of spines: mushroom, stubby and filopodium. Spine density is a marker of the number of excitatory inputs to pyramidal neurons (Mates and Lund 1983). Glutamate and dopamine afferents terminate on dendritic spines whereas, GABA terminals are often found on dendritic shafts and cell bodies (Levitt et al., 1993). Moreover, several hypotheses implicate one or more of these neurotransmitter systems in the pathophysiology of schizophrenia (Weickert et al., 1998; Haroutunian et al., 2003; Bergson et al., 2003). Somenarain 2005, have observed a decrease in spine density in both Layer III and V in Area 9. Layer III pyramidal neurons are the corticocortical projections (Lund et al., 1975); they play a critical role in information processing such as working memory. Layer V pyramidal neurons are the main projection cells from the cortex to other subcortical and cortical areas (Lewis 1997); therefore, changes in information in one cortical area could affect many brain regions. Additionally, a loss of spines reflects a loss of excitatory input to these neurons; therefore, it is expected that cognitive information processing might be disturbed as seen in schizophrenia. This is consistent with previous reports of decrease synaptophysin, a 38-kd integral membrane protein of small synaptic vesicles, which is important in calcium-dependent synaptic transmission (Glantz and Lewis 1997). Moreover, the spines of basal dendrites receive both dopamine and glutamate afferents (Smiley et al., 1992); thus, this give credence to possible disturbances in these transmitter systems in schizophrenia. Additionally, the basal dendrites are the site for afferents from the MD nucleus of the thalamus, an area of the brain that has consistently shown neuroanatomical deficits in schizophrenia (Andreasen et al., 1994; Buchsbaum et al., 1996; Byne et al., 1997, 2001, 2002; Jones 1997, Popken et al., 2000; Young et al., 2000).

4. Decreases in neurogranin

Recently, studies from the Jones group have reported significant decreases in neurogranin, a protein found in dendrites and spines (Broadbelt et al., 2006; Somenarain, 2005). Neurogranin (RC3), a postsynaptic calpacitin, was first identified in a hybridization study designed to isolate mRNAs enriched in the rat forebrain but absent in the cerebellum. As the name indicated, it was rat cortex-enriched cDNA clone number 3 (Watson et al., 1990). Neurogranin was independently purified by Baudier et al., (1991) from brain based on its affinity for calmodulin (CaM) and as a substrate for protein kinase C (PKC). Neurogranin is only 78 amino acids long and has sequence similarity to neuromodulin, a protein associated with axonal growth cone development and maturation (Baudier et al., 1991). Interestingly, both neurogranin and neuromodulin share a 20 amino acid sequence, AAAAKIQASFRGHMARKKIK, designated as the IQ motif (Apel and Storm 1992). This sequence contains a binding domain for CaM and a PKC phosphorylation site (Baudier et al., 1991). Neurogranin however, is found abundantly in neuronal cell bodies, dendrites and dendritic spines. In areas such as the frontal parietal cortex, granular cells of the dentate gyrus, apical dendrites of pyramidal cells of the CA1 and CA3 regions of the hippocampus, and the striatal cortex (Chicurel et al., 1993, Neuner-Jehle et al., 1996). Immunoelectron microscopic studies in the cerebral cortex, hippocampus and neostriatum in rats showed that neurogranin exists in the perinuclear and dendritic cytosol. It concentrates in dendritic spines in close proximity with postsynaptic densities and subsynaptic membranes (Watson et al 1992, Neuner-Jehle et al., 1996). This position is quite interesting, because neurogranin is a PKC substrate that interacts with CaM and both PKC and CaM are required for the induction of long term potentiation (Gerendasy and Sutcliffe 1997). Much research suggest that neurogranin might be involved in Ca^{2+}/CaM and PKC-dependent cascades that guide dendritic spine development and remodeling, as well as long-term potentiation (LTP) and long-term depression (LTD). Neurogranin binds calmodulin and, therefore, renders it unable to interact with free calcium (Ho et al, 2000; Prichard et al, 1999). Knockout mice lacking neurogranin exhibit problems with spatial learning and long-term potentiation (Ho et al, 2000); suggesting a role for neurogranin in processing and transmission of information and suggesting a possible role in schizophrenia. Gerendasy and Sutcliffe (1997) postulated that neurogranin regulate Ca^{2+} fluxes in dendritic spines by releasing CaM to bind Ca^{2+}. The size and duration of Ca^{2+} fluxes determine which Ca^{2+}-dependent enzymes are stimulated and ultimately, which second messenger cascades are activated for LTP or LTD. Enzymes such as CaM kinase II and adenylate clyclase favours LTP; whereas, calcineurin and cyclic nucleotide phosphodiesterase, favors LTD (For review see Gerendasy and Sutcliffe 1997). The binding of calmodulin by neurogranin is abrogated by phosphorylation by PKC, oxidation by nitric oxide or large concentration of Ca^{2+} (Ho Pak et al., 2000 and Prichard et al., 1999). Most recently, a study by Broadbelt et al., 2008 showed a decrease in calmodulin in the prefrontal cortex suggesting that the calcium calmodulin dependent pathway may be altered in the PFC.

Immunohistochemical studies in rats and mice showed that peak expression of the neurogranin protein postnatally coincides with developmental periods of rapid dendritic growth and the formation of 80% of cortical synapses (Alvarez-Bolado et al., 1996, Uylings et al., 1990). Suggesting therefore, an increase in neurogranin concentration coincides with the onset of synaptogenesis. The number and size of spines on dendrites is mediate by calcium-dependent mechanisms that are initiated by glutamate receptor-mediated influx of Ca^{++} ions (Gerendasy and Sutcliffe 1997). Proteins involved in Ca^{++} signaling, such as neurogranin, therefore may play a major role in spine morphology and number and as such cell signaling.

A loss of neurogranin is suggestive of both morphological and functional alterations in the prefrontal cortical area 9. Much evidence has pointed to morphological changes in the pyramidal cells in the prefrontal cortex. Recent data have shown functional alterations in these cells as well. This data represent the first link between morphological alterations and functional alterations in pyramidal cells in the prefrontal cortex. Future work needs clarify the significance of these alterations and how they contribute to the behavioral and cognitive problems observed in patients with schizophrenia.

5. The role of antipsychotic drugs

Since their introduction in 1959, neuroleptic drugs have been used extensively in the treatment of schizophrenia and other neuropsychiatric diseases, such as bipolar disease, depression and schizoaffective disease (Harrison et al., 2000). Most of the patients in recent neuropathological studies in schizophrenia have received neuroleptic medication. In recent years a battery of treatments have become available that treat the symptoms of schizophrenia and attempt to improve the quality of life of patients. The conventional or older typical antipsychotic medication (phentothiazines, butyrophenones, and thioxanthenes) e.g., chlorpromazine, haloperidol, fluphenazine and molindone are used to reduce the positive symptoms of schizophrenia and have a strong affinity for dopamine and serotonin receptors (Hirsch and Weinberger 2003).

The recently developed medications e.g., clozapine, risperidone, olanzapine, quetiapine and sertindole are more effective against the negative symptoms of schizophrenia (Hirsch and Weinberger 2003). The newer medications, often called atypical because they have a different mechanism of action than the older medications, are more effective against negative symptoms and show fewer side effects, and are effective against treatment-resistant patients. The therapeutic effects of the major neuroleptics, typical or atypical, are based on their ability to bind neurotransmitter receptors like dopamine and serotonin (Harrison 1999a). There are five classes of dopamine receptors D_1-D_5; all are seven transmembrane domain G protein-coupled receptors linked to adenyl cyclase (Harrison 1999a). The serotonin 5-HT receptors are divided in seven branches 5-$HT_{1\text{-}7}$. The 5-HT_3 is an ion channel and all the others are coupled to G protein linked to adenyl cyclase or the phosphor-inositol system. The 5-HT_{2a} is of particular relevance in schizophrenia because of it affinity for atypical neuroleptics (Harrison 1999a). Though, D_2 blockade has been central to the antipsychotic activity of typical neuroleptics. The atypical neuroleptics such as clozapine bind to D_1, D3, D_4 and D_5 as well as 5-HT_{2a} and noradrenergic receptors; however, D_4 shows the strongest affinity (Harrison 1999a). Recently, the dopamine D_4 and 5-HT_{2a} receptors are of particular importance in schizophrenia due to their binding mechanisms with atypical neuroleptics. The exact mechanisms of how these interactions operate are still under investigation.

Although they are treasured for their therapeutic significance, neuroleptics are known to produce structural brain changes in areas such as the striatum, where there are increases in the number of symmetric and axodendritic synapses relative to asymmetric and axospinous synapses (Benes et al., 1985, Klinzova et al., 1989, Meshul et al., 1992). Suggesting that antipsychotics induce an altered numerical balance in favor of inhibitory synapses, given that asymmetric and axospinous synapses are mostly glutamatergic and as such excitatory (Benes et al., 1985). Some reports suggest a correlation of antipsychotic dosage and increase brain atrophy and decrease thalamic volume (Gur et al., 1998). These macroscopic studies suggest that neuroleptic exposure is a potential confounding variable in most morphological and neurochemical findings reported in schizophrenia. Several studies have suggested that long-term treatment with antipsychotics might cause the morphological changes observed in schizophrenia (Benes et al., 1985; Klinzova et al., 1989; Meshul et al., 1992). Although these studies were done in rodents with normal brains, together the data provide good evidence that chronic antipsychotic treatment induces synaptic plasticity and alters the synaptic ultrastructure.

A study on rhesus monkeys demonstrated long-term haloperidol exposure can increase phosphorylation of MAP2 and down regulate spinophilin, a dendritic spine associated protein (Lidow et al., 2001). A study in rat showed treatment with antipsychotics can modulate the expression of MAP2 genes (Law et al., 2004). This is different from what is shown for MAP2 in schizophrenia (Somenarain et al., 2010); therefore, animal studies may not be the best indicator of neuroleptic effect. Additionally, animal studies are based on normal neural networks so the neuroleptic drugs may not have the same effect as altered neural networks. Because antipsychotic drugs can affect many neurotransmitter systems (Harrison et al., 2000), they have the ability to regulate the activity of kinases and phosphatases via second messengers (Lidow et al., 2001). These enzymes regulate phosphorylation states of many proteins, one such is MAP2 (Diaz-Nido et al., 1990). MAP2 is found in dendrites and cell bodies and is an important protein in formation and stabilization of microtubules (Matus 1988). Phosphorylation of MAP2 can destabilize dendritic microtubules because it is a sensitive cross-linker and adjustable spacer in the polymerization of tubulin in microtubules, and as such the cytoskeletal processes of the cell (Boyne et al., 1995).

In order to correctly interpret the morphological data it is important to know what alterations are due to neuroleptics and which are not. A comparison of drug-naïve and treated subjects in contemporary postmortem studies is not feasible since nearly all patients with schizophrenia use neuroleptics. The use of animals to study the effects of antipsychotics has some attraction; however, there are problems when extrapolating results between species. First, the cerebral cortex in animals and humans vary in terms of size and the distribution of neurotransmitter receptors. For example, rodent's cerebrum is a thousand times smaller than humans (Harrison et al., 2000). Secondly, there are marked differences in organization of the PFC. For example, in primate PFC there is a distinct layer IV which is absent in rat (Harrison et al., 2000). Lastly, rodents metabolize antipsychotics differently than humans, and might respond neuropathologically in different ways; moreover, animal brains are normal (Harrison et al., 2000).

Thus, researchers have devised other means to control for neuroleptic exposure. The use of a non-schizophrenic group treated with antipsychotics, such as bipolar disease, schizoaffective and depression often produced mixed results (Harrison et al., 2000). This is attributed to the fact that a significant number of patients who were first diagnosed as schizoaffective or for depression are later diagnosed with schizophrenia, which suggest that they share intrinsic pathological features with schizophrenia (Harrison et al., 2000). Therefore, it is foreseeable why when used as controls for neuroleptic exposure the results are overlapping. Somenarain (2005, 2010) have used a cohort of Huntington Chorea brains to determine if neuroleptic drugs can cause morphological changes in the brain and confound the results reported in schizophrenia. Although there are reports of cortical changes in Huntington Chorea (Harrison et al., 2000), the main deficit is a loss of neurons in the striatum (Harrison et al., 2000). Huntington's patients experience some psychiatric symptoms, like hallucinations and delusions, similarly to schizophrenics; therefore, many are given neuroleptic drugs to control those symptoms. A comparison of schizophrenic and Huntington Chorea is a more meaningful assessment in determining if neuroleptic drugs could be responsible for some of the morphological changes reported in schizophrenia. Somenarain (2005) have done an exhaustive study comparing MAP2, Neurogranin, dendrites and spines in schizophrenia, Huntington Chorea and normal controls. All of the above parameters were shown to be decreased in schizophrenia; however, there were no significant differences seen between Huntington Chorea and controls. We believe that this is strong support that neuroleptic drugs may not be responsible for some of the changes seen in DLPFC neuropil in schizophrenia.

6. Conclusion

The loss of dendritic material on the pyramidal cells in the DLPFC may have an indelible impact on the functional capacity of these neurons. These neurons are the primary cortical as well as subcortical projection neurons; therefore, they play a very important role in information processing. Functionally, the DLPFC is involved in attention, memory, orderly thinking and planning, functions that have been shown to be disturbed in schizophrenia. The loss of MAP2 may have a detrimental impact on the structural integrity of neurons. MAP2 proteins play a very important role in the regulation of the functional organization of the cytoskeletal network of neurons. The loss of this protein supports the studies that showed loss of dendrites and spines. Whether the loss of MAP2 is the cause or as a result is not known. The loss of neurogranin provides additional support that there is a loss of dendritic material on the pyramidal cells of the DLPFC. Neurogranin postnatally coincides with developmental periods of rapid dendritic growth and the formation of cortical synapses. The loss of neurogranin is suggestive of both morphological and functional alterations in the prefrontal cortex. There is strong support that the losses of these substances is real and are probably not due to neuroleptic exposure. This is supported by the fact that Somenarain (2005) did an extensive study using Huntington chorea brains which showed no changes due to neuroleptic exposure compared to controls. Together, these studies provide very strong support that the DLPFC neuropil is reduced in schizophrenia.

7. References

Alvarez-Bolado G, Rodriguez-Sanchez P, Tejero-Diez P, Fairen A, Diez-Guerra F (1996) Neurogranin in the development of the rat telencephalon. Neuroscience 73:565-580.

Andreasen NC, Ehrhardt JC, Swayze VW, Alliger RJ, Yuh WTC, Cohen G, Ziebell S (1990) MRI of the brain in schizophrenia: The pathological significance of structural abnormalities. Archives of General Psychiatry 47:35-44.

Andreasen NC, Swayze N, Flaum M, Yates WR, Amdt S, McChesney C (1990) Ventricular enlargement in schizophrenia evaluated with CT scanning: effects of gender, age and stage of illness. Archives of General Psychiatry 47:1054-9.

Andreasen NC, Flashman L, Flaum M, Arndt S, Swayze V, O'Leary DS, Ehrhardt JC, Yuh WTC (1994) Regional brain abnormalities in schizophrenia measured with MRI. JAMA 272:1763-69.

Andreasen NC, Arndt S, Swayze V 2nd, Cizadlo T, Flaum M, O'Leary D (1994) Thalamic abnormalities in schizophrenia visualized through magnetic resonance image averaging. Science 266:294-8.

Andreasen NC (1988) Brain Imaging: Applications in psychiatry. Science 239:1381-88.

Andreasen NC (2000) Schizophrenia: the fundamental questions. Brain Research Reviews 31:106-112.

Apel ED, Storm DR (1992) Functional domains of neuromodulin (GAP)-43. Perspectives Development. Neurobiology 1:3-11.

Audesirk G, Cabell L, Kern M (1997) Modulation of neurite branching by protein phosphorylation in cultured rat hippocampal neurons. Developmental Brain Research 102: 247-260.

Baddeley A (1986) Working Memory, Oxford University Press.

Barbas H, Pandya DN (1989) Architecture and intrinsic connections of the prefrontal cortex in the rhesus monkey. Journal of Comparative Neurology 286: 353-375.

Barbas H (1992) Architecture and cortical connections of the prefrontal cortex in the rhesus monkey. Advance Neurology 57: 91-115.

Baudier J, Delouime JC, Van Dorsselaer A, Black D and Matthes HW (1991) Purification and characterization of a brain-specific protein kinase C substrate, neurogranin (p17). Identification of a consus amino acid sequence between neurogranin and neuromodulin (GAP43) that corresponds to the protein kinase C phosphorylation site and the calmodulin-binding domain. Journal of Biological Chemistry 266:229-237.

Beasley CL, Reynolds GP (1997) Parvalbumin-immunoreactive neurons are reduced in the prefrontal cortex of schizophrenics. Schizophrenia Research 24:349-355.

Benes FM, Paskevich PA, Davidson J, Domesik VB (1985) Synaptic rearrangements in medial prefrontal cortex of haloperidol-treated rats. Brain Research 348:15-20

Benes FM (1991) Toward a neurodevelopmental understanding of schizophrenia and other psychiatric disorders. In Cicchetti D, Toth SL (eds), Models and Integrations:

Rochester Symposium on Developmental Psychopathology, vol 3, Rochester, NY, Univ of Rochester Press, pp 161-184.

Bergson C, Levenson R, Goldman-Rakic P, Lidow MS (2003) Dopamine receptor-interacting proteins: the Calcium connection in dopamine signaling. Trends in Pharmacological Sciences 24:486-492.

Boyne LJ, Martin K, Hockfield S, Fischer I (1995) Expression and distribution of phosphorylated MAP1b in growing axons of cultured hippocampal neurons. Journal of Neuroscience Research 40:439-450.

Brickman AM, Bushbaum MS, Shihabuddin L, Byne W, Newmark R, Brand J, Ahmed S, Mitelman SA, Hazlett EA (2004) Thalamus size and outcome in schizophrenia. Schizophrenia Research 71:473-484.

Broadbelt K, Jones LB (2008) Evidence of altered calmodulin immunoreactivity in areas 9 and 32 0f schizophrenic prefrontal cortex. Journal of Psychiatric Research 42(8):612-21.

Broadbelt K, Rampersaud A, Jones LB (2006) Evidence of altered neurogranin immunoreactivity in areas 9 and 32 of schizophrenic prefrontal cortex. Schizophrenia Research 87 (1-3):6-14.

Broadbelt K, Byne WB, Jones LB (2002) Evidence for a decrease in primary and secondary basilar dendrites on pyramidal cells in area 32 of schizophrenic prefrontal cortex. Schizophrenia Research 58:75-81.

Buchanan RW, Vladar K, Barta PE, and Pearlson GD (1998) Structural evaluation of the prefrontal cortex in schizophrenia. American Journal of Psychiatry 155:1049-1055.

Buchsbaum MS, Nuechterlein KH, Haier RJ, WU J, Sicotte N, Hazlett E, Asarnow R, Potkin S, Guich S (1990) Glucose metabolic rate in normals and schizophrenics during the Continuous Performance Test assessed by PET. British Journal of Psychiatry 156:216-27.

Buchsbaum MS, Someya T, Teng CY, Abel L, Chin S, Najafi A (1996) PET and MRI of the thalamus in never-medicated patients with schizophrenia. American Journal of Psychiatry 153:191-9.

Buxhoeveden D, Ror E, Switala A (2000) Reduced interneuronal space in schizophrenia. Biological Psychiatry 47(7):681.

Byne W, Jones L, Kemether E, Haroutunian V, Davis KL (1997) Towards localization of thalamic pathology in schizophrenia. APA Abstract NR544.

Byne W, Buchsbaum MS, Kemether E, Hazlett EA, Shinwari A, Mitropoulou V, Siever LJ (2001) Magnetic resonance imaging of the thalamic mediodorsal nucleus and pulvinar in schizophrenia and schizotypal personality disorder. Archives of General Psychiatry 58:133-140.

Byne W, Buchsbaum MS, Mattiace LA, Hazlett EA, Kemether E, Elhakem SL, Purohit DP, Haroutunian V, and Jones L (2002) Postmortem assessment of thalamic nuclear volumes in subjects with schizophrenia. American Journal of Psychiatry 159:59-65.

Chicurel ME, Terrian DM, Potter H (1993) mRNA at the synapse: analysis of a synaptosomal preparation enriched in hippocampal dendritic spines. Journal of Neuroscience 13:4054-4063.

Chugani HT, Phelps ME, Mazziotta JC (1987) Positron emission tomography study of human brain functional development. Annals of Neurology 22:487-497

Daniel DG, Goldberg TE, Gibbons RD, Weinberger DR (1991) Lack of a bimodal distribution of ventricular size in schizophrenia: a Gaussian mixture of 1056 cases and controls. Biological Psychiatry 30:887-903.

Daviss SR, Lewis DA (1995) Local circuit neurons of the prefrontal cortex in schizophrenia: Selective increase in the density of calbindin-immunoreactive neurons. Psychiatric Research 59:81-96.

Diaz-Nido J, Serrano L, Hernandez MA, Avila J (1990) Phosphorylation of microtubule proteins in rat brain at different development stages: comparison with that found in neuronal cultures. Journal of Neurochemistry 54:211-222.

Fuster JM (1989) The prefrontal cortex: Anatomy, Physiology and Neurophysiology of the Frontal lobe. New York, Raven Press.

Garey LJ, Ong WY, Barnes TRE (1993) Dendritic spine loss on pyramidal cells of temporal cortex of schizophrenia. Neuropathology Applied Neurobiology 19:186-7.

Garey LJ, Ong WY, Patel TS, Kanani M, Davis A, Mortimer AM (1998) Reduced dendritic spine density on cerebral cortical pyramidal neurons in schizophrenia. Journal of Neurology and Neurosurgery Psychiatry 65:446-53.

Gerendasy D, Sutcilffe G (1997) RC3/Neurogranin, a Postsynaptic Calpacitin for setting the response threshold to calcium influxes. Molecular Neurobiology 15:131-163.

Glantz LA, Lewis DA (1997) Reduction of synaptophysin immunoreactivity in the prefrontal cortex of subjects with schizophrenia. Archives General Psychiatry 54:943-52.

Glantz LA, Lewis DA (2000) Decrease dendritic spine density on prefrontal cortical pyramidal neurons in schizophrenia. Archives General Psychiatry 57:65-73.

Goldberg TE, Gold JM (1995) Neurocognitive deficits in schizophrenia. In Hirsch SR, Weinberger DR (eds): Schizophrenia. Oxford, Blackwell Science Limited. pp 146-162.

Goldman-Rakic PS (1995) Dissolution of cerebral cortical mechanisms in subjects with schizophrenia. In: Watson SJ. Ed. Biology of Schizophrenia and Affective Disease. Washington, DC: American Psychiatric Press pp. 113-27.

Goldman-Rakic PS, Selemon LD (1997) Functional and anatomical aspects of prefrontal pathology in schizophrenia. Schizophrenia Bulletin 23(3):437-458.

Gur RE, Maany V, Mozley PD, Swanson C, Bilker W, Gur RC (1998) Subcortical MRI volumes in neuroleptic-naïve and treated patients with schizophrenia. American Journal of Psychiatry 155:1711-17.

Haroutunian V, Dracheva S, Davis K (2003) Neurobiology of glutamatergic abnormalities in schizophrenia. Neuroscience 3:67-76.

Harrison PJ (1999) The neuropathology of schizophrenia. A critical review of the data and their interpretation. Brain 122:593-624.

Harrison PJ (1999a) Neurochemical alterations in schizophrenia affecting the putative receptor targets of atypical antipsychotics. British Journal of Psychiatry 174 (Suppl. 38), 12-22.

Harrison PJ, Roberts GW (2000) The neuropathology of schizophrenia. Progress and interpretations. Oxford University Press pp 150-185.

Hely TA, Graham B, Van Ooyen A (2001) A computational model of dendrite elongation and branching based on MAP2 phosphorylation. Journal of Theoretical Biology 210:375-384.

Herzog W. and Weber K.(1978) Fractionation of brain microtubule-associated proteins. Isolation of two different proteins which stimulate tubulin polymerization in Vitro. European Journal of Biochemistry 92:1-8.

Hirokawa N, Hisanaga S, Shiomura Y (1988) Map2 is a component of cross bridges between microtubules and neurofilament in the neuronal cytoskeleton. Journal of Neuroscience 8: 2769-2779.

Hirsch and Weinberger (2003) Schizophrenia 2nd Edition. Blackwell Publishing.

Honer WG, Bassett AS, Smith GN, Lapointe JS, Kalkai P (1994) Temporal lobe abnormalities in multigenerational families with schizophrenia. Biological Psychiatry 36:737-43.

Honer WG, Falkai P, Young C, Wang T, Xie J, Bonner J, Hu L, Boulianne GL, Luo Z, Trimble WS (1997) Cingulate cortex synaptic terminal proteins and neural cell adhesive molecule in schizophrenia. Neuroscience 78: 99-110.

Ho Pak J, Huang FL, Li J, Balschun D, Reymann KG, Westphal H, Huang KP (2000) Involvement of neurogranin in the modulation of calcium/calmodulin-dependent protein kinase II, synaptic plasticity, and spatial learning: a study with knockout mice. PNAS 97:11232-11237.

Huntington's Disease Collaborative Research Group (1993) A novel gene containing a trinucleotide repeat that is expanded and unstable on Huntington's disease chromosomes. Cell 72:971-983.

Johnstone EC, Crow TJ, Frith CD, Stevens M, Kreel L, Husband J (1976) Cerebral ventricular size and cognitive impairment in chronic schizophrenia. Lancet ii: 924-926.

Jones GE (1997) Cortical development and thalamic pathology in schizophrenia. 23(3):483-501.

Jones L, Johnson N, Byne W (2002) Alterations in MAP2 immunocytochemistry in area 9 and 32 of schizophrenic prefrontal cortex. Psychiatry Research Neuroimaging 9:3621-3625.

Kalus P, Muller TJ, Zuschratter W, Senitz D, (2000) The dendritic architecture of prefrontal pyramidal neurons in schizophrenic patients. Neuroreport 9:3621-3625.

Karson CN, Griffin WS, Mrak RE, Sturner WQ, Shillutt S, Guggenheim FG (1996) Reduced levels of synaptic proteins in the prefrontal cortex in schizophrenia. Neuroscience Abstract 22:1677.

Kindermann SS, Brown G, Zorrilla LE, Olsen RK, Jeste DV (2004) Spatial working memory among middle aged and older patients with schizophrenia and volunteers using fMRI. Schizophrenia Research 68:203-216.

Klinzova AJ, Haselhorst U, Uranova NA, Schenk H, Isomin VV (1989) The effect of haloperidol on synaptic plasticity in rat medial prefrontal cortex. J Hirnforsch 30:51-57.

Kolluri N, Sun Z, Sampson AR, Lewis DA (2005) Lamina-specific reductions in dendritic spine density in the prefrontal cortex of subjects with schizophrenia. American Journal of Psychiatry 162(6):1200-2.

Law AJ, Hutchinson LJ, Burnet OWJ, Harrison PJ (2004) Antichotics increase MAP2 mRNA but not spinophilin mRNA in rat hippocampus and cortex. Inter Science 76:3, 376-382.

Lawrie SM, Abukmeil SS (1998) Brain abnormality in schizophrenia. A systematic and quantitative review of volumetric magnetic resonance imaging studies. British Journal of Psychiatry 172:110-120.

Leonard C M (1972) The connections of the dorsomedial nuclei. Brain Behavior and Evolution 6:524-541.

Levitt J, Lewis DA, Yoshioka T, Lund JS (1993) Topography of pyramidal neuron intrinsic connections in macaque monkeys prefrontal cortex (areas 9 & 46). Journal of Comparative Neurology 338:360-76.

Lewis DA, Anderson SA (1995) The functional architecture of the prefrontal cortex and schizophrenia. Psychology Medicine 25: 887-894.

Lewis DA (1997) Development of the prefrontal cortex during Adolescence: Insights into Vulnerable neural circuits in schizophrenia. Neuropsychopharmacology 16:385-89.

Lewis DA, Cruz DA, Melchitzky DS, Pierri JN (2001) Lamina-specific decifits in parvalbumin-immunoreactive varicosities in the prefrontal cortex of subjects with schizophrenia: Evidence for fewer projections from the thalamus. The American Journal of Psychiatry 158:1411-22.

Lidow MS, Songa Z, Castnerb SA, Allenc PB, Greengarde P, Goldman-Rakic PS (2001) Antipsychotic treatment induces alterations in dendrite and spine-associated proteins in dopamine-rich areas of the primate cerebral cortex. Biological Psychiatry 49:1-12.

Lund JS, Lund RD, Hendrickson AE, et al. (1975) The origin of efferent pathways from the primary visual cortex, area 17, of the macaque monkey as shown by retrograde transport of horseradish peroxidase. Journal of Comparative Neurology 164:287-303.

Maccioni R and Cambiazo V (1995) Role of microtubule-associated proteins in the control of microtubule assembly. Physiological Reviews 75:835-864.

Mates SL, Lund JS (1983) Spine formation and maturation of type I synapses on spiny stelate neurons in primary visual cortex. Journal of Comparative Neurology 221:91-97.

Matus A, (1988) Microtubule-associated proteins: their potential role in determining neuronal cytoarchitecture. Brain Research Reviews 13:179-212.

Matus A, Bernhardt R, Bodmer R, and Alaimos D (1986) Microtubule-associated protein 2 and tubulin are differentially distributed in the dendrites of developing neurons. Neuroscience 17:371-389.

Meshul CK, Janowsky A, Casey DE, Stallbaumer RK, Taylor B (1992) Effects of haloperidol and clozapine on the density of "perforated" synapses in caudate, nucleus accumbens, and medial prefrontal cortex. Psychopharmacology 106:45-52.

Melchitcky DS, Sesack SR, Pucak ML, Lewis DA (1995) Synaptic targets of pyramidal neuron axon collaterals providing horizontal connections in monkey prefrontal cortex. Society of Neuroscience Abstract 21: 409.

Miguel-Hidalgo JJ, Dubay P, Shao Q, Stockmeier C, Rajkowska G. (2005) Unchanged packing density but altered size of neurofilament immunoreactive neurons in the orefrontal cortex in schizophrenia and major depression. Schizophrenia Research 76 (2-3): 159-71.

Murphy, DB, Boresy BB (1975) Association of high molecular weight proteins with microtubules and their role in microtubule assembly in vitro. Proceedings of the National Academy of Science USA 72:2696-2700.

Neuner-Jehle M, Denizot J P, and Mallet (1996) Neurogranin is locally concentrated in rat cortical and hippocampal neurons. Brain Research 733:149-154.

Noga JT, Bartley AJ, Jones DW, Torrey EF, Weinberger DR. (1996) Cortical gyral anatomy and gross brain dimensions in monozygotic twins discordant for schizophrenia. Schizophrenia Research 22:27-40.

Norman DA (1970) Models of human memory (New York: Academic Press).

Pakkenberg B (1993) Total nerve cell number in neocortex in chronic schizophrenics and controls estimated using optical dissectors. Biological Psychiatry 34:768-772.

Perrone-Bizzozero NI, Sower AC, Bird ED, Benowitz LI, Ivins KJ, Neve RL (1996) Levels of the growth-associated protein GAP-43 are selectively increased in association cortices in schizophrenia. Proceedings of the National Academy of Science USA 93:14182-87.

Pierri JN, Volk Cl, Auh S, Sampson A, Lewis DA, (2001) Decreased somal size of deep layer 3 pyramidal neurons in the prefrontal cortex of subjects with schizophrenia. Archives of General Psychiatry 58,466-473.

Pierri JN, Volk Cl, Auh S, Sampson A, Lewis DA, (2003) Somal size of prefrontal cortical pyramidal neurons in schizophrenia: differential effects across neuronal subpopulations. Biological Psychiatry 54 (2), 111-20..

Popken JG, Bunney EW, Potkin GS, Jones GE (2000) Subnucleus-specific loss of neurons in medial thalamus of schizophrenics. PNAS 97(15):9276-80.

Powell TPS (1981) Certain aspects of the intrinsic organization of the cerebral cortex. pp1-19. Raven press. New York.

Price J L, Amaral D G (1981) Journal of Neuroscience 1:1242–1259.

Prichard L, Deloulmes JC, Storm DR (1999) Interactions between neurogranin and calmodulin *in vivo*. Journal of Biological Chemistry 274:7689-7694.

Reveley AM, Riveley MA, Clifford CA, Murray RM (1982) Cerebral ventricular size in twins discordant for schizophrenia. Lancet 1:540-1.

Selemon LD, Rajkowska G, Goldman-Rakic PS (1995) Abnormally high neuronal density in the schizophrenic cortex: A morphometric analysis of prefrontal area 9 and occipital area17. Archives of General Psychiatry 52:805-818.

Selemon LD, Goldman-Rakic (1999) The reduced neuropil hypothesis: A circuit based model of schizophrenia. Biological Psychiatry 45:17-25.

Shapiro RM (1993) Regional neuropathology in schizophrenia: Where are we? Where are we going? Schizophrenia Research 10:187-239.

Sharma T, Lancaster E, Lee D, Lewis S, Sigmundsson T, Takei N (1998) Brain changes in schizophrenia. British Journal of Psychiatry 173:132-8.

Silverman JM, Smith CJ, Guo SL, Mohs RC, Siever LJ, Davis KL (1998) Lateral ventricular enlargement in schizophrenic probands and their siblings with schizophrenia-related disorders. Biological Psychiatry 43:97-106.

Smiley JF, Williams SM, Szigeti K (1992) Light electron microscopic characterization of dopamine-immunoreactive axons in human cerebral cortex. Comparative Neurology 321:325-35.

Somenarain L, Jones L (2010) A comparative study of MAP2 immunostaining in areas 9 and 17 in schizophrenia and Huntington chorea. Journal of Psychiatric Research 44:694-699.

Somenarain L (2005) Morphological changes in schizophrenia: Fact or neuroleptic exposure. ProQuest Dissertations & Theses 3187402.

Subroto G, Gleason K, Potts B, Amezcua K, Tamminga C (2009) Differential expression of metabotropic glutamate receptor 2 and 3 in schizophrenia: A mechanism for antipsychotic drug action. American Journal of Psychiatry 166:812-820.

Suddath RL, Christison GW, Torrey EF, Casanova MF, Weinberger DR (1990) Anatomical abnormalities in the brains of monozogotic twins discordant for schizophrenia. Journal of Medicine 322:789-94.

Takagi SF (1980) Trends Neuroscience 13:313–315.

Thune JJ, Uylings HBM, Pakkenberg B (2001) No deficit in total number of neurons in the prefrontal cortex in schizophrenics. Journal of Psychiatric Research 35:15-21.

Uylings H B M, Van Eden C G, Parnavelas J G, Kalsbeek A (1990) The prenatal and postnatal development of rat cerebral cortex. The Cerebral Cortex of the Rat MIT Press, Cabbridge, MA, pp. 35-76.

Van Horn JD, McManus IC (1992) Ventricular enlargement in schizophrenia. American Journal of Psychiatry 160:687-697.

Van Ooyen A, van Pelt J, Corner MA. (1995) Implication of activity dependent neurite outgrowth for neuronal morphology and network development. Journal of Theoretical. Biology 172:63-82.

Van Pelt J, van Ooyen A, Corner MA. (1996) Growth cone dynamics and activity-dependent processes in neuronal network development. Progress in Brain Research 108:333-46.

Vostrikov V, Orlovskaya D, Uronova N (2007) Deficit of pericapillary oligodendrocytes in the prefrontal cortex in schizophrenia. World Journal of Biological Psychiatry 8:1-9.

Watson J B, Battenberg E F, Wong K K, Bloom F and Sutcliffe J G (1990) Subtractive cDNA cloning of RC3, a rodent cortex-enriched mRNA encoding a novel 78 residue protein. Journal Neuroscience Research 26:397-408.

Watson J B, Sutcliffe J G, Fisher R S (1992) Localization of the protein kinase C phosphorylation/calmodulin-binding substrate RC3 in dendritic spines of neostriatal neurons. Proceedings of the National Academy of Science USA 89:8581-8585.

Weickert CS, Kleinman JE (1998) The neuroanatomy and neurochemistry of schizophrenia. Schizophrenia 21:57-75.

Weinberger DR, Berman KF, Zec RF (1986) Physiologic dysfunction of dorsolateral prefrontal cortex in schizophrenia: I. Regional cerebral blood flow (rCBF) evidence. Archives of General Psychiatry 43:114-25.

Weinberger DR (1988) Schizophrenia and the frontal lobe. Trends in Neuroscience 11:367-70.

Yarita H, Iino M, Tanabe T, Kogure S, Takagi S F. Journal of Neurophysiology 1980;43:69–85.

Young K, Manaye KF, Liang C, Hicks PB, German DC (2000) Reduced number of MD and anterior thalamic neurons in schizophrenia. Biological Psychiatry 47:944-53.

2

Electrophysiological Deficits in Schizophrenia: Models and Mechanisms

Catherine R. Jutzeler, Michael E. McMullen, Robert F. Featherstone, Valerie M. Tatard-Leitman, Michael J. Gandal, Gregory C. Carlson and Steven J. Siegel
Translational Neuroscience Program, Department of Psychiatry, University of Pennsylvania, Philadelphia, PA USA

1. Introduction

Schizophrenia a complex neuropsychiatric disorder, is characterized by core impairments including positive symptoms (hallucinations, delusions), negative symptoms (blunted affect, alogia, social deficits, anhedonia, avolition), as well as persistent neurocognitive deficits (memory, concentration, and learning). Positive symptoms usually show good response to currently approved medications, all of which act exclusively by blocking D2 receptors. Alternatively, the negative and neurocognitive symptoms respond poorly to D2 antagonists, and therefore persist even in treated patients. Developing new therapies to target treatment-resistant symptoms requires identification of neural endophenotypes associated with these deficits (Braff and Light, 2005). Additionally, neurophysiological biomarkers may be objective indices of prominent features in schizophrenia patients such as cognitive dysfunction (Javitt et al., 2008). The brain processes underlying neurocognitive symptoms can be investigated using various neurophysiological measures such as event related potentials (ERP) and electroencephalography (EEG). Event-related potentials and EEG oscillations represent coordinated neuronal activity and are thought to be a means to assess fundamental mechanisms of memory, attention, learning, and other cognitive functions. Consequently, these measures are likely to be an appropriate biomarker for brain abnormalities in schizophrenia. As such, great effort has been made to link particular electrophysiological features with relevant aspects of schizophrenia including psychopathology, clinical outcome, genetics, and pharmacology.
First, we will introduce the reader to the human EEG by giving an overview of the different components, highlighting each component's clinical relevance, as well as addressing its limitations. Subsequently, we highlight the characteristics of ERPs of schizophrenia. In the second part of the review, current preclinical models (i.e., transgenic, pharmacological, and environmental approaches) of EEG abnormalities in schizophrenia will be discussed. We then discuss potential requirements of future model and methods in order to provide further insight into the pathophysiological disease mechanism and thus allow the development and evaluation of new treatments.

2. Human electroencephalogram (EEG)

Electroencephalography was the first physiological technique used to examine the brain by recording electric field potentials with the capability to reflect both the normal and abnormal electrical activity of the brain. EEG evolved into an indispensable method for studying cerebral information processing, particularly due to the introduction of source localization techniques and the decomposition of event-related activity into its frequency components (Winterer, 2011). Conventionally, EEG is recorded from the scalp using numerous electrodes affixed to specific scalp locations and is represented as changes in potential difference. The scalp EEG reflects the summated potentials from a large synchronously activated population of pyramidal cells in the cerebral cortex. These potentials are thought to originate primarily from excitatory and inhibitory neural electric activity, including action potential (AP) and postsynaptic potentials (Dietrich and Kanso, 2010). A small subset of EEG applications (e.g. epilepsy and neurooncology) makes use of implanting the electrodes directly inside the brain. In this section, we will refer only to EEG measured from the scalp surface.

Recording paradigms. The pattern of the electrical brain activity is generally investigated in three different paradigms 1) at rest, 2) during sensory stimulation (tone, flash light), or 3) during a cognitively driven task. Oscillatory activity during the resting-state (baseline oscillations) is acquired while the subject lies still without engaging in a task. Irregularities in baseline oscillations are important indicators for non-physiological brain activity. Internal as well as external events (tone, flash light) induce changes in oscillatory activity, which are observable in the EEG. Commonly, the evoked EEG is assessed by engaging the patient in a research specific task (e.g. listening to tones, sort pictures, remember numbers). These complimentary techniques can be used to determine alterations in default as well as specific networks, and as such have been used to define measures of signal to noise processing in schizophrenia and related disorders.

Advantages and limitations. Compared to in vivo ligand binding and hemodynamic measures including positron emission tomography (PET) and functional magnetic resonance imaging (fMRI) respectively, the greatest advantage of the EEG is the high degree of temporal resolution, which is typically 1ms or less. Such rapid data acquisition allows one to record complex pattern of neural interactions occurring within a physiological time range. Alternatively, hemodynamic and ligand binding measures provide a higher degree of spatial resolution than is possible using EEG techniques. Currently, the signal source localization for EEG lacks millimeter scale resolution due to blurring through the skull and scalp. Additionally, inverse source localization techniques are not suitable for deep structures and reply heavily on the constraints and assumptions of the models used. Consequently many possible EEG generator configurations may explain any given pattern of scalp EEG. Therefore, good spatial and temporal resolution is typically obtained by combining EEG with fMRI imaging (Javitt et al., 2008).

2.1 Event-related Potentials (ERP)

Electroencephalography provides a method to investigate general function of the brain including its reaction to particular stimuli that will be represented as changes in the EEG, globally known as event-related potentials (ERP) or evoked potentials (EP). These event-related potentials are defined as the oscillatory brain responses that are triggered by the occurrence of particular stimuli (auditory, visual, somatosensory).

Auditory evoked potential. Significant voltage fluctuations are detectable resulting from evoked neural activity and allow one to measure distinct stages in neural information processing. Moreover, ERPs reflect sub-cortical and cortical information processing in real time and thus they provide a useful tool for examine cognitive mechanisms in both normal brain function and disorder-related impairments. Each acoustic stimulus consists of the three primary components frequency, intensity, and time (Weber et al., 1981). Frequency refers to the spectrum of sound in hertz (Hz) and relates to the location of physical stimulation along the basilar membrane of the cochlea and along the tonotopic representation of the central auditory pathways (G. Celesia, 2005). Relative to a control the intensity refers to a stimulus loudness which is expressed in decibels (dB). The third component time, commonly measured in either microseconds (μs) or milliseconds (ms), comprises duration, repetition rate, and phase of onset of the stimulus.

The flow of information through the brain is reflected by the sequence of ERPs peaks. Human auditory evoked potential consists of three subsets of latency-defined components corresponding to progression of brain activity related to the auditory stimulus through the auditory pathway: brainstem auditory-evoked potentials (BAEP), middle-latency auditory-evoked potentials (MLAEP), and long-latency auditory-evoked potentials (LLAEP). Early sensory responses characteristically occur within a 10-milisecond time period after the presentation of an auditory stimulus at high intensities (70-90 dB normal hearing level [nHL]). A cascaded activation of the brainstem nuclei along the auditory pathway generates six waves starting at the cochlear nuclear complex - in this regard, these responses are called brainstem evoked potentials (BAEP) or auditory brainstem potentials (ABP) and are represented by the roman numerals I-VI (Buchwald and Huang, 1975, Bolz and Giedke, 1982). The I to V interpeak latency represents the brainstem transmission time as well as the brainstem auditory process. BAEP have been shown to be effective in the evaluation of integrity of the peripheral and central auditory pathways (G. Celesia, 2005). Clinical applications of BAEP are suitable in hearing assessment, determination of hearing loss, evaluation of brainstem function, and diagnosis of neurological disorders. Although BAEP are widely applied in clinical practice, concerns about the quality, comparability, and reproducibility have been raised (Chiappa and Young, 1985). In fact, the BAEP varies considerably in relation to changing aforementioned auditory stimulus parameters. Standardization of recordings techniques with respect to variables such as the positioning of the electrodes, stimulus characteristics, and click presentation time is important to obtain reproducible BAEPs.

Middle-latency auditory evoked potentials (MLAEP), defined as responses between 10 and 50ms (including the peaks N0, P0, N20, P50), are thought to correspond to the stimulus transduction in the auditory thalamus and auditory cortex (Picton et al., 1974). Most likely, these responses are originated from the medial geniculate nucleus and the primary auditory cortex (Woods et al., 1987). Middle-latency potentials find clinical application in the assessment of hearing threshold and identification of auditory perception (G. Celesia, 2005). Additionally, MLAPs provide a reliable method to asses thresholds to low frequencies that are crucial for speech perception (G. Celesia, 2005). However, contrary findings have been reported regarding to the reliability of the MLAP which arises questions about their clinical use. For instance, there is no consensus in terms of the presence of MLAPs in children. Several studies report the MLAP to be reliably recordable (Mendel et al., 1977, Mendelson and Salamy, 1981), others found the MLAP to be absent or unstable (Skinner and Glattke, 1977, Davis et al., 1983). While present, MLAP may serve as an indicator of hearing sensitivity, an absence of MLAP cannot be taken as an indication of hearing loss. Furthermore, in the normal population, the MLAP varies considerably, especially across age groups (Kraus et al., 1985). The difference in MLAP in normal subjects compared to MLAP in patients with neurological, cognitive, and speech disorders is also noted to be too small to equal an absent or abnormal MLAP with auditory pathway dysfunction. Longer latency components typically occur more than 50ms after acoustic stimulation reflecting the neural activity in the frontal cortex and cortical association areas (Gallinat et al., 2002). These potentials are predominately classified into obligate (N1, P1, P2) and task related components (P300, N400, MMN) referring to the dependence on characteristics of external (visual and acoustic) and internal stimuli, respectively. Thus, human LLAEP are mainly characterized by two major deflections, specifically the negative deflection N100, and the positive deflection P300 with latencies of 100 ms and 300 ms post, respectively. Abnormalities in LLAEP have been related with various type of psychopathology.

2.2 Components of the human ERP

The stages of information processing are mainly represented by following ERP components: P50, N100, P200, P300, and the mismatch negativity. P50 reflects the pre-attentive, N100 and P200 the early stages and P300 the late stage of information processing.

Sensory gating denotes the ability of the central nervous system (CNS) to inhibit or suppress the response to irrelevant or distracting sensory input in order to focus on task-relevant sensory information. Habituation following repeated exposure to the same sensory stimulus is an essential protective mechanism of the brain against flooding of the higher cortical centers with unnecessary information (Venables, 1964). A commonly used electrophysiological procedure to assess sensory gating in humans is the paired-click paradigm (PCP) (Adler et al., 1982, Boutros et al., 1993). During this task, a pair of identical brief auditory stimuli is presented at an interval of 500ms. Additionally, an interpair interval of 8-10s assure that the effects of one pair of stimuli do not carry over to the next pair (Zouridakis and Boutros, 1992). If inhibitory pathways are functioning normally, the amplitude of the response to the second stimulus (test response) is decreased because of inhibition pathways that are activated in response to a first (conditioning) stimulus. The quality of the sensory gating mechanism is expressed as the ratio of the two amplitudes (second amplitude/ first amplitude times 100)(Mazhari et al., 2011). Hence, low ratios indicate better sensory gating capability due to a stronger inhibition of irrelevant input.

Mainly, three evoked potential components are used to examine the sensory gating: P50, N100, and P200. Under physiological conditions the amplitudes of P50, N100, and P200 to the second stimulus (S2) in the pair are significantly reduced compared to the first stimulus (S1) reflecting an inhibitory mechanism to minimize the disruptive effects of the second repeating and therefore irrelevant stimulus (Williams et al., 2011). Peaking between 15 and 80 msec following stimulus presentation, P50 is the earliest major component that habituates to stimulus repetition. Attentional influences are minimal at this early stage of information processing making the P50 component optimal for the investigation of pre-attentive sensory mechanism (Grunwald et al., 2003). The N100, the largest component of the auditory evoked potential, has a peak latency of about 100ms and is a neurophysiological parameter reflecting arousal and attention (Strik et al., 1992). Its generation is conducted by a complex network of cortical areas (Rosburg et al., 2008). The amplitude of N100 is sensitive a long-list of individual related factors (e.g. attention, hearing threshold, motivation, drug and smoking history) and physical characteristics of the stimulus (e.g., duration, intensity, rise time). N100 is primarily an exogenous component which is elicited by any discernible auditory stimulus, irrespective of attention. However, distinct differences between attended and unattended stimuli are observed (Rosburg et al., 2008). For example, the level of arousal has a modulating effect on the amplitude of the N100 evoked by unattended stimuli while the degree of selective attention influences the N100 amplitude evoked by attended stimulus. Auditory P200 is a positive event-related positive deflection automatically peaking roughly 200ms after stimulus presentation regardless of attention and task variables. However, its latency and amplitude co-vary with aspects of selective attention and stimulus encoding processes. P200 is reported to index early information processing, selective attention, and stimulus encoding (Shenton et al., 1989, Polich and Squire, 1993). Thus, the auditory temporal cortex has been highly implicated in P200 generation (Shenton et al., 1989). It is noteworthy that brain regions that are not primary sources of P200 may modify the response as a function of experimental conditions (e.g., attentive versus inattentive).

Mismatch Negativity. The ability to detect changes in auditory stimulus characteristics and adapt thereafter are basic neuronal functions that can be measured with ERPs in both, humans and animals. Mismatch negativity (MMN) reflects the context-dependent information processing which is required to compare a deviant incoming stimulus with the neural representation already stored in the transient auditory memory (Bomba and Pang, 2004). When a string of tones with a specific regularity (sequence of homogenous tones) is presented, the brain stores the features of this auditory stimulation in a short-duration neural memory trace (Ulanovsky et al., 2004). While this echoic memory is still active, each new auditory input is compared to the existing trace for a break of regularity (deviant tone), which generates a neuronal adaptation giving rise to the MMN (Naatanen, 2000). MMN is most frequently elicited in an auditory oddball paradigm. A sequence of repetitive standard stimuli is randomly interrupted by a deviant oddball stimulus which may differ in stimulus characteristics such as pitch, intensity, or duration. Generators are located in the auditory and frontal cortices (Giard et al., 1990, Alho, 1995). Of particular importance, MMN is evoked irrespective of attention (e.g. present in comatose patients) (Fischer et al., 2000). Peaking between 100 and 225ms, MMN is a difference wave between responses to frequent and deviant stimuli. In clinical neurosciences, MMN has been widely used in various applications, in particular in schizophrenia research, due to its good reproducibility and the ability to assess it without a task (Garrido et al., 2009).

P300. Probably the most extensive studied long-latency ERP component is the P300 (also termed P3), a time-locked positive deflection emerging 250 ms to 500 ms after attending stimulus. First described by Sutton et al. in 1965, P300 is thought to reflect an information processing cascade when attentional and memory mechanisms are engaged (Polich, 2007). Although related to the process of sensory stimulus mismatch detection, the P300 component represents an attention-driven memory comparison process in which every incoming stimulus will be revised to detect possible stimulus feature modifications. According to whether changes are present or absent, the electrophysiological recordings will differ. If no change can be detected, only sensory evoked potentials are recorded (N100, P200, N200). If a new stimulus is presented and the subject allocates attentional resources to the target, the neural stimulus representation is altered and the consequent update leads to the generation of P300 (Polich, 2007). Similar to the MMN, the auditory P300 is elicited in context of an oddball paradigm, but in contrast to MMN elicitation the generation of P300 requires the test-taking person to be attentive and respond physically or mentally to the presented target. Commonly, subjects are instructed to either push a button following the infrequent target or to count deviants. The P300 is measured by quantifying its amplitude and its latency within a time window which varies (e.g. 250-500ms) as a function of the subjects age stimulus mode, and task conditions (Singh and Basu, 2009). P300 amplitude is also considered to index brain activity reflecting attention to incoming stimulus information when representations are updated (Polich, 2007, Turetsky et al., 2007b). The P300 latency is thought to be a measure of perceptual processing speed (Polich, 2007). The P300 consists of two subcomponents, an early potential P3a and a later component P3b. While P3a is evoked by any novel stimulus, the task-relevant P3b potential is only elicited during target stimulus processing (Javitt et al., 2008). P3a is hypothesized to be generated by stimuli which change the content of the working memory. This attentional-driven neural activity may then be transmitted to brain areas associated with memory storage and subsequently generate the P3b. Supportively, time frequency analyses indicate that theta and alpha activity govern the relationship of the P3a to attention and P3b to memory processing (Intriligator and Polich, 1994, Spencer and Polich, 1999, Polich, 2007). The P3a appears to be sensitive to specific neurotransmitters; in particular dopamine and glutamate have been implicated in the mediation of P3a. Specifically, clinical populations associated with reduced dopamine levels (e.g., Parkinson's disease, rest-less leg syndrome) exhibited deficient P3a (Hansch et al., 1982, Stanzione et al., 1991). Conversely, pharmacological enhancement of dopamine level was shown to increase P3a in patients with low baseline amplitudes (Takeshita and Ogura, 1994). In addition, glutamatergic and GABAergic disequilibrium impair the generation of P3a. Watson found both the NMDA receptor antagonist ketamine and the GABA-A receptor agonist thiopental to reduce P3a amplitude, while ketamine also shortened the P3a latency (Watson et al., 2009). The second P300 subcomponent, P3b, is thought to serve as a measure of evaluation of environmental signals including contextual information (Squires et al., 1976, Barcelo and Knight, 2007). Furthermore, perceptual analysis and response initiation are suggested to be reflected by P3b. The locus coeruleus–norephedrine system (LC-NE) is of importance for the regulation of sensory signal transmission and was suggested to underlie the generation of P3b (Nieuwenhuis et al., 2005). Pharmacological evidence emerges from studies in which subjects were exposed to nicotine, a NE-release mediating agent, inducing a significant increase in P3b amplitude (Polich and Criado, 2006).

In summary, P300 and its subcomponents may provide an insight to the mechanisms and pathways of various cognitive processes. However, the understanding and investigation of these coponents is coined by some noteworthy limitations. Studies of the differences in the P300 observed across various patient populations have been highly variable (Polich, 2007). Specifically, in only 10-15% of normal young adults the P3a can readily be observed. Despite simplicity of the task situation and the reliability of observing ERPs in the oddball paradigm, the cerebral mechanisms producing the P300 remain elusive. As such, the neural generators of P300 are imprecisely delineated (Soltani and Knight, 2000, Eichele et al., 2005, Linden, 2005).

2.3 ERP measurements and analysis

The primary step of all ERP analysis is to extract the event-related portion of the recorded field potentials. Detecting ERP activity within ongoing activity is a general problem since brain responses to individual sensory, cognitive, or motor events are relatively small compared to the steadily ongoing background activity, also called noise, (i.e., the activity not related to the stimulus). Thus, to enhance the responses in contrast to the background noise (i.e., improve signal-to-noise ratio) the analysis of ERP is done by averaging the oscillatory activity of a series of trials.

Power measure. Power reflects the amplitude of an oscillation. Amplitude (μV) is defined as difference between the mean pre-stimulus baseline voltage and the largest positive or negative going peak of the ERP waveform with in a time window. Its latency (ms) defines the time from stimulus onset to the point of maximum amplitude (Polich, 2007). For a stationary signal, in which the EEG does not change over time, the Fast-Fourier Transform (FFT) is used to spectrally decompose the time-invariant signal into component frequencies. The power spectrum yielded by FFT analysis is used for resting-state tasks. The analysis of non-stationary neural activity requires signal-processing methods that compute changes in oscillatory activity at a particular frequency across time. Oscillatory responses can be categorized by their phase- and temporal-relationship to repeated trials of a sensory or cognitive event (Galambos and Makeig, 1992, Tallon-Baudry et al., 1998). Oscillations directly in phase with a stimulus (i.e., phase- and time-locked) are called evoked oscillations. Induced oscillatory activity is modulated by a stimulus but is not strictly phase-locked to event onset (i.e., time- but not phase-locked). Oscillatory activity that is in-phase with a stimulus averages across trials to produce an evoked-response assuming that (1) the delay of the electrical brain responses relative to the stimulus is invariable across the testing trial; and (2) the ongoing background activity is steady (Da Silva, 2005). In the time domain, induced oscillations tend to average out and thus require different single-trial signal processing methods for identification. Finally, total power refers to the sum of evoked and induced power and is typically represented as difference from or a percentage change from pre-stimulus baseline power at each frequency (Gandal et al., 2010).

Phase measures. The main approach is to decompose a neural time series into phase information at a given frequency. Applying time-frequency transforms, one can investigate changes in frequency-specific measures during a given task with millisecond precision. **Event-related spectral perturbation (ERSP)** is a measure of change of power from baseline associated with a stimulus presentation, and includes both phase locked and non-phase locked activity (Shin et al., 2010). Time-frequency transforms also provide measures of the phase of oscillations, allowing for investigation of phase-synchrony. **Phase-synchrony** is independent of oscillatory amplitude and is therefore thought to be a more direct measure of the synchronization of neural signals. The phase locking factor (PLF) (i.e., intertrial coherence, ITC) describes the similarity in phase at a given point in time across trials at a single electrode site. This measure is unitless, ranging from 0 to 1.

Auditory Steady State Responses (ASSR) are middle-latency auditory evoked potentials triggered by presentation of auditory stimuli at rates between 1 and 200 Hz or by continuous tones modulated in amplitude and or frequency. The responses from both types of stimuli are a metric for looking at synchronous neuronal activity in the brain's auditory processing. Conventionally, values of 0.5, 1, 2 and 4 kHz are used for the continuous carrier tone whereas repetitive stimulus trains are often presented around 40 Hz (Galambos et al., 1981, Herdman and Stapells, 2001, Luts and Wouters, 2005). The modulation of the carrier tone occurs in amplitude or frequency at a set rate. The response to these periodic modulations or stimulation trains is measured for phased locking and amplitude. ASSR stimuli contrast with the broadband clicks delivered with Auditory Brain Responses (ABRs). Whereas the auditory stimulus of the ABRs consist of a spectrum of tones in one stimulus click, the ASSR stimulations (especially with continuous tone amplitude modulation) can target specific tones, giving ASSRs a level of frequency-specific information sensitivity that is not present in the ABR metric (Roeser, 2007). ASSRs therefore give a consistent measurement of brain responses reflective of information processing and hearing thresholds without the need of subject involvement.

Frequencies. Oscillatory activity is generally evaluated within EEG frequency ranges: delta (0–4 Hz), theta (4–8 Hz), alpha (8–12 Hz), beta (12–30 Hz), and gamma (>30 Hz). Furthermore, each range is linked to specific perceptual and cognitive processes as well as behavioral states (Table 1) (Basar et al., 2001). In 1929, Hans Berger first depicted measurable brain activity at a frequency of ~10Hz and termed this oscillation **alpha** (Berger, 1929). Alpha oscillations are correlated to brain function such as inhibition, attention, consciousness and primarily generated in thalamus, hippocampus, and cortical regions (Uhlhaas and Singer, 2010). The **theta** range is associated with perceptual processing, learning, memory, and synaptic plasticity (Huerta and Lisman, 1993). Cortico-hippocampal circuits have been found as key generators of the rhythm (Ehrlichman et al., 2009a). **Beta** oscillations are believed to be generated in overall cortical structures and are involved in sensory gating, attention, and long-term synchronization (Kopell et al., 2000, Gross et al., 2004, Hong et al., 2008a). **Gamma** oscillations have received special attention in the research of neuropsychiatric disorders due to their alleged role in sensory binding, selective attention, associative and perceptual learning, encoding and retrieval of memory traces (Singer, 1993, Bragin et al., 1995, Chrobak and Buzsaki, 1998, Miltner et al., 1999, Fries et al., 2001). Gamma-band oscillations depend on intact function of the fast-spiking GABAergic (parvalbumin containing) interneurons (Fuchs et al., 2001). These subsets of inhibitory GABAergic interneurons, located in hippocampal and cortical areas, are proposed to play a primary role in the generation of the gamma oscillations (Uhlhaas and Singer, 2010).

Frequency range	Primary generators	Function
Alpha (8-12 Hz)	Thalamus, hippocampus, cortical regions	Inhibition, attention, consciousness
Theta (4-7 Hz)	Cortico-hippocampal circuits	Perceptual processing, learning, memory, synaptic plasticity
Beta (13-10 Hz)	Overall cortical structures	sensory gating, attention, and long-term synchronization
Gamma (30-200 Hz)	Hippocampal and cortical	Perception, selective attention, consciousness, encoding and retrieval of memory traces

Table 1. Functional correlates of neural oscillations

3. EEG abnormalities in schizophrenia

3.1 Abnormalities in obligate ERP

Neurophysiological measures have been widely applied with regard to schizophrenia since they provide the ability to index abnormalities in information processing, to localize involved brain regions and correlate well with negative and cognitive deficits. Supporting evidence from EEG studies suggest that the core pathophysiology of schizophrenia is related to abnormal brain dynamics, neural synchronization, and connectivity. Schizophrenia patients exhibit deficits in amplitude and/or gating of the P50, N100, and P200 obligate components, as well as reductions in task related mismatch negativity, P3a, and P3b. Thus, this section will introduce readers to the characteristic ERPs of schizophrenia, which are typified by alterations in all amplitude, latency, and gating of several key components relative to healthy population.

Mismatch negativity provides a useful tool for investigating mechanism underlying cognitive dysfunction in patients suffering from schizophrenia as well as autism, dyslexia, and dementia. Initially, Shelley and colleagues found abnormalities of MMN in individuals with schizophrenia (Shelley et al., 1991). Similarly, more than 30 studies report a significant attenuated MMN amplitude in patients with schizophrenia, for both frequency and latency (Umbricht and Krljes, 2005). Thus, these findings are believed to reflect the degraded auditory perception, a feature linked with schizophrenia (Naatanen, 2003). For instance according to Javitt, schizophrenia subjects exhibit impairments not only in generation of frequency-MMN, but also in tone-matching performance (Javitt, 2000). Additionally, studies have noted a correlation between the magnitude of the MMN and disease severity (Catts et al., 1995). However, it is necessary to note that changes of MMN parameters (e.g., prolongation of latency and reduction of amplitude) are not sufficiently specific to diagnose particular disease. Disturbances in the glutamatergic system, more specifically the inadequate NMDA-receptor neurotransmission, have been implicated in neurocognitive deficits of schizophrenia (Javitt and Zukin, 1991). Thus, the assumption that MMN depends on intact NMDA receptor signaling makes MMN a particularly interesting paradigm for schizophrenia research. NDMAR antagonists, such as ketamine and phencyclidine (PCP), have been shown to selectively abolish the MMN suggesting the NMDAR-dependent neurotransmission to underlie deficits in MMN generation and echoic memory (Javitt, 2000, Umbricht et al., 2000, Naatanen, 2003). Furthermore, MMN has been proved useful in clinical investigations of schizophrenia patients due to its robustness to changes in attention and performance (Garrido et al., 2009). Intrestingly, also siblings of schizophrenia patients have been reported to exhibit impaired working memory reflected in a reduction of the MMN amplitude (Sevik et al., 2011). Although the literature contains conflicting results, MMN may serve as an index of genetic predisposition to schizophrenia and disease progression (Jessen et al., 2001, Michie et al., 2002, Shinozaki et al., 2002).

Disturbances in information processing are key features of schizophrenia (Braff, 1993). Insufficient inhibitory processing of repetitive, irrelevant acoustic stimuli has been reported in patients as well as their first-degree relatives (Bramon et al., 2004, de Wilde et al., 2007). Using a double-click auditory paradigm, Adler and others have noted that schizophrenia patients have a diminished **gating** of the auditory P50 (Adler et al., 1982) (Judd et al., 1992, Olincy and Martin, 2005). While in healthy subjects a repeated presentation of an auditory stimulus causes a >60% reduction in S2 amplitude, schizophrenia patients routinely fail to suppress their response to the second click (Adler et al., 1982, Braff and Geyer, 1990, Stevens et al., 1991). Adler and colleagues also noted a diminishment of the amplitude and latency of the response to the first stimuli in unmedicated individuals with schizophrenia (Adler et al., 1986). Neuroleptics increase **P50** latency and amplitude, but do not normalize conditioning-testing ratios. As such, the observed gating deficits may actually result as an epiphenomenon of medication, rather than as part of the disease (Siegel et al., 2005). Despite this limitation, P50 gating has been interpreted by some to demonstrate reduced capability to extract relevant from irrelevant information, leading to an overload of information reaching consciousness and cognitive fragmentation (Venables, 1960, Patterson et al., 2008). This may contribute to many of the difficulties people suffering from struggle with including the inability to stay focused during conversation or the being overwhelmed by the physical environment (Freedman et al., 1996, Turetsky et al., 2007b, Williams et al., 2011). The brain regions and their neural dynamics that underlie the malfunctioning of inhibitory processes still remain to be determined. Furthermore, it should be noted that this P50 gating phenomenon has not been replicated outside a small number of institutions, suggesting a large impact of operator processing on the measure (de Wilde et al., 2007). As such, P50 gating is not an ideal measure of signal processing and should not be used in place of more robust and reproducible findings using other ERP measures and components.

Patients with schizophrenia exhibit deficits in **N100** generation, especially at long interstimulus intervals (ISI) and extremely short ISIs. Amplitude reduction and latency delay of the auditory N100 are robust physiological abnormalities in schizophrenia (Roth et al., 1981, Laurent et al., 1999). However, the findings are inconsistent and seem to depend on the experimental conditions used (Davis et al., 1966, Pritchard, 1986). Reduced N100 amplitude reflects deficits in mechanism involved in initial sensory processing and early selective attention, prominent features seen in schizophrenia (Strik et al., 1992, Frangou et al., 1997). Although N100 amplitude reduction is relatively independent of symptom severity, Ahveninen and colleagues proposed N100 reduction could serve as an endophenotypic trait marker of functional brain changes related to genetic predisposition to schizophrenia (Ahveninen et al., 2006). There is some evidence that N100 amplitude reduction is also seen in first-degree relatives (Blackwood et al., 1991, Turetsky et al., 2008). For instance, a combined EEG/MEG study on monozygotic and dizygotic twins discordant for schizophrenia revealed an N100 amplitude reduction in both schizophrenia patients and their unaffected siblings (Ahveninen et al., 2006). More evidence for the heritability of the N100 amplitude comes from similar twin studies (Blackwood et al., 1991, Frangou et al., 1997). Furthermore, a reduction in N100 amplitude appears not to be specific to schizophrenia in that it is also reported in patients with bipolar disorder, and hypothyroidism (Umbricht et al., 2003, Oerbeck et al., 2007). Reduced gating of the N100 response to repeated stimulation has also been demonstrated in schizophrenia (Turetsky et al., 2008).

The auditory **P200** indexes early stimulus processing and thus is informative to study in schizophrenia, which has been linked to deficits in early information processing. Numerous reports have demonstrated that amplitude and gating of the P200 are reduced in schizophrenia (Roth et al., 1981, Boutros et al., 2004a, Boutros et al., 2004b, Lijffijt et al., 2009a, Gjini et al., 2010). Moreover, reduced amplitude appears to be related to negative symptoms, in particular anhedonia and avolition (Shenton et al., 1989). P200 gating shows a positive relationship to attentional performance and the post-attentive cognitive P300 response (Boutros et al., 2004b, Lijffijt et al., 2009b). Pharmacological studies indicate various neurotransmitters, such as glutamate and dopamine, contribute to the generation of P200. As such, healthy people display schizophrenia-like decreases in P200 amplitude during acute exposure to ketamine (Murck et al., 2006). Moreover, amphetamine administration reduces P200 amplitude to the first stimulus in an auditory gating paradigm, suggesting that decreased NMDA-mediated transmission may produce the observed attenuation of the P200 through facilitation of dopamine release (Connolly et al., 2004). Various family studies indicate that there are abnormalities in P200 among relatives of schizophrenia patients, suggesting a substantial genetic component to this endophenotype (Frangou et al., 1997, Freedman et al., 1997). Similar to N100, the P200 has further been suggested as a measure for sensory gating since both components produce less inter-subject and inter-protocol variability as compared to P50.

In the oddball paradigm, the **P300** response indexes cortical responses related to recognizing and assessing the significance of rare stimuli. Meta-analysis has shown that schizophrenia patients have significantly reduced P300 amplitudes and that their P300 latency is significantly delayed compared to normal controls (Bramon et al., 2004). Diminished P300 may indicate the presence of unsteady background activity that interferes with detecting the identity and salience of the task-related stimulus (Pfefferbaum et al., 1989). Additionally, Pritchard suggested that P3 amplitude attenuation may potentially serve as a trait marker for the negative symptoms of schizophrenia (Pritchard, 1986). Several studies support a negative correlation between P3 amplitude and severity of negative symptoms, but emphasize its validity only in medicated patients (Roth et al., 1975, Pfefferbaum et al., 1989). Anti-psychotic medications were also shown to significantly affect the amplitude but not latency of P300 (Bramon et al., 2004). Interestingly, it has been proposed that the P300 waveform is a physiological correlate of an update in working memory related to changes in the environment (Donchin and Isreal, 1980). This idea is supported by the finding that P300 amplitude and latency correlate with neuropsychological performance scores in patients. Notably, there are correlations between decreased P300 amplitude, lower IQ and poorer memory performance as well as increased P300 latency and lower IQ, poorer total memory scores, and serial clustering (Shajahan et al., 1997). Evidence that P300 abnormalities may serve as an indicator for genetic vulnerability arises from recent studies which found similar P300 alteration in first-degree relatives including decreased amplitude and increased latency (Saitoh et al., 1984, Blackwood et al., 1991, Kidogami et al., 1991).

In addition to the task related P3, also known as the P3b, an automatic, task-independent portion of the P3 called the P3a is thought to be modulated by both glutamate and dopamine (Siegel et al., 2003). A growing body of evidence suggests that there is also a reduction in P3a amplitude in schizophrenia (Mathalon et al., , Mathalon et al., 2000, Alain et al., 2002, Devrim-Ucok et al., 2006, Ford et al., 2008, van der Stelt and van Boxtel, 2008, Mathalon et al., 2010). Prolongation of P3a latency is also observed in patients (Frodl et al., 2001). Within the schizophrenia population, patients with prominent auditory hallucinations manifest a P3a amplitude reduction compared to those without hallucinations (Fisher et al., 2010). This data has been interpreted to indicate that hallucinations reflect a preferential attention to internally generated brain activity, relative to incoming exogenous stimuli (Fisher et al., 2008). Furthermore, P3a has been linked to functional outcomes in schizophrenia in that reduced P3a amplitude is associated with extended illness duration and increased depression-anxiety symptoms (Mathalon et al., 2000, van der Stelt and van Boxtel, 2008).

Deficient processing of contextual information is a prominent feature of cognitive dysfunction in schizophrenia. Thus, P3b response has been extensively studied in schizophrenia and shows promise both as a measure of attentional processes during signal detection and as a predictor of performance on formal laboratory tests of cognition.

Suppressed P3b amplitude is a widely replicated finding in schizophrenia, while P3b latency elongation is less consistently reported (Blackwood et al., 1991, Ford et al., 1992, Roxborough et al., 1993, Coburn et al., 1998, Jeon and Polich, 2003). Most investigations of P3b have been conducted in chronic schizophrenia populations. Thus, it is of considerable interest to determine if these abnormalities are present at onset or are exacerbated by chronicity. To address this question, few studies have investigated the P3b component in first-episode schizophrenia (FES) and consistently report a reduction in P3b amplitude as well as prolonged latencies (Hirayasu et al., 1998, Brown et al., 2002, Demiralp et al., 2002, Wang et al., 2003). Furthermore, the P3b amplitude appears to correlate inversely with the disorder's duration (Olichney et al., 1998, Mathalon et al., 2000, Martin-Loeches et al., 2001). Brown and others identified similarities in P3b amplitudes in FES and CS patients (Hirayasu et al., 1998, Brown et al., 2002). Similarly, unaffected first-degree relatives of patients have frequently been reported to exhibit reduced P3b amplitudes (Blackwood et al., 1991, Kidogami et al., 1991, Roxborough et al., 1993). Additionally, most studies of P3 and its subcomponents have been performed in medicated patients. Thus, the effect of neuroleptics on these ERP components remains controversial. Some studies suggested that antipsychotic medication increases the P3b amplitude, in contrast to others which failed to replicate this finding (Pfefferbaum et al., 1989, Ford et al., 1994, Coburn et al., 1998, Umbricht et al., 1998). Lastly, it is important to note that the alterations of P3a and P3b are not specific to schizophrenia. For instance, bipolar depression is linked to similar impairments. Although the lack of specificity is a limitation with respect to addressing the unique pathophysiology of schizophrenia, the P3 family may still serve as a trait marker for schizophrenia vulnerability.

3.2 Event-related Spectral Perturbations (ERSP) abnormalities in schizophrenia

Neural oscillation and their synchronization are thought to reflect important mechanisms for interneural communication and binding of information that is processed in distinct brain areas (Roach and Mathalon, 2008). These oscillations are decomposed in order to examine individual frequency ranges. These frequency domains are linked to distinct cognitive and perceptual processes, some of which are known to be impaired in schizophrenia. Therefore, this section will discuss the schizophrenia-like alterations in time-frequency measures in baseline, evoked and non-evoked auditory responses across all frequency. Furthermore, a growing body of evidence indicates that people with schizophrenia also display abnormal EEG rhythms, in both high (beta and gamma) and low frequency bands (delta and theta). Contemporary EEG studies mainly focus on gamma oscillations because this range is thought to reflect a fundamental mechanism to integrate neural networks and play a critical role in cognitive function (Tiitinen et al., 1993, Gandal et al., 2010). Alternatively, earlier EEG studies in schizophrenia focused primarily on lower frequencies and found substantial evidence of abnormalities.

Increased pre-stimulus **theta-** and **delta**-band activity have consistently been observed in schizophrenia, occurring; 1) both locally and among distant electrodes; 2) regardless of medication history, and 3) in both first-episode and chronic patients (Morihisa et al., 1983, Morstyn et al., 1983, Sponheim et al., 1994). Converging evidence from magnetic resonance imaging studies supports that the default network in schizophrenia tends to be overactive (Fehr et al., 2003, Harrison et al., 2007). Positive symptoms were found to positively correlate with an elevated resting-state theta activity in certain brain areas (Garrity et al.,

2007). Contrary to resting-state activity, a number of studies using time-frequency measures revealed a reduction in theta and delta power of both phase locked and non-phase locked responses to an auditory stimulus in individuals with schizophrenia (Ford et al., 2008, Doege et al., 2009). Although a number of abnormal findings have been reported in the delta frequency range among people with schizophrenia, these data have been inconsistent across studies (Siekmeier and Stufflebeam, 2010).

Several investigators reported reduced or even absent power and coherence of **alpha** activity in schizophrenia during resting EEG and sustained attention (Itil, 1979, Merrin and Floyd, 1992). Also, Sponheim and others noted that individuals with schizophrenia exhibit reduced alpha activity, along with increased neighboring frequencies in the theta and beta bands. However, within the patient group no further differences were found between first-episode and chronic patients or between medication-naïve and medicated patients (Sponheim et al., 1994, Boutros et al., 2008). This consistency among clinical populations suggests that these abnormalities are a stable characteristic of schizophrenia and not treatment-related or duration-dependent. These EEG alpha alterations appear to correlate with the severity of negative symptoms. Indeed, repetitive transcranial magnetic stimulation was reported to improve negative symptoms and concomitantly to increase the alpha activity amplitude (Jin et al., 2006). As reviewed above, alpha oscillatory activity is associated with attention, which is impaired in schizophrenia. Investigation of evoked and induced alpha oscillations in schizophrenia revealed reduced alpha power and impaired ability to synchronize the phase of ongoing alpha activity. Greater trial-by-trial variability may be due the interference of ongoing background brain activity with the recruitment of neural systems which is indispensable for the processing of sensory information. For example, disturbed phase-locking leads to an increased trial-by-trial variability and diminished amplitude of certain ERP components, such as the N100 (Makeig et al., 2000, Gallinat et al., 2004, Haenschel et al., 2009, White et al., 2009). The influence of alpha oscillations on N100 is mirrored by a positive correlation between attention and N100 amplitude. Taken together, this may delineate the mechanism of impaired attention in schizophrenia. Furthermore, White proposed that an interaction between alpha and **gamma** oscillations is necessary for high fidelity and integrated communication within and across brain structures, facilitating coherent sensory registration (White et al., 2009). Given that a growing body of evidence also reveals disturbances in gamma oscillations in schizophrenia, it is possible that the interaction between early gamma and evoked alpha activity is diminished in schizophrenia. Gamma abnormalities have been reported in a variety of contexts, including in sensory-driven, cognitive, and resting-state paradigms. These deficits are present at first-episode psychosis, in unmedicated patients, and, to a lesser degree, in unaffected relatives, suggesting that abnormal gamma synchrony is a heritable feature of schizophrenia(Rodin et al., 1968b, Leicht et al., 2009)Symond et al., 2005). In resting-state paradigms, several studies reported elevated high-frequency EEG activity in schizophrenia (Finley, 1944, Itil et al., 1972, Fenton et al., 1980). Accordingly, two large studies found elevated pre-stimulus gamma power in schizophrenia patients during auditory paradigms (Winterer et al., 2004, Hong et al., 2008b). However, no group-differences in pre-stimulus gamma power were observed in smaller study, perhaps reflecting a need for larger sample sizes to detect subtle changes (Brockhaus-Dumke et al., 2008). Numerous studies have also investigated evoked and induced gamma oscillatory activity in schizophrenia. The overall findings suggest a reduction in stimulus-related gamma-band oscillations (Leicht et al., ,

Basar-Eroglu et al., 2009, Leicht et al., 2010a, Leicht et al., 2010b) (for review see (Gandal et al., 2010). However, not all studies found differences in evoked gamma-activity between patients and healthy comparison individuals, again suggesting that gamma band abnormalities may be subtle and require relatively large samples with sufficient power to detect population differences (Blumenfeld and Clementz, 2001, Brockhaus-Dumke et al., 2008).

Finally, lower levels of **beta** oscillatory activity have been observed in patients with schizophrenia (Rutter et al., 2009). In sleep studies, unmedicated patients had higher beta power at all stages of the sleep compared to healthy individuals (Tekell et al., 2005). Alternatively, deficient power and synchronization of evoked and induced EEG rhythms in the beta and gamma bands have frequently been reported (Clementz et al., 1997, Cho et al., 2006, Uhlhaas et al., 2006). Interestingly, these findings were replicated in medication-naïve and chronically medicated patients. However like other frequencies, contradictory and negative finding exists. Thus, few studies report an augmentation in evoked beta activity, which may be due to methodological or analytical differences (for review see (Uhlhaas and Singer, 2010).

3.3 Auditory steady-state response abnormalities in schizophrenia

Auditory steady-state auditory responses (ASSRs), in which the evoked potential entrains to stimulus frequency and phase, are reduced in amplitude and phase locking in patients with schizophrenia, particularly at 40 Hz (Kwon et al., 1999, Brenner et al., 2003, Light et al., 2006, Krishnan et al., 2009). Importantly, these deficits are present in schizophrenia patients during their first hospitalization. Several animal models of schizophrenia display similar ASSR disruption as those found in humans (Spencer et al., 2008, Vohs et al., 2010). These issues suggest deficiencies in the coordinated timing of neural populations within specific types of networks (Maharajh et al., 2010). The Gamma frequency has been correlated with many of the neuro-cognitive behaviors that are disrupted in schizophrenia (Haig et al., 2000). Thus, ASSR in the gamma spectrum may offer an objective biomarker of schizophrenia and provide further insight as to how disruptions in gamma affect neuronal processing and behavior. ASSRs have also been used to help elucidate potential mechanisms by which hallucinations in schizophrenia are associated with phase synchronization between the primary auditory cortices (Mulert et al., 2010).

4. Preclinical models of EEG abnormalities

4.1 Approaches to modeling EEG in mice

Historically, EEG and ERPs have been most commonly obtained from deeply anesthetized animals. In such preparations, the animal is typically placed within a stereotaxic apparatus and surgical procedures are used to remove the skull and expose the brain. A recording electrode is then lowered into the appropriate location in the brain and recordings are obtained. Typically, auditory stimuli are delivered through speakers located in the stereotaxic apparatus. There are several advantages to the use of this methodology. First, since the electrode is not permanently affixed to the skull, it can be moved around so as to obtain the best signal possible. This is especially true if the researcher is interested in obtaining ERP/EEG recordings within cell populations that can be easily identified according to a unique firing pattern. Second, since the auditory stimulus is presented at a very short and invariant distance from the auditory canal, the resulting EEG response will typically show low levels of variance across trials and across different animals, leading to very stable and reliable results. Third, since the animal is anesthetized the EEG/ERP is less likely to be influenced by such factors as state of arousal, movement or attention to extraneous stimuli. While less popular in recent years, this methodology is still widely used within some research communities and is especially useful when one is interested in studying EEG and electrophysiology primarily as an end in itself. A major drawback to recording EEG in this manner lies in the limited translatability to the types of EEG methodologies used in patient populations. If this is a goal of the study, recording EEG in awake and freely moving animals is the more optimal choice. While the results obtained using this methodology can indeed be confounded by extraneous factors, such factors may actually be useful to study within the context of translational research. For example, changes in arousal can occur following exposure to drugs that stimulate nicotinic receptors and EEG techniques could be used to examine the neural processes responsible for this change. It should be noted that these two techniques can produce very different results under some circumstances. For example, amphetamine increases theta oscillations in anesthetized animals, but decreases theta in awake animals. This difference could be due to the fact that the inherent state of arousal is greatly different in the two cases, or could be due to the locomotor enhancing effects of amphetamine, which could act to increase movement related theta in awake but not anesthetized animals.

A second consideration involves the question of electrode placement. In some cases, EEG and ERPs can be obtained from electrodes placed on the scalp (in humans) or the surface of the cortex (in animals). Alternatively, electrodes can be placed within a particular region of the brain, such as the hippocampus, that the researcher may be interested in. Superficially, recording from the surface of the cortex offers the greatest similarity to the scalp recordings ordinarily obtained in human subjects and, thus, may be of greatest interest to researchers interested in translational studies. However, it should be noted that there is often little overlap in organization and topography between human and animal cortices, and this could lead to divergent or erroneous results. Similarly, since the relative size of the cortex is much smaller in animals and since electrical activity can carry over great distances in the brain it is quite likely that surface recordings in animals are strongly influenced by electrical activity occurring in sub-cortical areas. This is much less likely to be an issue in humans, given the much greater size of the cortex in this species. Traditionally, depth recordings have been the exclusive domain of animal researchers, due to the difficulty of obtaining depth recordings in human subjects (although such recordings have been obtained in humans during surgical intervention to reduce epileptic seizures). In general, depth recordings have been most widely used by researchers interested in studying the function of particular brain regions and offer a great opportunity to study neural activity within isolated brain regions. It should be noted that there are some EEG phenomena that are only see during depth recordings in isolated regions. A primary example of this is movement-induced increases in hippocampal theta, which are only observed when recording EEG directly in the hippocampus (Krause et al., 2003). Nonetheless, depth recordings offer many advantages over surface electrodes. First, since depth electrodes are located within the neural tissue, as opposed to being on top of the brain or on the scalp, signals obtained with depth recordings usually have much greater amplitude than those obtained from the surface. As a consequence, there is typically less variance across trials and across animals in depth recordings. Second, depth recordings are less susceptible to the confounding effects of muscle activity or movement that often occur when recording from the scalp. Finally, due to the emergence of deep brain stimulation as a method to improve brain function in various disease states, it is becoming increasingly possible to record from within particular brain regions in humans as well, suggesting that the results from depth recordings done in rodents may become increasingly translatable to human studies (McCracken and Grace, 2009).

4.1.1 EEG from human to mouse

In addition to human studies, the neural information processing has been investigated with auditory evoked potentials in cats, rats, mice, and monkeys (Cook et al., 1968, Javitt et al., 1996, de Bruin et al., 1999, Javitt et al., 2000, de Bruin et al., 2001, Pincze et al., 2001, Ehlers and Somes, 2002). Rodents were shown to share many similarities with humans for specific portions of the ERP, including mouse analogs of the P50, N100, P200, and P300 components. These components are named the P20, N40, P80, and P120 in mice according to the time point the deflection takes place. They occur at approximately 40% of the latency of the human components and share similar overall morphology with the human components in response to parametric manipulation and pharmacological agents (Iwanami et al., 1994, Siegel et al., 2003, Hajos, 2006). The latency shift may be explained by the difference in brain size. As such, shorter distances allow faster progression of neural activity. However, the literature about the analogy of humans and rodent ERP is controversial and highly debated (Ehlers et al., 1997, Miyazato et al., 1999).

4.1.2 Mouse correlates of the human ERP waveform

The human P50 component is a positive deflection that occurs approximately 50 milliseconds following the onset of sensory stimulation. Mice show a similar early positive ERP component that emerges roughly 20 milliseconds after stimulus onset (Siegel et al., 2003, Maxwell et al., 2004, Umbricht et al., 2004). The mouse P20 shows a number of similarities to the human P50, including inter-stimulus interval (ISI) and intensity functions (Onitsuka et al., 2000, Maxwell et al., 2004), as well as pharmacological response to a wide variety of agents including amphetamine, ketamine, nicotine and neuroleptics (Stevens et al., 1995, Maxwell et al., 2004, Halene and Siegel, 2008, Rudnick et al., 2009). These factors have led to the suggestion that the P50 could potentially serve as a useful biomarker for detecting disease presence and for assessing treatment response. Several studies have shown correlations between reduced P50 (gating and amplitude) and impaired performance on measures of sustained attention and speed of processing (Cullum et al., 1993, Erwin et al., 1998, Potter et al., 2006, Smith et al., 2010). Decreases in P50 gating and amplitude are related to reduced working memory performance in schizophrenia (Cullum et al., 1993, Smith et al., 2010). Furthermore, mice show a negative deflection in the ERP around 40 milliseconds that shares a remarkable similarity with the human N100. For example, both the mouse N40 and human N100 show decreased amplitude during acute exposure to ketamine (Maxwell et al., 2006a, Murck et al., 2006, Lazarewicz et al., 2010). Furthermore, the mouse N40 has been shown to be sensitive to changes in stimulus novelty (MMN). Ketamine administration attenuates this sensitivity (Siegel et al., 2003, Ehrlichman et al., 2008).

Following the N100, the human ERP contains a second positive deflection termed P200. Mice show a clear P200-like response that appears around 80 milliseconds following stimulus onset. Several lines of evidence have proposed a relationship between the mouse P80 and cognitive function. Example given, P80 amplitude and gating are reduced in mice exposed to ketamine but are increased following nicotine treatment (Connolly et al., 2004, Amann et al., 2009). The P300 component is seen during cognitive processing of stimuli or during departures from a frequently occurring stimulus (Linden, 2005). Corresponding to the human P3a, an augmentation in the mouse P120 has been shown following a novel stimulus (Siegel et al., 2003). However, there has not been a clearly defined demonstration of a P3b-like response in rodents. The lack of evidence for a P3b type component in rodents may be due to fact that the methodology required to produce such a response has not been pursued (Figure 1).

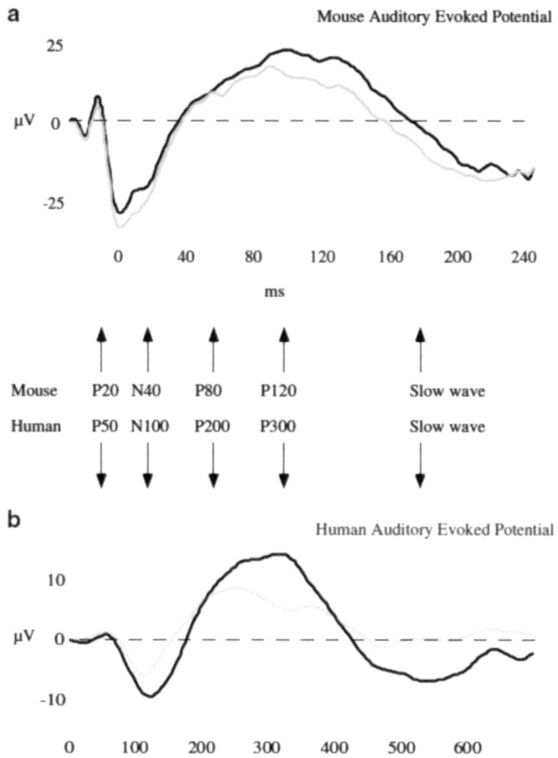

Fig. 1. (a) Mouse ERP to novel (black) and standard (gray) across all strains and drug treatment conditions. (b) Human ERP responses to novel (black) and standard (gray). Note that the human P300 and mouse P120 display increased amplitude following novel stimuli. As in Figure3, the timescale for mice is 40% that in humans and the amplitude of evoked potentials is greater in mice due to the use of intracranial electrodes as compared to scalp electrodes in humans. Reproduced with permission from Siegel (Siegel et al., 2003).

Mismatch negativity is elicited when the monotony or repetitive stimulation is interrupted by a deviant stimulus. Although deviant stimuli result in ERPs with similar morphology to that elicited by the repetitive stimulus, the negative deflection is enhanced in amplitude and latency. While mismatch negativity is simple to evoke and constitutes a robust finding in humans, dichotomy exists between the studies in rodents. The most contentious point is the existence of MMN in mice. As the human MMN temporally follows the N100, the MMN-like activity in rodents appears as a negative deflection after the N40 component. Furthermore, similar to human, ketamine abolished the generation of MMN-like activity in mice (Ehrlichman et al., 2008). However, mismatch negativity-like activity observed in mice generates an ERP with increased amplitude in N40, but contradictory findings of the latency changes exits. Among others, Sambeth and Ruusuvirta did not observe any significant differences in the deviance-related activity compared to the standard-related activity (Ruusuvirta et al., 1998, Sambeth et al., 2003). However, a number of other studies have confirmed the presence of evoked potential components that are similar to MMN observed in humans (Ehlers and Somes, 2002, Siegel et al., 2003, Umbricht et al., 2005). Umbricht demonstrated that the deviant manipulation (e.g., frequency, probability, duration) has to be well chosen in that only deviants differing in stimulus duration from standard stimuli were shown to successfully induce the MMN in mice. Alternatively, Ehrlichman and others have shown frequency elicited MMN in mice (Ehrlichman et al., 2009a). In summary, although several approaches in mouse have succeeded to induce ERP activity corresponding to the human MMN, further studies are needed to establish this endophenotype as a robust model.

4.2 Model systems

Animal models are extremely useful and serve as an essential tool for investigating mechanisms and treatments for a variety of human disorders including schizophrenia.

Similar to human evoked-potential studies, rodents can be examined for endophenotypes of pre-attentive auditory processing, the ability to discriminate between tones presented at different frequencies or temporal proximity. Auditory evoked responses have been extensively explored in rats and mice (Simpson and Knight, 1993, Siegel et al., 2003, Umbricht et al., 2004), with highly analogous waveforms observed across species. The following section provides an overview of currently used approaches to model particular aspects or endophenotypes of schizophrenia, highlighting the advantages and limitations of each model. In particular, transgenic, pharmacological, and environmental models are reviewed.

4.2.1 Pharmacological approaches

Pharmacological models of schizophrenia are based on the current understanding of the alterations in various neurotransmitter systems. They rely on the observation that certain drugs induce prominent behaviors and features mimicking aspects of schizophrenia. The lack of efficacy for antipsychotics with respect to negative symptoms and cognitive deficits is a significant obstacle for the treatment of schizophrenia. Developing new drugs to target these symptoms requires appropriate neural biomarkers that can be investigated in model organisms, be used to track treatment response, and provide insight into pathophysiological disease mechanisms.

This section reviews the extent to which EEG studies in pharmacological model systems have helped to understand the contributions of dopamine, glutamate (e.g. NMDA receptors), and nicotine in both disease and therapy.

Dopamine. Schizophrenia has traditionally been linked to dysfunctional dopamine neurotransmission (Carlsson, 1977, Bennett et al., 1998). The dopamine hypothesis postulates dopaminergic hyperfunction in schizophrenia. Among other neurotransmitters, dopamine is involved in the sensory gating (Javanbakht, 2006). For instance, the indirect dopamine agonist, amphetamine, produces a psychotic state in healthy individuals and exacerbates the symptoms of psychosis in patients (Angrist et al., 1970, Levy et al., 1993). Amphetamine became one of the most used models for schizophrenia, largely because it reproduces fairly well positive symptoms (e.g., hallucinations, paranoia, and psychosis) in humans. In addition to studies in humans, auditory gating has also been frequently demonstrated in laboratory animals (Shaywitz et al., 1976, Adler et al., 1988, Stevens et al., 1991). As such, amphetamine-induced alterations of the auditory processing abnormalities common to schizophrenia are well characterized in rodents and applied in multiple studies to investigate the amphetamine effect on rodent ERP. It has been repeatedly reported that amphetamine significantly disturbs ERP amplitude and gating, in particular diminishing N40 and P80 components (Stevens et al., 1991, Stevens et al., 1996, de Bruin et al., 1999, Maxwell et al., 2004). Furthermore, normal gating in rats is disrupted following amphetamine administration. Decreased N50, the rat correlate of the human P50, amplitude and abolished suppression of the neural response to the second stimulus resemble the gating disturbances seen in acutely psychotic, unmedicated patients (Adler et al., 1986). Ehrlichman and colleagues found amphetamine to reduce theta power following a stimulus which is consistent with other animal models and also with studies in humans suffering from schizophrenia (Yamamoto, 1997, Koukkou et al., 2000, Krause et al., 2003, Ehrlichman et al., 2009a). However, amphetamine did not significantly change basal power (theta, gamma) and evoked gamma power which is inconsistent with common findings in schizophrenia. Suggesting, while dopamine plays a key role in the generation of theta oscillations, its involvement in generating gamma oscillations is marginal (Kocsis et al., 2001, Kirk and Mackay, 2003). Amphetamine has been a heuristic model of positive psychosis fundamental to schizophrenia. However, amphetamine poorly mimics negative and cognitive symptoms of the disorder (Angrist et al., 1974). Moreover, chronic, stabilized patients generally exhibit a diminished response when exposed to amphetamine and also of the show a paradoxical behavioral improvement (Kornetsky, 1976, Angrist et al., 1982). Consequently, amphetamine has been proposed to constitute a model of positive psychosis in general, not specifically to schizophrenia. Finally, increased dopamine activity seems to play a limited role in the generation of negative and cognitive symptoms. Conclusively, amphetamine-treated animals provide only a limited representation of the traits of schizophrenia (i.e., positive symptoms).

Glutamate. Considerable evidence implicates reduced glutamatergic N-methyl-D-aspartate receptor (NMDAR) mediated signaling as the core pathophysiologic deficit of schizophrenia (i.e., the Glutamate Hypothesis) (Goff and Coyle, 2001, Coyle, 2006). Pharmacological evidence emerges from the effects NMDA receptor antagonists such as PCP, ketamine, and dizocilpine (MK801). Specifically, in healthy subjects aforementioned NMDAR antagonists were shown to induce a transient state characterized by symptoms associated with schizophrenia (Pearlson, 1981, Krystal et al., 1994). NMDAR antagonists as model of schizophrenia became of great interest because these antagonists cover the complete spectrum of symptoms: 1) positive (paranoia, agitation, and auditory hallucinations), 2) negative (apathy, though disorder, social withdrawal) and 3) cognitive symptoms (impaired working memory) (Becker et al., 2003). NMDA receptor antagonizing drugs have also been reported to induce schizophrenia-like alteration of event-related potentials, such as reduced P300 and impaired MMN (Oranje et al., 2000, Umbricht et al., 2000). As reviewed above, NMDARs are critically involved in the generation of human MMN making them a fortiori interesting as a target to model schizophrenia. In line with human studies, animals treated with NMDAR antagonists exhibit similar electrophysiological shifting. Taken together, all these aspects prompted researchers to increasingly employ pharmacological NMDAR blockade as a disease model (Olney et al., 1999). Thus, the following section reasons approaches using ketamine, PCP, and MK801 to model the glutamatergic theories of schizophrenia.

Patients treated with **ketamine** experience an exacerbation of positive and negative system, suggesting that NMDAR antagonists affect a brain system that is already vulnerable in schizophrenia (Javitt, 2010). Similar to healthy humans, animals treated with ketamine exhibit behavioral and electrophysiological features that closely resemble schizophrenia. Consistent with results in human, studies have demonstrated that acute ketamine administration decreases the amplitude and latency of the mouse N40 and P80 mimicking schizophrenia-like abnormalities on those components (Connolly et al., 2004, Maxwell et al., 2006a). However, a study by de Bruin and colleagues (de Bruin et al., 1999) reported that acute ketamine had no effect on gating of the N40 and P80 components. However, De Bruin confirmed that ketamine selectively decreased the amplitude of P80 in awake rats (de Bruin et al., 1999). Furthermore, mice undergoing 14 days of chronic ketamine (daily acute administration) showed lasting effects of long-term ketamine exposure such as decreased N40 amplitude (Maxwell et al., 2006a). Reduced ability to detect changes in the auditory environment is a further characteristic of schizophrenia which can be addressed by administering ketamine to rodents. Ketamine has been reported to impair gating of responses to repeated clicks presented at 100ms intervals (Boeijinga et al., 2007). While some studies have reported ketamine to disrupt MMN (Connolly et al., 2004, Bickel and Javitt, 2009, Ehrlichman et al., 2009a), others observed no significant effects (de Bruin et al., 1999, Connolly et al., 2004, Heekeren et al., 2008). In animals, ketamine disrupted the auditory gating and MMN with deficits similar to those seen in schizophrenia (Miller et al., 1992, Tikhonravov et al., 2008). Thus, deviance-elicited changes in N40 amplitude and in the subsequent temporal region between 50-75 msec (late N40 negativity) are observable, which displays characteristics similar to those seen with MMN in humans. Ehrlichman and others have found that ketamine attenuates both of these responses (Ehrlichman et al., 2008). These findings are important for several reasons. (1) They bolster the link between deviance detection and the NMDA receptor system. (2) They support the hypothesis that mouse N40 is the analogous to the human N100 which finally (3) demonstrates the feasibility of ketamine as a NMDAR antagonist to be a model of schizophrenia. Using the auditory click paradigm, Lazarewicz and others investigated the effect of ketamine on background, evoked, and induced power (Lazarewicz et al.). While low dose of ketamine (5mg/kg) only affected background power in the theta range, the higher dose (20mg/kg) significantly increased background power in theta and gamma range. Additionally, they observed a decrease in evoke theta power (3-12Hz) and an increase in evoked gamma power. Similar findings were replicated in rats as well as in humans (Hahn et al., 2006, Hong et al.). The reports of gamma power abnormalities highly diverge. Reduction on gamma power and synchronization are frequently reported in schizophrenia (Haig et al., 2000, Gallinat et al., 2004, Uhlhaas and Singer). However, inconsistent data exist (Lee et al., 2003, Spencer et al., 2003). Acute brain slice preparations have also been used to investigate gamma synchrony in pharmacologic models of schizophrenia. Such paradigms have demonstrated strikingly divergent results from the in vivo studies described above. Whereas in vivo studies demonstrated consistent brain-region independent increases in gamma activity with ketamine, slice studies reported increased gamma power only in auditory cortex with no changes in other cortical regions.

Phencyclidine (PCP) and other dissociative PCP-like drugs (e.g., MK801) are extensively applied to model schizophrenia, in particular due to its ability to mirror the symptomatology of schizophrenia including positive, negative, and cognitive symptoms (Bodi et al., 1959, Javitt et al., 1987). Especially, psychosis induced by PCP gained great interest since it reflects fairly well clinical features of the schizophrenia psychosis. Rats exposed to acute PCP display an impaired sensory gating, in particular of N2. Furthermore, Dissanayake and others found PCP to disrupt the gating of N2 in cortical and hippocampal areas (Miller et al., 1992, Mears et al., 2006, Dissanayake et al., 2009). Clozapine, an atypical neuroleptic, prevented the disruption in gating which stands in agreement with human studies demonstrating successful reversal of sensory gating deficits in schizophrenia (Nagamoto et al., 1996, Adler et al., 2004). Furthermore, schizophrenia-like abnormalities in MMN generation have been demonstrated by exposing monkeys to PCP (Javitt et al., 2000). Notably, PCP inhibited the N1 and P1 generation at long inter-stimulus-intervals (ISI), while at short ISI their generation was unaffected. Further, phencyclidine increases gamma frequency power, in particular in the hippocampus (Ma and Leung, 2000). Furthermore, an elevation in hippocampal theta power is observable following PCP administration. In contrary, total cortical power was reported to be decreased. Perinatal PCP exposure was found to result in long-lasting deficits in sensory gating, cognitive, and executive functioning in adult mice. Furthemore, atypical antispsychotics reverse these impairments. These biochemical and behavioral changes phenotipically resemble observations seen in schizophrenia and may serve as a model of the development of schizophrenia (Broberg et al., 2008, Wang et al., 2008).

Finally, **Dizocilpine (MK801)** is frequently used as an animal model of schizophrenia (Fletcher et al., 1989). However, in human research ketamine/PCP are used instead of MK801 due to its severe neurotoxicity. A single injection of MK801 is sufficient to model positive and negative symptoms. Animals treated acutely with MK801 mimic successfully the features of psychosis. Higher doses of MK-801 produce changes in brain activity accompanied by strong behavioral effects involving impaired locomotor control (Kovacic and Somanathan). Specifically, MK801 significantly augments low frequencies (1-6Hz) in cortical and amygdalar areas, while it concomitantly reduces higher frequencies (16-32Hz) (Ehlers et al., 1992). Also, the deficit in P200 gating seen in schizophrenia can be mimicked in the mouse correlate P80 by administrating MK801 (Ehlers et al., 1992). Finally, MK801 was shown to dose-dependently block the generation of MMN in unanesthetized monkeys and anesthetized rats (Javitt et al., 1996, Tikhonravov et al., 2008).

In summary, pharmacological approaches targeting NMDAR are effective tools in examining the pathophysiology of schizophrenia. Compared to other pharmacological animal models of schizophrenia, the NMDAR antagonist model provides clinical parallels allowing researchers to translate findings and treatment strategies from animal into human studies. A further advantage is the fact that acute exposures of above reviewed NMDAR antagonist induce schizophrenia-like symptomatology in healthy individuals lasting several hours up to days (Bakker and Amini, 1961). However, NMDAR antagonists produce acute receptor hypofunction and therefore fail to reflect chronic, developmental disruption in glutamatergic signaling that may underlie schizophrenia pathogenesis. Collectively, these virtues exemplify reasons for NMDA model in providing useful strategies to identify neural endophenotypes in regard to development of new therapies to target treatment-resistant symptoms.

Nicotine. Nicotine has generated interest as a candidate for therapeutic use in alleviating schizophrenia symptoms. Individuals with schizophrenia are three times more likely to smoke and have high nicotine dependence compared to the general population (Hughes et al., 1986, de Leon and Diaz, 2005). They also have lower smoking cessation rates and self-administer more nicotine during cigarette smoking than control patients, a finding supported by measuring cotinine, a nicotine metabolite used as a biomarker of tobacco exposure (Olincy et al., 1997, de Leon and Diaz, 2005). This, along with the known prevalence of genotype differences leading to the loss of function in the alpha 7 nicotinic receptor found in individuals with schizophrenia, (Adler et al., 1998, Leonard et al., 2001, Picciotto and Zoli, 2008) supports the idea that individuals with schizophrenia self-administer nicotine as a form of self-medication to rectify deficits in neurocognitive performance and alleviate symptoms associated with the disease (Dalack and Meador-Woodruff, 1996, Kumari and Postma, 2005, Kumari et al., 2006)(Dalack and Meador-Woodruff, 1996).As mentioned previously, individuals with schizophrenia exhibit a higher ratio between the second and first stimulus in the auditory gating paradigm reflecting a dysfunction in stimulus processing. Acute nicotine in humans transiently normalizes the P50 gating deficit. This is observed with cigarette smoking in schizophrenia patients (Adler et al., 1993)as well as in studies using nicotine-containing gum in non-smoking family members of schizophrenia patients who exhibited P50 gating deficits (Adler et al., 1992). Mice undergoing 14 days of chronic nicotine increased both in the amplitude and gating of the P20, while having only acute nicotine decrease the amplitude and gating of N40(Metzger et al., 2007). A variety of pharmacological models further demonstrate the importance of the nAChr in stimulus gating. nAChR agonists display similar affects to nicotine. Acute administration of DMXB-A, a nicotinic agonist specifically targeting the alpha7 nicotinic, significantly suppressed the P50 of the test stimulus in subjects with schizophrenia, bringing the gating of the schizophrenia patients into the range of controls (Meyer et al., 1997, Olincy et al., 2006). These results were consistent with animal model studies testing the same drug(Stevens et al., 1998). Administration of 5-I A-85380, an alpha4beta2 nAChR agonist, in DBA/2 mice also significantly reduced the second to first stimulus response ratio (Wildeboer and Stevens, 2008). Tropisetron, a partial alpha7 agonist significantly improves gating in schizophrenia patients (Koike et al., 2005). Luntz-Leybman (Luntz-Leybman et al., 1992) showed that alpha-bungarotoxin, an alpha-7 nAChR antagonist, disrupts P20 and P40 gating in rats while mecamylamine showed no affect. Physiostigmine, a drug that deters the breakdown of endogenous cholinergic drug in the body by inhibiting acetylcholinesterase, normalizes P50 gating in a schizophrenia-free individual that exhibited gating deficits in the P50 gating, further supporting nicotine's role in modulating sensory gating (Adler et al., 1992). Direct pharmacological targeting of the nAChR directly is not necessarily the only way to trigger the receptors effects. In animal models, Siegel demonstrated that dopamine reuptake inhibition and nicotine antagonism both contribute to the observed phenotype of gating impairment in both the P20 and P40 gating in mice (Siegel et al., 2005). Nicotine and haloperidol increased P20 amplitude, supporting a role for nicotine agonists in pre-attentive sensory encoding deficits. While it remains elusive, the mechanism of action underlying the gating difference could be critical to understanding and treating the physiological disturbances that cause the phenotype of schizophrenia, and nicotine is shown to affect this mechanism.

Since MMN deficits are thought to indicate degraded auditory perception experienced by schizophrenia patients, it follows that the effect of nicotine administration on schizophrenia symptoms be assessed using this measure. In the schizophrenia-free population, nicotine has been shown to enhance MMN amplitudes and shorten MMN latencies (Inami et al., 2005, Martin et al., 2009). Further evidence for the role of nicotine in ameliorating the MMN deficit emerges from the administration of the nicotinic agonist AZD3480, selective for the alpha-4-beta-2 subtype. As such, AZD3480 significantly increases the MMN amplitude and reduces the MMN latency, at the same time significantly enhancing scores in cognitive tests of attention and episodic memory when administered chronically for ten days (Dunbar et al., 2007). Human studies directly assessing the effects of nicotine on individuals with schizophrenia are few in number and exhibit mixed results. Acute nicotine transiently normalized the amplitude of MMN in response to duration but not frequency changes in auditory stimuli (Dulude et al., 2010). Inami found that acute transdermal nicotine in non-smokers reduces the MMN latency in healthy subjects, but not in patients with schizophrenia (Inami et al., 2007). This finding could be unique to the schizophrenia population that refrains from smoking and may reflect either differential drives to smoke based on symptom alleviation or be affected by the myriad of neuronal adaptations that chronic nicotine exposure induces, creating two distinct populations in schizophrenia. More studies are needed to elucidate the role of nicotinic receptors on MMN performance. There are several issues that limit nicotine being used as therapeutic drug. The ubiquity of nicotine receptors in the CNS and PNS make it difficult for a drug to target a specific region of the brain. A therapeutic drug's binding specificity and route of administration would therefore have to be optimized so as to minimize drug side affects. Nicotine itself has a short half-life. The rapid metabolism of the drug and its transient effects would mean that a mechanism of sustained release would need to be employed for the agent to remain active for an extended period of time. However, a direct impediment to this therapeutic modification is that nicotinic receptors exhibit quick desensitization. This would mean target receptors might not be available for binding and drug efficacy. These factors must be addressed before nicotine can be seriously considered as a candidate as a therapeutic drug for schizophrenia patients. There are currently several drugs that act at the nAChR that show promise. Agonists like DMXBA have been shown to successfully overcome several of these pharmacological challenges and stand as contenders for therapeutic relief (Martin and Freedman, 2007). Other options include the use of a positive allosteric modulator to enhance the efficacy of the receptor without directly activating it (Gronlien et al., 2007).

4.2.2 Transgenic approaches

Schizophrenia carries an important genetic contribution with a heritability of approximately 80% (Sullivan et al., 2003). ERPs deficits, particularly of the P50, N100, P300 and MMN components are among the most heritable (approximately 70%) and reproducible phenotypes of schizophrenia (Frangou et al., 1997, Ahveninen et al., 2006, Hall et al., 2006, Turetsky et al., 2007a). Whereas the number of candidate genes for schizophrenia is estimated to be over 1000, a subset of specific genetic contributions have been directly associated with ERPs. These genes are mostly involved in dopaminergic, nicotinic and glutamatergic mechanisms. For example, P50 gating deficits have been linked to the alpha-7 nicotinic acetylcholine receptor as well as the Catechol-O-methyltransferase (COMT) genes (Lu et al., 2007), although the later result was not replicated in a recent study (Shaikh et al., , Freedman et al., 1997, Leonard et al., 1998, Shaikh et al., 2011). Also, P300 amplitude decrease is associated with COMT and Disrupted in schizophrenia-1 (DISC1) genes while P300 increased latency is significantly influenced by the dopamine D2/D3 receptor as well as the Neuregulin-1 (NRG1) genes (Hill et al., 1998, Anokhin et al., 1999, Blackwood et al., 2001, Gallinat et al., 2003, Blackwood and Muir, 2004, Berman et al., 2006, Mulert et al., 2006, Bramon et al., 2008). Finally, whereas MMN is most extensively investigated in regard to glutamatergic mechanisms, no study has genetically linked both. However, a genetic association between MMN and the COMT gene has been shown (Baker et al., 2005). Those reports, combined with the aforementioned pharmacological studies, demonstrate the importance of investigating ERPs in specific transgenic (Tg) mouse models of schizophrenia. To date, the Tg mouse models that have been used to study ERPs components can be separated in 3 main groups based on the molecular pathway in which the target gene is involved: 1) Dopamine (COMT and G_sa Tg mice), 2) glutamate (NRG1 and NMDA receptor-1 (NR1)) Tg mice and 3) nicotine (C3H α 7 receptor Tg mice).

Dopamine. *COMT Tg mice:* The Catechol-O-methyltransferase (COMT) is a key regulatory enzyme that degrades dopamine and thus controls dopamine availability (Axelrod and Tomchick, 1958, Goldberg and Weinberger, 2004). In humans, a single nucleotide polymorphism leads to the substitution of a Valine in place of a Methionine at the 158/108 locus (Lachman et al., 1996). This modification results in a two-fold increase of its activity thereby reducing dopamine levels (Chen et al., 2004). A recent study from our laboratory using COMT-Val-tg mice (Papaleo et al., 2008) shows a lack of change in P20 amplitude but a trend of P20 latency increase (unpublished data). These results are consistent with the human data mentioned above, which show both significant and non-significant genetic linkage between the COMT gene and P50 gating deficits. We also observed increased N40 latency and decreased P80 amplitude as well as reduced baseline theta and gamma power.

G_sa Tg mice: G_sa Tg mice express an isoform of the G-protein subunit G_sa that is constitutively active due to a point mutation (Q227L) that prevents hydrolysis of bound GTP (Wand et al., 2001, Gould et al., 2004). G_sa Tg mice displayed decreased amplitude of cortically-generated N40 that is reversed by the Gi-coupled dopamine D2-receptor antagonist haloperidol (Maxwell et al., 2006b). This result is consistent with the amplitude reduction of the N100 observed in patients with schizophrenia (Frangou et al., 1997, Ahveninen et al., 2006).

Glutamate. *NRG1 Tg mice:* NRG-1 is a high-risk gene for schizophrenia that has been associated with NMDA receptor hypofunction (Gu et al., 2005, Hahn et al., 2006, Bjarnadottir et al., 2007, Li et al., 2007). Although several Tg mice for NRG1 have been engineered, to our knowledge, only one study has tested auditory ERPs (Ehrlichman et al., 2009b). This study has used the NRG1 model in which all three major types of NRG1 have a partial deletion of the EGF like domain. These NRG1 heterozygote mice did not show deficits in P20 amplitude or gating. Nevertheless, they showed disrupted mismatch negativity similar to what is observed in schizophrenia. It would be interesting to investigate ERPs in the other NRG1 Tg mouse lines as it may help to identify which form of NRG1 mutant are most closely associated with the electrophysiological abnormalities commonly found in schizophrenia.

NR1 Tg mice: NR1 hypomorphic mice express 5-10% of the normal NR1 protein (Mohn et al., 1999). Several studies have reported behavioral abnormalities in these mice that are also found in schizophrenia. Since then, NR1 hypomorphic mice have been considered as a translation model for the disease. Measure of auditory and visual event related potentials showed significant increased amplitudes of P20 and N40 in NR1 hypomorphic mice, suggesting decreased inhibitory tone (Bodarky et al., 2009, Halene et al., 2009). Indeed, auditory gating for the P20 and the N40 peak is significantly impaired in these mice compared to their wild-type littermates (Bickel et al., 2007, 2008). Those results correlate with the pathophysiology of the observed gating and ERPs generation alterations in schizophrenia (Javitt et al., 2000).

Nicotine. *C3H α7 Tg mice* (Adams et al., 2008)**:** C3Há7 null mutant heterozygote mice exhibit significant reduction of the alpha-7 nicotinic receptor in the hippocampus. In these mice, the auditory gating for P20 and N40 was decreased compare to the wild type mice. This result is consistent with the deficit of P50 gating reported for schizophrenia patients. These data reinforce the idea of a genetic linkage between the alpha-7 nicotinic receptor and this phenotype observed in human.

4.2.3 Environmental approaches

The notion that schizophrenia occurs as a result of problems in neurodevelopment is strongly suggested by the appearance of a number of gross alterations in the brain inn schizophrenia, including enlargement of the cerebral ventricles, decreased cortical volume, and hippocampal cellular pathology (Harrison, 1999). That these alterations have occurred early in development can be assumed given that they occur largely in areas of the brain, such as the hippocampus, that complete the developmental process long before the typical onset of the disease. Although the full emergence of schizophrenia symptoms usually does not occur until late-adolescence or early-adulthood, people who subsequently go on to develop schizophrenia often show numerous deficits in cognitive and social function indicative of problems early in the developmental process. Given the importance of identifying the potential mechanisms that underlie such developmental changes, numerous neurodevelopmental models have been proposed in animals that presume to replicate the conditions leading to schizophrenia-like brain dysfunction.

NNVHL. Lesioning of the ventral hippocampal area during early life has been shown to reproduce in rodents many of the symptoms observed in schizophrenia. Important features of this model are: 1) post-pubertal emergence of behavioral changes 2) schizophrenia-like deficits in cognition 3) schizophrenia-like changes on putative positive symptom measures, such as amphetamine-induced locomotor activity and pre-pulse inhibition 4) schizophrenia-like cellular and neuroanatomical changes, including reductions in parvalbumin expressing GABAergic interneurons 5) exaggerated response to glutamate agonist and antagonists, suggestive of a hypoglutamatergic state. Importantly, most of these changes occur only when the lesion is induced during the neonatal period and do not occur in adult animals given similar lesions of the ventral hippocampus, suggesting that it is the altered neurodevelopmental environment that is the source of the changes observed in the model.

Methylazoxymethanol. Embryonic exposure to methylazoxymethanol acetate (MAM), an inhibitor of cell division, is currently a popular animal model of schizophrenia. Exposure to MAM at embryonic day 17 produces a pattern of brain atrophy in adult animals similar to that seen in human schizophrenia (i.e. cortical and hippocampal atrophy) (Talamini et al., 1998). Importantly, these neural changes overlap with dysfunctions across a wide range of behavioral and cognitive domains known to be affected in humans with schizophrenia, including measures sensitive to mesolimbic dopamine function and cognitive performance. Thus, MAM treated animals display impaired long-term memory, working memory and attentional flexibility, as well as increased responsiveness to amphetamine as adults (Fiore et al., 2002, Gourevitch et al., 2004, Moore et al., 2006, Featherstone et al., 2007). The enhanced response to amphetamine is not seen when animals are tested during the pre-pubescent period, suggesting that the behavioral changes induced by MAM follow the same developmental time course seen in the human disease (Moore et al., 2006). Parvalbumin (PV) expressing GABAergic interneurons are dramatically reduced in both the hippocampus and PFC following embryonic MAM treatment, suggesting that these cells may be especially vulnerable to the effects of MAM. Moreover, it is possible that the loss of such cells could be responsible for many of the cognitive and behavioral changes that occur following MAM treatment (Penschuck et al., 2006). For example, PV expressing GABAergic interneurons are known to be the primary source of high frequency gamma oscillations. In a latent inhibition procedure, MAM treated animals showed reduced gamma power during pre-exposure to a tone and this was shown to correspond with impaired development of latent inhibition (Lodge et al., 2009). In contrast, exposure to MAM did not alter activity in the lower frequency theta band, suggesting a high degree of specificity in the underlying change induced by MAM treatment. Additionally, MAM treated animals show an enhanced locomotor response to NMDA antagonists such as ketamine and PCP, and this also appears to correspond strongly and specifically with a reduced ability for these drugs to alter activity within the gamma frequency range. Both studies suggest that MAM treatment results in a decreased inhibitory tone consistent with the proposed role of GABAergic interneurons in inhibitory function.

4.3 Limitation and future models

ERPs and ERSPs have been widely used to examine neural activity in normal individuals and those suffering from schizophrenia. The high degree of similarity between the methods used to assess these measures in humans and laboratory animals has made these techniques very valuable for studying normal and abnormal brain function. Presently, however, it is unclear how such measures relate to clinical symptoms or cognitive impairments, although evidence for a link between these measures and cognition is beginning to emerge. Future studies will need to assess the degree to which ERP and EEG measures relate to cognitive performance on tasks in mice that more closely replicate those used in humans. Establishment of such a link could provide a novel means for assessing cognition in mice and for testing potential pharmaceutical interventions for schizophrenia. Much work has been done assessing EEG during cognitive performance in humans, as well as in non-human primates, which has typically focused on sophisticated analyses of neural oscillations and synchrony. While such measures are interesting, ERP measures are also useful candidates for translational biomarkers of cognition, since they do not require extensive expertise to analyze and there are years of human data using these measures. Further, mice are excellent subjects for translational research, given the wide range of genetically modified mice available to researchers.

5. References

Adams CE, Yonchek JC, Zheng L, Collins AC, Stevens KE (Altered hippocampal circuit function in C3H alpha7 null mutant heterozygous mice. Brain Res 1194:138-145.2008).

Adler LE, Hoffer LD, Wiser A, Freedman R (Normalization of auditory physiology by cigarette smoking in schizophrenic patients. The American journal of psychiatry 150:1856-1861.1993).

Adler LE, Hoffer LJ, Griffith J, Waldo MC, Freedman R (Normalization by nicotine of deficient auditory sensory gating in the relatives of schizophrenics. Biological psychiatry 32:607-616.1992).

Adler LE, Olincy A, Cawthra EM, McRae KA, Harris JG, Nagamoto HT, Waldo MC, Hall MH, Bowles A, Woodward L, Ross RG, Freedman R (Varied effects of atypical neuroleptics on P50 auditory gating in schizophrenia patients. The American journal of psychiatry 161:1822-1828.2004).

Adler LE, Olincy A, Waldo M, Harris JG, Griffith J, Stevens K, Flach K, Nagamoto H, Bickford P, Leonard S, Freedman R (Schizophrenia, sensory gating, and nicotinic receptors. Schizophrenia bulletin 24:189-202.1998).

Adler LE, Pachtman E, Franks RD, Pecevich M, Waldo MC, Freedman R (Neurophysiological evidence for a defect in neuronal mechanisms involved in sensory gating in schizophrenia. Biological psychiatry 17:639-654.1982).

Adler LE, Pang K, Gerhardt G, Rose GM (Modulation of the gating of auditory evoked potentials by norepinephrine: pharmacological evidence obtained using a selective neurotoxin. Biological psychiatry 24:179-190.1988).

Adler LE, Rose G, Freedman R (Neurophysiological studies of sensory gating in rats: effects of amphetamine, phencyclidine, and haloperidol. Biological psychiatry 21:787-798.1986).

Ahveninen J, Jaaskelainen IP, Osipova D, Huttunen MO, Ilmoniemi RJ, Kaprio J, Lonnqvist J, Manninen M, Pakarinen S, Therman S, Naatanen R, Cannon TD (Inherited auditory-cortical dysfunction in twin pairs discordant for schizophrenia. Biol Psychiatry 60:612-620.2006).

Alain C, Bernstein LJ, Cortese F, Yu H, Zipursky RB (2002) Deficits in automatically detecting changes in conjunction of auditory features in patients with schizophrenia. In: Psychophysiology, vol. 39, pp 599-606.

Alho K (Cerebral generators of mismatch negativity (MMN) and its magnetic counterpart (MMNm) elicited by sound changes. Ear and hearing 16:38-51.1995).

Amann LC, Halene TB, Ehrlichman RS, Luminais SN, Ma N, Abel T, Siegel SJ (Chronic ketamine impairs fear conditioning and produces long-lasting reductions in auditory evoked potentials. Neurobiology of disease 35:311-317.2009).

Angrist B, Peselow E, Rubinstein M, Corwin J, Rotrosen J (Partial improvement in negative schizophrenic symptoms after amphetamine. Psychopharmacology 78:128-130.1982).

Angrist B, Sathananthan G, Wilk S, Gershon S (Amphetamine psychosis: behavioral and biochemical aspects. Journal of psychiatric research 11:13-23.1974).

Angrist BM, Schweitzer JW, Friedhoff AJ, Gershon S (Investigation of p-methoxyamphetamine excretion in amphetamine induced psychosis. Nature 225:651-652.1970).

Anokhin AP, Todorov AA, Madden PA, Grant JD, Heath AC (Brain event-related potentials, dopamine D2 receptor gene polymorphism, and smoking. Genet Epidemiol 17 Suppl 1:S37-42.1999).

Axelrod J, Tomchick R (Enzymatic O-methylation of epinephrine and other catechols. J Biol Chem 233:702-705.1958).

Baker K, Baldeweg T, Sivagnanasundaram S, Scambler P, Skuse D (COMT Val108/158 Met modifies mismatch negativity and cognitive function in 22q11 deletion syndrome. Biol Psychiatry 58:23-31.2005).

Bakker CB, Amini FB (Observations on the psychotomimetic effects of Sernyl. Comprehensive psychiatry 2:269-280.1961).

Barcelo F, Knight RT (An information-theoretical approach to contextual processing in the human brain: evidence from prefrontal lesions. Cereb Cortex 17 Suppl 1:i51-60.2007).

Basar-Eroglu C, Schmiedt-Fehr C, Mathes B, Zimmermann J, Brand A (Are oscillatory brain responses generally reduced in schizophrenia during long sustained attentional processing? Int J Psychophysiol 71:75-83.2009).

Basar E, Basar-Eroglu C, Karakas S, Schurmann M (Gamma, alpha, delta, and theta oscillations govern cognitive processes. Int J Psychophysiol 39:241-248.2001).

Becker A, Peters B, Schroeder H, Mann T, Huether G, Grecksch G (Ketamine-induced changes in rat behaviour: A possible animal model of schizophrenia. Progress in neuro-psychopharmacology & biological psychiatry 27:687-700.2003).

Bennett BA, Hollingsworth CK, Martin RS, Harp JJ (Methamphetamine-induced alterations in dopamine transporter function. Brain research 782:219-227.1998).

Berger H (Ueber das Electrocephalogramm des Menschen. Arch Psychiatr Nervenkr 527-570.1929).

Berman SM, Noble EP, Antolin T, Sheen C, Conner BT, Ritchie T (P300 development during adolescence: effects of DRD2 genotype. Clin Neurophysiol 117:649-659.2006).

Bickel S, Javitt DC (Neurophysiological and neurochemical animal models of schizophrenia: focus on glutamate. Behavioural brain research 204:352-362.2009).

Bickel S, Lipp HP, Umbricht D (Impaired attentional modulation of auditory evoked potentials in N-methyl-D-aspartate NR1 hypomorphic mice. Genes Brain Behav 6:558-568.2007).

Bickel S, Lipp HP, Umbricht D (Early auditory sensory processing deficits in mouse mutants with reduced NMDA receptor function. Neuropsychopharmacology 33:1680-1689.2008).

Bjarnadottir M, Misner DL, Haverfield-Gross S, Bruun S, Helgason VG, Stefansson H, Sigmundsson A, Firth DR, Nielsen B, Stefansdottir R, Novak TJ, Stefansson K, Gurney ME, Andresson T (Neuregulin1 (NRG1) signaling through Fyn modulates NMDA receptor phosphorylation: differential synaptic function in NRG1+/- knock-outs compared with wild-type mice. J Neurosci 27:4519-4529.2007).

Blackwood DH, Fordyce A, Walker MT, St Clair DM, Porteous DJ, Muir WJ (Schizophrenia and affective disorders--cosegregation with a translocation at chromosome 1q42 that directly disrupts brain-expressed genes: clinical and P300 findings in a family. Am J Hum Genet 69:428-433.2001).

Blackwood DH, Muir WJ (Clinical phenotypes associated with DISC1, a candidate gene for schizophrenia. Neurotox Res 6:35-41.2004).

Blackwood DH, St Clair DM, Muir WJ, Duffy JC (Auditory P300 and eye tracking dysfunction in schizophrenic pedigrees. Archives of general psychiatry 48:899-909.1991).

Blumenfeld LD, Clementz BA (Response to the first stimulus determines reduced auditory evoked response suppression in schizophrenia: single trials analysis using MEG. Clin Neurophysiol 112:1650-1659.2001).

Bodarky CL, Halene TB, Ehrlichman RS, Banerjee A, Ray R, Hahn CG, Jonak G, Siegel SJ (Novel environment and GABA agonists alter event-related potentials in N-methyl-D-aspartate NR1 hypomorphic and wild-type mice. J Pharmacol Exp Ther 331:308-318.2009).

Bodi T, Share I, Levy H, Moyer JH (Clinical trial of phencyclidine (sernyl) in patients with psychoneurosis. Antibiotic medicine & clinical therapy 6:79-84.1959).

Boeijinga PH, Soufflet L, Santoro F, Luthringer R (Ketamine effects on CNS responses assessed with MEG/EEG in a passive auditory sensory-gating paradigm: an attempt for modelling some symptoms of psychosis in man. Journal of psychopharmacology (Oxford, England) 21:321-337.2007).

Bolz J, Giedke H (Brain stem auditory evoked responses in psychiatric patients and healthy controls. Journal of neural transmission 54:285-291.1982).

Bomba MD, Pang EW (Cortical auditory evoked potentials in autism: a review. Int J Psychophysiol 53:161-169.2004).

Boutros N, Zouridakis G, Rustin T, Peabody C, Warner D (The P50 component of the auditory evoked potential and subtypes of schizophrenia. Psychiatry research 47:243-254.1993).

Boutros NN, Arfken C, Galderisi S, Warrick J, Pratt G, Iacono W (The status of spectral EEG abnormality as a diagnostic test for schizophrenia. Schizophrenia research 99:225-237.2008).

Boutros NN, Korzyuko O, Oliwa G, Feingold A, Campbell D, McClain-Furmanski D, Struve F, Jansen BH (Morphological and latency abnormalities of the mid-latency auditory evoked responses in schizophrenia: a preliminary report. Schizophrenia research 70:303-313.2004a).

Boutros NN, Korzyukov O, Jansen B, Feingold A, Bell M (Sensory gating deficits during the mid-latency phase of information processing in medicated schizophrenia patients. Psychiatry research 126:203-215.2004b).

Braff DL (Information processing and attention dysfunctions in schizophrenia. Schizophrenia bulletin 19:233-259.1993).

Braff DL, Geyer MA (Sensorimotor gating and schizophrenia. Human and animal model studies. Archives of general psychiatry 47:181-188.1990).

Braff DL, Light GA (The use of neurophysiological endophenotypes to understand the genetic basis of schizophrenia. Dialogues in clinical neuroscience 7:125-135.2005).

Bragin A, Jando G, Nadasdy Z, Hetke J, Wise K, Buzsaki G (Gamma (40-100 Hz) oscillation in the hippocampus of the behaving rat. J Neurosci 15:47-60.1995).

Bramon E, Dempster E, Frangou S, Shaikh M, Walshe M, Filbey FM, McDonald C, Sham P, Collier DA, Murray R (Neuregulin-1 and the P300 waveform--a preliminary association study using a psychosis endophenotype. Schizophr Res 103:178-185.2008).

Bramon E, Rabe-Hesketh S, Sham P, Murray RM, Frangou S (Meta-analysis of the P300 and P50 waveforms in schizophrenia. Schizophrenia research 70:315-329.2004).

Brenner CA, Wilt MA, Lysaker PH, Koyfman A, O'Donnell BF (Psychometrically matched visual-processing tasks in schizophrenia spectrum disorders. Journal of abnormal psychology 112:28-37.2003).

Broberg BV, Dias R, Glenthoj BY, Olsen CK (Evaluation of a neurodevelopmental model of schizophrenia--early postnatal PCP treatment in attentional set-shifting. Behavioural brain research 190:160-163.2008).

Brockhaus-Dumke A, Mueller R, Faigle U, Klosterkoetter J (Sensory gating revisited: relation between brain oscillations and auditory evoked potentials in schizophrenia. Schizophrenia research 99:238-249.2008).

Brown KJ, Gonsalvez CJ, Harris AW, Williams LM, Gordon E (Target and non-target ERP disturbances in first episode vs. chronic schizophrenia. Clin Neurophysiol 113:1754-1763.2002).

Buchwald JS, Huang C (Far-field acoustic response: origins in the cat. Science (New York, NY 189:382-384.1975).

Carlsson A (Does dopamine play a role in schizophrenia? Psychological medicine 7:583-597.1977).

Catts SV, Shelley AM, Ward PB, Liebert B, McConaghy N, Andrews S, Michie PT (Brain potential evidence for an auditory sensory memory deficit in schizophrenia. The American journal of psychiatry 152:213-219.1995).

Chen J, Lipska BK, Halim N, Ma QD, Matsumoto M, Melhem S, Kolachana BS, Hyde TM, Herman MM, Apud J, Egan MF, Kleinman JE, Weinberger DR (Functional analysis of genetic variation in catechol-O-methyltransferase (COMT): effects on mRNA, protein, and enzyme activity in postmortem human brain. Am J Hum Genet 75:807-821.2004).

Chiappa KH, Young RR (Evoked responses. Overused, underused, or misused? Archives of neurology 42:76-77.1985).

Cho RY, Konecky RO, Carter CS (Impairments in frontal cortical gamma synchrony and cognitive control in schizophrenia. Proceedings of the National Academy of Sciences of the United States of America 103:19878-19883.2006).

Chrobak JJ, Buzsaki G (Gamma oscillations in the entorhinal cortex of the freely behaving rat. J Neurosci 18:388-398.1998).

Clementz BA, Blumenfeld LD, Cobb S (The gamma band response may account for poor P50 suppression in schizophrenia. Neuroreport 8:3889-3893.1997).

Coburn KL, Shillcutt SD, Tucker KA, Estes KM, Brin FB, Merai P, Moore NC (P300 delay and attenuation in schizophrenia: reversal by neuroleptic medication. Biological psychiatry 44:466-474.1998).

Connolly PM, Maxwell C, Liang Y, Kahn JB, Kanes SJ, Abel T, Gur RE, Turetsky BI, Siegel SJ (The effects of ketamine vary among inbred mouse strains and mimic schizophrenia for the P80, but not P20 or N40 auditory ERP components. Neurochemical research 29:1179-1188.2004).

Cook JD, Ellinwood EH, Jr., Wilson WP (Auditory habituation at primary cortex as a function of stimulus rate. Experimental neurology 21:167-175.1968).

Coyle JT (Glutamate and schizophrenia: beyond the dopamine hypothesis. Cellular and molecular neurobiology 26:365-384.2006).

Cullum CM, Harris JG, Waldo MC, Smernoff E, Madison A, Nagamoto HT, Griffith J, Adler LE, Freedman R (Neurophysiological and neuropsychological evidence for attentional dysfunction in schizophrenia. Schizophrenia research 10:131-141.1993).

Da Silva F (2005) Event-related potentials: Methodology and Quantification. In: Electroencephalography: Basic principles, clinical applications, and related fields, vol. 1 (E.Niedermeyer, F. D. S., ed), pp 991-1001 Philadelphia: Lippincott Williams & Wilkins.

Dalack GW, Meador-Woodruff JH (Smoking, smoking withdrawal and schizophrenia: case reports and a review of the literature. Schizophrenia research 22:133-141.1996).

Davis H, Hirsh SK, Turpin LL (Possible utility of middle latency responses in electric response audiometry. Advances in oto-rhino-laryngology 31:208-216.1983).

Davis H, Mast T, Yoshie N, Zerlin S (The slow response of the human cortex to auditory stimuli: recovery process. Electroencephalography and clinical neurophysiology 21:105-113.1966).

de Bruin NM, Ellenbroek BA, Cools AR, Coenen AM, van Luijtelaar EL (Differential effects of ketamine on gating of auditory evoked potentials and prepulse inhibition in rats. Psychopharmacology 142:9-17.1999).

de Bruin NM, Ellenbroek BA, van Schaijk WJ, Cools AR, Coenen AM, van Luijtelaar EL (Sensory gating of auditory evoked potentials in rats: effects of repetitive stimulation and the interstimulus interval. Biological psychology 55:195-213.2001).

de Leon J, Diaz FJ (A meta-analysis of worldwide studies demonstrates an association between schizophrenia and tobacco smoking behaviors. Schizophrenia research 76:135-157.2005).

de Wilde OM, Bour LJ, Dingemans PM, Koelman JH, Linszen DH (A meta-analysis of P50 studies in patients with schizophrenia and relatives: differences in methodology between research groups. Schizophrenia research 97:137-151.2007).

Demiralp T, Ucok A, Devrim M, Isoglu-Alkac U, Tecer A, Polich J (N2 and P3 components of event-related potential in first-episode schizophrenic patients: scalp topography, medication, and latency effects. Psychiatry research 111:167-179.2002).

Devrim-Ucok M, Keskin-Ergen HY, Ucok A (Novelty P3 and P3b in first-episode schizophrenia and chronic schizophrenia. Progress in neuro-psychopharmacology & biological psychiatry 30:1426-1434.2006).

Dietrich A, Kanso R (A review of EEG, ERP, and neuroimaging studies of creativity and insight. Psychological bulletin 136:822-848.2010).

Dissanayake DW, Zachariou M, Marsden CA, Mason R (Effects of phencyclidine on auditory gating in the rat hippocampus and the medial prefrontal cortex. Brain research 1298:153-160.2009).

Doege K, Bates AT, White TP, Das D, Boks MP, Liddle PF (Reduced event-related low frequency EEG activity in schizophrenia during an auditory oddball task. Psychophysiology 46:566-577.2009).

Donchin E, Isreal JB (Event-related potentials and psychological theory. Progress in brain research 54:697-715.1980).

Dulude L, Labelle A, Knott VJ (Acute nicotine alteration of sensory memory impairment in smokers with schizophrenia. J Clin Psychopharmacol 30:541-548.2010).

Dunbar G, Boeijinga PH, Demazieres A, Cisterni C, Kuchibhatla R, Wesnes K, Luthringer R (Effects of TC-1734 (AZD3480), a selective neuronal nicotinic receptor agonist, on cognitive performance and the EEG of young healthy male volunteers. Psychopharmacology 191:919-929.2007).

Ehlers CL, Kaneko WM, Wall TL, Chaplin RI (Effects of dizocilpine (MK-801) and ethanol on the EEG and event-related potentials (ERPS) in rats. Neuropharmacology 31:369-378.1992).

Ehlers CL, Somes C (Long latency event-related potentials in mice: effects of stimulus characteristics and strain. Brain research 957:117-128.2002).

Ehlers CL, Somes C, Thomas J, Riley EP (Effects of neonatal exposure to nicotine on electrophysiological parameters in adult rats. Pharmacology, biochemistry, and behavior 58:713-720.1997).

Ehrlichman RS, Gandal MJ, Maxwell CR, Lazarewicz MT, Finkel LH, Contreras D, Turetsky BI, Siegel SJ (N-methyl-d-aspartic acid receptor antagonist-induced frequency oscillations in mice recreate pattern of electrophysiological deficits in schizophrenia. Neuroscience 158:705-712.2009a).

Ehrlichman RS, Luminais SN, White SL, Rudnick ND, Ma N, Dow HC, Kreibich AS, Abel T, Brodkin ES, Hahn CG, Siegel SJ (Neuregulin 1 transgenic mice display reduced mismatch negativity, contextual fear conditioning and social interactions. Brain Res 1294:116-127.2009b).

Ehrlichman RS, Maxwell CR, Majumdar S, Siegel SJ (Deviance-elicited changes in event-related potentials are attenuated by ketamine in mice. Journal of cognitive neuroscience 20:1403-1414.2008).

Eichele T, Specht K, Moosmann M, Jongsma ML, Quiroga RQ, Nordby H, Hugdahl K (Assessing the spatiotemporal evolution of neuronal activation with single-trial event-related potentials and functional MRI. Proceedings of the National Academy of Sciences of the United States of America 102:17798-17803.2005).

Erwin RJ, Turetsky BI, Moberg P, Gur RC, Gur RE (P50 abnormalities in schizophrenia: relationship to clinical and neuropsychological indices of attention. Schizophrenia research 33:157-167.1998).

Featherstone RE, Rizos Z, Nobrega JN, Kapur S, Fletcher PJ (Gestational methylazoxymethanol acetate treatment impairs select cognitive functions: parallels to schizophrenia. Neuropsychopharmacology 32:483-492.2007).

Fehr T, Kissler J, Wienbruch C, Moratti S, Elbert T, Watzl H, Rockstroh B (Source distribution of neuromagnetic slow-wave activity in schizophrenic patients--effects of activation. Schizophrenia research 63:63-71.2003).

Fenton GW, Fenwick PB, Dollimore J, Dunn TL, Hirsch SR (EEG spectral analysis in schizophrenia. Br J Psychiatry 136:445-455.1980).

Finley KH (ON THE OCCURRENCE OF RAPID FREQUENCY POTENTIAL CHANGES IN THE HUMAN ELECTROENCEPHALOGRAM. The American journal of psychiatry 194-200.1944).

Fiore M, Korf J, Antonelli A, Talamini L, Aloe L (Long-lasting effects of prenatal MAM treatment on water maze performance in rats: associations with altered brain development and neurotrophin levels. Neurotoxicology and teratology 24:179-191.2002).

Fischer C, Morlet D, Giard M (Mismatch negativity and N100 in comatose patients. Audiology & neuro-otology 5:192-197.2000).

Fisher DJ, Labelle A, Knott VJ (Auditory hallucinations and the mismatch negativity: processing speech and non-speech sounds in schizophrenia. Int J Psychophysiol 70:3-15.2008).

Fisher DJ, Labelle A, Knott VJ (Auditory hallucinations and the P3a: attention-switching to speech in schizophrenia. Biological psychology 85:417-423.2010).

Fletcher EJ, Millar JD, Zeman S, Lodge D (Non-competitive antagonism of N-methyl-d-aspartate by displacement of an endogenous glycine-like substance. The European journal of neuroscience 1:196-203.1989).

Ford JM, Pfefferbaum A, Roth W (P3 and schizophrenia. Annals of the New York Academy of Sciences 658:146-162.1992).

Ford JM, Roach BJ, Hoffman RS, Mathalon DH (The dependence of P300 amplitude on gamma synchrony breaks down in schizophrenia. Brain research 1235:133-142.2008).

Ford JM, White PM, Csernansky JG, Faustman WO, Roth WT, Pfefferbaum A (ERPs in schizophrenia: effects of antipsychotic medication. Biological psychiatry 36:153-170.1994).

Frangou S, Sharma T, Alarcon G, Sigmudsson T, Takei N, Binnie C, Murray RM (The Maudsley Family Study, II: Endogenous event-related potentials in familial schizophrenia. Schizophrenia research 23:45-53.1997).

Freedman R, Adler LE, Myles-Worsley M, Nagamoto HT, Miller C, Kisley M, McRae K, Cawthra E, Waldo M (Inhibitory gating of an evoked response to repeated auditory stimuli in schizophrenic and normal subjects. Human recordings, computer simulation, and an animal model. Archives of general psychiatry 53:1114-1121.1996).

Freedman R, Coon H, Myles-Worsley M, Orr-Urtreger A, Olincy A, Davis A, Polymeropoulos M, Holik J, Hopkins J, Hoff M, Rosenthal J, Waldo MC, Reimherr F, Wender P, Yaw J, Young DA, Breese CR, Adams C, Patterson D, Adler LE, Kruglyak L, Leonard S, Byerley W (Linkage of a neurophysiological deficit in schizophrenia to a chromosome 15 locus. Proceedings of the National Academy of Sciences of the United States of America 94:587-592.1997).

Fries P, Reynolds JH, Rorie AE, Desimone R (Modulation of oscillatory neuronal synchronization by selective visual attention. Science (New York, NY 291:1560-1563.2001).

Frodl T, Meisenzahl EM, Muller D, Greiner J, Juckel G, Leinsinger G, Hahn H, Moller HJ, Hegerl U (Corpus callosum and P300 in schizophrenia. Schizophrenia research 49:107-119.2001).

Fuchs EC, Doheny H, Faulkner H, Caputi A, Traub RD, Bibbig A, Kopell N, Whittington MA, Monyer H (Genetically altered AMPA-type glutamate receptor kinetics in interneurons disrupt long-range synchrony of gamma oscillation. Proceedings of the National Academy of Sciences of the United States of America 98:3571-3576.2001).

G. Celesia MB (2005) Auditory Evoked Potentials. In: Electroencephalography: Basic principles, clinical applications, and related fields, vol. 1 (E.Niedermeyer, F. D. S., ed), pp 1045-1065 Philadelphia: Lippincott Williams & Wilkins.

Galambos R, Makeig S (Physiological studies of central masking in man. I: The effects of noise on the 40-Hz steady-state response. The Journal of the Acoustical Society of America 92:2683-2690.1992).

Galambos R, Makeig S, Talmachoff PJ (A 40-Hz auditory potential recorded from the human scalp. Proceedings of the National Academy of Sciences of the United States of America 78:2643-2647.1981).

Gallinat J, Bajbouj M, Sander T, Schlattmann P, Xu K, Ferro EF, Goldman D, Winterer G (Association of the G1947A COMT (Val(108/158)Met) gene polymorphism with prefrontal P300 during information processing. Biol Psychiatry 54:40-48.2003).

Gallinat J, Mulert C, Bajbouj M, Herrmann WM, Schunter J, Senkowski D, Moukhtieva R, Kronfeldt D, Winterer G (Frontal and temporal dysfunction of auditory stimulus processing in schizophrenia. NeuroImage 17:110-127.2002).

Gallinat J, Winterer G, Herrmann CS, Senkowski D (Reduced oscillatory gamma-band responses in unmedicated schizophrenic patients indicate impaired frontal network processing. Clin Neurophysiol 115:1863-1874.2004).

Gandal MJ, Edgar JC, Klook K, Siegel SJ (Gamma synchrony: Towards a translational biomarker for the treatment-resistant symptoms of schizophrenia. Neuropharmacology.2010).

Garrido MI, Kilner JM, Stephan KE, Friston KJ (The mismatch negativity: a review of underlying mechanisms. Clin Neurophysiol 120:453-463.2009).

Garrity AG, Pearlson GD, McKiernan K, Lloyd D, Kiehl KA, Calhoun VD (Aberrant "default mode" functional connectivity in schizophrenia. The American journal of psychiatry 164:450-457.2007).

Giard MH, Perrin F, Pernier J, Bouchet P (Brain generators implicated in the processing of auditory stimulus deviance: a topographic event-related potential study. Psychophysiology 27:627-640.1990).

Gjini K, Arfken C, Boutros NN (Relationships between sensory "gating out" and sensory "gating in" of auditory evoked potentials in schizophrenia: a pilot study. Schizophrenia research 121:139-145.2010).

Goff DC, Coyle JT (The emerging role of glutamate in the pathophysiology and treatment of schizophrenia. The American journal of psychiatry 158:1367-1377.2001).

Goldberg TE, Weinberger DR (Genes and the parsing of cognitive processes. Trends Cogn Sci 8:325-335.2004).

Gould TJ, Bizily SP, Tokarczyk J, Kelly MP, Siegel SJ, Kanes SJ, Abel T (Sensorimotor gating deficits in transgenic mice expressing a constitutively active form of Gs alpha. Neuropsychopharmacology 29:494-501.2004).

Gourevitch R, Rocher C, Le Pen G, Krebs MO, Jay TM (Working memory deficits in adult rats after prenatal disruption of neurogenesis. Behavioural pharmacology 15:287-292.2004).

Gronlien JH, Hakerud M, Ween H, Thorin-Hagene K, Briggs CA, Gopalakrishnan M, Malysz J (Distinct profiles of alpha7 nAChR positive allosteric modulation revealed by structurally diverse chemotypes. Mol Pharmacol 72:715-724.2007).

Gross J, Schmitz F, Schnitzler I, Kessler K, Shapiro K, Hommel B, Schnitzler A (Modulation of long-range neural synchrony reflects temporal limitations of visual attention in humans. Proceedings of the National Academy of Sciences of the United States of America 101:13050-13055.2004).

Grunwald T, Boutros NN, Pezer N, von Oertzen J, Fernandez G, Schaller C, Elger CE (Neuronal substrates of sensory gating within the human brain. Biological psychiatry 53:511-519.2003).

Gu Z, Jiang Q, Fu AK, Ip NY, Yan Z (Regulation of NMDA receptors by neuregulin signaling in prefrontal cortex. J Neurosci 25:4974-4984.2005).

Haenschel C, Bittner RA, Waltz J, Haertling F, Wibral M, Singer W, Linden DE, Rodriguez E (Cortical oscillatory activity is critical for working memory as revealed by deficits in early-onset schizophrenia. J Neurosci 29:9481-9489.2009).

Hahn CG, Wang HY, Cho DS, Talbot K, Gur RE, Berrettini WH, Bakshi K, Kamins J, Borgmann-Winter KE, Siegel SJ, Gallop RJ, Arnold SE (Altered neuregulin 1-erbB4 signaling contributes to NMDA receptor hypofunction in schizophrenia. Nat Med 12:824-828.2006).

Haig AR, Gordon E, De Pascalis V, Meares RA, Bahramali H, Harris A (Gamma activity in schizophrenia: evidence of impaired network binding? Clin Neurophysiol 111:1461-1468.2000).

Hajos M (Targeting information-processing deficit in schizophrenia: a novel approach to psychotherapeutic drug discovery. Trends Pharmacol Sci 27:391-398.2006).

Halene TB, Ehrlichman RS, Liang Y, Christian EP, Jonak GJ, Gur TL, Blendy JA, Dow HC, Brodkin ES, Schneider F, Gur RC, Siegel SJ (Assessment of NMDA receptor NR1 subunit hypofunction in mice as a model for schizophrenia. Genes Brain Behav 8:661-675.2009).

Halene TB, Siegel SJ (Antipsychotic-like properties of phosphodiesterase 4 inhibitors: evaluation of 4-(3-butoxy-4-methoxybenzyl)-2-imidazolidinone (RO-20-1724) with auditory event-related potentials and prepulse inhibition of startle. The Journal of pharmacology and experimental therapeutics 326:230-239.2008).

Hall MH, Schulze K, Rijsdijk F, Picchioni M, Ettinger U, Bramon E, Freedman R, Murray RM, Sham P (Heritability and reliability of P300, P50 and duration mismatch negativity. Behav Genet 36:845-857.2006).

Hansch EC, Syndulko K, Cohen SN, Goldberg ZI, Potvin AR, Tourtellotte WW (Cognition in Parkinson disease: an event-related potential perspective. Annals of neurology 11:599-607.1982).

Harrison BJ, Yucel M, Pujol J, Pantelis C (Task-induced deactivation of midline cortical regions in schizophrenia assessed with fMRI. Schizophrenia research 91:82-86.2007).

Harrison PJ (The neuropathology of schizophrenia. A critical review of the data and their interpretation. Brain 122 (Pt 4):593-624.1999).

Heekeren K, Daumann J, Neukirch A, Stock C, Kawohl W, Norra C, Waberski TD, Gouzoulis-Mayfrank E (Mismatch negativity generation in the human 5HT2A agonist and NMDA antagonist model of psychosis. Psychopharmacology 199:77-88.2008).

Herdman AT, Stapells DR (Thresholds determined using the monotic and dichotic multiple auditory steady-state response technique in normal-hearing subjects. Scandinavian audiology 30:41-49.2001).

Hill SY, Locke J, Zezza N, Kaplan B, Neiswanger K, Steinhauer SR, Wipprecht G, Xu J (Genetic association between reduced P300 amplitude and the DRD2 dopamine receptor A1 allele in children at high risk for alcoholism. Biol Psychiatry 43:40-51.1998).

Hirayasu Y, Asato N, Ohta H, Hokama H, Arakaki H, Ogura C (Abnormalities of auditory event-related potentials in schizophrenia prior to treatment. Biological psychiatry 43:244-253.1998).

Hong LE, Buchanan RW, Thaker GK, Shepard PD, Summerfelt A (Beta (~16 Hz) frequency neural oscillations mediate auditory sensory gating in humans. Psychophysiology 45:197-204.2008a).

Hong LE, Summerfelt A, Buchanan RW, O'Donnell P, Thaker GK, Weiler MA, Lahti AC (Gamma and delta neural oscillations and association with clinical symptoms under subanesthetic ketamine. Neuropsychopharmacology 35:632-640.2008b).

Huerta PT, Lisman JE (Heightened synaptic plasticity of hippocampal CA1 neurons during a cholinergically induced rhythmic state. Nature 364:723-725.1993).

Hughes JR, Hatsukami DK, Mitchell JE, Dahlgren LA (Prevalence of smoking among psychiatric outpatients. The American journal of psychiatry 143:993-997.1986).

Inami R, Kirino E, Inoue R, Arai H (Transdermal nicotine administration enhances automatic auditory processing reflected by mismatch negativity. Pharmacology, biochemistry, and behavior 80:453-461.2005).

Inami R, Kirino E, Inoue R, Suzuki T, Arai H (Nicotine effects on mismatch negativity in nonsmoking schizophrenic patients. Neuropsychobiology 56:64-72.2007).

Intriligator J, Polich J (On the relationship between background EEG and the P300 event-related potential. Biological psychology 37:207-218.1994).

Itil TM (1979) Computer analyzed EEG findings in adult schizophrenics, psychotic children and 'high risk' children for schizophrenia.

In: Biological Psychiatry Today(Obiols, J., Ballus, C., Gonzalez Monclus, E. et al. (Eds),, ed), pp 1239-1308 Amsterdam: ElsevieriNorth Holland Biomedical Press.

Itil TM, Saletu B, Davis S (EEG findings in chronic schizophrenics based on digital computer period analysis and analog power spectra. Biological psychiatry 5:1-13.1972).

Iwanami A, Shinba T, Sumi M, Ozawa N, Yamamoto K (Event-related potentials during an auditory discrimination task in rats. Neuroscience research 21:103-106.1994).

Javanbakht A (Sensory gating deficits, pattern completion, and disturbed fronto-limbic balance, a model for description of hallucinations and delusions in schizophrenia. Medical hypotheses 67:1173-1184.2006).

Javitt DC (Intracortical mechanisms of mismatch negativity dysfunction in schizophrenia. Audiology & neuro-otology 5:207-215.2000).

Javitt DC (Glutamatergic theories of schizophrenia. The Israel journal of psychiatry and related sciences 47:4-16.2010).

Javitt DC, Jayachandra M, Lindsley RW, Specht CM, Schroeder CE (Schizophrenia-like deficits in auditory P1 and N1 refractoriness induced by the psychomimetic agent phencyclidine (PCP). Clin Neurophysiol 111:833-836.2000).

Javitt DC, Jotkowitz A, Sircar R, Zukin SR (Non-competitive regulation of phencyclidine/sigma-receptors by the N-methyl-D-aspartate receptor antagonist D-(-)-2-amino-5-phosphonovaleric acid. Neuroscience letters 78:193-198.1987).

Javitt DC, Spencer KM, Thaker GK, Winterer G, Hajos M (Neurophysiological biomarkers for drug development in schizophrenia. Nature reviews 7:68-83.2008).

Javitt DC, Steinschneider M, Schroeder CE, Arezzo JC (Role of cortical N-methyl-D-aspartate receptors in auditory sensory memory and mismatch negativity generation: implications for schizophrenia. Proceedings of the National Academy of Sciences of the United States of America 93:11962-11967.1996).

Javitt DC, Zukin SR (Recent advances in the phencyclidine model of schizophrenia. The American journal of psychiatry 148:1301-1308.1991).

Jeon YW, Polich J (Meta-analysis of P300 and schizophrenia: patients, paradigms, and practical implications. Psychophysiology 40:684-701.2003).

Jessen F, Fries T, Kucharski C, Nishimura T, Hoenig K, Maier W, Falkai P, Heun R (Amplitude reduction of the mismatch negativity in first-degree relatives of patients with schizophrenia. Neuroscience letters 309:185-188.2001).

Jin Y, Potkin SG, Kemp AS, Huerta ST, Alva G, Thai TM, Carreon D, Bunney WE, Jr. (Therapeutic effects of individualized alpha frequency transcranial magnetic stimulation (alphaTMS) on the negative symptoms of schizophrenia. Schizophrenia bulletin 32:556-561.2006).

Judd LL, McAdams L, Budnick B, Braff DL (Sensory gating deficits in schizophrenia: new results. The American journal of psychiatry 149:488-493.1992).

Kidogami Y, Yoneda H, Asaba H, Sakai T (P300 in first degree relatives of schizophrenics. Schizophrenia research 6:9-13.1991).

Kirk IJ, Mackay JC (The role of theta-range oscillations in synchronising and integrating activity in distributed mnemonic networks. Cortex; a journal devoted to the study of the nervous system and behavior 39:993-1008.2003).

Kocsis B, Di Prisco GV, Vertes RP (Theta synchronization in the limbic system: the role of Gudden's tegmental nuclei. The European journal of neuroscience 13:381-388.2001).

Koike K, Hashimoto K, Takai N, Shimizu E, Komatsu N, Watanabe H, Nakazato M, Okamura N, Stevens KE, Freedman R, Iyo M (Tropisetron improves deficits in auditory P50 suppression in schizophrenia. Schizophrenia research 76:67-72.2005).

Kopell N, Ermentrout GB, Whittington MA, Traub RD (Gamma rhythms and beta rhythms have different synchronization properties. Proceedings of the National Academy of Sciences of the United States of America 97:1867-1872.2000).

Kornetsky C (Hyporesponsivity of chronic schizophrenic patients to dextroamphetamine. Archives of general psychiatry 33:1425-1428.1976).

Koukkou M, Federspiel A, Braker E, Hug C, Kleinlogel H, Merlo MC, Lehmann D (An EEG approach to the neurodevelopmental hypothesis of schizophrenia studying schizophrenics, normal controls and adolescents. Journal of psychiatric research 34:57-73.2000).

Kovacic P, Somanathan R (Clinical physiology and mechanism of dizocilpine (MK-801): electron transfer, radicals, redox metabolites and bioactivity. Oxidative medicine and cellular longevity 3:13-22.2010).

Kraus N, Smith DI, Reed NL, Stein LK, Cartee C (Auditory middle latency responses in children: effects of age and diagnostic category. Electroencephalography and clinical neurophysiology 62:343-351.1985).

Krause M, Hoffmann WE, Hajos M (Auditory sensory gating in hippocampus and reticular thalamic neurons in anesthetized rats. Biological psychiatry 53:244-253.2003).

Krishnan GP, Hetrick WP, Brenner CA, Shekhar A, Steffen AN, O'Donnell BF (Steady state and induced auditory gamma deficits in schizophrenia. NeuroImage 47:1711-1719.2009).

Krystal JH, Karper LP, Seibyl JP, Freeman GK, Delaney R, Bremner JD, Heninger GR, Bowers MB, Jr., Charney DS (Subanesthetic effects of the noncompetitive NMDA antagonist, ketamine, in humans. Psychotomimetic, perceptual, cognitive, and neuroendocrine responses. Archives of general psychiatry 51:199-214.1994).

Kumari V, Aasen I, ffytche D, Williams SC, Sharma T (Neural correlates of adjunctive rivastigmine treatment to antipsychotics in schizophrenia: a randomized, placebo-controlled, double-blind fMRI study. NeuroImage 29:545-556.2006).

Kumari V, Postma P (Nicotine use in schizophrenia: the self medication hypotheses. Neurosci Biobehav Rev 29:1021-1034.2005).

Kwon JS, O'Donnell BF, Wallenstein GV, Greene RW, Hirayasu Y, Nestor PG, Hasselmo ME, Potts GF, Shenton ME, McCarley RW (Gamma frequency-range abnormalities to auditory stimulation in schizophrenia. Archives of general psychiatry 56:1001-1005.1999).

Lachman HM, Papolos DF, Saito T, Yu YM, Szumlanski CL, Weinshilboum RM (Human catechol-O-methyltransferase pharmacogenetics: description of a functional polymorphism and its potential application to neuropsychiatric disorders. Pharmacogenetics 6:243-250.1996).

Laurent A, Garcia-Larrea L, d'Amato T, Bosson JL, Saoud M, Marie-Cardine M, Maugiere F, Dalery J (Auditory event-related potentials and clinical scores in unmedicated schizophrenic patients. Psychiatry research 86:229-238.1999).

Lazarewicz MT, Ehrlichman RS, Maxwell CR, Gandal MJ, Finkel LH, Siegel SJ (Ketamine modulates theta and gamma oscillations. Journal of cognitive neuroscience 22:1452-1464.2010).

Lee KH, Williams LM, Breakspear M, Gordon E (Synchronous gamma activity: a review and contribution to an integrative neuroscience model of schizophrenia. Brain Res Brain Res Rev 41:57-78.2003).

Leicht G, Karch S, Karamatskos E, Giegling I, Moller HJ, Hegerl U, Pogarell O, Rujescu D, Mulert C (Alterations of the early auditory evoked gamma-band response in first-degree relatives of patients with schizophrenia: hints to a new intermediate phenotype. Journal of psychiatric research 45:699-705.2010a).

Leicht G, Kirsch V, Giegling I, Karch S, Hantschk I, Moller HJ, Pogarell O, Hegerl U, Rujescu D, Mulert C (Reduced early auditory evoked gamma-band response in patients with schizophrenia. Biological psychiatry 67:224-231).

Leicht G, Kirsch V, Giegling I, Karch S, Hantschk I, Moller HJ, Pogarell O, Hegerl U, Rujescu D, Mulert C (Reduced early auditory evoked gamma-band response in patients with schizophrenia. Biological psychiatry 67:224-231.2010b).

Leonard S, Adler LE, Benhammou K, Berger R, Breese CR, Drebing C, Gault J, Lee MJ, Logel J, Olincy A, Ross RG, Stevens K, Sullivan B, Vianzon R, Virnich DE, Waldo M,

Walton K, Freedman R (Smoking and mental illness. Pharmacology, biochemistry, and behavior 70:561-570.2001).

Leonard S, Gault J, Moore T, Hopkins J, Robinson M, Olincy A, Adler LE, Cloninger CR, Kaufmann CA, Tsuang MT, Faraone SV, Malaspina D, Svrakic DM, Freedman R (Further investigation of a chromosome 15 locus in schizophrenia: analysis of affected sibpairs from the NIMH Genetics Initiative. Am J Med Genet 81:308-312.1998).

Levy DL, Smith M, Robinson D, Jody D, Lerner G, Alvir J, Geisler SH, Szymanski SR, Gonzalez A, Mayerhoff DI, et al. (Methylphenidate increases thought disorder in recent onset schizophrenics, but not in normal controls. Biological psychiatry 34:507-514.1993).

Li B, Woo RS, Mei L, Malinow R (The neuregulin-1 receptor erbB4 controls glutamatergic synapse maturation and plasticity. Neuron 54:583-597.2007).

Light GA, Hsu JL, Hsieh MH, Meyer-Gomes K, Sprock J, Swerdlow NR, Braff DL (Gamma band oscillations reveal neural network cortical coherence dysfunction in schizophrenia patients. Biological psychiatry 60:1231-1240.2006).

Lijffijt M, Lane SD, Meier SL, Boutros NN, Burroughs S, Steinberg JL, Moeller FG, Swann AC (P50, N100, and P200 sensory gating: relationships with behavioral inhibition, attention, and working memory. Psychophysiology 46:1059-1068.2009a).

Lijffijt M, Moeller FG, Boutros NN, Steinberg JL, Meier SL, Lane SD, Swann AC (Diminished P50, N100 and P200 auditory sensory gating in bipolar I disorder. Psychiatry research 167:191-201.2009b).

Linden DE (The p300: where in the brain is it produced and what does it tell us? Neuroscientist 11:563-576.2005).

Lodge DJ, Behrens MM, Grace AA (A loss of parvalbumin-containing interneurons is associated with diminished oscillatory activity in an animal model of schizophrenia. J Neurosci 29:2344-2354.2009).

Lu BY, Martin KE, Edgar JC, Smith AK, Lewis SF, Escamilla MA, Miller GA, Canive JM (Effect of catechol O-methyltransferase val(158)met polymorphism on the p50 gating endophenotype in schizophrenia. Biol Psychiatry 62:822-825.2007).

Luntz-Leybman V, Bickford PC, Freedman R (Cholinergic gating of response to auditory stimuli in rat hippocampus. Brain research 587:130-136.1992).

Luts H, Wouters J (Comparison of MASTER and AUDERA for measurement of auditory steady-state responses. International journal of audiology 44:244-253.2005).

Ma J, Leung LS (Relation between hippocampal gamma waves and behavioral disturbances induced by phencyclidine and methamphetamine. Behavioural brain research 111:1-11.2000).

Maharajh K, Teale P, Rojas DC, Reite ML (Fluctuation of gamma-band phase synchronization within the auditory cortex in schizophrenia. Clin Neurophysiol 121:542-548.2010).

Makeig S, Enghoff S, Jung TP, Sejnowski TJ (A natural basis for efficient brain-actuated control. IEEE Trans Rehabil Eng 8:208-211.2000).

Martin-Loeches M, Molina V, Munoz F, Hinojosa JA, Reig S, Desco M, Benito C, Sanz J, Gabiri A, Sarramea F, Santos A, Palomo T (P300 amplitude as a possible correlate of frontal degeneration in schizophrenia. Schizophrenia research 49:121-128.2001).

Martin LF, Davalos DB, Kisley MA (Nicotine enhances automatic temporal processing as measured by the mismatch negativity waveform. Nicotine Tob Res 11:698-706.2009).

Martin LF, Freedman R (Schizophrenia and the alpha7 nicotinic acetylcholine receptor. Int Rev Neurobiol 78:225-246.2007).

Mathalon DH, Ford JM, Rosenbloom M, Pfefferbaum A (P300 reduction and prolongation with illness duration in schizophrenia. Biological psychiatry 47:413-427.2000).

Mathalon DH, Hoffman RE, Watson TD, Miller RM, Roach BJ, Ford JM (Neurophysiological Distinction between Schizophrenia and Schizoaffective Disorder. Frontiers in human neuroscience 3:70).

Mathalon DH, Hoffman RE, Watson TD, Miller RM, Roach BJ, Ford JM (Neurophysiological Distinction between Schizophrenia and Schizoaffective Disorder. Frontiers in human neuroscience 3:70.2010).

Maxwell CR, Ehrlichman RS, Liang Y, Trief D, Kanes SJ, Karp J, Siegel SJ (Ketamine produces lasting disruptions in encoding of sensory stimuli. The Journal of pharmacology and experimental therapeutics 316:315-324.2006a).

Maxwell CR, Liang Y, Kelly MP, Kanes SJ, Abel T, Siegel SJ (Mice expressing constitutively active Gsalpha exhibit stimulus encoding deficits similar to those observed in schizophrenia patients. Neuroscience 141:1257-1264.2006b).

Maxwell CR, Liang Y, Weightman BD, Kanes SJ, Abel T, Gur RE, Turetsky BI, Bilker WB, Lenox RH, Siegel SJ (Effects of chronic olanzapine and haloperidol differ on the mouse N1 auditory evoked potential. Neuropsychopharmacology 29:739-746.2004).

Mazhari S, Price G, Waters F, Dragovic M, Jablensky A (Evidence of abnormalities in mid-latency auditory evoked responses (MLAER) in cognitive subtypes of patients with schizophrenia. Psychiatry research 187:317-323.2011).

McCracken CB, Grace AA (Nucleus accumbens deep brain stimulation produces region-specific alterations in local field potential oscillations and evoked responses in vivo. J Neurosci 29:5354-5363.2009).

Mears RP, Klein AC, Cromwell HC (Auditory inhibitory gating in medial prefrontal cortex: Single unit and local field potential analysis. Neuroscience 141:47-65.2006).

Mendel MI, Adkinson CD, Harker LA (Middle components of the auditory evoked potentials in infants. The Annals of otology, rhinology, and laryngology 86:293-299.1977).

Mendelson T, Salamy A (Maturational effects on the middle components of the averaged electroencephalic response. Journal of speech and hearing research 24:140-144.1981).

Merrin EL, Floyd TC (Negative symptoms and EEG alpha activity in schizophrenic patients. Schizophrenia research 8:11-20.1992).

Metzger KL, Maxwell CR, Liang Y, Siegel SJ (Effects of nicotine vary across two auditory evoked potentials in the mouse. Biological psychiatry 61:23-30.2007).

Meyer EM, Tay ET, Papke RL, Meyers C, Huang GL, de Fiebre CM (3-[2,4-Dimethoxybenzylidene]anabaseine (DMXB) selectively activates rat alpha7 receptors and improves memory-related behaviors in a mecamylamine-sensitive manner. Brain research 768:49-56.1997).

Michie PT, Innes-Brown H, Todd J, Jablensky AV (Duration mismatch negativity in biological relatives of patients with schizophrenia spectrum disorders. Biological psychiatry 52:749-758.2002).
Miller CL, Bickford PC, Luntz-Leybman V, Adler LE, Gerhardt GA, Freedman R (Phencyclidine and auditory sensory gating in the hippocampus of the rat. Neuropharmacology 31:1041-1048.1992).
Miltner WH, Braun C, Arnold M, Witte H, Taub E (Coherence of gamma-band EEG activity as a basis for associative learning. Nature 397:434-436.1999).
Miyazato H, Skinner RD, Garcia-Rill E (Sensory gating of the P13 midlatency auditory evoked potential and the startle response in the rat. Brain research 822:60-71.1999).
Mohn AR, Gainetdinov RR, Caron MG, Koller BH (Mice with reduced NMDA receptor expression display behaviors related to schizophrenia. Cell 98:427-436.1999).
Moore H, Jentsch JD, Ghajarnia M, Geyer MA, Grace AA (A neurobehavioral systems analysis of adult rats exposed to methylazoxymethanol acetate on E17: implications for the neuropathology of schizophrenia. Biological psychiatry 60:253-264.2006).
Morihisa JM, Duffy FH, Wyatt RJ (Brain electrical activity mapping (BEAM) in schizophrenic patients. Archives of general psychiatry 40:719-728.1983).
Morstyn R, Duffy FH, McCarley RW (Altered topography of EEG spectral content in schizophrenia. Electroencephalography and clinical neurophysiology 56:263-271.1983).
Mulert C, Juckel G, Giegling I, Pogarell O, Leicht G, Karch S, Mavrogiorgou P, Moller HJ, Hegerl U, Rujescu D (A Ser9Gly polymorphism in the dopamine D3 receptor gene (DRD3) and event-related P300 potentials. Neuropsychopharmacology 31:1335-1344.2006).
Mulert C, Kirsch V, Pascual-Marqui R, McCarley RW, Spencer KM (Long-range synchrony of gamma oscillations and auditory hallucination symptoms in schizophrenia. Int J Psychophysiol 79:55-63.2010).
Murck H, Spitznagel H, Ploch M, Seibel K, Schaffler K (Hypericum extract reverses S-ketamine-induced changes in auditory evoked potentials in humans - possible implications for the treatment of schizophrenia. Biological psychiatry 59:440-445.2006).
Naatanen R (Mismatch negativity (MMN): perspectives for application. Int J Psychophysiol 37:3-10.2000).
Naatanen R (Mismatch negativity: clinical research and possible applications. Int J Psychophysiol 48:179-188.2003).
Nagamoto HT, Adler LE, Hea RA, Griffith JM, McRae KA, Freedman R (Gating of auditory P50 in schizophrenics: unique effects of clozapine. Biological psychiatry 40:181-188.1996).
Nieuwenhuis S, Gilzenrat MS, Holmes BD, Cohen JD (The role of the locus coeruleus in mediating the attentional blink: a neurocomputational theory. Journal of experimental psychology 134:291-307.2005).
Oerbeck B, Reinvang I, Sundet K, Heyerdahl S (Young adults with severe congenital hypothyroidism: cognitive event related potentials (ERPs) and the significance of an early start of thyroxine treatment. Scandinavian journal of psychology 48:61-67.2007).

Olichney JM, Iragui VJ, Kutas M, Nowacki R, Morris S, Jeste DV (Relationship between auditory P300 amplitude and age of onset of schizophrenia in older patients. Psychiatry research 79:241-254.1998).

Olincy A, Harris JG, Johnson LL, Pender V, Kongs S, Allensworth D, Ellis J, Zerbe GO, Leonard S, Stevens KE, Stevens JO, Martin L, Adler LE, Soti F, Kem WR, Freedman R (Proof-of-concept trial of an alpha7 nicotinic agonist in schizophrenia. Archives of general psychiatry 63:630-638.2006).

Olincy A, Martin L (Diminished suppression of the P50 auditory evoked potential in bipolar disorder subjects with a history of psychosis. The American journal of psychiatry 162:43-49.2005).

Olincy A, Young DA, Freedman R (Increased levels of the nicotine metabolite cotinine in schizophrenic smokers compared to other smokers. Biological psychiatry 42:1-5.1997).

Olney JW, Newcomer JW, Farber NB (NMDA receptor hypofunction model of schizophrenia. Journal of psychiatric research 33:523-533.1999).

Onitsuka T, Ninomiya H, Sato E, Yamamoto T, Tashiro N (The effect of interstimulus intervals and between-block rests on the auditory evoked potential and magnetic field: is the auditory P50 in humans an overlapping potential? Clin Neurophysiol 111:237-245.2000).

Oranje B, van Berckel BN, Kemner C, van Ree JM, Kahn RS, Verbaten MN (The effects of a sub-anaesthetic dose of ketamine on human selective attention. Neuropsychopharmacology 22:293-302.2000).

Papaleo F, Crawley JN, Song J, Lipska BK, Pickel J, Weinberger DR, Chen J (Genetic dissection of the role of catechol-O-methyltransferase in cognition and stress reactivity in mice. J Neurosci 28:8709-8723.2008).

Patterson JV, Hetrick WP, Boutros NN, Jin Y, Sandman C, Stern H, Potkin S, Bunney WE, Jr. (P50 sensory gating ratios in schizophrenics and controls: a review and data analysis. Psychiatry research 158:226-247.2008).

Pearlson GD (Psychiatric and medical syndromes associated with phencyclidine (PCP) abuse. The Johns Hopkins medical journal 148:25-33.1981).

Penschuck S, Flagstad P, Didriksen M, Leist M, Michael-Titus AT (Decrease in parvalbumin-expressing neurons in the hippocampus and increased phencyclidine-induced locomotor activity in the rat methylazoxymethanol (MAM) model of schizophrenia. The European journal of neuroscience 23:279-284.2006).

Pfefferbaum A, Ford JM, White PM, Roth WT (P3 in schizophrenia is affected by stimulus modality, response requirements, medication status, and negative symptoms. Archives of general psychiatry 46:1035-1044.1989).

Picciotto MR, Zoli M (Neuroprotection via nAChRs: the role of nAChRs in neurodegenerative disorders such as Alzheimer's and Parkinson's disease. Front Biosci 13:492-504.2008).

Picton TW, Hillyard SA, Krausz HI, Galambos R (Human auditory evoked potentials. I. Evaluation of components. Electroencephalography and clinical neurophysiology 36:179-190.1974).

Pincze Z, Lakatos P, Rajkai C, Ulbert I, Karmos G (Separation of mismatch negativity and the N1 wave in the auditory cortex of the cat: a topographic study. Clin Neurophysiol 112:778-784.2001).

Polich J (Updating P300: an integrative theory of P3a and P3b. Clin Neurophysiol 118:2128-2148.2007).

Polich J, Criado JR (Neuropsychology and neuropharmacology of P3a and P3b. Int J Psychophysiol 60:172-185.2006).

Polich J, Squire LR (P300 from amnesic patients with bilateral hippocampal lesions. Electroencephalography and clinical neurophysiology 86:408-417.1993).

Potter D, Summerfelt A, Gold J, Buchanan RW (Review of clinical correlates of P50 sensory gating abnormalities in patients with schizophrenia. Schizophrenia bulletin 32:692-700.2006).

Pritchard WS (Cognitive event-related potential correlates of schizophrenia. Psychological bulletin 100:43-66.1986).

Roach BJ, Mathalon DH (Event-related EEG time-frequency analysis: an overview of measures and an analysis of early gamma band phase locking in schizophrenia. Schizophrenia bulletin 34:907-926.2008).

Roeser RJ, Valente, M., & Dunn, H.H. (2007) Audiology diagnosis New York: Thieme Medical publishers.

Rosburg T, Boutros NN, Ford JM (Reduced auditory evoked potential component N100 in schizophrenia--a critical review. Psychiatry research 161:259-274.2008).

Roth WT, Kopell BS, Tinklenberg JR, Huntsberger GE, Kraemer HC (Reliability of the contingent negative variation and the auditory evoked potential. Electroencephalography and clinical neurophysiology 38:45-50.1975).

Roth WT, Pfefferbaum A, Kelly AF, Berger PA, Kopell BS (Auditory event-related potentials in schizophrenia and depression. Psychiatry research 4:199-212.1981).

Roxborough H, Muir WJ, Blackwood DH, Walker MT, Blackburn IM (Neuropsychological and P300 abnormalities in schizophrenics and their relatives. Psychological medicine 23:305-314.1993).

Rudnick ND, Koehler C, Picciotto MR, Siegel SJ (Role of beta2-containing nicotinic acetylcholine receptors in auditory event-related potentials. Psychopharmacology 202:745-751.2009).

Rutter L, Carver FW, Holroyd T, Nadar SR, Mitchell-Francis J, Apud J, Weinberger DR, Coppola R (Magnetoencephalographic gamma power reduction in patients with schizophrenia during resting condition. Human brain mapping 30:3254-3264.2009).

Ruusuvirta T, Penttonen M, Korhonen T (Auditory cortical event-related potentials to pitch deviances in rats. Neuroscience letters 248:45-48.1998).

Saitoh O, Niwa S, Hiramatsu K, Kameyama T, Rymar K, Itoh K (Abnormalities in late positive components of event-related potentials may reflect a genetic predisposition to schizophrenia. Biological psychiatry 19:293-303.1984).

Sambeth A, Maes JH, Van Luijtelaar G, Molenkamp IB, Jongsma ML, Van Rijn CM (Auditory event-related potentials in humans and rats: effects of task manipulation. Psychophysiology 40:60-68.2003).

Sevik AE, Anil Yagcioglu AE, Yagcioglu S, Karahan S, Gurses N, Yildiz M (Neuropsychological performance and auditory event related potentials in schizophrenia patients and their siblings: A family study. Schizophrenia research.2011).

Shaikh M, Hall MH, Schulze K, Dutt A, Walshe M, Williams I, Constante M, Picchioni M, Toulopoulou T, Collier D, Rijsdijk F, Powell J, Arranz M, Murray RM, Bramon E

(Do COMT, BDNF and NRG1 polymorphisms influence P50 sensory gating in psychosis? Psychol Med 41:263-276).
Shaikh M, Hall MH, Schulze K, Dutt A, Walshe M, Williams I, Constante M, Picchioni M, Toulopoulou T, Collier D, Rijsdijk F, Powell J, Arranz M, Murray RM, Bramon E (Do COMT, BDNF and NRG1 polymorphisms influence P50 sensory gating in psychosis? Psychological medicine 41:263-276.2011).
Shajahan PM, O'Carroll RE, Glabus MF, Ebmeier KP, Blackwood DH (Correlation of auditory 'oddball' P300 with verbal memory deficits in schizophrenia. Psychological medicine 27:579-586.1997).
Shaywitz BA, Yager RD, Klopper JH (Selective brain dopamine depletion in developing rats: an experimental model of minimal brain dysfunction. Science (New York, NY 191:305-308.1976).
Shelley AM, Ward PB, Catts SV, Michie PT, Andrews S, McConaghy N (Mismatch negativity: an index of a preattentive processing deficit in schizophrenia. Biological psychiatry 30:1059-1062.1991).
Shenton ME, Faux SF, McCarley RW, Ballinger R, Coleman M, Duffy FH (Clinical correlations of auditory P200 topography and left temporo-central deficits in schizophrenia: a preliminary study. Journal of psychiatric research 23:13-34.1989).
Shin YW, Krishnan G, Hetrick WP, Brenner CA, Shekhar A, Malloy FW, O'Donnell BF (Increased temporal variability of auditory event-related potentials in schizophrenia and Schizotypal Personality Disorder. Schizophrenia research 124:110-118.2010).
Shinozaki N, Yabe H, Sato Y, Hiruma T, Sutoh T, Nashida T, Matsuoka T, Kaneko S (The difference in Mismatch negativity between the acute and post-acute phase of schizophrenia. Biological psychology 59:105-119.2002).
Siegel SJ, Connolly P, Liang Y, Lenox RH, Gur RE, Bilker WB, Kanes SJ, Turetsky BI (Effects of strain, novelty, and NMDA blockade on auditory-evoked potentials in mice. Neuropsychopharmacology 28:675-682.2003).
Siegel SJ, Maxwell CR, Majumdar S, Trief DF, Lerman C, Gur RE, Kanes SJ, Liang Y (Monoamine reuptake inhibition and nicotine receptor antagonism reduce amplitude and gating of auditory evoked potentials. Neuroscience 133:729-738.2005).
Siekmeier PJ, Stufflebeam SM (Patterns of spontaneous magnetoencephalographic activity in patients with schizophrenia. J Clin Neurophysiol 27:179-190.2010).
Simpson GV, Knight RT (Multiple brain systems generating the rat auditory evoked potential. II. Dissociation of auditory cortex and non-lemniscal generator systems. Brain research 602:251-263.1993).
Singer W (Synchronization of cortical activity and its putative role in information processing and learning. Annual review of physiology 55:349-374.1993).
Singh SM, Basu D (The P300 event-related potential and its possible role as an endophenotype for studying substance use disorders: a review. Addiction biology 14:298-309.2009).
Skinner P, Glattke TJ (Electrophysiologic response audiometry: state of the art. The Journal of speech and hearing disorders 42:179-198.1977).
Smith AK, Edgar JC, Huang M, Lu BY, Thoma RJ, Hanlon FM, McHaffie G, Jones AP, Paz RD, Miller GA, Canive JM (Cognitive abilities and 50- and 100-msec paired-click

processes in schizophrenia. The American journal of psychiatry 167:1264-1275.2010).

Soltani M, Knight RT (Neural origins of the P300. Critical reviews in neurobiology 14:199-224.2000).

Spencer KM, Nestor PG, Niznikiewicz MA, Salisbury DF, Shenton ME, McCarley RW (Abnormal neural synchrony in schizophrenia. J Neurosci 23:7407-7411.2003).

Spencer KM, Polich J (Poststimulus EEG spectral analysis and P300: attention, task, and probability. Psychophysiology 36:220-232.1999).

Spencer KM, Salisbury DF, Shenton ME, McCarley RW (Gamma-band auditory steady-state responses are impaired in first episode psychosis. Biological psychiatry 64:369-375.2008).

Sponheim SR, Clementz BA, Iacono WG, Beiser M (Resting EEG in first-episode and chronic schizophrenia. Psychophysiology 31:37-43.1994).

Squires KC, Wickens C, Squires NK, Donchin E (The effect of stimulus sequence on the waveform of the cortical event-related potential. Science (New York, NY 193:1142-1146.1976).

Stanzione P, Fattapposta F, Giunti P, D'Alessio C, Tagliati M, Affricano C, Amabile G (P300 variations in parkinsonian patients before and during dopaminergic monotherapy: a suggested dopamine component in P300. Electroencephalography and clinical neurophysiology 80:446-453.1991).

Stevens KE, Fuller LL, Rose GM (Dopaminergic and noradrenergic modulation of amphetamine-induced changes in auditory gating. Brain research 555:91-98.1991).

Stevens KE, Kem WR, Mahnir VM, Freedman R (Selective alpha7-nicotinic agonists normalize inhibition of auditory response in DBA mice. Psychopharmacology 136:320-327.1998).

Stevens KE, Luthman J, Lindqvist E, Johnson RG, Rose GM (Effects of neonatal dopamine depletion on sensory inhibition in the rat. Pharmacology, biochemistry, and behavior 53:817-823.1996).

Stevens KE, Meltzer J, Rose GM (Nicotinic cholinergic normalization of amphetamine-induced loss of auditory gating in freely moving rats. Psychopharmacology 119:163-170.1995).

Strik WK, Dierks T, Boning J, Osterheider M, Caspari A, Korber J (Disorders of smooth pursuit eye movement and auditory N100 in schizophrenic patients. Psychiatry research 41:227-235.1992).

Sullivan PF, Kendler KS, Neale MC (Schizophrenia as a complex trait: evidence from a meta-analysis of twin studies. Arch Gen Psychiatry 60:1187-1192.2003).

Takeshita S, Ogura C (Effect of the dopamine D2 antagonist sulpiride on event-related potentials and its relation to the law of initial value. Int J Psychophysiol 16:99-106.1994).

Talamini LM, Koch T, Ter Horst GJ, Korf J (Methylazoxymethanol acetate-induced abnormalities in the entorhinal cortex of the rat; parallels with morphological findings in schizophrenia. Brain research 789:293-306.1998).

Tallon-Baudry C, Bertrand O, Peronnet F, Pernier J (Induced gamma-band activity during the delay of a visual short-term memory task in humans. J Neurosci 18:4244-4254.1998).

Tekell JL, Hoffmann R, Hendrickse W, Greene RW, Rush AJ, Armitage R (High frequency EEG activity during sleep: characteristics in schizophrenia and depression. Clin EEG Neurosci 36:25-35.2005).

Tiitinen H, Sinkkonen J, Reinikainen K, Alho K, Lavikainen J, Naatanen R (Selective attention enhances the auditory 40-Hz transient response in humans. Nature 364:59-60.1993).

Tikhonravov D, Neuvonen T, Pertovaara A, Savioja K, Ruusuvirta T, Naatanen R, Carlson S (Effects of an NMDA-receptor antagonist MK-801 on an MMN-like response recorded in anesthetized rats. Brain research 1203:97-102.2008).

Turetsky BI, Calkins ME, Light GA, Olincy A, Radant AD, Swerdlow NR (Neurophysiological endophenotypes of schizophrenia: the viability of selected candidate measures. Schizophr Bull 33:69-94.2007a).

Turetsky BI, Greenwood TA, Olincy A, Radant AD, Braff DL, Cadenhead KS, Dobie DJ, Freedman R, Green MF, Gur RE, Gur RC, Light GA, Mintz J, Nuechterlein KH, Schork NJ, Seidman LJ, Siever LJ, Silverman JM, Stone WS, Swerdlow NR, Tsuang DW, Tsuang MT, Calkins ME (Abnormal auditory N100 amplitude: a heritable endophenotype in first-degree relatives of schizophrenia probands. Biological psychiatry 64:1051-1059.2008).

Turetsky BI, Kohler CG, Indersmitten T, Bhati MT, Charbonnier D, Gur RC (Facial emotion recognition in schizophrenia: when and why does it go awry? Schizophrenia research 94:253-263.2007b).

Uhlhaas PJ, Linden DE, Singer W, Haenschel C, Lindner M, Maurer K, Rodriguez E (Dysfunctional long-range coordination of neural activity during Gestalt perception in schizophrenia. J Neurosci 26:8168-8175.2006).

Uhlhaas PJ, Singer W (Abnormal neural oscillations and synchrony in schizophrenia. Nat Rev Neurosci 11:100-113.2010).

Ulanovsky N, Las L, Farkas D, Nelken I (Multiple time scales of adaptation in auditory cortex neurons. J Neurosci 24:10440-10453.2004).

Umbricht D, Javitt D, Novak G, Bates J, Pollack S, Lieberman J, Kane J (Effects of clozapine on auditory event-related potentials in schizophrenia. Biological psychiatry 44:716-725.1998).

Umbricht D, Koller R, Schmid L, Skrabo A, Grubel C, Huber T, Stassen H (How specific are deficits in mismatch negativity generation to schizophrenia? Biological psychiatry 53:1120-1131.2003).

Umbricht D, Krljes S (Mismatch negativity in schizophrenia: a meta-analysis. Schizophrenia research 76:1-23.2005).

Umbricht D, Schmid L, Koller R, Vollenweider FX, Hell D, Javitt DC (Ketamine-induced deficits in auditory and visual context-dependent processing in healthy volunteers: implications for models of cognitive deficits in schizophrenia. Archives of general psychiatry 57:1139-1147.2000).

Umbricht D, Vyssotki D, Latanov A, Nitsch R, Lipp HP (Deviance-related electrophysiological activity in mice: is there mismatch negativity in mice? Clin Neurophysiol 116:353-363.2005).

Umbricht D, Vyssotky D, Latanov A, Nitsch R, Brambilla R, D'Adamo P, Lipp HP (Midlatency auditory event-related potentials in mice: comparison to midlatency auditory ERPs in humans. Brain research 1019:189-200.2004).

van der Stelt O, van Boxtel GJ (Auditory P300 and mismatch negativity in comatose states. Clin Neurophysiol 119:2172-2174.2008).

Venables PH (The effect of auditory and visual stimulation on the skin potential response of schizophrenics. Brain 83:77-92.1960).

Venables PH (Performance and Level of Activation in Schizophrenics and Normals. Br J Psychol 55:207-218.1964).

Vohs JL, Chambers RA, Krishnan GP, O'Donnell BF, Berg S, Morzorati SL (GABAergic modulation of the 40 Hz auditory steady-state response in a rat model of schizophrenia. The international journal of neuropsychopharmacology / official scientific journal of the Collegium Internationale Neuropsychopharmacologicum (CINP) 13:487-497.2010).

Wand G, Levine M, Zweifel L, Schwindinger W, Abel T (The cAMP-protein kinase A signal transduction pathway modulates ethanol consumption and sedative effects of ethanol. J Neurosci 21:5297-5303.2001).

Wang CZ, Yang SF, Xia Y, Johnson KM (Postnatal phencyclidine administration selectively reduces adult cortical parvalbumin-containing interneurons. Neuropsychopharmacology 33:2442-2455.2008).

Wang J, Hirayasu Y, Hiramatsu K, Hokama H, Miyazato H, Ogura C (Increased rate of P300 latency prolongation with age in drug-naive and first episode schizophrenia. Clin Neurophysiol 114:2029-2035.2003).

Watson TD, Petrakis IL, Edgecombe J, Perrino A, Krystal JH, Mathalon DH (Modulation of the cortical processing of novel and target stimuli by drugs affecting glutamate and GABA neurotransmission. The international journal of neuropsychopharmacology / official scientific journal of the Collegium Internationale Neuropsychopharmacologicum (CINP) 12:357-370.2009).

Weber BA, Seitz MR, McCutcheon MJ (Quantifying click stimuli in auditory brainstem response audiometry. Ear and hearing 2:15-19.1981).

White TP, Joseph V, O'Regan E, Head KE, Francis ST, Liddle PF (Alpha-gamma interactions are disturbed in schizophrenia: a fusion of electroencephalography and functional magnetic resonance imaging. Clin Neurophysiol 121:1427-1437.2009).

Wildeboer KM, Stevens KE (Stimulation of the alpha4beta2 nicotinic receptor by 5-I A-85380 improves auditory gating in DBA/2 mice. Brain research 1224:29-36.2008).

Williams TJ, Nuechterlein KH, Subotnik KL, Yee CM (Distinct neural generators of sensory gating in schizophrenia. Psychophysiology 48:470-478.2011).

Winterer G, Coppola R, Goldberg TE, Egan MF, Jones DW, Sanchez CE, Weinberger DR (Prefrontal broadband noise, working memory, and genetic risk for schizophrenia. The American journal of psychiatry 161:490-500.2004).

Winterer GaM, R. W. (2011) Electrophysiology of Schizophrenia. In: Schizophrenia(Harrison, D. R. W. a. P. J., ed), pp 311-333 Oxford, UK: Wiley-Blackwell.

Woods DL, Clayworth CC, Knight RT, Simpson GV, Naeser MA (Generators of middle- and long-latency auditory evoked potentials: implications from studies of patients with bitemporal lesions. Electroencephalography and clinical neurophysiology 68:132-148.1987).

Yamamoto J (Cortical and hippocampal EEG power spectra in animal models of schizophrenia produced with methamphetamine, cocaine, and phencyclidine. Psychopharmacology 131:379-387.1997).

Zouridakis G, Boutros NN (Stimulus parameter effects on the P50 evoked response. Biological psychiatry 32:839-841.1992).

3

State of Art of Serum Brain-Derived Neurotrophic Factor in Schizophrenia

Davide Carlino[1], Monica Baiano[2],
Maurizio De Vanna[1] and Enrico Tongiorgi[3]
[1]*Psychiatric Clinic, BRAIN Centre for Neuroscience, Department of Medical, Technological and Tralsational Sciences, University of Trieste*
[2]*Center for Weight and Eating Disorders – Veneto Orientale – Portogruaro (VE)*
[3]*BRAIN Centre for Neuroscience, Department of Life Sciences, University of Trieste*
Italy

1. Introduction

Schizophrenia is a common severe psychiatric disorder which affects approximately 1% of the world population. Imaging studies and postmortem analysis have clearly shown that schizophrenia is not a mere functional disorder, but rather includes several histological abnormalities in various areas of the brain. Today, deficits in brain development or a malfunction in the dopaminergic system are considered the leading hallmarks of schizophrenia (Fatemi & Folsom, 2009; Howes & Kapur, 2009; Iritani, 2007).

Although the pathogenesis of schizophrenia remains still unresolved, it is now clear that this disorder is the result of a complex interplay between inheritable genetic mutations in a large number of genes (a few common mutations with a small effect combined with many rare ones with a stronger effect), various environmental influences and epigenetic effects (van OS & Kapur, 2009; Owen et al., 2009; O'Donnel et al., 2009; Psychiatric GWAS Consortium [PGC], 2009; Roth et al., 2009). Over the years, multiple theories have been proposed to explain how these factors may generate schizophrenia. The different models proposed include principally the neurodevelopmental and the dopaminergic hypotheses which have been reviewed elsewhere (Fatemi & Folsom, 2009; Howes & Kapur, 2009). These two hypotheses may not necessarily be mutually exclusive as, for instance, a local dysfunction in dopaminergic neurotransmission may be the result of a failed development. Moreover, a number of studies pointed to the role of neurotrophins in the pathogenesis of schizophrenia.

Neurotrophins are a small group of secreted dimeric proteins that affect the development of the nervous system in all vertebrates' species and are involved in the development and maturation of several brain networks including the dopaminergic system (Buckley et al. 2007; Shoval & Weizman, 2005; Thome et al. 1998). Brain-Derived Neurotrophic Factor (BDNF) is the most widely distributed neurotrophin in the central nervous system (CNS) and is known to exert growth and trophic effects able to support many aspects of neuronal development including axonal growth and connectivity (Segal et al., 1995), neuronal survival and apoptosis (Segal et al., 1997), and formation of dopaminergic-related systems. Furthermore, BDNF has a dynamic effect on synaptic organization, promoting long-term changes of synaptic transmission (Shen et al., 1997), as well as learning and memory processes (Yamada et al., 2002). For these reasons many studies investigated the role of BDNF in the pathophysiology of schizophrenia but their findings resulted contradictory. For example, some postmortem studies conducted on schizophrenia brains showed elevated BDNF levels in the anterior cingulate, hippocampus (Takahashi et al., 2000) and cerebral cortex (Durany et al., 2001), whereas others found decreased BDNF levels in the hippocampus (Durany et al., 2001) and prefrontal cortex (Weickert et al., 2003, 2005).

Interestingly, in both humans and rodents, BDNF is present not only in the brain but also in peripheral tissues and especially, in the blood (Pruunsild et al., 2007; Aid et al., 2007). The origin of circulating BDNF has been debated as this neurotrophin is produced by many different body tissues and epithelia, including smooth muscle cells of blood vessels (Donovan et al., 1995). However, it has been demonstrated that radiolabeled BDNF injected in the jugular vein or in the brain ventricle readily crosses the blood-brain barrier in both directions (Pan et al., 1998) and can be taken up by platelets that function as storage and release system (Karege et al., 2005). In addition, it has been shown that physical exercise induces an increase of serum BDNF levels which is contributed by 70% from the brain (Rasmussen et al., 2009). Thus, measurement of circulating BDNF is very attractive, because it may provide information on brain functioning and blood samples are largely available and may be drawn non-invasively from living subjects as frequently as necessary. BDNF can be measured using simple enzyme linked immunoadsorbent assays (ELISA) that are commercially available and recent methodological studies have pointed out the possibility to obtain reliable measures of BDNF in serum preparations with stable values over several months of serum storage at -20°C, while in contrast, there is high variability in the measures of BDNF in whole blood or plasma because of the presence of release from platelets and degradation processes that are active even during storage (Elfving et al, 2009; Trajkovska et al., 2007). For these reasons, there is currently a great interest to validate the use of serum BDNF as possible biomarker in brain diseases, including psychiatric illnesses (for a recent meta-analisis of serum BDNF in depression see: Sen et al., 2008).

To assess if BDNF can represent a good biomarker in schizophrenia, a growing number of studies compared BDNF serum levels between patients with schizophrenia and healthy control subjects but unfortunately, with controversial results. Indeed, several investigators found a significant decrease in serum BDNF concentrations (Carlino et al., 2011; Chen et al., 2009; Grillo et al., 2007; Ikeda et al., 2008, Jindal et al., 2010; Pirildar et al., 2004; Rizos et al., 2008; Shimizu et al., 2002; Tan et al., 2005a, 2005b; Toyooka et al., 2002; Xiu et al., 2009; Zhang et al., 2007, 2008); while other studies documented normal (Shimizu et al., 2003; Jockers-Schrubl et al. 2004; Huang et al. 2006) or even increased circulating BDNF (Gama et al., 2007; Reis et al., 2008). Because of these discrepancies, we decided to perform a systematic review and a meta-analysis of studies measuring serum concentrations of BDNF to elucidate whether or not this neurotrophin is abnormally produced in patients with schizophrenia. Additionally, we were interested in identifying factors that might contribute to the different findings in literature, as to improve the design of future investigations in this field.

2. Methods

2.1 Search strategy

The PUBMED, OVID MEDLINE, PSYCHINFO and EMBASE databases were searched using the following medical subject headings (MeSH): "Brain-Derived Neurotrophic Factor" OR

"BDNF" AND "schizophrenia". In addition, all reference lists of the selected papers were examined for studies not indexed electronically. The search aimed to find all papers published through January 2011.We used the PRISMA guidelines to carry out this review (Figure 1).

2.2 Inclusion/exclusion criteria for both the systematic review and meta-analysis

Studies had to fulfill the following inclusion criteria :

1. Investigation of serum BNDF levels in patients with schizophrenia and healthy comparison subjects.
2. Mean serum BDNF reported (ng/ml or pg/ml).
3. Clinical characterization of patients with schizophrenia according to DSM-IV, ICD-10 or an equivalent system employed as a diagnostic tool. Study samples including some schizoaffective or schizophreniform subjects were also considered.
4. Published in English.

Exclusion criteria comprised:

1. Samples including non-schizophrenia psychosis or other schizophrenia spectrum disorders.
2. Plasma BDNF levels were measured.
3. Publications describing case reports or case series.
4. Patients or comparison subjects with neurological or medical disorders or substance or alcohol abuse.
5. Comparison subjects screened for psychiatric disorders.

In addition, in the studies exploring the same subject population or part of it, only the publication with the largest sample size was selected. When necessary, study Authors were contacted and asked to supply for missing or incomplete information.

2.3 Data abstraction and quality rating

Each paper was scrutinized by two independent reviewers (D.C. and M.B.) separately, and the following data from the article was obtained: age, gender, education, age at onset, duration of illness, number of hospitalizations, medications used (type, dosage and duration of treatment) and laboratory parameters. Mean serum BDNF levels (expressed in ng/ml) and the methods used for statistical analyses were also extracted from the article. Furthermore, the reviewers rated the quality of each study using a modified version of the quality rating check-list reported on Baiano et al. (2007).

Category 1: subjects

1. Prospective evaluation of patients, use of specific diagnostic criteria and description of demographic data;
2. Prospective evaluation of healthy control subjects, description of demographic data, exclusion of psychiatric and medical illnesses;
3. Presentation of significant variables (e.g. age, gender, age at onset, duration of illness, number of hospitalizations, medications used);

Category 2: methods for sampling and analysis

1. Clear description of laboratory technique and measurements, such in a way to be reproducible;
2. Blindness of investigators to experimental setup;
3. Report of intra and inter-assay reliability;

Category 3: results and conclusions

- Use of appropriate statistical tests;
- Presentation of main results and parameters for statistical significance;
- Consistence of conclusions with the results and discussion of study limits.

Each item was scored 1, 0.5 or 0 if criteria were completely met, partly met or unmet, respectively. This procedure was performed to evaluate the completeness of the available publications and not to criticize the investigations *per se*.

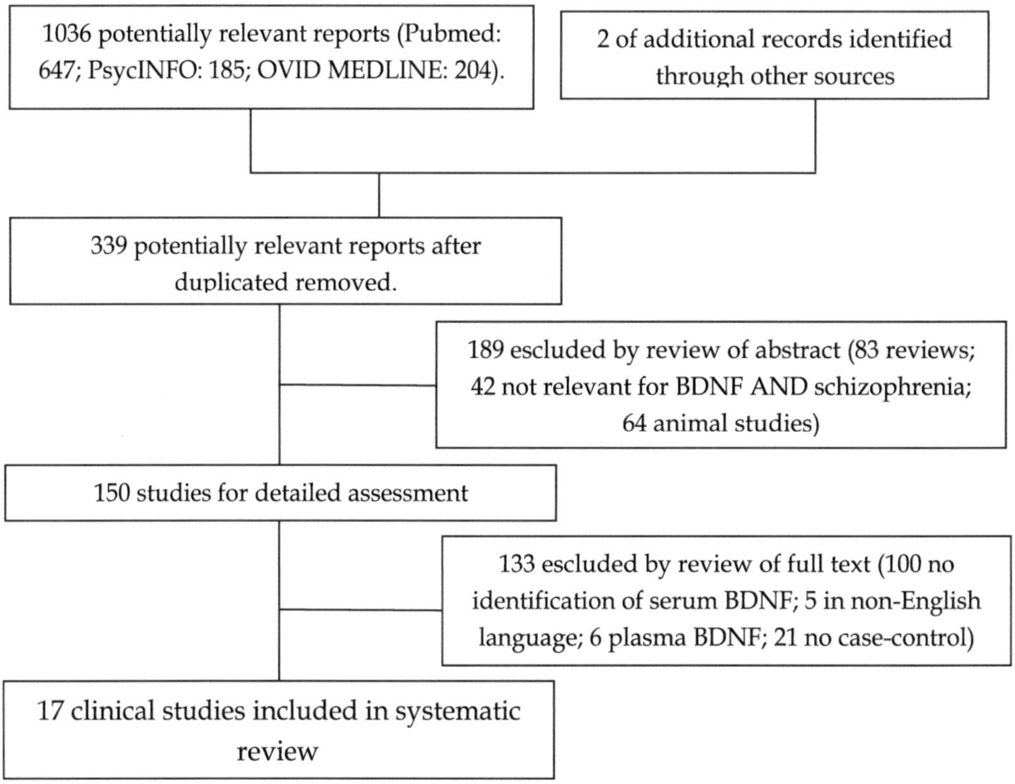

Fig. 1. Flowchart of results of systematic review and meta-analysis search strategy.

2.4 Statistical analysis

The calculations were performed by means of the statistical software package STATA 8.0 (StataCorp LP, Texas). Data were analyzed by using a random effects model (*Metan command*), which typically takes into account the between study variability, leading to wider confidence intervals than those obtained by a fixed effects model. Thus, studies were weighted for the inverse variance, obtaining the DerSimonian-Laird's effect size (Deeks et al., 2001). Heterogeneity between studies was explored using the Q-test. Since we hypothesized a statistically significant heterogeneity, a meta-regression analysis was planned to assess the effects of selected factors (i.e.: gender distribution, ethnicity, ELISA kit used and average age) on results between studies (*Metareg command*). Publication bias was assessed by Egger's tests (Egger et al., 1997) (*Metabias command*). All p values were two sided and the cutoff for statistical significance was 0.05.

3. Results

3.1 Systematic review

A total of 334 references were obtained. All the studies found in PUBMED database overlapped with those retrieved using OVID MEDLINE and PSYCHINFO databases. A total of 1036 references were identified. All the studies found in PUBMED database overlapped with those retrieved using OVID MEDLINE, EMBASE, PSYCHINFO lists. Most of them (322) did not meet the inclusion criteria, most analyzing *val66met* BDNF polymorphism, mRNA expression or post-mortem studies.

Thus, 17 were finally considered but 16 were actually included in the systematic review (Carlino et al., 2011; Chen et al., 2009; Gama et al., 2007; Grillo et al., 2007; Huang et al., 2006; Ikeda et al., 2008; Jindal et al., 2010; Jockers-Schrübl et al., 2004; Pirildar et al., 2004; Reis et al., 2008; Rizos et al., 2008; Shimizu et al., 2003; Tan et al., 2005a; Toyooka et al., 2002; Xiu et al., 2009; Zhang et al., 2008). Indeed, as per Authors suggestion, we excluded the study by Zhang et al. (2007) (124 patients and 50 controls) since the patients' sample consistently overlapped with that of the study published by Zhang and co-workers in the 2008 (196 patients and 50 controls).

3.1.1 Findings

Most of the studies (12/16) measuring serum BDNF documented lower concentrations of this neurothropin in patients with schizophrenia (Carlino et al., 2011; Chen et al., 2009; Grillo et al., 2007; Ikeda et al., 2008; Jindal et al., 2010; Jockers-Schrübl et al., 2004; Pirildar et al., 2004; Rizos et al., 2008; Tan et al., 2005a; Toyooka et al., 2002; Xiu et al., 2009; Zhang et al., 2008); however, in other studies, BDNF concentrations were either increased (Gama et al., 2007; Reis et al., 2008); or normal (Huang et al., 2006; Shimizu et al., 2003) (Table 1).

Five out of the 16 researches investigated gender effects, demonstrating either significantly lower (Xiu et al., 2009) or higher serum BDNF levels in males suffering from schizophrenia (Gama et al., 2007). Conversely, no gender effect emerged in Carlino et al., (2011), Huang et al. (2006) and Rizos et al. (2008) and in all healthy control subjects.

3.1.2 Clinical features of patients

15/16 studies reported on the mean age of the patients with schizophrenia (mean: 37.22±9.48 SD years; range: 22.4-52.3). Nine studies provided data for age of onset of schizophrenia (mean: 25.70±4.86 SD years; range: 19.93-33.8) and 13 for length of illness (mean: 180.13±127.65 SD months; range 8.8-388.8). Six out of 16 papers reported on the mean dosage of antipsychotic medications, expressed as chlorpromazine equivalents (mean: 581.12±219.90 SD; range:330.4-936.6). In one paper (Zhang et al., 2008), data for other psychopharmacological treatment (lithium, valproic acid) were included, but there were no details about the role of these drugs on serum BDNF levels.

Only Jockers- Schrübl et al. (2004) evaluated the role of substance abuse (cannabis) in serum BDNF levels: the Authors found significantly elevated BDNF serum concentrations (by up to 34%) in patients with chronic cannabis abuse or multiple substance abuse prior to disease onset. Drug-naïve schizophrenic patients without cannabis consumption showed similar results to normal controls and cannabis controls without schizophrenia.

In relation to the source of recruitment, 6/16 studies included only inpatients (Chen et al., 2009; Reis et al., 2008; Rizos et al., 2008; Tan et al., 2005a; Xiu et al., 2009; Zhang et al., 2008), 1/16 included only outpatients (Gama et al., 2007), 3/16 considered both in-patients and out-patients (Carlino et al., 2011; Huang et al., 2006; Ikeda et al., 2008) and 6/16 publications did not provide data (Grillo et al., 2007; Jindal et al., 2010; Jockers-Schrübl et al., 2004; Pirildar et al., 2004; Shimizu et al., 2003; Toyooka et al., 2002). In our research, we found that Japanese subjects were investigated in three studies (Ikeda et al., 2008; Shimizu et al., 2003; Toyooka et al., 2002), Caucasians in another four studies (Carlino et al., 2011; Jockers-Schrübl et al., 2004; Pirildar et al., 2004, Rizos et al., 2008) and Asians in five studies (Chen et al., 2009; Huang et al., 2006; Tan et al., 2005a, Xiu et al., 2009, Zhang et al., 2008). In four studies, ethnicity was unspecified (Gama et al., 2007; Grillo et al., 2007, Reis et al., 2008; Jindal et al., 2010).

Six studies reported no diagnostic subtypes of schizophrenia (Ikeda et al., 2008; Gama et al., 2007; Jockers- Schrübl et al., 2004; Pirildar et al., 2004;Reis et al., 2008; Rizos et al., 2008; Toyooka et al., 2002) while in seven studies it was assessed the differences in serum BDNF levels among diagnostic subtypes (Chen et al., 2009; Grillo et al., 2007; Huang et al., 2006; Shimizu et al., 2003; Tan et al., 2005a; Xiu et al., 2009; Zhang et al., 2008). Different forms of schizophrenia had no association with BDNF serum levels in 5 papers (Grillo et al., 2007, Shimizu et al., 2003; Tan et al., 2005a; Xiu et al., 2009; Zhang et al., 2008), while Chen et al. (2009) showed significantly higher BDNF levels in paranoid (10.4 ± 4.3 ng/ml) compared to undifferentiated (8.0 ± 3.9 ng/ml) and other combined subtypes (7.5± 4.1 ng/ml). Huang et al. (2006) showed that patients with catatonic schizophrenia had lower serum BDNF protein levels than patients with paranoid schizophrenia and residual schizophrenia.

In a second step, phase of illness and use of antipsychotic drugs were considered. We found that four studies enrolled only drug-naïve first-episode patients (Chen et al., 2009; Jindal et al., 2010; Jockers-Schrübl et al., 2004; Rizos et al., 2008), eight studies recruited only chronic, medicated patients (Carlino et al., 2011; Gama et al., 2007; Ikeda et al., 2008; Reis et al, 2008; Tan et al., 2005a; Toyooka et al., 2002; Xiu et al., 2009; Zhang et al., 2008) and two studies included medicated patients with unclear phase of illness (Grillo et al., 2007; Huang et al., 2006). Notably, the study by Pirildar et al. (2004) and Shimizu et al. (2003) investigated both chronically antipsychotic-treated and drug-naïve patients; in particular, in Pirildar et al. (2004) some first episode medicated subjects were included. All the 16 studies excluded patients with a history of neurological disease, physical illness, and alcohol or substance abuse. Clinical data are summarized in Table 2.

3.1.3 Serum BDNF concentrations and laboratory procedures

Among studies, laboratory procedures were comparable with some minor variations. Sera were centrifuged to eliminate the blood clot with a mild centrifugation at 2000, 3000 or 3500 rpm for 5-15min at room temperature or 15°C); then, they were stored frozen at -70/-80°C until used. Serum BDNF concentrations were measured using sandwich ELISA assays (see Table 1 for full detail). Finally, all the studies except one (Gama et al., 2007) reported clearly on mean BDNF concentrations. Specifically, mean serum BDNF values were 14.43±10.24 SD ng/ml (range: 0.098-37.1) for patients and 17.99±13.41 SD ng/ml, (range: 0.12-52.2) for healthy blood donors.

3.1.4 Study quality

The mean total quality scores for the reports were 7.63±1.17 SD (min.:5.5; max.: 9). We correlated total and partial quality scores of studies on serum BDNF with the year of publication, which was significantly positively correlated to total quality score (r=0.53) and study methodology score (Category 2) (r=0.59) but not to study design score (Category 1) (r= -0.20) or study consistency score (Category 3) (r=0.27).

Authors	ELISA kit	Quality of rating (QR)	Control	Schizophrenic patients	
			Serum BDNF (mean ng/ml ± SD)	Serum BDNF (mean ng/ml ± SD)	Medication
Toyoka et al., 2002	Sigma Chemical	6.5	11.4 ± 7.7	6.3 ± 3.4	29=haloperidol, 5=chlorpromazine, 31=levomepromazine, 2=zotepin, 3=bromperidol, 1=risperidone, 9=other
Ikeda et al., 2003	Promega	9	52.2 ± 25.3	37.1 ± 20.4	Typical and atypical (dose not available)
Shimizu et al., 2003 (part I)	Promega	6.5	28.5 ± 9.1	27.9 ± 12.3	----
Shimizu et al., 2003 (part II)		6.5	28.5 ± 9.1	23.8 ± 8.1	
Pirildar et al., 2004 (part I)	Promega	8	26.8 ± 9.3	14.4 ± 2.8	17=risperidone, 2=clozapine, 3=olanzapine
Pirildar et al., 2004 (part II)		8	26.8 ± 9.3	16.3 ± 4.0	
Jockers-Schrübl et al., 2004	Promega	6.5	13.2 ± 5.2	13.1 ± 5.9	----
Tan et al., 2005	BanDing Biomedical	9	9.1 ± 4.3	5.8 ± 2.1	38=clozapine, 19=risperidone, 12=haloperidol, 5=chlorpromazine, 5=perphenazine, 2=others (*n* = 2)
Huang et al., 2006	Promega	5.5	14.17 ± 6.9	14.2 ± 6.9	----
Grillo et al., 2007	Chemicon	8	0.17 ± 0.0	0.11 ± 0.1	20=Clozapine; 24=typical antipsychotics; 6=chlorpromazine; 15=levomepromazine; 5=haloperidol

Authors	ELISA kit	Quality of rating (QR)	Control	Schizophrenic patients	
			Serum BDNF (mean ng/ml ± SD)	Serum BDNF (mean ng/ml ± SD)	Medication
Zhang et al., 2008	BanDing Biomedical	7.5	9.4 ± 4.4	7.0 ± 3.1	98=clozapine, 36=risperidone, 20=perphenazine, 19=haloperidol, 14=chlorpromazine, 9=fluphenazine, 9=trifluperazine
Reis et al., 2008	R&D Systems	6	4.31 ± 2.1	7.75 ± 1.9	28=haloperidol, 3=chlorpromazine, 3=levoepromazine, 6=trifluorperazine
Rizos et al., 2008	R&D Systems	7	30.0 ± 8.4	23.9 ± 6.0	----
Xiu et al., 2009	BanDing Biomedical	9	11.9 ± 2.3	9.9 ± 2.0	157=Clozapine, 89=risperidone, 31=haloperidol, 21=chlorpromazine, 26=perphenazine, 27=sulpiride, 13=other
Chen et al., 2009	BanDing Biomedical	8.5	12.1±2.2	9.0±4.2	----
Jindal et al., 2010	Promega	9	116.78±38.42	97.58±31.41	----
Carlino et al., 2011	Promega	9	26.5 ± 4.22	25.3 ± 3.71	4=haloperidol, 2=zuclopenthixol, 2=haloperidol decanoate, 10= olanzapine, 6=risperidone, 8=quetiapine, 1=olanzapine +zuclopenthixol , 2=olanzapine +haloperidol, 2=quetiapine +haloperidol,2= quetiapine +zuclopenthixol, 3=risperidone+haloperidol

Table 1. Methodological aspects of the studies measuring serum BDNF in schizophrenia. *

3.1.5 Meta-analysis

Fifteen out of the 16 publications considered for the systematic review were used for the meta-analysis (Carlino et al., 2011; Chen et al., 2009; Grillo et al., 2007; Huang et al., 2006; Ikeda et al., 2008; Jindal et al., 2010; Jockers-Schrübl et al., 2004; Pirildar et al., 2004; Reis et al., 2008; Rizos et al., 2008; Shimizu et al., 2003; Tan et al., 2005a; Toyooka et al., 2002; Xiu et al., 2009; Zhang et al., 2008). The study by Gama et al., (2007) was eliminated, as it was the only one to report serum BDNF in pg/µg of total protein while in all other studies serum BDNF concentration was given in ng or pg/ml serum and therefore, no comparison between the Gama's and the other studies was possible. Since the studies by Shimizu et al., (2003) and Pirildar et al., (2004) reported on separate data for both medicated and unmedicated patients, we performed calculations considering patients' subgroups as follows: Shimizu et al., 2003 part I and Pirildar et al., 2004 part I = medicated patients; Shimizu et al., 2003 part II and Pirildar et al., 2004 part II = unmedicated patients. Therefore, we carried out calculations on 17 samples of patients.

Authors	Stages of disease	Ethnicity *	Control			Schizophrenic patients			
			N	Age (mean ± SD)	M/F	N	Age (mean ± SD)	M/F	Illness duration (mean-months ± SD)
Toyoka et al., 2002	Chronic	JPT	35	45.6 ± 11.3	14/21	34	48.6 ± 14.0	17/17	25±12.3
Ikeda et al., 2003	Chronic	JPT	87	39.8 ± 10.7	47/40	74	41.9 ± 11.1	39/35	19.6±11.2
Shimizu et al.,2003 (part I)	Chronic	JPT	40	36.5 ± 11.3	20/20	25	36.0 ± 13.2	13/12	Med scz: 14.1±9.87; FEP: 1.09±1.36
Shimizu et al.,2003 (part II)	First episode/ drug naïve	JPT	40	36.5 ± 10.7	20/20	15	34.7 ± 16.0	7/8	
Pirildar et al., 2004 (part I)	Chronic	CEU	22	25.7 ± 5.8	7/15	12	29.8 ± 9.3	5/7	15.2±13.04
Pirildar et al., 2004 (part II)	First episode/ drug naïve	CEU	22	25.7 ± 5.8	7/15	10	25.1 ± 9.1	2/8	
Jockers-Schrübl et al., 2004	First episode/ drug naïve	CEU	61	32.3	28/33	102	33.3	50/52	----
Tan et al., 2005	Chronic	CHB	45	45.6 ± 6.3	34/11	125	18.3 ± 6.3	93/32	22.6±7.7
Huang et al., 2006	Chronic	CHB	96	29.1 ± 10.0	36/60	126	34.0 ± 10.0	72/54	6.0±5.0
Grillo et al., 2007	Chronic	YRI/CEU (ratio not specified)	25	34.1 ± 7.2	12/13	44	35.5 ± 7.2	19/25	

Authors	Stages of disease	Ethnicity *	Control			Schizophrenic patients			
			N	Age (mean ± SD)	M/F	N	Age (mean ± SD)	M/F	Illness duration (mean-months ± SD)
Zhang et al., 2008	Chronic	CHB	50	----	34/16	196	----	130/66	22 ± 7
Reis et al., 2008	Chronic	YRI/CEU (ratio not specified)	20	----	20/0	40	52.3 ± 9.8	40/0	32.4 ± 9.2
Rizos et al., 2008	First episode/ drug naïve	CEU	15	26.6 ± 5.8	6/9	14	25.4 ± 5.8	10/4	----
Xiu et al., 2009	Chronic	CHB	323	50.9 ± 9.2	228/95	364	51.3 ± 9.2	281/83	27.0 ± 10.1
Chen et al., 2009	First episode/ drug naïve	CHB	90	29.9 ± 9.8	49/41	88	29.2 ± 9.6	47/41	23.4 ± 19.1
Jindal et al., 2010	First episode/ drug naïve	CEU	41	22.31 ± 5.67	25/16	24	22.4 ± 5.47	17/10	----
Carlino et al., 2011	Chronic	CEU	40	46.78 ± 10.79	20/20	40	49.23 ± 9.03	20/20	23.05 ± 10.99

Table 2. Clinical characteristics of studies included in the meta-analysis. International HapMap Project: YRI: Yoruba in Ibadan, Nigeria; JPT: Japanese in Tokyo; CHB: Han Chinese in Beijing, China; CEU: CEPH (Utah residents with ancestry from Northern and Western Europe).

Raw total serum BDNF levels (ng/ml) were used to calculate the related effect sizes. The overall estimate of SMD (*standardized mean differences*) in serum BDNF levels between patients with schizophrenia and healthy controls was significant ($z=4.14$; $p<0.001$) but considerable heterogeneity emerged from publications ($Q=139.15$; d.f.=16; $p<0.001$; $\tau^2= 0.2826$) (Figure 2).
Therefore, we regressed the SMD against potential sources of heterogeneity (i.e.: gender, age, ethnicity and ELISA kit used). This analysis demonstrated a significant association of BDNF levels with all these variables (age: $z=15.28$; gender: $z=10.92$ for males; $z=4.60$ for females; ethnicity: $Z=9.37$ and ELISA kit: $z=8.55$; $p<0.001$). Moreover, to determine if this systematic review and meta-analyses was subjected to publication bias (i.e. the presence of asymmetrical collection of data due to the missing of studies reporting negative results, or to the tendency of small studies to show greater effects than larger studies), we carried out the Egger's weighted regression and evidence of significant publication bias was found ($p<0.001$). Subsequently, the eleven studies investigating chronic, medicated patients with schizophrenia were considered (Carlino et al., 2011; Grillo et al., 2007; Huang et al., 2006; Ikeda et al., 2008; Pirildar et al., 2004 part I; Reis et al, 2008; Shimizu et al., 2003 part I; Tan et al., 2005a; Toyooka et al., 2002; Xiu et al., 2009; Zhang et al., 2008). Significant heterogeneity was found ($Q=120.85$, d.f=10, $p<0.001$, $\tau^2=0.3545$) and patients and healthy control subjects differed for serum BDNF levels, as demonstrated by the SMD test ($z=2.69$; $p=0.007$) (Figure 3).

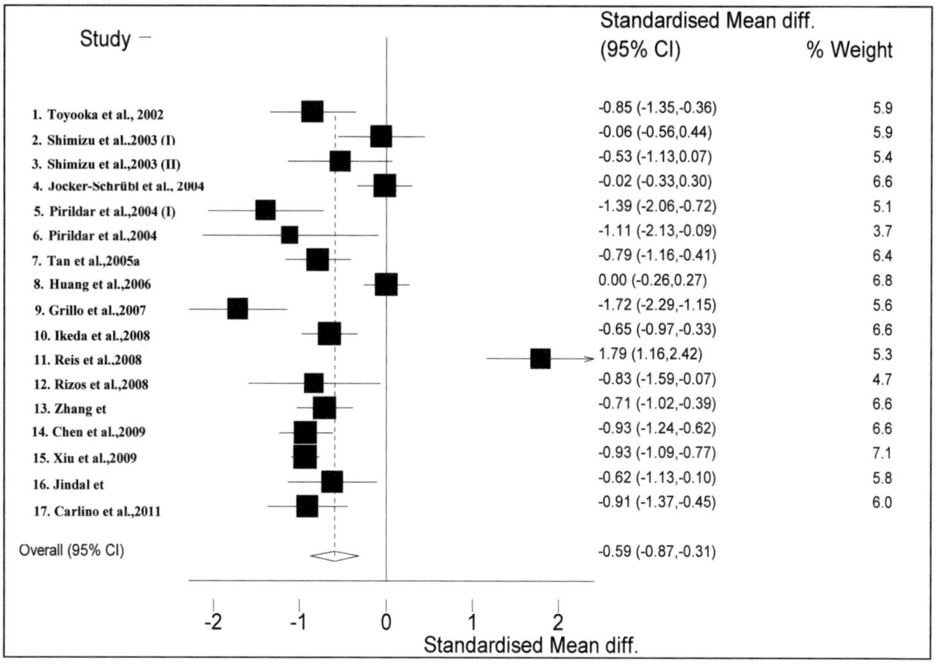

Fig. 2. Forrest plot depicting the meta-analysis of serum BDNF levels in patients with schizophrenia.

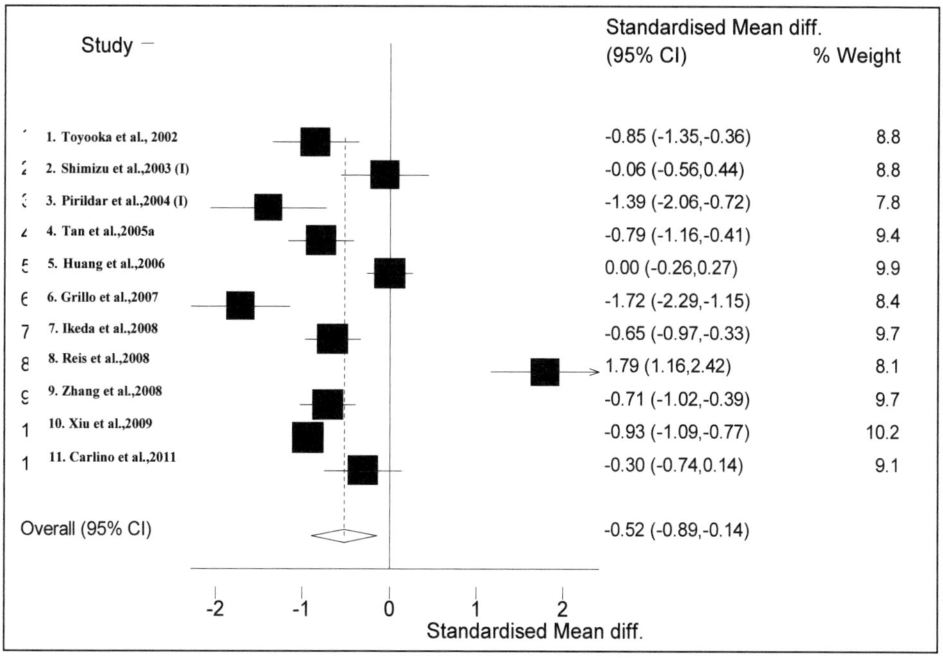

Fig. 3. Forrest plot presenting the meta-analysis of serum BDNF in chronic medicated patients with schizophrenia.

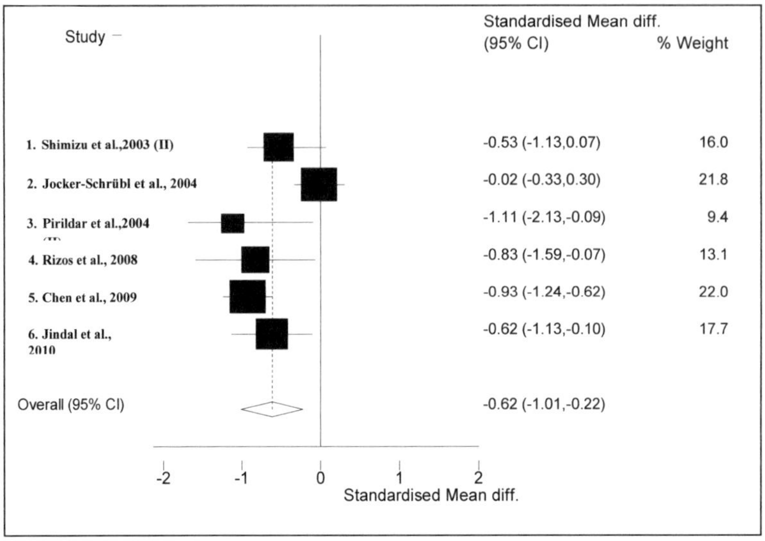

Fig. 4. Forrest plot presenting the meta-analysis of serum BDNF in unmedicated patients with schizophrenia.

The meta-regression analysis showed that age (z=13.89), gender (z=11.09 for males; z=7.36 for females), ethnicity (z=6.76), type of ELISA kit (z=6.67), chlorpromazine equivalents' medication dosage (z=5.97) and duration of illness (z=7.03) may all explain heterogeneity ($p<0.001$). Similar results were obtained by meta-analyzing the six studies including first-episode unmedicated patients (Chen et al., 2009; Jindal et al., 2010; Pirildar et al., 2004; Rizos et al., 2008; Shimizu et al., 2003 part II) (Figure 4). Indeed, we found that both the Q test for heterogeneity (Q=18.30; d.f =5; p=0.003; τ^2=0.1595) and Dersimonian and Laird pooled effect size (z=3.06, p=0.002) were significant. As previously demonstrated, heterogeneity may be due to age (z=15.33), gender (z=4.55 for males; z=4.84 for females), ethnicity (z=5.47), type of ELISA kit (z=4.45).

4. Conclusion

Our systematic review and meta-analysis showed that lower serum BDNF levels were detected in patients with schizophrenia in comparison to healthy controls in most even if not in all studies. Interestingly, reduced serum BDNF levels were found both in drug-naïve first episode and chronic medicated schizophrenia patients, as also found in studies investigating plasma BDNF concentrations (Buckely et al., 2007; Palomino et al., 2006; Tan et al., 2005b). These findings show that reduced serum BDNF levels are associated with schizophrenia but also suggest that serum BDNF is not a crucial biological marker of the clinical state in schizophrenia or a marker of antipsychotic medication efficacy, in agreement with a recent meta-analysis (Green et al., 2010).

The serum BDNF concentration in healthy populations, varied from a minimum of 0.17 ng/ml (Grillo et al., 2007) to a maximum of 52.2 ng/ml (Ikeda et al., 2003), the mean value among the thirteen paper analysed was 16.2 ng/ml (SD=14.59). Although we observed variability between studies using the same commercial ELISA, differences in serum BDNF concentration appeared mainly due to the different kit used. For example the three studies which used the kit purchased from BanDing Biomed reported values of serum BDNF in Chinese healthy donors of 11.9 ± 2.3 ng/ml (Xiu et al., 2009); 9.4 ± 4.4 ng/ml (Zhang et al., 2008); 9.1 ± 4.3 ng/ml (Tan et al., 2005) while higher levels of serum BDNF were detected with the kit from Promega in healthy donors from Japan, 28.5 ± 9.1 ng/ml (Shimizu et al., 2003); Turkey 26.8 ± 9.3 ng/ml (Pirildar et al., 2004) and Taiwan 14.17 ± 6.9 ng/ml (Huang et al., 2006). Finally, two studies using the R&D System ELISA assay showed very distant results because Rizos et al. (2008) detected 30.0 ± 8.4 ng/ml of serum BDNF in healthy controls from Greece while Reis et al., (2008) in Brazil, found 4.31 ± 2.1 ng/ml. Two other studies from Brazil also showed particularly low levels using the assay from another company (Chemicon), i.e. 0.19 ± 0.1 ng/ml (Gama et al., 2007) and 0.17 ± 0.0 ng/ml (Grillo et al., 2007). It is possible that this finding might reflect reduced amounts of serum BDNF in the Brazilian population. Another interpretation suggests a very low sensitivity of the ELISA kit from Chemicon. In conclusion, the most likely range of concentrations of serum BDNF in the World healthy population is 9-30 ng/ml with some possible specific regional variations.

However, the great heterogeneity between studies and the presence of a publication bias may limit the interpretation of these results. Firstly, the phenotypic complexity, together with the multifarious nature of the so-called "schizophrenic psychoses", limits our ability to form a simple and logical, biologically-based hypothesis for the disease group. Secondly, all studies used ELISA assays that have different sensitivity and cannot distinguish between the three different protein forms of BDNF consisting in the precursor pro-BDNF (of 32 KDA) and its two proteolytic products mature BDNF (mBDNF of 14KDa) and truncated BDNF (truncBDNF of 28 KDa). Since pro-BDNF and mBDNF elicit opposing actions on synaptic plasticity and cell survival, their distinction could be essential to determine the role of BDNF in specific aspects of schizophrenia's neurobiology.

4.1 The role of proBDNF in patients with schizophrenia

BDNF is initially synthesized as a 32 KDa precursor protein (prepro-BDNF) in endoplasmic reticulum, and then processed into two isoforms (as the truncated-BDNF 28 KDa and mature 14 kDa BDNF) by two different proteolitic cleavages. Mature BDNF (mBDNF) is generated either intracellularly in the trans-Golgi by furin (Mowla et al., 2001, Matsumoto et al., 2008), or extracellularly by plasmin or matrixmetalloprotease-7 (Lee et al., 2001, Yang et al. 2009; Nagappan et al., 2009). Truncated-BDNF is cleaved by the Membrane-Bound Transcription Factor Site-1 protease (MBTFS-1), also identified as Subtilisin/kexin-isozyme 1 (Seidah et al., 1999). This isoform is not further processed into mBDNF and its function has not been elucidated yet.

According to the "Ying and Yang" hypothesis (Lu et al., 2005), both mBDNF and proBDNF have particular neurobiological properties. In particular, proBDNF regulate neuronal survival (Teng et al., 2005; Koshimizu et al., 2009; Woo et al., 2005) and boosts synaptic pruning whereas mBDNF improves the differentiation of new neurons. Also, the conversion of proBDNF into mBDNF seems to be decisive for signal transmission and synaptic plasticity. Indeed, mBDNF and the Tissue Plasminogen Activator (TPA) but not proBDNF are essential in late-phase long-term potentiation (L-LTP) and long-term memory (Pang et al., 2004). These results underscore that a wrong matching of the proBDNF/mBDNF ratio may alter neuroplastic mechanisms, corresponding to the neurobiological substrate of impaired cognitive performance.

An increasing number of postmortem researches have been carried out to measure the expression of proBDNF and mBDNF isoforms in animal models and in healthy human volunteers or subjects affected by neuropsychiatric disorders. Reduced mBDNF levels were found in three studies (Karege et al., 2005; Weickert et al., 2003; Wong et al., 2010), particularly in the dorsolateral prefrontal cortex (DLPFC) of patients with schizophrenia compared to healthy controls. Weickert et al. (2003) found that mBDNF protein levels were not associated with post-mortem interval (PMI), tissue pH, age, or storage time of the serum. There were no significant main influences of gender or brain hemisphere, nor significant correlations between diagnosis and gender or diagnosis and brain hemisphere. On the other hand, Chen et al. (2001) showed that there was no significant variation for mBDNF among patients with schizophrenia and those with a diagnosis of affective disorders (unipolar and bipolar disorders) and Dunham et al., (2009) detected no difference for preproBDNF (35KDa) between patients with schizophrenia and those with unipolar depression and bipolar disorder. In contrast, Wong et al. (2010) found reduced truncated BDNF and preproBDNF proteins in the DLPFC of patients with schizophrenia, even if the reduction in preproBDNF protein did not achieve statistical significance.

In a previous study (Carlino et al., 2011), we provided evidence of variation in serum levels of different BDNF isoforms in patients with chronic schizophrenia. Particularly, we showed that reduced levels of serum truncated-BDNF/total BDNF ratio correlate with worst PANSS negative and positive symptoms and poorer neurocognitive functions. Instead, measurement of total serum BDNF levels resulted scarcely useful, even if we found a small decline in the whole population of schizophrenic patients. We further highlighted that when using a cut-off at the mean value of the healthy group + 2SD, the measurement of serum truncated-BDNF represents a useful empirical test to recognize schizophrenic patients with high cognitive impairment, with sensitivity = 67.5%, Specificity = 97.5%, PPV = 96.4% and NPV = 75%.

Regulated proteolysis of one inactive precursor to make active peptides and proteins is a general biological mechanism to generate different products from a single gene. Mammalian pro-BDNF precursor is processed to generate truncated-BDNF 28 KDa or mature 14 kDa BDNF by two dissimilar proteolitic cleavages. Mature BDNF is created intracellularly by furin (Mowla et al., 2001), or extracellularly, by plasmin or matrixmetalloprotease-7 (Lee et al., 2001), whereas truncated-BDNF is generated by a specific Ca^{2+}dependent serine proteinase known as Membrane-bound transcription factor site-1 protease (MBTFS-1), also identified as Subtilisin/Kexin-Isozyme 1 (SKI-1) (Seidah et al., 1999); it is not further processed into the mature 14 kDa BDNF form representing a final proteolytic product whose role is ambiguous. Recent findings have established that mature and pro-BDNF elicit opposite biological functions (Teng et al., 2005; Woo et al., 2005), leading to the hypothesis that from an incorrect balancing of the diverse isoforms may origin a pathological consequence. In recent times, Koshimizu et al. (2009) pointed out that overexpression of pro-BDNF leads to apoptosis of cultured cerebellar granule neurons and produce a striking decrease in the number of cholinergic fibers of basal forebrain neurons and hippocampal dendritic spines, without disturbing the survival of these neurons. Blockade of activation of p75 receptor did not permit spine number to fall. Importantly, the pro-BDNF preparation used in this paper contained a large amount of truncated-BDNF, although at a much lesser extent than pro-BDNF. It is therefore possible that truncated-BDNF may have a similar outcome than pro-BDNF through activation of the same signalling pathways. Alternatively, truncated-BDNF may be an inactive variety of pro-BDNF or operate as a quencher of pro-BDNF by producing inactive heterodimers. The latter possibility reminds the supposed function for truncated-TrkB. Hence, a clear decrease in truncated-BDNF may direct to pathologically amplified signalling of pro-BDNF. Further studies will be necessary to clarify the biological characteristics of truncated-BDNF.

Chronic patients with schizophrenia are often characterized to suffer progressive significant intellectual decline (Heinrichs, 2006). In our study, schizophrenic patients with reduced truncated-BDNF had worse efficency in all neurocognitive tests in relationship to the other patients with normal levels of truncated-BDNF, although the correlation between Trail Making Test Part A score and truncated- BDNF abundance do not reach the statistically significance. Our results further enlarge a recent research telling that evaluation of total serum BDNF may be useful to predict for a good outcome in neurocognitive enhancement sessions in schizophrenic patients (Vinogradov et al., 2009). Importantly, we also underline that four healthy subjects with low truncated-BDNF had poor scores in Trail Making Test B and Symbol Digit Coding attention test. So we can hypothesize that schizophrenic patients with low serum truncated-BDNF and worse cognitive functioning are likely to be more resistant to a non-psychopharmacological neurocognitive training.

On the basis of these findings, we sharpen the role of evaluation of serum BDNF as an empirical system to estimate cognitive defects related to proBDNF processing as a potential biological system basic in the pathophysiology of schizophrenia.

4.2 The role of ethnic differences in serum BDNF levels in patients with schizophrenia

An element of heterogeneity that emerges from this meta-analysis is represented by the ethnic differences amongst the samples. In this context it is of great interest to note that there are divergent findings of the positive or negative associations between BDNF *val66met* polymorphism and schizophrenia, especially in Caucasian and Asian participants. These differences may partially explain the differences in serum BDDNF levels among papers. Studies in *in vitro* and in animal models have shown that Met allele alters both sorting and secretion of proBDNF, such that less regulated (activity dependent) secretion is likely to occur in carriers of at least one Met allele. Several genetic associational studies have shown that SNPs in BDNF are associated with schizophrenia (Nanko et al., 2003; Szekeres et al., 2003), and a meta-analysis study also illustrated an association between C270T and schizophrenia (Zintzaras, 2007), but not between Val66Met and schizophrenia (Kanazawa et al., 2007; Naoe et al., 2007; Xu et al., 2007; Zintzaras, 2007).

Great differences in the allelic frequencies for the BDNF Val66Met polymorphism between populations of different ethnic origins have been reported in public databases (http://www.hapmap.org) for the same populations (Tables 3 and 4). In Caucasian subjects, the frequency of the Met allele is 25–32%, whereas in Asian peoples the Met allele is more frequent, around 40–50% (Pivac et al., 2009; Verhagen et al., 2010). These variations among different ethnic groups in the allelic frequencies of the BDNF polymorphism may be caused by either the natural selection of an advantageous allele by unknown environmental issues or through a founder effect.

However, we advise prudence in the analysis of these facts, also because despite this obvious difference in outcomes of schizophrenia across ethnicities, cross-cultural research in psychiatry focuses on similarities rather than differences. For example, subtypes of schizophrenia may have different prevalence across countries: in the International Pilot

Study of Schizophrenia (1973) and the Determinants of Outcome of Severe Mental Disorders study (1992), catatonia was identified in 10% of cases in developing countries respect to less than 1% in developed countries. Hebephrenia was found in 13% of cases in developed countries and 4% in developing countries. Currently, we have not sufficient data about the role of diagnostic subtypes and serum BDNF levels or BDNF polymorphisms.

Genotype - Population descriptors	Genotype frequencies
G/G – YRI	0.683
G/G – JPT	0.190
G/G – CHB	0.488
G/G – CEU	1.000
A/G- YRI	0.283
A/G- JPT	0.357
A/G- CHB	0.349
A/G- CEU	n.a.
A/A- YRI	0.033
A/A- JPT	0.452
A/A- CHB	0.163
A/A- CEU	0

Table 3. YRI: Yoruba in Ibadan, Nigeria; JPT: Japanese in Tokyo, Japan; CHB: Han Chinese in Beijing, China; CEU: CEPH (Utah residents with ancestry from northern and western Europe). G/G = Met/Met; A/G =Val/Met; A/A = Val/Val.

Allele - Population descriptors	Allele frequencies
G- YRI	0.825
G- JPT	0.369
G- CHB	0.663
G- CEU	1.000
A- YRI	0.175
A – JPT	0.631
A- CHB	0.337
A- CEU	0

Table 4. YRI: Yoruba in Ibadan, Nigeria; JPT: Japanese in Tokyo, Japan; CHB: Han Chinese in Beijing, China; CEU: CEPH (Utah residents with ancestry from northern and western Europe).

Another diagnostic caveats regards the Caucasian studies that often investigated not only patients with schizophrenia, but also subjects with schizophrenia spectrum disorders such as schizophreniform disorder or schizoaffective disorder, while Asian and other studies investigated only patients with schizophrenia. This difference in methodology might also have contributed to the inconsistent findings between the Caucasian and the Asian studies.

The substantial variation in the Val66Met frequencies between Asian and Caucasian samples indicates that ethnicity may be of importance in the issue, because if the association among Caucasians reflects linkage disequilibrium with another gene variant, the extent of linkage may vary between populations. A recent study focused on the complex microsatellite polymorphism BDNF-LCPR located ~1.0 kbp upstream of the translation initiation site of BDNF (Okada et al., 2006); this polymorphism contained 23 novel allelic variants, including four major alleles (A1–A4). Kawashima et al. (2009) consider that if BDNF is indeed associated with schizophrenia, the A1 allele in BDNF-LCPR would be a hopefully useful marker in the Japanese population.

Also, we must not forget the interchange between genetic and environmental issues, that may essentially vary for men and women. In this regard, it would be interesting to evalute if gender-related epistatic effects pertaining to the *Val66Met* polymorphism subsist. Literature data showed that gender differences in schizophrenia reproduce divergences in neurodevelopmental mechanisms and social influences on illness risk and course. Men have poorer premorbid functioning and have worse negative and less depressive manifestations than women. Substance abuse is more frequent in male. Results of gender variations in brain morphology (e.g. hippocampal volume) are conflicting but refer to matter of sexual dimorphism, meaning that the same elements are significant to explain sex disparities in both normal neurodevelopment and those in relationship with schizophrenia.

Another factor to consider is the epigenetic influence. "Epigenetic" refers to the covalent modifications of chromatin. Epigenetic machinery not only is responsible for lasting differences in gene activity in the CNS but also controls gene expression necessary for cognition. Thus, the likelihood of an epigenetic involvement in schizophrenia is an interesting hypothesis. In fact, epidemiological studies have identified several environmental risk factors for schizophrenia, counting marijuana consumption and obstetric complications. A recent study by Nicodemus and colleagues (2008) showed a significant association between four candidate genes for schizophrenia which are likely to have a role in hypoxic situations, including BDNF detecting significant evidence for gene x environment interaction in schizophrenic patients with or without obstetric complications. Recently, several studies underline that DNA methylation contributing to ongoing regulation of BDNF transcription in the CNS to control synaptic plasticity and memory mechanism (for e review, see Roth et al., 2009a). In addition, BDNF DNA methylation has also been found to play a part in altered gene expression in response to environmental pressure, such as social experiences (Roth et al., 2009). Indeed, stressful social experiences early in life have long-lasting consequences such as increased anxiety, drug-seeking behavior, cognitive impairment, and altered affiliative behaviours (Branchi et al., 2004; Fumagalli et al., 2007; Lippmann et al., 2007). Finally, it was recently revealed that social experiences early during the first postnatal week generate lasting changes in DNA methylation in BDNF gene in relationship with reduction of BDNF gene expression in the adult prefrontal cortex (Roth et al., 2009b).

Overall, the available data suggest that DNA methylation may indeed be an epigenetic mechanism that contributes to the aberrant regulation of genes associated with schizophrenia. The hard work to recognize vulnerability genes for multifactorial disorders such as schizophrenia, has inspired the development of alternative methodologies. Since genetic heterogeneity has been a major dilemma in complex disorders, investigators have attempted to increase homogeneity in their samples. Recently, alternative phenotypic definitions have been defined that might be more closely linked to biological pathway (*endophenotypes*), for example sensory gating deficits or working memory dysfunction (Gottesman and Gould, 2003).

Another advance to decrease basic genetic complexity is the utilization of genetic isolates. Isolated populations originated from a small number of founder couples. Throughout history, many populations, counting isolated as well as outbred populations, undergo

alternating era of adversities (e.g. war, epidemics, or famine) with period characterized by rapid growth of the population. Due to increased inbreeding and genetic drift in isolates, certain alleles will be present more frequently in the population, while others are lost, increasing genetic homogeneity. Additionally, due to geographic, cultural, or religious barriers, isolated populations did not experience a large degree of admixture with adjacent peoples for many generations, ensuing in a relatively small gene pool ("founder effect").
So the recognition of a gene or allele that clinically and/or genetically is not as important in outbred populations as in isolated populations might untangle molecular pathways and find out new candidate genes, which might have a higher involvement on illness risk in general. Several studies highlight susceptibility loci for schizophrenia in isolated populations (Venken et al., 2007).

4.3 Future research proposals

The hypothesis that relapse could be predicted by low neurotrophin levels is consistent with the neurobiology of relapse and with preliminary data in first episode psychosis patients (Parikh et al., 2003). Therefore, large populations of high-risk subjects or untreated first episode patients need to be longitudinally investigated to improve the statistical importance of the analysis (Pantelis et al., 2003). In fact, in the absence of a neuroleptic naïve cohort followed longitudinally to evaluate pattern of neurotrophins over time, it is difficult to determine whether any relationship between relapse and low neurotrophins would be due to an underlying neurobiological vulnerability to relapse, an inadequate therapeutic response to antipsychotics, or inadequate antipsychotic exposure due to medication noncompliance. In the first part of the meta-analysis, serum BDNF levels were shown to be reduced in patients with schizophrenia even if the difference was moderately significant ($p<0.05$). However, considerable statistical heterogeneity was detected between studies. In the second part of the meta-analysis, we found that serum BDNF levels in patients with drug free/first episode psychosis were significantly lower in patients compared to healthy control subjects, but we could not detect any significant alteration in serum BDNF levels in patients with chronic schizophrenia. In both cases, a high heterogeneity was between the studies was highlighted and it is still unclear whether the reduction in serum BDNF levels observed in drug naïve/first episode patients with schizophrenia is due more to antipsychotic treatment or toxic effect of psychosis in itself. Therefore, future biochemical studies should longitudinally investigate larger samples of high-risk individuals, drug free first-episode patients and unaffected family members. Such populations are crucial to systematically examine whether serum BDNF levels changes are already present before the appearance of symptoms, or whether they develop afterwards, as a result of the course of illness. Such biochemical studies, should be crossed with MRI, genetic and metabolism investigations data, in order to further investigate whether serum BDNF levels represent an indicator of vulnerability to the disease and to better understand the functional expression of serum BDNF levels abnormalities in schizophrenia.

5. References

Aid. T.; Kazantseva, A., Piirsoo, M., Palm, K. & Timmusk, T. (2007). Mouse and rat BDNF gene structure and expression revisited. *Journal of Neuroscience Research,* Vol.85, No.3, (February 2007), pp. 525-535, ISSN 0360-4012

Baiano, M.; David, A., Versace, A., Churchill, R., Balestrieri, M. & Brambilla, P. (2007). Anterior cingulate volumes in schizophrenia: a systematic review and a meta-analysis of MRI studies. *Schizophrenia Research,* Vol.93, No.1-3, (July 2007), pp. 1-12, ISSN 0920-9964

Bowie, C.R.; Leung, W.W., Reichenberg, A., McClure, M.M., Patterson, T.L., Heaton, R.K. & Harvey, P.D. (2008). Predicting schizophrenia patients' real-world behavior with specific neuropsychological and functional capacity measures. *Biological Psychiatry,* Vol.63, No.5, (March 2008), pp. 505-511, ISSN 0006-3223

Branchi, I.; Francia, N. & Alleva E. (2004). Epigenetic control of neurobehavioural plasticity: The role of neurotrophins. *Behavioral Pharmacology,* Vol.15, No.5-6, (September 2004), pp. 353-362, ISSN 0955-8810

Buckley, P.F.; Pillai, A., Evans, D., Stirewalt, E. & Mahadik, S. (2007). Brain Derived Neurotropic Factor in First -Episode Psychosis. *Schizophrenia Research,* Vol.91, No.1-3, (March 2007), pp. 1-5, ISSN 0920-9964

Carlino, D.; Leone, E., Di Cola, F., Baj, G., Marin, R., Dinelli, G., Tongiorgi, E. & De Vanna, M. (2011). Low serum truncated-BDNF isoform correlates with higher cognitive impairment in schizophrenia. *Journal of Psychiatric Research,* Vol.45, No.2, (February 2011), pp. 273-279, ISSN 0022-3956

Chen, D.C.; Wang, J., Wang, B., Yang, S.C., Zhang, C.X., Zheng, Y.L., Li, Y.L., Wang, N., Yang, K.B., Xiu, M.H., Kosten, T.R. & Zhang, X.Y. (2009). Decreased levels of serum brain-derived neurotrophic factor in drug-naïve first-episode schizophrenia: relationship to clinical phenotypes. *Psychopharmacology,* Vol.207, No.3, (December 2009), pp. 375-380, ISSN 0033-3158

Dickinson, D.; Ramsey, M.E. & Gold, J.M. (2007). Overlooking the obvious: a meta-analytic comparison of digit symbol coding tasks and other cognitive measures in schizophrenia. *Archives of General Psychiatry,* Vol.64, No.5, (May 2007), pp. 532-542, ISSN 0003-990X

Donovan, M.J.; Miranda, R.C., Kraemer, R., McCaffrey, T.A., Tessarollo, L., Mahadeo, D., Sharif, S., Kaplan, D.R., Tsoulfas, P. & Parada, L. (1995). Neurotrophin and neurotrophin receptors in vascular smooth muscle cells. Regulation of expression in response to injury, *American Journal of Pathology,* Vol.147, No.2, (August 1995), pp. 309-324, ISSN 0002-9440

Durany, N.; Michel, T., Zöchling, R., Boissl, K.W., Cruz-Sánchez, F.F., Riederer, P. & Thome, J. (2001). Brain-derived neurotrophic factor and neurotrophin 3 in schizophrenic psychoses. *Schizophrenia Research,* Vol.52, No.1-2, (October 2001), pp. 79-86, ISSN 0920-9964

Elfving, B.; Plougmann, P.H. & Wegener, G. (2010). Detection of brain-derived neurotrophic factor (BDNF) in rat blood and brain preparations using ELISA: pitfalls and solutions. *Journal of Neuroscience Methods,* Vol.187, No.1, (March 2010), pp. 73-77, ISSN 0165-0270

Fatemi, S.H. & Folsom, T.D. (2009). The neurodevelopmental hypothesis of schizophrenia, revisited. *Schizophrenia Bulletin,* Vol.35, No.3, (May 2009), pp. 528-548, ISSN 1787-9965

Fumagalli, A.; Molteni, R., Racagni, G. & Riva, M.A. (2007). Stress during development: Impact on neuroplasticity and relevance to psychopathology. *Progress in Neurobiology,* Vol.81, No.4, (March 2007), pp. 197–217, ISSN 0555-4047

Gama, C.S.; Andreazza, A.C., Kunz, M., Berk, M, Belmonte-de-Abreu, P.S. & Kapczinski, F. (2007). Serum levels of brain derived neurotrophic factor in patients with schizophrenia and bipolar disorder. *Neuroscience Letters*, Vol.420, No.1, (June 2007), pp. 45-48, ISSN 0304-3940

Gottesman, I.I. & Gould, T.D. (2003). The endophenotype concept in psychiatry: etymology and strategic intentions. *American Journal of Psychiatry*, Vol.160, No.4, (April 2003), pp. 636-645, ISSN: 0002-953X

Green, M.J.; Matheson, S.L., Shepherd, A., Weickert, C.S. & Carr, V.J. (2010). Brain-derived neurotrophic factor levels in schizophrenia: a systematic review with meta-analysis. Molecular Psychiatry, Vol.24, (August 2010), [Epub ahead of print], ISSN 1359-4184

Grillo, R.W.; Ottoni, G.L., Leke, R., Souza, D.O., Portela, L.V. & Lara, D.R. (2007). Reduced serum BDNF levels in schizophrenic patients on clozapine or typical antipsychotics. *Journal of Psychiatric Research*, Vol.41, No.1-2, (January-February 2007), pp. 31–35, ISSN 0022-3956

Harvey, P.D.; Keefe, R.S., Patterson, T.L., Heaton, R.K. & Bowie, C.R. (2009). Abbreviated neuropsychological assessment in schizophrenia: prediction of different aspects of outcome. *Journal of Clinical and Experimental Neuropsychology*, Vol.31, No.4, (May 2009), pp. 462-471, ISSN 1380-3395

Heinrichs, R.W. (2005). The primacy of cognition in schizophrenia. *American Psychologist*, Vol.60, No.3, (April 2005), pp. 229-242, ISSN 0003-066X

Howes, O.D. & Kapur, S. (2009). The dopamine hypothesis of schizophrenia: version III--the final common pathway. *Schizophrenia Bulletin*, Vol.35, No.3, (May 2009), pp. 549-562, ISSN 1787-9965

Huang, T.L. & Lee, C.T. (2006). Associations between serum brain-derived neurotrophic factor levels and clinical phenotypes in schizophrenia patients. *Journal of Psychiatric Research*, Vol.40, No.7, (October 2006), pp. 664–668, ISSN 0022-3956

Ikeda, Y.; Yahata, N., Ito, I., Nagano, M., Toyota, T., Yoshikawa, T., Okubo, Y. & Suzuki, H. (2008). Low serum levels of brain-derived neurotrophic factor and epidermal growth factor in patients with chronic schizophrenia. *Schizophrenia Research*, Vol.101, No.1-3, (April 2008), pp. 58–66, ISSN 0920-9964

Iritani, S. (2007). Neuropathology of schizophrenia: a mini review. *Neuropathology*, Vol.27, No.6, (December 2007), pp. 604-8, ISSN 0919-6544

Jablensky, A.; Sartorius, N., Ernberg, G., Anker, M., Korten, A., et al (1992) Schizophrenia: manifestations, incidence and course in different cultures. A World Health Organization ten-country study. *Psychological Medicine. Monograph Supplement*, Vol.20, (November 1992), pp. 1–97. ISSN 0264-1801

Jindal, R.D.; Pillai, A.K., Mahadik, S.P., Eklund, K., Montrose, D.M. & Keshavan, M.S. (2010). Decreased BDNF in patients with antipsychotic naïve first episode schizophrenia. *Schizophrenia Research*, Vol.119, No.1-3, (June 2010), pp. 47–51, ISSN 0920-9964

Jockers-Scherübl, M.C.; Danker-Hopfe, H., Mahlberg, R., Selig, F., Rentzsch, J., Falk Schürer, F., Lang, U.E. & Hellweg, R. (2004). Brain-derived neurotrophic factor serum concentrations are increased in drug-naïve schizophrenic patients with chronic cannabis abuse and multiple substance abuse. *Neuroscience Letters*, Vol.371, No.1, (November 2004), pp. 79–83, ISSN 0304-3940

Kanazawa, T.; Glatt, S.J., Kia-Keating, B., Yoneda, H. & Tsuang, M.T. (2007). Metaanalysis reveals no association of the Val66Met polymorphism of brainderived neurotrophic factor with either schizophrenia or bipolar disorder. *Psychiatric Genetics*, Vol.17, No.3, (June 2007), pp. 165–170, ISSN 0955-8829

Karege, F.; Bondolfi, G., Gervasoni, N., Schwald, M., Aubry, J.M. & Bertschy, G. (2005). Low brain-derived neurotrophicfactor (BDNF) levels in serum of depressed patients probably results from lowered platelet BDNF release unrelated to platelet reactivity. *Biological Psychiatry*, Vol.57, No.9, (May 2005), pp. 1068-72, ISSN 0006-3223

Kawashima, K.; Ikeda, M., Kishi, T., Kitajima, T., Yamanouchi, Y., Kinoshita, Y., Okochi, T., Aleksic, B., Tomita, M., Okada, T., Kunugi, H., Inada, T., Ozaki, N. & Iwata, N. (2009). BDNF is not associated with schizophrenia: data from a Japanese population study and meta-analysis. *Schizophrenia Research*, Vol.112, No.1-3, (July 2009), pp. 72-79, ISSN 0920-9964

Keefe, R.S.; Bilder, R.M., Harvey, P.D., Davis, S.M., Palmer, B.W., Gold, J.M., Meltzer, H.Y., Green, M.F., Miller, D.D., Canive, J.M., Adler, L.W., Manschreck, T.C., Swartz, M., Rosenheck, R., Perkins, D.O., Walker, T.M., Stroup, T.S., McEvoy, J.P. & Lieberman J.A. (2006). Baseline neurocognitive deficits in the CATIE schizophrenia trial. *Neuropsychopharmacology*, Vol.31, No.9, (September 2006), pp. 2033-2046, ISSN 0893-133X

Keefe, R.S.; Mohs, R.C., Bilder, R.M., Harvey, P.D., Green, M.F., Meltzer, H.Y., Gold, J.M. & Sano, M. (2003). Neurocognitive assessment in the Clinical Antipsychotic Trials of Intervention Effectiveness (CATIE) project schizophrenia trial: development, methodology, and rationale. *Schizophrenia Bulletin*, Vol.29, No.1, (2003), pp. 45-55, ISSN 0586-7614

Koshimizu, H., Kiyosue, K., Hara, T., Hazama, S., Suzuki, S., Uegaki, K., Nagappan, G., Zaitsev, E., Hirokawa, T., Tatsu, Y., Ogura, A., Lu, B. & Kojima, M. (2009). Multiple functions of precursor BDNF to CNS neurons: negative regulation of neurite growth, spine formation and cell survival. *Molecular Brain*, Vol.13, No.2, (August 2009), pp. 27, ISSN 17566606

Lee, R.; Kermani, P., Teng, K.K. & Hempstead, B.L. (2001). Regulation of cell survival by secreted proneurotrophins. *Science*, Vol.294, No.5548, (November 2001), pp. 1945-1948, ISSN 0193-4511

Lippmann, M.; Bress, A., Nemeroff, C.B., Plotsky, P.M. & Monteggia LM. (2007). Long-term behavioural and molecular alterations associated with maternal separation in rats. *European Journal Neuroscience*, Vol.25, No.10, (May 2007), pp. 3091–3098, ISSN 0953-816X

Matsumoto, T.; Rauskolb, S., Polack, M., Klose, J., Kolbeck, R., Korte, M. & Barde, Y.A. (2008). Biosynthesis and processing of endogenous BDNF: CNS neurons store and secrete BDNF, not pro-BDNF. *Nature Neuroscience*, Vol.11, No.2, (February 2008), pp. 131-133, ISSN 1097-6256

Mowla, S.J.; Farhadi, H.F., Pareek, S., Atwal, J.K., Morris, S.J., Seidah, N.G. & Murphy, R.A. (2001). Biosynthesis and post-translational processing of the precursor to brain-derived neurotrophic factor. *The Journal of Biological Chemistry*, Vol.276, No.16, (April 2001), pp. 12660-12666, ISSN 0021-9258

Nagappan, G.; Zaitsev, E., Senatorov, V.V. Jr, Yang, J., Hempstead, B.L. & Lu, B. (2009) Control of extracellular cleavage of ProBDNF by high frequency neuronal activity.

Proc Natl Acad Sci U S A, Vol.106, No.4, (January 2009), pp. 1267-1272, ISSN 0027-8424

Nanko, S.; Kunugi, H., Hirasawa, H., Kato, N., Nabika, T. & Kobayashi, S. (2003). Brain-derived neurotrophic factor gene and schizophrenia: polymorphism screening and association analysis. *Schizophrenia Research*, Vol.62, No.3, (August 2003), pp. 281–283, ISSN 0920-9964

Naoe, Y.; Shinkai, T., Hori, H., Fukunaka, Y., Utsunomiya, K., Sakata, S., Matsumoto, C., Shimizu, K., Hwang, R., Ohmori, O. & Nakamura, J. (2007). No association between the brain derived neurotrophic factor (BDNF) Val66Met polymorphismand schizophrenia in Asian populations: evidence from a case-control study and meta-analysis. *Neuroscience Letters*, Vol.415, No.2, (March 2007), pp. 108–112, ISSN 0304-3940.

Nicodemus, K.K.; Marenco, S., Batten, A.J., Vakkalanka, R., Egan, M.F., Straub, R.E. & Weinberger, D.R. (2008).Serious obstetric complications interact with hypoxia-regulated/vascularexpression genes to influence schizophrenia risk. *Molecular Psychiatry* Vol.13, No.9, (September 2008), pp. 873–877, ISSN 1359-4184

O'Donnell K.; O'Connor TG & Glover V. (2009). Prenatal stress and neurodevelopment of the child: focus on the HPA axis and role of the placenta. *Developmental Neuroscience*, Vol.31, No.4, (June 2009), pp. 285-292, ISSN 0378-5866

Okada, T.; Hashimoto, R., Numakawa, T., Iijima, Y., Kosuga, A., Tatsumi, M., Kamijima, K., Kato, T. & Kunugi, H., (2006). A complex polymorphic region in the brain-derived neurotrophic factor (BDNF) gene confers susceptibility to bipolar disorder and affects transcriptional activity. Molecular Psychiatry, Vol.11, No.7, (July 2006), pp. 695–703, ISSN 1359-4184

Owen M.J.; Williams H.J. & O'Donovan M.C. (2009). Schizophrenia genetics: advancing on two fronts. *Current Opinionin Genetics & Development*, Vol.19, No.3, (June 2009), pp. 266-270, ISSN 0959-437X

Palomino, A.; Vallejo-Illarramendi, A., González-Pinto, A., Aldama, A., González-Gómez, C., Mosquera, F., González-García, G. & Matute, C. (2006). Decreased levels of plasma BDNF in first-episode schizophrenia and bipolar disorder patients. *Schizophrenia Research*, Vol.86, No.1-3, (September 2006), pp. 321-322, ISSN 0920-9964

Pan, W.; Banks, W.A., Fasold, M.B., Bluth, J. & Kastin, A.J. (1998). Transport of brain-derived neurotrophic factor acrossthe blood-brain barrier. *Neuropharmacology*, Vol.37, No.12, (December 1998), pp. 1553-1561, ISSN 0028-3908

Pantelis, C.; Velakoulis, D., McGorry, P.D., Wood, S.J., Suckling, J., Phillips, L.J., Yung, A.R., Bullmore, E.T., Brewer, W., Soulsby, B., Desmond, P. & McGuire, P.K. (2003). Neuroanatomical abnormalities before and after onset ofpsychosis: a cross-sectional and longitudinal MRI comparison. *Lancet*, Vol.361, No.9354, (January 2003), pp. 281-288, ISSN 0140-6736

Parikh, V.; Evans, D.R., Khan, M.M. & Mahadik, S.P. (2003). Nerve growth factor in never-medicated first-episode psychotic and medicated chronic schizophrenic patients: possible implications for treatment outcome. *Schizophrenia Research*, Vol.60, No.2-3, (April 2003), pp. 117-123, ISSN 0920-9964

Pirildar, S.; Gönül, A.S., Taneli, F. & Akdeniz, F. (2004). Low serum levels of brain-derived neurotrophic factor in patients with schizophrenia do not elevate after antipsychotic treatment. *Progress in Neuro-Psychopharmacology & Biological Psychiatry*, Vol.28, No.4, (July 2004), pp. 709- 713, ISSN 0278-5846

Pivac, N.; Kim, B., Nedić, G., Joo, Y.H., Kozarić-Kovacić, D., Hong, J.P.& Muck-Seler, D. (2009). Ethnic differences in brain-derived neurotrophic factor Val66Met polymorphism in Croatian and Korean healthy participants. *Croatian Medical Journal*, Vol.50, No.1, (February 2009), pp. 43-48, ISSN 0353-9504

Pruunsild, P.; Kazantseva, A., Aid, T., Palm, K. & Timmusk, T. (2008). Dissecting the human BDNF locus: bidirectional transcription, complex splicing, and multiple promoters. *Genomics*, Vol.90, No.3, (September 2008), pp. 397-406, ISSN 0888-7543

Psychiatric GWAS Consortium Coordinating Committee, Cichon, S.; Craddock, N., Daly, M., Faraone, S.V., Gejman, P.V., Kelsoe, J., Lehner, T., Levinson, D.F., Moran, A., Sklar, P. & Sullivan, P.F. (2009). Genomewide association studies: history, rationale, and prospects for psychiatric disorders. *American Journal of Psychiatry*, Vol.166, No.5, (May 2009), pp. 540-556, ISSN 0002-953X

Rasmussen, P.; Brassard, P., Adser, H., Pedersen, M.V., Leick, L., Hart, E., Secher, N.H., Pedersen, B.K. & Pilegaard, H. (2009). Evidence for a release of brain-derived neurotrophic factor from the brain during exercise. *Experimental Physiology*, Vol.94, No.10, (October 2009), pp. 1062-1069, ISSN 0958-0670

Reis, H.J.; Nicolato, R., Guimarães Barbosa, I., Teixeira do Prado, P.H., Romano-Silva, M.A. & Teixeira, A.L. (2008). Increased serum levels of brain-derived neurotrophic factor in chronic institutionalized patients with schizophrenia. *Neuroscience Letters*, Vol.439, No.2, (July 2008), pp. 157–159, ISSN 0304-3940

Rizos, E.N.; Rontos, I., Laskos, E., Arsenis, G., Michalopoulou, P.G., Vasilopoulos, D., Gournellis, R. & Lykouras, L. (2008). Investigation of serum BDNF levels in drug-naive patients with schizophrenia. *Progress in Neuro-Psychopharmacology & Biological Psychiatry*, Vol.32, No.5, (July 2008), pp. 1308–1311, ISSN 0278-5846

Roth T.L.; Lubin, F.D., Sodhi, M. & Kleinman, J.E. (2009a). Epigenetic mechanisms in schizophrenia. *Biochimica et Biophysica Acta*, Vol.1790; No.9, (September 2009), pp. 869–877, ISSN 0006-3002

Roth, T.L.; Lubin, F.D., Funk, A,J. & Sweatt, J.D. (2009b). Lasting epigenetic influence of early- life adversity on the bdnf gene. Biological Psychiatry, Vol.65, No.9, (May 2009), pp. 760–769, ISSN 0006-3223

Segal, R.A.; Pomeroy, S.L. & Stiles, C.D. (1995). Axonal growth and fasciculation linked to differential expression of BDNF and NT3 receptors in developing cerebellar granule cells. *Journal of Neuroscience*, Vol.15, No.7 Pt 1, (July 1995), pp. 4970-4981, ISSN 0270-6474

Segal, R.A.; Rua, L. & Schwartz, P. (1997). Neurotrophins and programmed cell death during cerebellar development. *Advances in Neurology*, Vol.72, pp. 79-86 , ISSN 0091-3952

Seidah, N.G.; Mowla, S.J., Hamelin, J., Mamarbachi, A.M., Benjannet, S., Toure, B.B., Basak, A., Munzer, J.S., Marcinkiewicz, J., Zhong, M., Barale, J.C., Lazure, C., Murphy, R.A., Chrétien, M. & Marcinkiewicz, M.(1999). Mammalian subtilisin/kexin isozyme SKI-1: a widely expressed proprotein convertase with a unique cleavage specificity and cellular localization. *Proceedings of the National Academy of Sciences*, Vol.96, No.4, (February 1999), pp. 1321-1326, ISSN 0027-8424

Sen, S.; Duman, R. & Sanacora, G. (2008). Serum brain-derived neurotrophic factor, depression, and antidepressant medications: meta-analyses and implications. *Biological Psychiatry,* Vol.64, No.6, (September 2008), pp. 527-532, ISSN 0006-3223

Shen, L.; Figurov, A. & Lu, B. (1997). Recent progress in studies of neurotrophic factors and their clinical implications.*Journal of Molecular Medicine,* Vol.75, No.9, (September 1997), pp. 637-644, ISSN 0377-046X

Shimizu, E.; Hashimoto, K., Watanabe, H., Komatsu, N., Okamura, N., Koike, K., Shinoda, N., Nakazato, M., Kumakiri, C., Okada, S. & Iyo, M. (2003). Serum brain-derived neurotrophic factor (BDNF) levels in schizophrenia are indistinguishable from controls. *Neuroscience Letters,* Vol.351, No.2, (November 2003), pp. 111–114, ISSN 0304-3940

Shoval, G. & Weizman, A. (2005). The possible role of neurotrophins in the pathogenesis and therapy of schizophrenia. *European Neuropsychopharmacology,* Vol.15, No.3, (May 2005), pp. 319-329, ISSN 0924-977X

Szekeres, G.; Juhasz, A., Rimanoczy, A., Keri, S. & Janka, Z., (2003). The C270T polymorphism of the brain-derived neurotrophic factor gene is associated with schizophrenia. *Schizophrenia Research,* Vol.65, No.1, (December 2003), pp. 15–18, ISSN 0920-9964

Takahashi, M.; Shirakawa, O., Toyooka, K., Kitamura, N., Hashimoto, T., Maeda, K., Koizumi, S., Wakabayashi, K., Takahashi, H., Someya, T. & Nawa, H. (2000). Abnormal expression of brain-derived neurotrophic factor and its receptor in the corticolimbic system of schizophrenic patients. *Molecular Psychiatry,* Vol.5, No.3, (May 2000), pp. 293-300, ISSN 1359-4184

Tan, Y.L.; Zhou, D.F. & Zhang, X.Y. (2005b). Decreased plasma brain-derived neurotrophic factor levels in schizophrenic patients with tardive dyskinesia: association with dyskinetic movements. *Schizophrenia Research,* Vol.77, No.2-3, (September 2005), pp. 263– 270, ISSN 0920-9964

Tan, Y.L.; Zhou, D.F., Cao, L.Y., Zou, Y.Z. & Zhang, X.Y. (2005a). Decreased BDNF in serum of patients with chronic schizophrenia on long-term treatment with antipsychotics. *Neuroscience Letters,* Vol.382, No.1-2, (July 2005), pp. 27–32, ISSN 0304-3940

Teng, H.K.; Teng, K.K., Lee, R., Wright, S., Tevar, S., Almeida, R.D., Kermani, P., Torkin, R., Chen, Z.Y., Lee, F.S., Kraemer, R.T., Nykjaer, A. & Hempstead, B.L. (2005). Pro-BDNF induces neuronal apoptosis via activation of a receptor complex of p75NTR and sortilin. *The Journal of Neuroscience,* Vol.25, No.22, (June 2005), pp. 5455-5463, ISSN 0270-6474

Thome, J., Foley, P. & Riederer, P. (1998). Neurotrophic factors and the maldevelopmental hypothesis of schizophrenic psychoses. *Journal of Neural Transmission,* Vol.105, No,1, (March 1998) pp.85-100. ISSN:0300-9564

Toyooka, K.; Asama, K., Watanabe, Y., Muratake, T., Takahashi, M., Someya, T. & Nawa, H. (2002). Decreased levels of brain-derived neurotrophic factor in serum of chronic schizophrenic patients. *Psychiatry Research,* Vol.110, No.3, (July 2002), pp. 249–257, ISSN 0165-1781

Trajkovska, V., Marcussen, A.B., Vinberg, M., Hartvig, P., Aznar, S. & Knudsen, G.M. (2007). Measurements of brain-derived neurotrophic factor: methodological aspects and demographical data. *Brain Research Bulletin,* Vol.73, No.1-3, (June 2007), pp. 143-149, ISSN 0361-9230

Van Os, J. & Kapur, S. (2009). Schizophrenia. *Lancet* Vol. 374, No. 9690, (August 2009), pp. 635-645, ISSN 0140-6736

Venken, T. & Del-Favero, J. (2007). Chasing Genes for Mood Disorders and Schizophrenia in Genetically Isolated Populations. Human Mutation Vol.28, No.12, (December 2007), pp. 1156-1170, 2007 ISSN 1059-7794

Verhagen, M.; van der Meij, A., van Deurzen, P.A., Janzing, J.G., Arias-Vásquez, A., Buitelaar, J.K. & Franke, B. (2010). Meta-analysis of the BDNF Val66Met polymorphism in major depressive disorder: effects of gender and ethnicity. *Molecular Psychiatry,* Vol.15, No.3, (March 2010), pp. 260-271, ISSN 1359-4184

Vinogradov, S.; Fisher, M., Holland, C., Shelly, W., Wolkowitz, O. & Mellon, S.H. (2009). Is Serum Brain-Derived Neurotrophic Factor a Biomarker for Cognitive Enhancement in Schizophrenia? *Biological Psychiatry,* Vol.66, No.6, (September 2009), pp. 549-553, ISSN 0006-3223

Weickert, C.S.; Hyde, T.M., Lipska, B.K., Herman, M.M., Weinberger, D.R. & Kleinman, J.E. (2003). Reduced brain-derived neurotrophic factor in prefrontal cortex of patients with schizophrenia. *Molecular Psychiatry,* Vol.8, No.6, (June 2003), pp. 592-610, ISSN 1359-4184

Weickert, C.S.; Ligons, D.L., Romanczyk, T., Ungaro, G., Hyde, T.M., Herman, M.M., Weinberger, D.R. & Kleinman, J.E. (2005). Reductions in neurotrophin receptor mRNAs in the prefrontal cortex of patients with schizophrenia. *Molecular Psychiatry,* Vol.10, No.7, (July 2005), pp. 637-650, ISSN 1359-4184

Wong, J., Hyde, T.M., Cassano, H.L., Deep-Soboslay, A., Kleinman, J.E., & Weickert, C.S. (2010). Promoter specific alterations of brain-derived neurotrophic factor mRNA in schizophrenia. *Neuroscience,* Vol.169, No.3, (Sep 2010), pp:1071-84. ISSN 0306-4522

Woo, N.H.; Teng, H.K., Siao, C.J., Chiaruttini, C., Pang, P.T., Milner, T.A., Hempstead, B.L. & Lu, B. (2005). Activation of p75NTR by pro-BDNF facilitates hippocampal long-term depression. *Nature Neuroscience,* Vol.8, No.8, (August 2005), pp. 1069-1077. ISSN 1097-6256

World Health Organization (1973) International pilot study of schizophrenia. Geneva: World Health Organization, p. 427

Xiu, M.H.; Hui, L., Dang, Y.F., Hou, T.D., Zhang, C.X., Zheng, Y.L., Chen, D.C., Kosten, T.R. & Zhang, X.Y. (2009). Decreased serum BDNF levels in chronic institutionalized schizophrenia on long-term treatment with typical and atypical antipsychotics. *Progress in Neuro-Psychopharmacology & Biological Psychiatry,* Vol.33, No.8, (November 2009), pp. 1508–1512, ISSN 0278-5846

Xu, M.Q.; St Clair, D., Ott, J., Feng, G.Y. & He, L., (2007). Brain-derived neurotrophic factor gene C-270T and Val66Met functional polymorphisms and risk of schizophrenia: a moderate-scale population-based study and metaanalysis. *Schizophrenia Research,* Vol.91, No.1-3, (March 2007), pp. 6–13, ISSN 0920-9964

Yamada, M.K.; Nakanishi, K., Ohba, S., Nakamura, T., Ikegaya, Y., Nishiyama, N. & Matsuki, N. (2002). Brain-derived neurotrophic factor promotes the maturation of GABAergic mechanisms in cultured hippocampal neurons. *Journal of Neuroscience,* Vol.22, No.17, (September 2002), pp. 7580-7585, ISSN 0270-6474

Yang, J.; Siao, C.J., Nagappan, G., Marinic, T., Jing, D., McGrath, K., Chen, Z.Y., Mark, W., Tessarollo, L., Lee, F.S., Lu, B. & Hempstead, B.L. (2009). Neuronal release of proBDNF. *Nature Neuroscience,* Vol.12, No.2, (February 2009), pp. 113-115, ISSN 1097-6256

Yoshimura, R.; Hori, H., Sugita, A., Ueda, N., Kakihara, S., Umene, W., Nakano, Y., Shinkai, K., Mitoma, M., Ohta, M., Shinkai, T. & Nakamura, J. (2007). Treatment with risperidone for 4 weeks increased plasma 3-methoxy-4-hydroxypnenylglycol (MHPG) levels, but did not alter plasma brain-derived neurotrophic factor (BDNF) levels in schizophrenic patients. *Progress in Neuro-Psychopharmacology & Biological Psychiatry,* Vol.31, No.5, (June 2005), pp. 1072–1077, ISSN 0278-5846

Zhang, X.Y.; Tan, Y.L., Zhou, D.F., Cao, L.Y., Wu, G.Y., Xu, Q., Shen, Y., Haile, C.N., Kosten TA, Kosten TR. (2007). Serum BDNF levels and weight gain in schizophrenic patients on long-term treatment with antipsychotics. *Journal of Psychiatric Research,* Vol.41, No.12, (December 2007), pp. 997–1004, ISSN 0022-3956

Zhang, X.Y.; Zhou, D.F., Wu, G.Y., Cao, L.Y., Tan, Y.L., Haile, C.N., et al. (2008). BDNF levels and genotype are associated with antipsychotic-induced weight gain in patients with chronic schizophrenia. *Neuropsychopharmacology,* Vol.33, No.9, (August 2008), pp. 2200–2205, ISSN 0893-133X

Zintzaras, E. (2007). Brain-derived neurotrophic factor gene polymorphisms and schizophrenia: a meta-analysis. *Psychiatric Genetics*, Vol.17, No.2, (April 2007), pp. 69–75, ISSN 0955-8829

4

Neurocognitive Expression of Hypofrontality in Long Term Schizophrenia

Marek Krzystanek[1], Irena Krupka-Matuszczyk[1] and Adam Klasik[2]
[1]*Department of Psychiatry and Psychotherapy, Medical University of Silesia in Katowice*
[2]*The Institute of Psychology, Opole University*
Poland

1. Introduction

Despite over a century of studies on schizophrenia, its pathogenesis still remains unexplained. In particular, cognitive dysfunctions, related to a decrease of prefrontal cortex activity in the human brain represent one of the main symptoms of schizophrenia. The cognitive dysfunctions usually precede, by a few years, the first acute episode of the disease. These dysfunctions are present in approximately 70% of persons suffering from schizophrenia, and can be maintained at a stable level over the rest of their lifetime (Rund et al., 2006). For instance, majority of patients enrolled in the CATIE study suffered from the cognitive disorders (Lieberman et al., 2005a).

According to Javitt (2010), the cognitive deficits are the key symptoms of schizophrenia, which usually precede an onset of some other symptoms of this disease. Due to that, the cognitive disorders can represent the leading concept among hypotheses, related to etiology of schizophrenia. The main component of these disorders is the deterioration of attention concentration and operative memory deficits, including the difficulty of holding some elements in short-term memory (Goldman-Rakic, 1999) that in turn translates into some cognitive dysfunctions. These disorders include also memory, learning abilities, and executive functions (Meltzer & McGurk, 2004). The cognitive dysfunctions related to hypofrontality consist of deterioration of the activity of prefrontal brain cortex (Carter et al., 1998).

In majority of patients, the cognitive deficits begin prior to their first disease episode, in the prodromal stage (Fuller et al., 2002). Individuals with prodromal schizophrenia symptoms often present deficits, ranging in intensity from almost normal conditions to the ones, resembling mental status of patients with the first episode of their disease (Lencz et al., 2006). In this aspect, neurocognitive disorders can be considered as the initial schizophrenia symptoms (Javitt, 2010). Due to these reasons, the cognitive disorders appear to be closely connected with the etiology of schizophrenia (Kantrowitz & Javitt, 2010b).

In schizophrenia, the cognitive dysfunctions and hypofrontality are associated with hypofunction of NMDA receptors (NMDA-R) (Marek et al., 2010), and according to Carlsson (2006), an abnormal function of NMDA-R is the main cause of schizophrenia. These cognitive disorders, mostly in form of concentration deterioration, and deficits of operative memory are results of prefrontal cortex dysfunctions, which are related to the deficit of glutamergic transmission, caused by the NMDA-R hypofunction (Thomsen et al., 2009).

There are two pharmacological models of the NMDA-R (receptor) hypofunction - acute and chronic (Pratt et al., 2008). Acute receptor antagonist model relates to a short-term administration of the NMDA-R antagonist. In this situation, blocking the NMDA-R causes disinhibition of neurotransmission and so called hyperfrontality that means increased glutamergic activity in the areas of prefrontal cortex (Homayoun & Moghaddam, 2007). There is indirect evidence that some cerebral metabolic disorders, in the acute phase of schizophrenia, resemble the changes that were observed experimentally, during administration of the NMDA-R antagonists, directly to different areas of the brain (Bubeníková-Valesová et al., 2008). Also, a significant increase of the glutaminic acid concentration in the cingular area has been noted both in patients with an early psychosis (Théberge et al., 2002), and with prodromal schizophrenia symptoms (Stone et al., 2009).

Pratt et al. (2008) proposed a chronic psylocybine (PCP) model, which explains a relation between the NMDA receptors hypofunction and hypofrontality. Chronic administration of the PCP to rats caused a reduction of glucose metabolism in their prefrontal cortex, and a decrease in the expression of protein marker of gamma aminobutyric acid (GABA) interneuron's' activity. In schizophrenia patients, similarly to chronic PCP abusers, the hypofrontality symptoms and GABA interneuron's deficits have been noted. According to the Pratt's model, hypofrontality represents neuroadaptation, created during a period of long-term glutamergic hyperfunction, caused by a chronic blockage of the NMDA-R, related to GABA interneurons.

Based on some studies, the cognitive deficits appear a few years prior to the onset of schizophrenia (Fuller et al., 2002; Kantrowitz et Javitt, 2010b), but there is no convincing evidence that they are present since early childhood (Paz et al., 2008; Perkins et al., 2005). A 28-year observational study by Seidman et al. (2006) has revealed that the patients with schizophrenia displayed some minor concentration disorders already at the age of 7 years. These disorders are subsequently aggravated, with the development of the disease. However, the exact moment of aggravation is still unknown. It is possible that the disorders' exacerbation can occur just before the first schizophrenia episode.

2. Study design

Our unpublished study results indicate the persistence of cognitive dysfunctions in schizophrenia, and are convergent with some recent research data in this area.

In our study, cognitive functioning was assessed with neuropsychological tests, included in the Vienna System Tests. Functions of attention, operational memory, learning and motor reactions were also examined. A battery of Cognition (COG), Block Taping Test (CORSI), SIGNAL and Reaction Test (RT) tests was performed in all of our paranoid schizophrenia patients.

3. Study group

We studied a group of 162 paranoid schizophrenics, treated with 3 different neuroleptics, or treatment-resistant patients (Figure 1).

Patients who were recruited to this study were diagnosed with paranoid schizophrenia, and treated in monotherapy with one of the following neuroleptics: haloperidol, clozapine or olanzapine. Subjects in the study group met the contemporary criteria of symptomatic remission in schizophrenia. The study covered also a group of chronically ill schizophrenic subjects, who were resistant to the pharmacologic treatment, and did not have the remission.

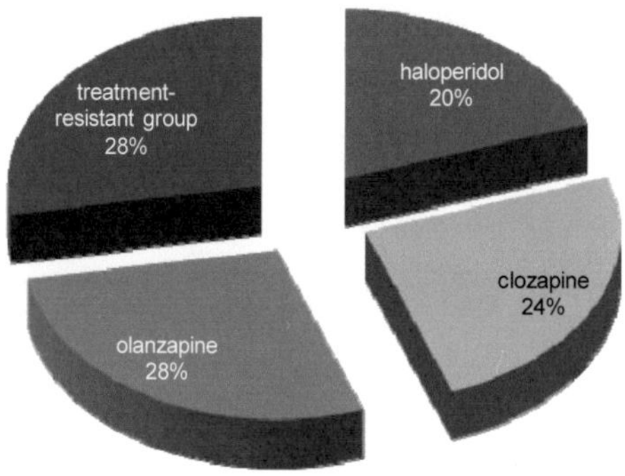

Fig. 1. Percentages of paranoid schizophrenia patient's sub-groups, treated with haloperidol, clozapine, olanzapine, and treatment-resistant. Results are shown as percentages (%) of the entire study group.

The gender characteristics of the study patients are shown in Figure 2.

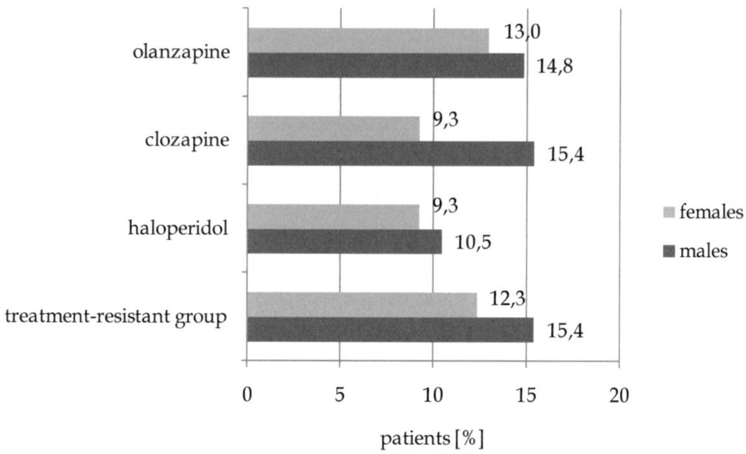

Fig. 2. Gender of patients in the study groups. Results are expressed as percentages (%) of the entire study group.

The mean age of patients was 46.1 years. The age of patients in the study groups is shown in Figure 3.

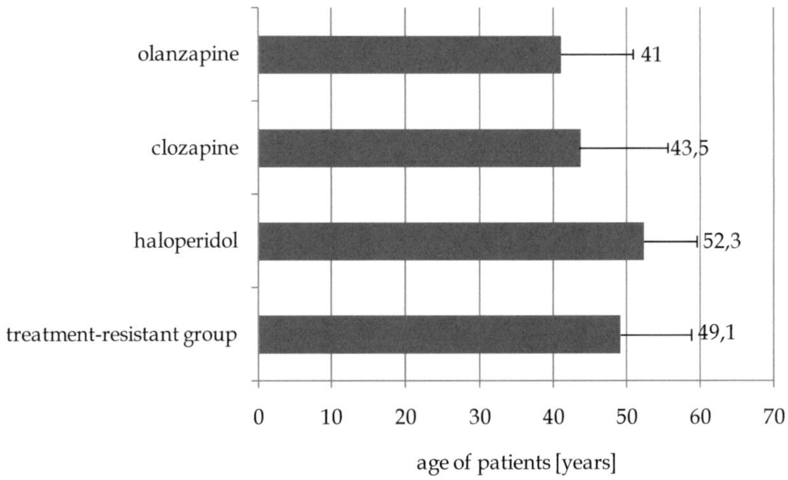

Fig. 3. Age of patients in the study groups. Results are expressed as the mean ± standard deviation (SD).

An average disease onset was at the age of 27.4 years (mean age) (Figure 4), and the mean period of the disease duration was 19.3 years (Figure 5).

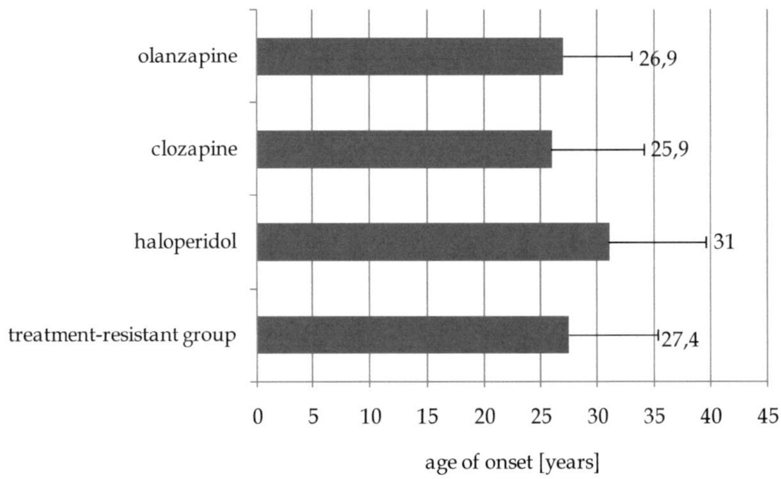

Fig. 4. The age of schizophrenia onset in the study groups of patients. The results are shown as means ± standard deviation (SD).

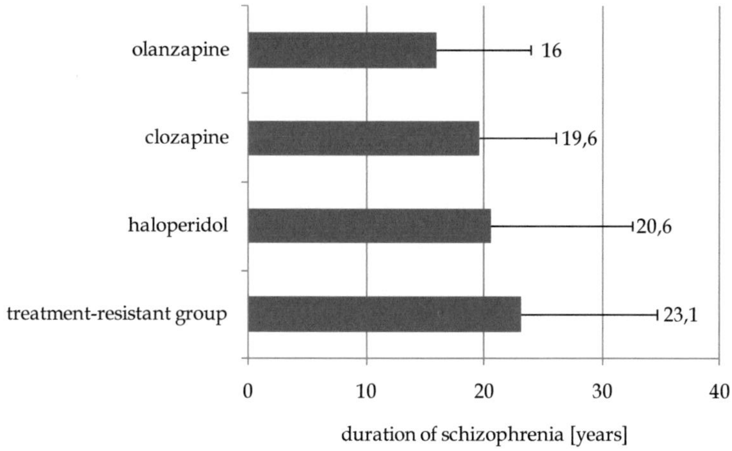

Fig. 5. The duration of the disease in the study groups of patients. The results are shown as means ± standard deviation (SD).

The mean numbers of hospitalizations of the study patients are shown in Figure 6.

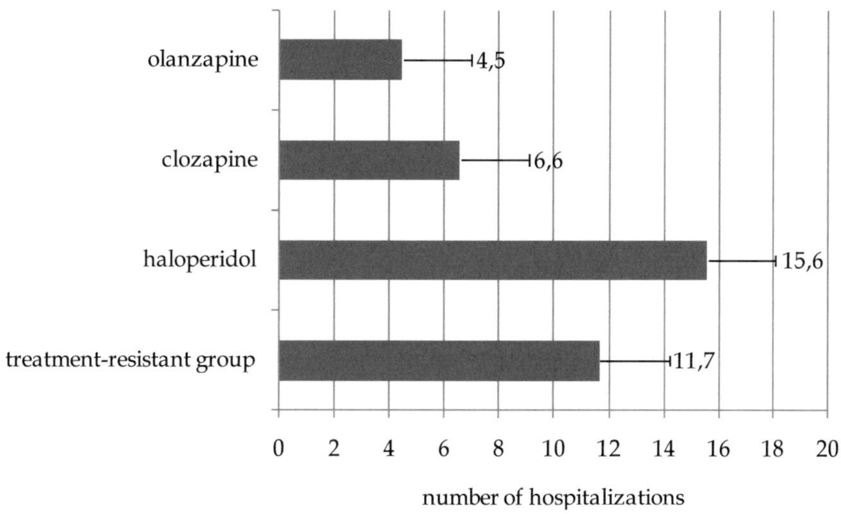

Fig. 6. The number of hospitalizations in the study groups of patients. The results are shown as means ± standard deviation (SD).

The results were analyzed statistically using non-parametric Kruskal-Wallis test and Tukey HSD test for unequal sample sizes. NIR post-hoc test was also applied. Confidence interval (CI) was established at the level of 95%. The results were established as statistically significant at $p<0,05$.

4. Results

The intensity of negative symptoms was significantly below, as compared to the results of patients treated with neuroleptics. It was shown both in the global results of Negative Symptom Assessment Scale (NSA-16) (Figure 7) and in its sub-scales assessing alogy (Figure 8), blunted affect (Figure 9), asociality-anhedonia (Figure 10) and avolition-apathy (Figure 11).
The intensity of negative symptoms, measured with NSA-16 was 32% lower in the group of patients treated with neuroleptics, as compared with the treatment resistant subjects (Figure 7).

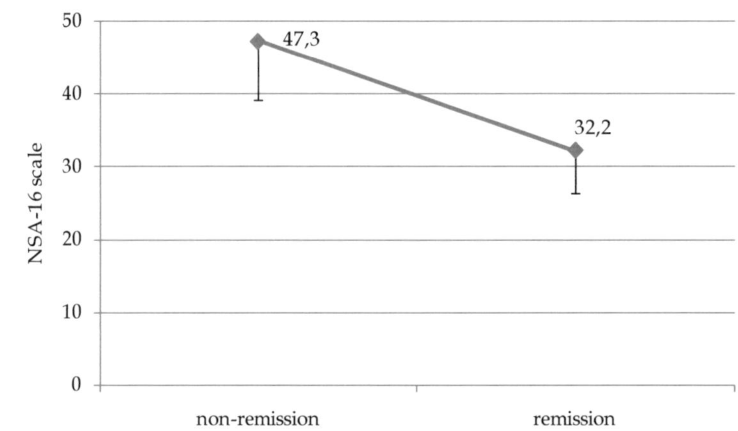

Fig. 7. Results of NSA-16 scale, in paranoid schizophrenia study groups of patients. Results are shown as means with standard deviation (SD). $H_{3,162}=84,7$, p=0,00001, $\eta^2_P=0,53$.

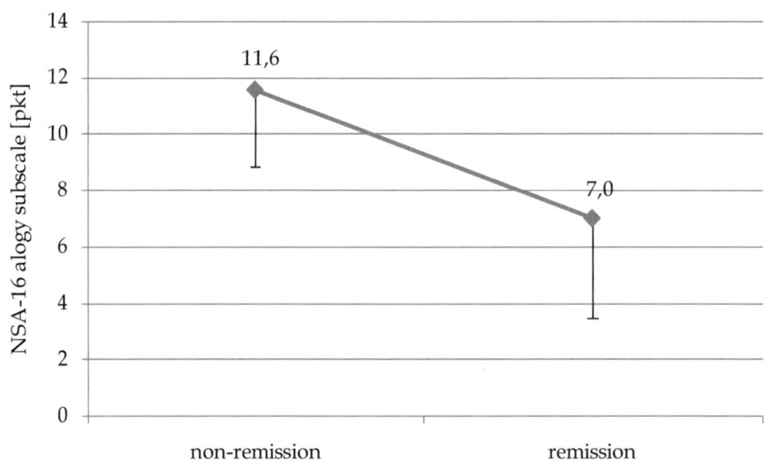

Fig. 8. Results of NSA-16 alogy subscale, in paranoid schizophrenia study groups of patients. Results are shown as means with standard deviation (SD). $H_{3,162}=70,7$, p=0,00001, $\eta^2_P=0,43$.

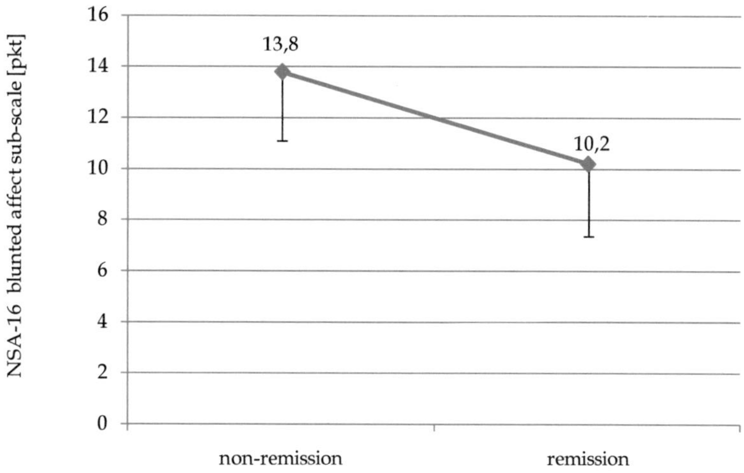

Fig. 9. Results of NSA-16 blunted affect subscale, in paranoid schizophrenia study groups of patients. Results are shown as the means with standard deviation (SD). $H_{3,162}$=65,6, p=0,00001, η^2_P=0,49.

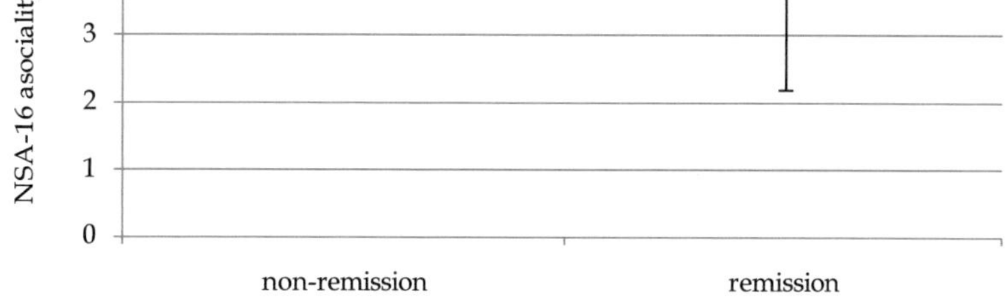

Fig. 10. Results of NSA-16 asociality-anhedonia subscale in paranoid schizophrenia study groups of patients. Results are shown as the means with standard deviation (SD). $H_{3,162}$=60,3, p=0,00001, η^2_P=0,35.

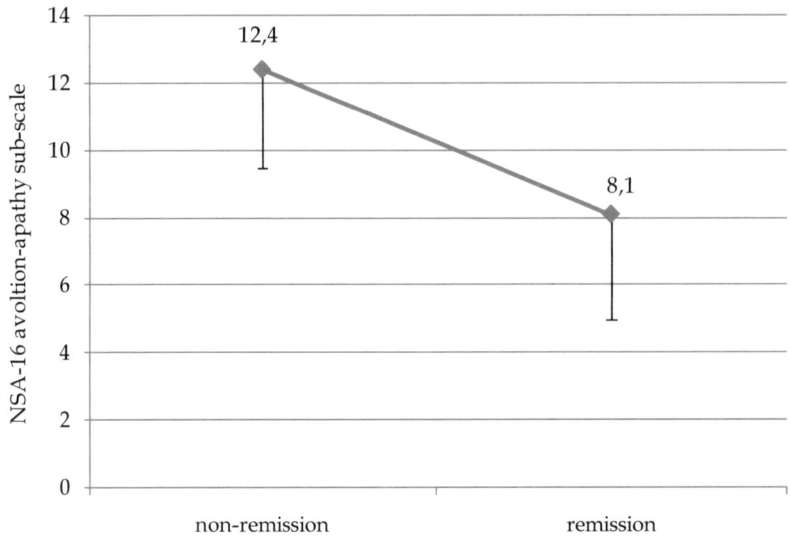

Fig. 11. Results of NSA-16 avolition-apathy subscale in paranoid schizophrenia study groups of patients. Results are shown as the means with standard deviation (SD). $H_{3,162}$=77,5, p=0,00001, η^2_P=0,46.

In the alogy subscale of NSA-16, the intensity of symptoms was 39,7% lower in the group of treatment resistant schizophrenic patients (Figure 8).

In the blunted affect subscale of NSA-16, the intensity of symptoms was 26,1% lower in the patients treated with neuroleptics (Figure 9).

The intensity of symptoms, according to asociality-anhedonia subscale of NSA-16, was 35,3 % higher in the treatment resistant schizophrenic patients group (Figure 10).

An analysis of the avolition-apathy subscale of NSA-16 revealed that the intensity of symptoms was 34,7% higher in the treatment resistant schizophrenia patients (Figure 11).

A clinical state of the study patients was assessed with the Clinical Global Impression–Severity (CGI-S) scale. Comparison of global clinical picture between the patients without remission and the patients effectively treated with neuroleptics revealed the significant difference (Figure 12).

In patients with remission, the intensity of the disease was assessed as minimal, but in the group of patients with residual symptoms, the intensity measured with CGI-S was moderate to severe.

An analysis of Person's correlation coefficient has revealed that in the group of patients without remission, the severity of the symptoms correlated with the intensity of negative symptoms, measured with NSA-16 scale (R=0,65, p=0.0001). The intensity of both positive (R=0,58, p=0.0001) and negative (R=0,37, p=0.0001) symptoms, in the study groups of patients was assessed, according to Positive and Negative Syndrome Scale (PANSS).

In patients treated with haloperidol, the severity of the disease correlated significantly (R=0,33, p=0,03) with the intensity of extrapyramidal symptoms, assessed with Simpson-Angus Extrapyramidal Symptoms Scale.

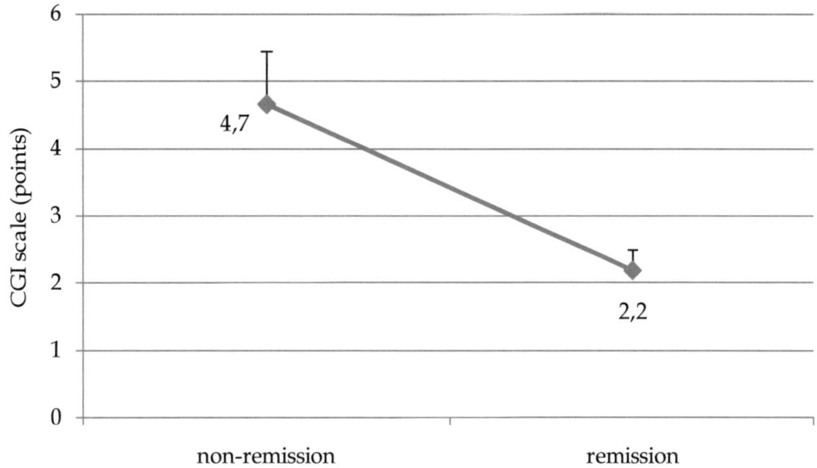

Fig. 12. Assessment of clinical state of paranoid schizophrenia, in study groups of patients, with Clinical Global Impression–Severity (CGI-S) scale. Results are shown as means with standard deviation (SD). $H_{3,162}$=117,3, p=0,0001, η^2_P=0,82.

Cognitive dysfunctions of various intensity were present in all groups of the study patients. They included disturbances of: attention, operational memory, learning mechanisms, and reaction time. These dysfunctions were present, even though the patients met the criteria of functional remission, and were treated with neuroleptics.

An analysis of logistic regression has indicated that the cognitive deficits in subjects with schizophrenia depended on the intensity of negative symptoms and are related to the schizophrenic process. However, these symptoms did not depend on the duration of the disease, and on the age of schizophrenia onset.

5. Discussion

Many authors indicate the steady persistence of cognitive dysfunctions, during the entire schizophrenia course.

In the study by Klingberg et al. (2008), alterations of cognitive functioning among schizophrenia patients were noted over the period of 15 months. Despite improvement of memory and concentration, comparing to the beginning of the disease, after a successful treatment of the acute episode, the patient's cognitive functioning, during the entire observation period did not return to normal level.

Also, in their 5-year study, Albus et al. (2006) indicated that the cognitive dysfunctions in schizophrenia were present from the beginning of the disease, and then, they remained stable, over the consecutive years. Both classical and atypical neuroleptics did not have any significant influence on these cognitive deficits, except from verbal fluency.

Likewise, the study by Kurtz et al. (2005), conducted on a small group of patients, indicated the presence of persistent deficits of cognitive functioning in schizophrenia, during the observation period of 10 years.

Another 10-year observation conducted by Stirling et al. (2003) has revealed that the deterioration of cognitive functioning in schizophrenia remained at a similar level during the entire duration of the disease. According to the same author, the deficit of executive functions was present already at the onset of the disease, and did not increase over the next 10-12 years.

According to a 10-year observation by Hoff et al. (2005), it was fund that the cognitive deficits had arisen prior to the first hospitalization, and subsequently lasted, without any significant deterioration, over the entire disease period.

Based on the study by Øie et al. (2010), the cognitive disorders among schizophrenic patients, especially in the spectrum of verbal memory, attention, and information processing speed, remained almost unchanged, despite a 13-year period of treatment. These cognitive deficits were present, despite the improvement of clinical symptoms, over a few years, after the first schizophrenia episode (de Mello Ayres et al., 2010).

The above research findings indicate that the cognitive disorders among patients with schizophrenia appear at the beginning of the disease, or even before the stage of full-blown disease, and then, they can be stable chronically.

According to contemporary standards of schizophrenia treatment, neuroleptics play the main role in therapy. Treatment starts at the beginning of acute schizophrenia episode, when a patient meets diagnostic criteria of the disease, including fully expressed positive schizophrenia symptoms. A hypothesis of the NMDA receptors' hypofunction and the associated cognitive disorders in schizophrenia indicate that the moment of treatment initiation is delayed by a few years.

Contemporary knowledge about cognitive disorders in schizophrenia reveals that they arise approximately 3-4 years before the first schizophrenia episode, and then, they last over the entire lifespan, at a stable level. Our study findings have confirmed the above results. The intensity of cognitive disorders among our study patients was not related to the duration of the disease. Despite an effective treatment, in patients suffering from this disease for many years, the attention disorders, operative memory deficits, as well as learning and reaction speed abnormalities persisted.

It seems that the primary cause of schizophrenia is closely related to the hypofunction of NMDA receptors. Pathogenetic process, dependent on the hypofunction of these receptors is initiated by disinhibition of neurotransmission in the OUN and hyperfrontality. Long-term effects of the glutamergic hypofunction in the OUN lead to hypofrontality, through mechanisms of neuroadaptation. Chronic persistence of cognitive dysfunctions, despite the effective symptomatic treatment indicates that the currently used neuroleptics do not normalize functions of glutamergic system.

This lack of normalization of the glutamergic system activity with the neuroleptics, explains their unsatisfactory therapeutic effect on the cognitive dysfunctions in schizophrenia. Treatment of these symptoms represents a very important pharmacotherapy goal in psychiatry, because the patients' quality of life depends mostly on the level of cognitive deficits, and intensity of negative symptoms.

According to a model of hypofunction of the NMDA receptors in schizophrenia, the treatment should already be started at the stage, in which the first cognitive disorders appear. Since the primary cause of glutamergic malfunction in schizophrenia is the hypofunction of NMDA receptors, related to GABA-ergic interneurons, the initial stage of therapy should include their stimulation, which can cause the return of inhibition of this neurotransmission in OUN. One of the considered medications in this area is acamprosate – a GABA-ergic agent, which normalizes the NMDA receptor functions and the release of glutamate (De Witte et al., 2005). In the second stage of the disease, characterized by hypofrontality and cognitive dysfunctions, the treatment should be focused on increasing the activity of glutamergic system. In the meantime, as indicated by our study results, the neuroleptics, through altering composition of different subunits of the NMDA receptor, can reduce its activity.

It appears that the treatment strategy, which considers the model of NMDA receptor hypofunction, can create a new direction of research in psychiatry.

Some proglutamergic agents, which are now under clinical investigation, may become a new generation of anti-schizophrenic drugs, in the future. They may also, like D-cycloserine - act as agonists of the NMDA receptor, or like sarcosice - inhibit the reverse uptake of glycine (Krzystanek et al., 2009).

6. Conclusion

The presented results strongly support an argument that schizophrenia may not be related to a degenerative process. The cognitive dysfunctions, as the first line of schizophrenic symptoms, can remain in schizophrenic patients for their lifetime, despite achieving clinical remission.

7. Acknowledgment

The study was funded by grant for scientific research (No KNW6-272/06) from the Ministry of Science and Higher Education in Poland. The cost of the publication was sponsored by Polpharma Biuro Handlowe Sp. z o.o.

8. References

Albus, M.; Hubmann, W.; Mohr, F.; Hecht, S.; Hinterberger-Weber, P.; Seitz, NN. & Küchenhoff, H. (2006). Neurocognitive functioning in patients with first-episode schizophrenia: results of a prospective 5-year follow-up study. *European Archives of Psychiatry and Clinical Neuroscience*, Vol.256, No.7, (October 2006), pp.442-451, ISSN 0940-1334

Bubeníková-Valesová, V.; Horácek, J.; Vrajová, M. & Höschl, C. (2008). Models of schizophrenia in humans and animals based on inhibition of NMDA receptors. *Neuroscience and Biobehavioral Reviews*, Vol.32, No.5, (July 2008), pp.1014-1023, ISSN 0149-7634

Carlsson, A. (2006). The neurochemical circuitry of schizophrenia. *Pharmacopsychiatry*, Vol.39, Suppl.1, (February 2006), pp.10-14, ISSN 0176-3679

Carter, C.S.; Perlstein, W.; Ganguli, R.; Brar, J.; Mintun, M. & Cohen, J.D. (1998). Functional hypofrontality and working memory dysfunction in schizophrenia. *American Journal of Psychiatry*, Vol.155, No. 9, (September 1998), pp.1285-1287, ISSN. 0002-953X

de Mello Ayres, A.; Scazufca, M.; Menezes, P.R.; Nakano, E.Y.; Regina, A.C.; Schaufelberger, M.S.; Murray, R.M.; McGuire, P.K.; Rushe, T. & Busatto, G.F. (2010). Cognitive functioning in subjects with recent-onset psychosis from a low-middle-income environment: multiple-domain deficits and longitudinal evaluation. *Psychiatry Research*, Vol.179, No.2, (September 2010), pp.157-164, ISSN 0165-1781

Fuller, R.; Nopoulos, P.; Arndt, S.; O'Leary, D.; Ho, B.C. & Andreasen, N.C. (2002). Longitudinal assessment of premorbid cognitive functioning in patients with schizophrenia through examination of standardized scholastic test performance. *American Journal of Psychiatry*, Vol.159, No.7, (July 2002), pp.1183-1189, ISSN 0002-953X

Lencz, T.; Smith, C.W.; McLaughlin, D.; Auther, A.; Nakayama, E.; Hovey, L. & Cornblatt, B.A. (2006). Generalized and specific neurocognitive deficits in prodromal schizophrenia. *Biological Psychiatry*, Vol.59, No.9, (May 2006), pp.863-871, ISSN 0006-3223

Goldman-Rakic, P.S. (1999). The physiological approach: functional architecture of working memory and disordered cognition in schizophrenia. *Biological Psychiatry*, Vol.46, No.5, (September 1999), pp.650-661, ISSN 0006-3223

Hoff, A.L.; Svetina, C.; Shields, G.; Stewart, J. & DeLisi, L.E. (2005). Ten year longitudinal study of neuropsychological functioning subsequent to a first episode of schizophrenia. *Schizophrenia Research*, Vol.78, No.1, (October 2005), pp.27-34, ISSN 0006-3223

Homayoun, H. & Moghaddam, B. (2007). NMDA receptor hypofunction produces opposite effects on prefrontal cortex interneurons and pyramidal neurons. *Journal of Neuroscience*, Vol.27, No.43, (October 2007), pp.11496-11500, ISSN 0270-6474

Javitt, D.C. (2010). Glutamatergic theories of schizophrenia. *The Israel Journal of Psychiatry and Related Sciences*, Vol.47, No.1, (January 2010), pp.4-16, ISSN 0333-7308

Kantrowitz, J.T. & Javitt, D.C. (2010a). N-methyl-d-aspartate (NMDA) receptor dysfunction or dysregulation: the final common pathway on the road to schizophrenia? *Brain Research Bulletin*, Vol.83, No.3-4, (September 2010), pp.108-121, ISSN 0333-7308

Kantrowitz J.T. & Javitt, D.C. (2010b). Thinking glutamatergically: changing concepts of schizophrenia based upon changing neurochemical models. *Clinical Schizophrenia & Related Psychoses*, Vol.4, No.3, (October 2010), pp.189-200, ISSN 1935-1232

Klasik, A.; Janas-Kozik, M.; Krupka-Matuszczyk, I. & Augustyniak, E. (2006). Funkcje poznawcze, ich rozwój oraz nowoczesne metody diagnozowania. *Przeglad Lekarski*, Vol.63, Suppl.1, (January 2006), pp.29-34, ISSN 0033-2240

Klingberg, S.; Wittorf, A.; Sickinger, S.; Buchkremer, G. & Wiedemann, G. (2008). Course of cognitive functioning during the stabilization phase of schizophrenia. *Journal of Psychiatric Research*, Vol.42, No.4, (March 2008), pp.259-267, ISSN 0022-3956

Krzystanek, M.; Pałasz, A.; Krzystanek, E. & Krupka-Matuszczyk, I. (2009). Niedoczynność receptora NMDA w patogenezie schizofrenii. *Farmakoterapia w Psychiatrii i Neurologii*, Vol.25, No.3-4, (December 2009), pp.29-38, ISSN 1234-8279

Kurtz, M.M.; Seltzer, J.C.; Ferrand, J.L. & Wexler, B.E. (2005). Neurocognitive function in schizophrenia at a 10-year follow-up: a preliminary investigation. *CNS Spectrum*, Vol.10, No.4, (April 2005), pp.277-280, ISSN 1092-8529

Lieberman, J.A.; Stroup, T.S.; McEvoy, J.P.; Swartz, M.S.; Rosenheck, R.A.; Perkins, D.O.; Keefe, R.S.; Davis, S.M.; Davis, C.E.; Lebowitz, B.D.; Severe, J. & Hsiao, J.K. (2005). Clinical Antipsychotic Trials of Intervention Effectiveness (CATIE) Investigators. Effectiveness of antipsychotic drugs in patients with chronic schizophrenia. *The*

New England Journal of Medicine, Vol.353, No.12, (September 2005), pp.1209-1223, ISSN 0028-4793

Marek, G.J.; Behl, B.; Bespalov, A.Y.; Gross, G.; Lee, Y. & Schoemaker, H. (2010). Glutamatergic (N-methyl-D-aspartate receptor) hypofrontality in schizophrenia: too little juice or a miswired brain? *Molecular Pharmacology*, Vol.77, No.3, (March 2010), pp.317-326, ISSN 0026-895X

Meltzer, H.Y. & McGurk, S.R. (1999). The effects of clozapine, risperidone, and olanzapine on cognitive function in schizophrenia. *Schizophrenia Bulletin*, Vol.25, No.2 (March 1999), pp.233-255, ISSN 0026-895X

Øie, M.; Sundet, K. & Rund, B.R. (2010). Neurocognitive decline in early-onset schizophrenia compared with ADHD and normal controls: evidence from a 13-year follow-up study. *Schizophrenia Bulletin*, Vol.36, No.3, (May 2010), pp.557-565, ISSN 0026-895X

Paz, R.D.; Tardito, S.; Atzori, M.& Tseng, K.Y. (2008). Glutamatergic dysfunction in schizophrenia: from basic neuroscience to clinical psychopharmacology. *European Neuropsychopharmacology*, Vol.18, No.11, (November 2008), pp.773-786, ISSN 0924-977X

Perkins, D.O.; Gu, H.; Boteva, K. & Lieberman, J.A. (2005). Relationship between duration of untreated psychosis and outcome in first-episode schizophrenia: a critical review and meta-analysis. *American Journal of Psychiatry*, Vol.162, No.10 (October 2005), pp.1785-1804, ISSN 0002-953X

Pratt, J.A.; Winchester, C.; Egerton, A.; Cochran, S.M. & Morris, B.J. (2008). Modelling prefrontal cortex deficits in schizophrenia: implications for treatment. *British Journal of Pharmacology*, Vol.153, Suppl.1, (March 2008), pp.465-470, ISSN 0007-1188

Rund, B.R.; Sundet, K.; Asbjørnsen, A.; Egeland, J.; Landrø, N.I.; Lund, A.; Roness, A.; Stordal, K.I. & Hugdahl, K. (2006). Neuropsychological test profiles in schizophrenia and non-psychotic depression. *Acta Psychiatrica Scandinavica*, Vol.113, No.4, (April 2006), pp.350-359, ISSN 0001-690X

Seidman, L.J.; Buka, S.L.; Goldstein, J.M. & Tsuang, M.T. (2006). Intellectual decline in schizophrenia: evidence from a prospective birth cohort 28 year follow-up study. *Journal of Clinical and Experimental Neuropsychology*, Vol.28, No.2, (February 2006), pp.225-242, ISSN 1380-3395

Stirling, J.; White, C.; Lewis, S.; Hopkins, R.; Tantam, D.; Huddy, A. & Montague, L. (2003). Neurocognitive function and outcome in first-episode schizophrenia: a 10-year follow-up of an epidemiological cohort. *Schizophrenia Research*, Vol.65, No.2-3, (December 2003), pp.75-86, ISSN 0006-3223

Stone, J.M.; Day, F.; Tsagaraki, H.; Valli, I.; McLean, M.A.; Lythgoe, D.J.; O'Gorman, R.L.; Barker, G.J. & McGuire, P.K.; OASIS. (2009). Glutamate dysfunction in people with prodromal symptoms of psychosis: relationship to gray matter volume. *Biological Psychiatry*, Vol.66, No.6, (September 2009), pp.533-539, ISSN 0006-3223

Théberge, J.; Bartha, R.; Drost, D.J.; Menon, R.S.; Malla, A.; Takhar, J.; Neufeld, R.W.; Rogers, J.; Pavlosky, W.; Schaefer, B.; Densmore, M.; Al-Semaan, Y. & Williamson, P.C. (2002). Glutamate and glutamine measured with 4.0 T proton MRS in never-treated patients with schizophrenia and healthy volunteers. *American Journal of Psychiatry*, Vol.159, No.11, (November 2002), pp.1944-1946, ISSN 0002-953X

Thomsen, M.S.; Christensen, D.Z.; Hansen, H.H.; Redrobe, J.P. & Mikkelsen, J.D. (2009). Alpha(7) Nicotinic acetylcholine receptor activation prevents behavioral and molecular changes induced by repeated phencyclidine treatment. *Neuropharmacology*, Vol.56, No.6-7, (May-June 2009), pp.1001-1009, ISSN 0028-3908

5

Linking Stress and Schizophrenia: A Focus on Prepulse Inhibition

T.N. Douma[1,3], M.J. Millan[2], B. Olivier[1,3] and L. Groenink[1,3]
[1]*Div. of Pharmacology, Utrecht Institute for Pharmaceutical Sciences, Utrecht,*
[2]*Institute de Reserche Servier, Croissys/Seine,*
[3]*Rudolf Magnus Institute of Neuroscience*
[1]*the Netherlands*
[2]*France*

1. Introduction

Schizophrenia affects about 0.5-1.0% of people worldwide, occurring roughly equally in both men and women. The exact causes of schizophrenia are not fully understood, although the consensus of current research is that schizophrenia is a developmental disorder, caused by a genetic liability interacting with environmental and psychosocial stress. However, the possible neurobiological mechanisms underlying this gene-stress interaction are largely unknown.

To study the role of stress in the development of schizophrenia, it is useful to dissect this complex disease into specific symptoms. In this respect, a well-accepted model for psychotic-like behavior is prepulse inhibition (PPI) of the startle response. In an attempt to clarify the link between stress and schizophrenia, this chapter reviews experimental studies that determined the effect of acute and chronic stressors on PPI in humans and rodents. In section 2, studies that have focused on stress in adulthood will be discussed, and in section 3, studies that have addressed effects of early-life stress on PPI will be outlined. Together, the findings of these PPI studies support the neurodevelopmental theories of schizophrenia, which state that insults, including stress, experienced during early brain development could particularly increase the risk of developing schizophrenia.

1.1 Symptom dimensions in schizophrenia

Schizophrenia is a mental disorder, characterized by a mixture of symptoms that are generally divide into three major clusters: positive, negative, and cognitive symptoms (APA, 2000). The first category signifies symptoms that reflect excess in normal function, which comprises psychotic symptoms. These mental phenomena are often dramatic; the patient appears to have lost contact with reality. Hallucinations are one type of positive symptom; they are perceptions disconnected from external stimuli, which may occur in any sensory modality, however, auditory hallucinations (i.e. hearing voices) are the most common hallucinations in schizophrenia. Delusions are another type of positive symptom, which are fixed, false beliefs that are not shared by other people in the patient's neighborhood. The most common form is the paranoid delusion, such as the false belief that one is spied on, or being persecuted. However, a variety of other themes is also possible, for instance the belief that the fillings in one's teeth are radio transmitters receiving extraterrestrial messages, or the belief that some outside agency has added or removed thoughts in one's brain.

Negative symptoms, on the contrary, describe loss or significant impairment of normal psychological functions, such as blunted affect, emotional withdrawal, poor rapport, passivity and apathy, and anhedonia (APA, 2000). Although this reduction in normal functioning may seem less dramatic as positive symptoms, particularly negative symptoms are associated with long periods of hospitalization and poor social functioning. Indeed, a patient's degree of negative symptoms appears to determine whether a patient is still able to function in society. Last, cognitive symptoms of schizophrenia comprise 'executive dysfunctions', including problems in maintaining goals, allocating attentional resources, evaluating and monitoring performance, and utilizing these capacities to solve problems.

1.2 Diathesis-stress hypothesis of schizophrenia

Schizophrenia is a complex illness, and its possible causes are still subject of debate. However, according to a widely adopted view, both a biological predisposition, and exposure to environmental stress are necessary ingredients for schizophrenia to become manifest - the so-called diathesis stress model (Zubin & Spring, 1977). A classical example of the association between environmental stress and the risk of developing schizophrenia, comes from studies of the 1944-1945 Dutch Hunger Winter (Susser & Lin, 1992; Susser et al., 1996; Susser et al., 1998). In this discrete period during the Second World War, there was a serious decline in food intake in six cities of western Netherlands. Among people born in these cities between 1944 and 1946, the most exposed birth cohort (i.e., conceived at the height of the famine) showed a twofold and statistically significant increase in the risk for developing schizophrenia (Susser & Lin, 1992). Since this particular famine, many others occurred worldwide, but these were less suitable for epidemiological investigations due to more disorganized conditions (St Clair et al., 2005). However, several years after the Dutch Hunger Winter, a similar occasion occurred in China. Specifically, from 1959-1961, people in affected provinces were starving and died in large numbers due to bad weather (for refs see (St Clair et al., 2005)). Among births that occurred during the famine years, the risk of developing schizophrenia in later life was significantly increased when compared to those born before or afterwards (St Clair et al., 2005).

These 'natural experiments' suggest that prenatal stress, i.e., exposure to maternal nutritional deficiency, could increase the risk of schizophrenia in later life. However, evidence from many observational studies that have investigated the association between experience of stress in adulthood and acute onset of psychotic illness, has not been confirmative (Phillips et al., 2007). In particular, there is no consistent evidence that experience of stressful life events is able to trigger onset of psychosis. Findings from longitudinal studies on the other hand, are stronger in linking episodes of relapse in schizophrenia patients to an elevated rate of stressful life events (Phillips et al., 2007; Walker et al., 2008), thus providing additional evidence for a role of stress exposure in (the course of) schizophrenia.

1.3 Neurodevelopmental hypothesis of schizophrenia

As mentioned earlier, schizophrenia is generally not diagnosed before the third decade of life, suggesting that it is the end point of some pathological process acting on the immature brain. This observation has led to the formulation of the neurodevelopmental hypothesis of schizophrenia, which states that environmental disturbances during early brain development influence risk of developing schizophrenia (Harrison, 1997; Rehn & Rees, 2005; Fatemi & Folsom, 2009). Some candidates for these early disturbances are, for instance, prenatal influenza exposure, obstetric complications, prenatal maternal psychological stress, maternal and fetal nutritional deficiency, season of birth (for refs, see (St Clair et al., 2005)). However, obviously, not every individual will get ill if they experience stress. Consequently, it is thought that manifestation of disease originates through an interaction with the genetic make-up of an individual (Harrison, 1997; Rehn & Rees, 2005; Fatemi & Folsom, 2009). Several lines of evidence support the neurodevelopmental hypothesis, including epidemiological studies, premorbid history and neuropathological postmortem studies (Fatemi & Folsom, 2009). With respect to genetics, many susceptibility genes, found to be associated with a heightened risk for developing schizophrenia, have been linked to neurodevelopmental processes, such as synaptic connectivity, synaptogenesis, and growth factors (Stahl, 2008).

However, a remaining question is, whether one single intervention early in development is enough to explain occurrence of schizophrenia much later in life. An alternative hypothesis, that works within the framework of the neurodevelopmental theory, is referred to as the double-hit model (Keshavan & Hogarty, 1999; Keshavan, 1999; Maynard et al., 2001). According to this model, maldevelopment within 2 critical windows of vulnerability combines to lead to clinical manifestations of schizophrenia. First, early developmental risk factors (i.e. genetic predisposition, environmental stressor) will cause a heightened vulnerability to the illness through anomalous neural development and subtle changes in behavior. However, for schizophrenia to become manifest, an additional second hit (i.e. an environmental factor such as drug abuse or social stress) is considered necessary. Thus, in this view, early and late risk factors are not simply additive, but instead, the first hit will increase an individual's vulnerability for effects of a subsequent hit (Keshavan & Hogarty, 1999; Keshavan, 1999; Maynard et al., 2001).

1.4 Prepulse inhibition of the startle response

In order to test the above-mentioned theories, animal models could be used. However, due to the nature of the symptoms and the pathological complexity of schizophrenia, it is impossible to reproduce the disease in its entirety in an animal model. As a possible solution, one could model specific aspects or symptoms of the disorder. A highly validated model in this respect is the behavioral paradigm of prepulse inhibition (PPI) of the acoustic startle response, which is typically, but not exclusively, diminished in schizophrenic patients (Braff et al., 2001a; Geyer et al., 2001; Swerdlow et al., 2001; Swerdlow et al., 2008). As disrupted PPI is a trait marker of schizophrenia, which is also displayed by patients' unaffected relatives, as well as schizotypal (i.e., non-psychotic, unmedicated) patients, impaired sensorimotor gating is considered an endophenotype of schizophrenia (Braff et al., 2008).

PPI refers to the normal suppression of a startle response to a strong stimulus when it is preceded by a weaker stimulus (the prepulse). In rodents, PPI is commonly measured as whole-body startle responses, whereas in human experiments, generally eye-blink responses are used. In theory, deficient PPI in schizophrenic patients reflects a dysfunction in the gating of sensory and cognitive information, clinically manifesting as a patient's inability to filter irrelevant thoughts and sensory stimuli from intruding into awareness (Braff et al., 1978; Braff et al., 2008). Some cross-sectional and longitudinal studies demonstrate that in patients, deficits in sensorimotor gating are improved by atypical antipsychotics (Swerdlow et al., 2008; Aggernaes et al., 2010). Neurophysiologically, PPI is mediated via the brainstem, whereas it is regulated by an extensive set of interrelated projections from the forebrain (Swerdlow et al., 2001). Pharmacological interventions that diminish PPI are well characterized in animal models (Geyer et al., 2001) and also increasingly applied in healthy human subjects (Braff et al., 2001b; Oranje et al., 2004; Jensen et al., 2007; Oranje et al., 2011). In particular, PPI is disrupted by dopamine receptor agonists (e.g., apomorphine), serotonin receptor agonists (e.g., 8-OHDPAT), and NMDA receptor antagonists (e.g., PCP). Accordingly, the different models of disrupted PPI have been used in the search of novel antipsychotic treatments, and each of the models has proven to be sensitive to at least some antipsychotic medications (Geyer et al., 2001). Notably, concerning interventions in the dopaminergic system, application of receptor agonists into the (subcortically located) nucleus accumbens and receptor antagonists in the medial prefrontal cortex diminish PPI (Wan & Swerdlow, 1993; Ellenbroek et al., 1998), providing considerable construct validity to PPI as a model for deficient sensorimotor gating in schizophrenic patients. Thus, PPI is considered a robust, predictable and neurobiologically informative experimental measure, broadly used in translational models for schizophrenia research. While PPI is largely determined by anatomical and genetic traits (Swerdlow et al., 2008), it may also be sensitive to effects of stress - which may be even more relevant, considering the leading theories on the development of schizophrenia. Therefore, the aim of this chapter is to explore the studies that applied experimental stressors to investigate their influence on PPI.

2. Adult stress and gating mechanisms: Evidence from animal and human studies

2.1 Effects of acute stress on sensorimotor gating: Animal studies

In this section, we will review the existing literature on the effects of acute and chronic stress on PPI in adult rodents. For this purpose, some studies have pharmacologically interfered with a neural system that is fundamental to the biological stress response in mammals, the hypothalamic-pituitary-adrenal (HPA) axis, as discussed in section 2.1.1. Alternatively, external stressors have been artificially applied to rodents in the laboratory. In general, these stressors can be classified as either physical (i.e., nociceptive) or psychological, which will be outlined in sections 2.1.2. and 2.1.3., respectively.

2.1.1 HPA modulators

In a straightforward approach to address the link between stress in adulthood and PPI, some studies have pharmacologically interfered with the HPA axis, a major mammalian stress system. Physiologically, the function of the HPA-axis is to transduce neural signals that arise in response to any physical or psychological stressor, into an endocrine response; starting at the level of the brain's major integrating center: the hypothalamus. In this structure, the neuropeptide corticotrophin-releasing factor (CRF) is produced. When CRF is released into the hypophyseal portal system, it travels to the pituitary gland, where it binds to CRF_1 receptors. This, in turn, triggers the secretion of adrenocorticotropic hormone

(ACTH). Subsequently, ACTH is transported via the systemic circulatory system to the cortex of the adrenals, where it triggers the release of glucocorticoids. Through a negative feedback at the level of the hypothalamus and pituitary, glucocorticoids (cortisol in primates and corticosterone in rodents) ultimately inhibit their own release. For decades, the HPA-axis has been linked to schizophrenia (Yeap & Thakore, 2005; Phillips et al., 2006; Phillips et al., 2007; Walker et al., 2008). Notable findings in patients are elevated cortisol levels, especially shortly before onset of psychosis (reviewed by Walker & Diforio, 1997; Walker et al., 2008), and altered stress responsiveness, with cortisol responses being both enhanced (Walker et al., 2008) and blunted (Brenner et al., 2009; van Venrooij et al., 2010).

Some experimental animal studies have investigated the influence of HPA-axis manipulations on PPI. For instance, Van den Buuse and co-workers investigated the effects of a dopaminergic D2 receptor antagonist (i.e. haloperidol) on the PPI response in mice following adrenalectomy and corticosterone replacement (2, 10 or 50 mg) (van den Buuse et al., 2004). Subsequently, the animals were tested for PPI after injection of haloperidol. In adrenal-intact mice and in mice implanted with 10 mg corticosterone, haloperidol treatment increased PPI, while in both the 2 and 50 mg corticosterone-adrenalectomy groups, PPI was unchanged. The authors explained their results by postulating a corticosterone-dopamine interaction; moderate levels of corticosterone would be needed for a normal dopaminergic tone, while both low and high concentrations of corticosterone would induce reductions in dopaminergic activity (Van den Buuse et al., 2004). Indeed, an interaction between corticosteroids and central mesolimbic dopaminergic activity is suggested by several studies (Piacentini et al., 2004; Pruessner et al., 2004; Marinelli et al., 2006).

At the level of CRF, intraventricular brain injections with the neuropeptide lead to reliable alterations in PPI. This is not surprising, given the putative involvement of CRF in stress disorders and psychosis (Nemeroff et al., 1984; Charney et al., 1993; Sautter et al., 2003; Herringa et al., 2006) and the fact that CRF receptors are expressed in areas that modulate startle and PPI, including brainstem, limbic and cortical nuclei (Van Pett et al., 2000). In rodents, both acute central administration of CRF (Conti et al., 2002; Risbrough et al., 2004; Conti, 2005; Bakshi et al., 2011) and chronic CRF overexpression (Dirks et al., 2002) diminish PPI. However, unlike central CRF, peripherally injected CRF at doses that are known to cause the release of ACTH and corticosterone, did not reduce PPI in rats (Conti, 2005). Consequently, it was suggested that the effect of central CRF on PPI might be independent of its effects on the HPA axis. This finding is in agreement with a study of Groenink et al. (2008), which showed that neither glucocorticoid receptor antagonists nor adrenalectomy did improve perturbation of PPI in mice overexpressing CRF (CRF-OE mice). In addition, elevation of corticosterone levels by pellet implantation did not affect PPI in wild-type mice. In contrast, two different CRF_1 receptor antagonists significantly restored PPI in CRF-OE mice, based on which the authors concluded that chronic overactivation of CRF_1 receptors rather than excessive glucocorticoid receptor stimulation underlies PPI deficits in CRF-OE mice. Also in rats, neither acute, nor repeated administration of corticosterone decreased PPI (Czyrak et al., 2003). In the brain, CRF acts via CRF_1 and CRF_2 receptors. Risbrough et al. (2004) investigated the respective roles of these two receptor subtypes in the startle response and sensorimotor gating in mice. Regarding the magnitude of startle, they found that CRF_1 receptors are required for the effects of CRF, and CRF_2 receptors appear to have an auxiliary role. Furthermore, CRF_1 receptor blockade reversed CRF-induced deficits in PPI, whereas CRF_2 receptor blockade potentiated the latter effect. In addition, CRF_2 receptor activation increased PPI. Together, as was argued, these findings support the idea that CRF_1 and CRF_2 receptors exert opposing roles in inhibition of startle, with CRF_1 decreasing PPI and CRF_2 increasing it. Thus, the effect of central CRF on PPI is probably not mediated by corticosterone. However, as was mentioned before, corticosteroids could play a role in regulating PPI via an interaction with mesolimbic dopaminergic activity.

2.1.2 Physical stressors

From animal models, it has long been known that intermittent and inescapable foot-shock can induce a state of analgesia (stress-induced analgesia), which is reversed by the opiate receptor antagonist naloxone (Madden et al., 1977). Functionally, this anticipation response to upcoming aversive stimuli reduces their impact and is thought to help the organism cope with the stressor (Willer & Ernst, 1986). To examine whether exposure to a severe stressor induces changes in sensory functioning that accompany stress-induced analgesia, Leitner and co-workers measured PPI in rats shortly (i.e., 20 min) after exposure of cold swim stress (Leitner, 1986). Next to a reliable analgesia, the stressed animals exhibited decreased prepulse inhibition. In a subsequent study, this stress-induced PPI-deficit appeared to be of a multisensory nature, as reductions in PPI were found in reaction to both visual and acoustic prepulse stimuli (Leitner, 1989). The author interpreted these results as a general decrease in sensory sensitivity, which extends beyond the noxious stimulus (i.e., cold water). The finding supports a possible role for opiates in the PPI-disruptive effect of analgesia, in that opioid receptor agonists, which produce perceptual distortions in animals and humans, disrupt PPI in a dose-dependent fashion (Bortolato et al., 2005). However, another nociceptive stressor, i.e., repeated inescapable foot-shocks, slightly increases PPI (Pijlman et al., 2003), or has no effect (Bijlsma et al., 2010; Bakshi et al., 2011). Possibly, these conflicting findings can be partly explained by the longer stress-test intervals applied in the latter studies (see table 1). Lastly, the physical stressor referred to as restraint stress, comprises physically restraining a rodent in a narrow cylinder, usually for 15-20 minutes, sometimes on several subsequent days. Restraint stress has been shown to increase plasma ACTH, beta-endorphin, and corticosterone levels, and also brain levels of serotonin and norepinephrine (for refs, see (Acri, 1994)). However, the studies that examined the effects of restraint on PPI, have mostly reported inconsistent, or no effects of restraint (Acri, 1994; Faraday, 2002; Bijlsma et al., 2010), and one study showed that repeated, but not acute, restraint stress decreased PPI (Sutherland & Conti, 2011).

Thus, studies that have applied physical stressors in adult rodents have yielded inconsistent or no effects on PPI (table 1.a.). However, although some of these artificial stressors have been shown to be capable of producing elevated levels of stress hormones, the ethological validity of these stressors is not very high. In the next section, studies that examined the influence of ethologically more relevant psychological stressors will be discussed.

2.1.3 Psychological stressors

As opposed to physical stress, psychological stress does not involve a nociceptive component, as physical contact with the stressogenic stimulus is absent. This can be accomplished in several ways. One particularly simple method to induce emotional stress involves forcing rats to witness another rat being exposed to physical stress, such as repeated foot-shocks, or restraint. This observational stressor has been found to activate mesocortical dopamine systems (Kaneyuki et al., 1991). However, it is also proposed to represent a milder form of stress, as plasma corticosterone levels were found to be less elevated, compared to the concomitant physical stress condition (Acri, 1994). Studies that examined sensorimotor gating following witness stress, have reported no effects on PPI (Acri, 1994; Pijlman et al., 2003).

Another psychological stressor, that is considered more potent, is referred to as social defeat. In this paradigm, an animal is made an intruder, by placing it into the residential cage of an aggressive conspecific, where it is attacked, though, generally, the experimenter will protect it from suffering too much physical harm. After a few minutes, the intruder is placed in a small cage within the resident's cage. As a consequence, it is not exposed to further injuries and direct attacks, but still remains in an unfamiliar environment, with olfactory, visual and to some extent physical (only via vibrissae) contact with the resident. Social defeat may have some face validity with respect to schizophrenia, as high levels of social competition and migration are proposed as risk factors for developing schizophrenia (Selten & Cantor-Graae, 2007). In rodents, social defeat has been associated with dopaminergic hyperactivity and to behavioral sensitization, whereby the animal displays an enhanced response to dopamine receptor agonists (Selten & Cantor-Graae, 2007). With respect to PPI, significant impairments in the response were found following 3 weeks of daily social defeat in adult mice, which could be normalized by acute treatment with the cannabinoid receptor agonist WIN55212.2 (Brzozka et al., 2011).

Another ethologically valid psychological stressor involves exposure to a predator. Next to foot-shock stress (see section 2.1.2), Bakshi and co-workers also exposed their rats to ferrets, one of their natural predators (Bakshi et al., 2011). To make sure that the stressor would be entirely psychogenic, the rats were protected from injury by a protective cage. This kind of predator exposure has been shown to elicit acute HPA axis activation, freezing behavior and ultrasonic vocalizations (for refs, see Bakshi et al., 2011). When compared to foot-shock stress, predator exposure was found to be equipotent in terms of the amplitude of acute corticosterone release. However, foot shock stress had no effects on PPI at any measured time-point, while predator exposure significantly disrupted PPI at 24 hours after the stress; but not acutely, or 48 hours, or 9 days later (Bakshi et al., 2011).

In our laboratory, we examined the influence of psychological stress, i.e., the potential threat of bright light, on PPI in Wistar rats. In rodents, high illumination potentiates startle (light-enhanced-startle, LES), an anxiety response sensitive to clinically effective anxiolytics (de Jongh et al., 2002). As shown in figure 1, exposure to bright light significantly reduced PPI, whereas subsequent return to the safe condition enhanced PPI (for details see figure legend). These changes were most marked at lower prepulse intensities (interaction effect of prepulse intensity*phase $F_{4, 80}=4.57$, $p<0.005$).

Schmajuk and co-workers also reported diminished PPI induced by dark-to-light transitions, an effect that was blocked by haloperidol (Schmajuk et al., 2009). However, in addition to PPI, the animals also showed attenuated startle, which indicates that the (lower) illumination conditions used in the Schmajuk study did not induce anxiety. Accordingly, the authors explained their findings by stating that sudden changes in environment illumination (i.e. novelty) may evoke dynamic changes in dopaminergic circuits that modulate the startle response and prepulse inhibition (Schmajuk et al., 2009).

In conclusion, the currently available studies, although limited, demonstrate that psychological stress can indeed affect PPI (table 1.b.). However, results are not unequivocal. Due to considerable variation in duration and time course of effect, it is unclear how long the PPI-disruptions will last, once the stressors are terminated, and further studies are warranted to assess time-course and robustness and underlying mechanism involved in the observed alterations in gating mechanisms.

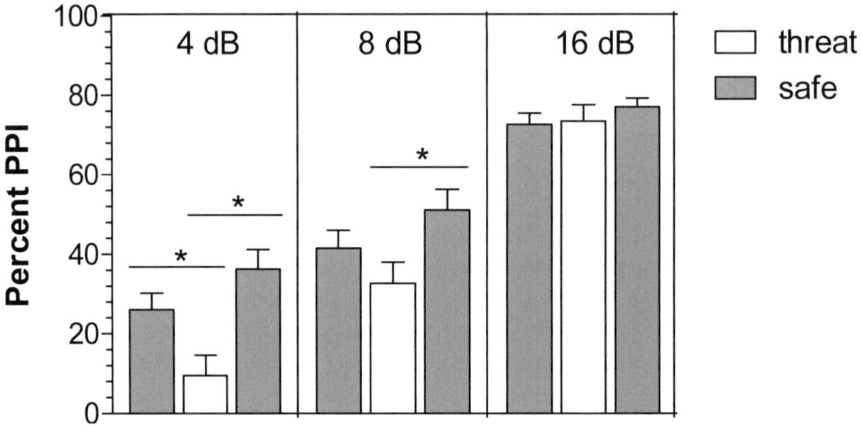

Fig. 1. PPI was measured under light-enhanced-startle conditions, with subsequent return to the dark (N=22). The test procedure was modified from de Jongh et al. (2002), and consisted of three phases. During phase 1 and 3 rats were tested in the dark, whereas during phase 2 the test cubicle was brightly lit (900 lux). Following a 5-min acclimatization period, each phase started and ended with five pulse alone trials. In between, five different trials were presented 10 times each: pulse alone (115 dB, 50 ms duration), pulse preceded by a 20 msec prepulse of either 74, 78 or 86 dB and no-stimulus trials, average inter trial interval 15 s. Shown is percent PPI (mean + S.E.M.) in safe (black bars) and threat (open bars) conditions. Potential threat (i.e. bright light) significantly reduced PPI, and subsequent return to the safe (i.e. dark) condition significantly enhanced PPI. * $P < 0.05$.

2.2 Effects of acute stress on sensorimotor gating: Human studies

In section 2.1. we have explored studies that investigated the influence of transient stress on the rodent PPI response. In the next sections, studies on human subjects are discussed, where stress has also been found to affect PPI. For instance, in a recent study, intravenous infusions of cortisol, in a dose resembling the physiological cortisol secretion in response to a moderate stressor, were shown to disrupt PPI in healthy participants (Richter et al., 2010). The disruptions reached a maximum at 20 minutes after administration, and returned to baseline another 20 minutes later. In an older study, Grillon and Davis investigated effects of stress and shock anticipation on PPI and startle in healthy subjects (Grillon & Davis, 1997). Basically, they measured PPI both when the subjects anticipated shocks (i.e. the threat condition) and when no shocks were anticipated (i.e. the safe condition). The authors argued that the fear induced by the threat condition would be superimposed on a generally stressful experience of the experiment. To distinguish effects of general alertness, they added a nonadversive control condition with a different group of participants. In this control experiment, participants were asked - and being paid for - to keep attention to auditory, visual and tactile stimuli in the test environment. As a result, both shock anticipation (i.e. fear) and attention to external stimuli significantly increased PPI. Regarding the increased PPI in the fear condition (later replicated by (Cornwell et al., 2008)), the authors suggested that threat of shock may have increased the general level of alertness,

which facilitates the processing of stimuli, thereby enhancing the effectiveness of the prepulse in inhibiting the startle response.
Repeated periods of shock anticipation however, were found to diminish PPI, an effect that was hypothesized to represent a progressive deficit in sensory functioning due to the prolonged stress of repeated shock anticipation. Apparently, this finding is not in agreement with animal work, where foot-shock stress had no effect on PPI (section 2.1.2). However, an important difference between human shock anticipation and the animal foot-shock paradigm is the physical component of the stress: during the entire experiment, human subjects only received a single shock, while animals were repeatedly exposed to shocks. In other words, the human threat-of-shock paradigm generally represented the psychological stress of potential threat, while the animal foot-shock stress had a large physical component of actual shocks, which might be less powerful. In this view, the human findings are consistent with the animal studies of (potential) threat, where diminished PPI was induced by the potential threat of bright light, and by the threat of predation (section 2.1.3.).

2.3 Effects of acute stress on sensory gating: Human studies

In addition to PPI, the brain's pre-attentive inhibitory functions are evaluated by an electrophysiological response-reduction paradigm, which is a paired-click test, wherein the P50 (or P1) wave of the vertex auditory event-related potential (i.e. computerized averages of the brain's electrical response to sound) is recorded. In healthy subjects, the P50 response to the second stimulus is generally attenuated (i.e. sensory gating), whereas in patients with schizophrenia and other psychiatric illnesses it is not suppressed (Adler et al., 1982; Adler et al., 1994), indexing deficits in filtering out irrelevant sensory stimuli (White & Yee, 1997). Like PPI, auditory sensory gating is influenced by stress. Note, that although the two experimental measures of brain inhibitory function are related, they are not identical in every respect, and partly regulated by different brain structures (Braff et al., 2001a). However, the fact that PPI and P50 gating are both measures of sensory gating that are influenced by stress, may point to possible common sources of functioning within the brain.
A few studies have reported decreased sensory gating following a stressful intervention. Effects of cold stress have been evaluated by the cold-pressor test, in which subjects have to submerge a hand to the wrist in cold water for a fixed period. To control for successful stress induction, subjective distress and arterial blood pressure were measured. With respect to PPI, the studies reported transient but significant deficits in response to cold stress, in addition to increased distress ratings and higher systolic arterial tension (Johnson & Adler, 1993; Ermutlu et al., 2005). Brief psychological stress has been found to exert similar effects. In a study by White and Yee (1997), subjects were administered an oral arithmetic task; this mentally stressful task resulted in reduced P50 suppression in the participants. Possible effects of attention were ruled out by adding an equally difficult, but non-stressful arithmetic task, which did not affect P50 suppression.

2.4 Conclusion section 2

In table 1.a. and 1.b., an overview is given of studies reporting on effects of acute stressors in adult life on measures of sensory gating. Available evidence, from both animal and human subjects, indicates that acute stress can modify sensory gating. However, underlying neurobiological mechanisms remain poorly understood. Possibly, in first instance, moderate threat or attention to the environment could facilitate processing of sensory stimuli, for instance, via increased cortical arousal. Indeed, substantial evidence confirms that directing attention to the prepulse signal enhances PPI in humans and, likewise, emotional learning has been shown to enhance PPI in rats (reviewed by Li et al., 2009a). Severe or prolonged stressors on the contrary, may cause (progressive) loss of sensory perception that functions to reduce the impact of impending aversive events (Grillon & Davis, 1997). Particularly, these perceptual changes may be mediated by cortisol and CRF-induced activation of the mesolimbic dopamine system, a neural circuitry implicated in both stress responsivity and PPI.

However, some studies do not find an effect at all. From the animal work under review, this appeared to be most often the case when physical stressors were used, as opposed to psychological stressors (compare, table 1.a. and 1.b.). Due to the small number of available studies, it is difficult to draw definite conclusion from this finding. Clearly, the rodent PPI response is strain, age and gender dependent (Palmer et al., 2000; Swerdlow et al., 2006; Pietropaolo & Crusio, 2009), and stress appears to differentially influence PPI across strains and sexes (Varty & Geyer, 1998; Faraday et al., 1999). Despite these limitations, it could be speculated that psychological stressors may have a higher ethological validity, which could produce more pronounced effects on PPI. In this respect, it is interesting to note that the stress that is associated with episodes of relapse in schizophrenia patients is often of a psychological nature (Walker & Diforio, 1997). However, more studies on the effects of different types of stress on PPI are needed to reach a conclusion at this point.

Physical stress						
Subject	**Intervention**	**Stress-test interval**	**PPI**	**Startle**	**P50**	**Reference**
Human	Cold stress	0	n.d.	n.d.	↓	Ermutlu et al., 2005; Johnson & Adler, 1993
Rat	Cold stress	20 min	↓	=	n.d.	Leitner, 1986
Rat	Foot-shock	5 days	↑	↑	n.d.	Pijlman et al., 2003
Rat	Foot-shock	0, 24 and 48 hr, 9 d	=	=	n.d.	Bakshi et al., 2011
Rat	Foot-shock	2 weeks	=	=	n.d.	Bijlsma et al., 2009
Rat	Restraint	0	=	=	n.d.	Acri, 1994
Rat	Restraint	5 min	↓ , =	=	n.d.	Faraday, 2002
Rat	Restraint	30 min	↓	=	n.d.	Sutherland & Conti, 2011
Rat	Restraint	3 weeks	=	=	n.d.	Bijlsma et al., 2009

Table 1.a Overview of animal and human studies on effects of physical stressors in adult life on measures of sensory gating. PPI, prepulse inhibition; P50; P50 wave of event-related potential; n.d., not determined; ↑, ↓, =, response is improved, diminished, unchanged, respectively, when compared to control conditions.

Emotional stress						
Subject	**Intervention**	**Stress-test interval**	**PPI**	**Startle**	**P50**	**Reference**
Human	Mental stress	0	n.d.	n.d.		White & Yee, 1997
Human	Attention Threat - brief prolonged	0	↑ ↑ ↓	= ↑ n.d.	n.d.	Grillon & Davis, 1997
Rat	Threat (intense light)	0	↓	↑	n.d.	Current chapter
Rat	Predator	24 hrs	↓	=	n.d.	Bakshi et al., 2011
Rat	Predator	0, 46 hrs, 9 d	=	=	n.d.	Bakshi et al., 2011
Rat	Novelty (light)	0	↓	↓	n.d.	Schmajuk et al., 2009
Mouse	Social defeat	24 hrs	↓	=	n.d.	Brzozka et al., 2011
Rat	Witness stress	0	=	=	n.d.	Acri, 1994
Rat	Witness stress	5 days	=	=	n.d.	Pijlman et al., 2003

Table 1.b Overview of animal and human studies on effects of emotional stressors in adult life on measures of sensory gating. PPI, prepulse inhibition; P50; P50 wave of event-related potential; n.d., not determined; ↑, ↓, =, response is improved, diminished, unchanged, respectively, when compared to control conditions.

Based on the available studies, it is suggested that in healthy organisms, alterations in PPI induced by acute stress in adulthood are probably reversible, not causing permanent break down of gating mechanisms. Considering the neurodevelopmental theory of schizophrenia (section 1.3), it may be more etiologically relevant to apply the experimental stressors in early life. Therefore, in the next section, the effects of neurodevelopmental interventions on the rodent PPI response will be discussed.

3. Early-life stress and prepulse inhibition: neurodevelopmental animal models

According to neurodevelopmental theories (section 1.3), schizophrenia is considered a developmental disorder, influenced by both genes and the (early) environment. To get more insight into the possible role of early risk factors in the development of schizophrenia, early-stress paradigms are applied to laboratory rodents. In the following section, some common approaches for introducing developmental stress are reviewed, with their subsequent impact on PPI in later life. Note that this section does not attempt to exhaustively cover all available types of early stress in relevant animal models. The interested reader is referred to more in-depth articles on this topic (Van den Buuse et al., 2003; Markham & Koenig, 2011).

3.1 Isolation rearing

One developmental manipulation that has received particular attention with respect to PPI is isolation-rearing. In this procedure, rats or mice are housed in single cages from the time of weaning (about 21 days after birth) until adulthood (Bakshi & Geyer, 1999; Varty et al., 1999; Varty et al., 2006; Pietropaolo et al., 2008), and thereby deprived of social contact with their peers during (neuro)development (Einon & Morgan, 1977). In comparison to group-housed controls, postweaning-isolated rodents exhibit a range of brain and behavioral changes, reminiscent to schizophrenia (Powell et al., 2003; Van den Buuse et al., 2003; Harte et al., 2007). Several studies have reported PPI deficits in isolation-reared rats (Geyer et al., 2001) and mice (Varty et al., 2006; Pietropaolo et al., 2008), which could be reversed by pretreatment with typical and atypical antipsychotics (Varty & Higgins, 1995). However, subsequent studies have indicated that the effect of isolation rearing is strain dependent (Weiss et al., 2000), sensitive to housing conditions (Weiss et al., 1999), developmental timing (Wilkinson et al., 1994), and could be prevented by handling the isolated rats (Krebs-Thomson et al., 2001). Moreover, in order to effectively disrupt PPI, isolation rearing has to be maintained until the moment of testing (Bakshi & Geyer, 1999; Varty et al., 1999). Based on these drawbacks, the validity of isolation rearing as possible animal model for early life effects on schizophrenia-related behaviors is considered questionable (Geyer et al., 2001; Varty et al., 1999).

3.2 Maternal separation

Since rats and mice are born at a more immature stage of development than humans, neonatal interventions in these animals are comparable with adverse events in mid-late gestation in humans (Van den Buuse et al., 2003). In this respect, maternal separation, being a neonatal neurodevelopmental model, differs fundamentally from isolation rearing (see previous section), which is a post weaning model. Maternal deprivation, or the temporary separation of rodent pups from their mother early in life, leads to various neurochemical changes, some with relevance to schizophrenia (Van den Buuse et al., 2003).

At the behavioral level, a single 24-hours period of maternal deprivation (at postnatal days 6 or 9) has been shown to induce deficits in PPI in a delayed fashion (i.e. arising after puberty), suggesting that certain long-term processes are set in motion by the early deprivation (Ellenbroek et al., 1998). These deficits could be reversed by pretreatment with typical and atypical antipsychotics (Ellenbroek et al., 1998). The fact that changes in PPI do not appear before adulthood, led Ellenbroek and co-workers to investigate whether the effect is unavoidable, or rather dependent on manipulations after the deprivation period (Ellenbroek & Cools, 2002). First, they combined maternal deprivation with the post weaning isolation rearing procedure (see section 3.1.). Surprisingly, whereas both procedures were found to reliably disrupt PPI when applied separately, together they had no effect. Furthermore, they investigated the role of the mother, as the deprivation procedure obviously affects the dam, as well as the pups. To do this, either half of the litters were maternally deprived (in this way, the mother had pups to nurse during the deprivation period), or maternally deprived mothers were cross fostered to non-deprived pups and vice versa. In all cases, the pups displayed small deficits in PPI, compared to fully deprived controls, suggesting that the behavior of the mother, and possibly, her milk production, is also affected by the deprivation period. Thus, the authors concluded that the post-deprivation period is of crucial importance for the development of prepulse inhibition deficits in maternally deprived rats. Also, methodological factors such as timing, duration, and number of deprivation episodes, could possibly explain a lack of effect of maternal deprivation (Ellenbroek & Cools, 2002). Thereby, the ability of maternal separation to produce PPI-disrupting effects appears to be dependent on genetic strain (Ellenbroek & Cools, 2000), and species under study (rat vs. mouse) (Millstein & Holmes, 2007; Groenink et al., 2011; Naert et al., 2011).

Thus, maternal separation seems to induce PPI-deficits in a delayed fashion; however, the effect could be influenced by various protecting or facilitating post-deprivational factors, which might be similar to the influence of early-life stressors in humans.

3.3 Prenatal maternal immune activation

Epidemiological, clinical and preclinical studies have provided evidence that gestational exposure to certain infections, such as influenza, contributes to the etiology of schizophrenia (see Introduction). Similarly, animal models of maternal immune activation have yielded behavioral, neurochemical and neurophysiological findings that are consistent with observations in schizophrenia patients (Brown & Derkits, 2010). Currently, specific candidate infections have been identified that appear to be associated with an increased risk of schizophrenia, including rubella, influenza, herpes simplex, toxoplasma gondii, measles, polio, and genital and/or reproductive infections (Meyer & Feldon, 2009). A mechanism common to the immune response accompanying these infections, is the release of inflammatory cytokines. Consequently, elevation of maternal cytokine levels during pregnancy is thought to alter the trajectory of brain development, resulting in the induction of pathophysiological processes associated with mental illness (Markham & Koenig, 2011). Animal models of maternal immune challenge have used different immunogenic agents, all inducing a cytokine-associated inflammatory response in the mothers. However, other factors could be of relevance as well, for instance, immune activation is associated with fever, weight loss and elevated corticosteroids, which might compromise the offspring's *in utero* metabolic needs, thereby possibly affecting fetal brain development (Markham & Koenig, 2011). The effects of maternal infection on PPI have been investigated in several studies.

Systemic administration of bacterial endotoxin lipopolysaccharide (LPS) is capable of inducing a powerful immune response in the exposed animal, as well as fever and weight loss (Markham & Koenig, 2011). While LPS can be detected in both maternal and placental tissues, it is not found in the fetus (Ashdown et al., 2006), indicating that LPS itself is not responsible for the effects of maternal infection on the fetal brain. Several studies reported PPI disruptions in adult rat offspring of LPS infected mothers (Borrell et al., 2002; Fortier et al., 2007; Romero et al., 2007; Romero et al., 2010). These PPI deficits were associated with changes in dopaminergic transmission, and could be reversed by adult treatment with antipsychotics (Borrell et al., 2002; Romero et al., 2007). Interestingly, next to LPS, also turpentine, i.e. an inducer of local inflammation, at doses known to produce fever, significantly decreased PPI in adult offspring (Fortier et al., 2007). In analogy to the human situation, the influence of prenatal human influenza virus exposure on later brain development and behavior has been studied. Respiratory infection of pregnant BALB/c and C57BL/6 mice with the human influenza virus resulted in various behavioral abnormalities in the adult offspring, among which deficits in PPI, which were sensitive for antipsychotics (Shi et al., 2003). In other studies, offspring of similarly infected mice displayed morphological and neurochemical changes reminiscent to schizophrenia, although the importance of these effects for the PPI deficits is unclear (Van den Buuse et al., 2003). Of note, however, is the large reduction in expression of the brain protein reelin in cortex en hippocampus (Fatemi et al., 1999), which is associated with both schizophrenia (Guidotti et al., 2000) and impaired PPI (Pappas et al., 2001). Lastly, viral infection is simulated in rats and mice by polyriboinosinic-polyribocytidilic acid (poly I:C), an agent structurally similar to double-stranded RNA, which forms the genetic material of some viruses. While administration of poly I:C to pregnant rodents can result in increased levels of cytokines in fetal brain, it only generates a non-specific immune response, without particular anti-viral antibodies (for references, see Markham & Koenig, 2011). With respect to PPI, treatment of pregnant mice or rats with poly I:C generates offspring that shows an impaired PPI response from post pubertal age (Ozawa et al., 2006; Li et al., 2009b; Piontkewitz et al., 2009; Vuillermot et al., 2010), which is presumably mediated by dopaminergic maldevelopment (Ozawa et al., 2006; Vuillermot et al., 2010).

Thus, animal models of prenatal maternal infection show altered fetal brain development and disrupted PPI in adult offspring, probably mediated by the maternal immune response. These findings are in line with epidemiologic and clinical investigations on infection as a risk factor of schizophrenia (Brown et al., 2010).

3.4 Multiple stressors

Based on the two-hit hypothesis of schizophrenia (see Introduction), several experimental animal studies have applied multiple interventions at different stages of development, to investigate their combined influence on schizophrenia-like behaviors. Possibly, this method may give additional mechanistic insights compared to single interventions alone. In the remaining part of this section, studies addressing the combined effects of multiple interventions on PPI will be discussed.

In one study, the interaction between stress and dopaminergic regulation of PPI was investigated (Choy & van den Buuse, 2008; Choy et al., 2009). After combining two subsequent stressors in neonatal and young-adult life (i.e., maternal deprivation and prolonged corticosterone treatment, respectively), PPI was tested in rats following acute injections with apomorphine. In controls and in rats that had undergone either one of the two stressors, the apomorphine treatment was found to disrupt PPI, while in the group that had experienced the multiple stress, no PPI-disruptions were observed in response to apomorphine (Choy & van den Buuse, 2008). According to the authors, their findings implicate an inhibitory interaction of early and late developmental stress, on dopaminergic regulation of PPI (Choy & van den Buuse, 2008). In a follow-up study, the authors suggested that this inhibitory interaction may be caused by receptor desensitization, because no changes were found in levels of dopamine D1 and D2 receptors (Choy et al., 2009). Notably, the finding that a subsequent stressor could reverse PPI-disruptive effects of a particular stressor, has been reported elsewhere (i.e., maternal separation and isolation rearing, (Ellenbroek & Cools, 2002). The above-mentioned experiments are in line with the idea that glucocorticoids could affect PPI by modulation of dopaminergic systems (see section 2.2.).

In most studies addressing the two-hit hypothesis, the first hit comprises a genetic predisposition. Consequently, it is investigated how genes interact with early stress to produce schizophrenia-like neurochemical and behavioral alterations. As the focus of this chapter lies on the effects of stress on PPI, we will not discuss the neurochemical findings from genetic animal models of schizophrenia. Genotypes that have been found to interact with early stress to influence PPI include, nuclear receptor Nurr1 heterozygosity (i.e., 12 weeks of isolation rearing - Eells et al., 2006), Snap-25 mouse mutant *blind-drunk* (i.e., variable prenatal stress - Oliver & Davies, 2009), and NMDA receptor hypofunction mouse mutant (predation stress - Duncan et al., 2004). Notably, the latter study made use of predator olfactory cues (i.e., rat odor), which normalized the reduced PPI that was observed under control conditions in male mutants only. This result is in contrast to the study of Bakshi (section 2.1.3.), where predator exposure was found to decrease PPI in rats. However, an important methodological difference should be noted. Bakshi and co-workers actually introduced a predator in their experiment, while Duncan et al. only exposed the animals to predator odor. This difference in approach might have implications for the level of threat perceived by the subjects. In particular, when solely olfactory cues signal predation risk, perceiving animals may become more vigilant, which is thought to facilitate processing of sensory stimuli, possibly increasing PPI. Proximal presence of the predator, on the other hand, is likely to represent a severe stressor, which may induce disruptions in PPI due to progressive loss of sensory perception (see section 2.4.). Possibly, the delayed stress effect observed in the Bakshi study could be accounted for by recruitment of central mediators of the stress response, such as CRF.

In conclusion, although limited, the studies mentioned in this section suggest that combining multiple stressors, or a genetic vulnerability and stress, may induce stronger alterations in sensorimotor gating, when compared to one single intervention. Further relevant studies are warranted to test this hypothesis.

4. General conclusions

In this chapter, we have discussed studies that investigated the association between experience of stress and PPI, the latter being a highly validated model for schizophrenia; a mental disorder that is thought to be caused by an interaction of a constitutional vulnerability with environmental stress (see Introduction). From both animal and human studies, it is found that - by an unknown mechanism - application of acute stressors in adulthood is able to affect PPI, at least, transiently (table 1). Possibly, on the short term, moderate threat or attention to the environment could facilitate processing of sensory stimuli via elevated cortical arousal, leading to increased information processing; while severe or prolonged stressors may cause progressive loss of sensory perception that functions to reduce the impact of impending aversive events (section 2.4.). These perceptual deteriorations may be mediated by, for instance, cortisol- and CRF-induced activation of the mesolimbic dopamine system, a neural system that is implicated in both stress responsivity and PPI. Also, it is suggested that alterations in PPI induced by the acute stressors under study are probably reversible, not causing permanent changes to brain structures important in the regulation of PPI. These results are in line with clinical and epidemiological findings, which suggest that experience of stressful life events does not trigger onset of psychotic illness in healthy individuals (see Introduction). However, clearly, the acute and chronic stressors applied in the laboratory do not mimic 'naturally occurring' transient stress in the real world. This type of stress may come and go, and, depending on how long it stays, it could ultimately cause permanent alterations in brain systems associated with psychosis in vulnerable individuals, as was observed in longitudinal studies (reviewed by Phillips et al., 2007; Walker et al., 2008).

The clinical observation that schizophrenia generally does not manifest until the third decade of life, suggests that it is the final outcome of pathological processes acting on the immature brain, and accordingly, it has led to formulation of the neurodevelopmental theory for the etiology of schizophrenia (see Introduction). In order to get more insight into the possible role of early environmental risk factors in illness development, early-stress paradigms are applied to rodents. Some developmental manipulations that have been shown to affect adult PPI include isolation rearing, maternal separation, and prenatal maternal immune activation (section 3). An alternative hypothesis within the framework of the neurodevelopmental theory of schizophrenia is referred to as the two-hit model. According to this model, early and late risk factors are not simply additive, but instead, the first hit will increase an individual's vulnerability for effects of a subsequent hit (see Introduction). Based on this theory, a few animal studies have applied multiple interventions at subsequent stages of development, to study their combined impact on schizophrenia-like behaviors, including PPI. Interestingly, although limited, results so far do not support the theory. Rather, instead of an augmentation, an inhibitory interaction of early and later developmental stress has been reported by two independent research groups. On the other hand, several studies have successfully identified candidate genes that could contribute to the induction of schizophrenia-like phenotypes in interaction with stress (section 3.4.). Possibly, investigating the interaction of these candidate genes with experimental stressors in animal studies, could represent a fruitful approach to model the link between stress and schizophrenia.

In humans, it is known that a wide variation exists in response to adversity, with some individuals being more stress-sensitive than others, and some individuals being more prone to developing an illness in response to environmental adversity than others (Kendler et al., 2005). Attempts have been made to explain the source of this variation; several studies have investigated the link between genetic polymorphisms and environmental stress in the etiology of schizophrenia. Some progress has been made, for instance, a recent genome-wide association study - contrasting large numbers of genetic variants in patients and controls - revealed significant associations between schizophrenia and polymorphisms in major histocompatibility complex (MHC), a region implicated in the bodily reactions to stress and infection (Stefansson et al., 2009). Also, although not yet replicated, the novel schizophrenia risk polymorphism ZNF804A was found to be associated with increased prefrontal-hippocampal and prefrontal-amygdala connectivity, possibly linking to increased sensitivity to stressful environments (Esslinger et al., 2009). In another study, the association between a serotonin transporter gene polymorphism (i.e. 5-HTTLPR), stress and disease characteristics was investigated in individuals diagnosed with psychotic disease (Goldberg et al., 2009). Therefore, symptoms occurring in the four-week period preceding hospitalization were evaluated in first-onset patients. As a result, stress (i.e. negative life-events preceding hospitalization) was found to be a predictor of depressive symptoms, but it did not interact with psychotic (or negative) symptoms. Together, the above-mentioned studies have genetically linked schizophrenia with several systems/brain structures important in stress regulation (e.g., MHC, amygdala, PFC). However, so far, no experimental studies have linked this gene-environment interaction with schizophrenia, which is probably caused by the fact that schizophrenia is a complex disorder, putatively determined by the sum of numerous small effects of individual genes; hence the importance of using endophenotypes such as PPI in association studies.

In conclusion, the link between stress and PPI appears to be in line with neurodevelopmental theories of schizophrenia; a single stressor in adult life does not seem to cause lasting alterations in PPI, however, when applied during a critical stage of neurodevelopment or in genetically vulnerable organisms, stress could be more powerful in robustly affecting PPI. It is suggested, that future animal studies aimed at investigating the role of stress in the development of information processing dysfunctions in schizophrenia, may benefit from implementing human risk gene polymorphisms that are associated with stress (e.g. by making use of inducible transgenic mouse models).

5. References

Acri J.B. (1994). Nicotine modulates effects of stress on acoustic startle reflexes in rats: dependence on dose, stressor and initial reactivity. *Psychopharmacology (Berl),* 116, No. 3, pp. 255-265, 0033-3158

Adler L.E., Hoffer L., Nagamoto H.T., Waldo M.C., Kisley M.A., & Giffith J.M. (1994). Yohimbine impairs P50 auditory sensory gating in normal subjects. *Neuropsychopharmacology,* 10, No. 4, pp. 249-257

Adler L.E., Pachtman E., Franks R.D., Pecevich M., Waldo M.C., & Freedman R. (1982). Neurophysiological evidence for a defect in neuronal mechanisms involved in sensory gating in schizophrenia. *Biol Psychiatry,* 17, No. 6, pp. 639-654, 0006-3223

Aggernaes B., Glenthoj B.Y., Ebdrup B.H., Rasmussen H., Lublin H., & Oranje B. (2010). Sensorimotor gating and habituation in antipsychotic-naive, first-episode schizophrenia patients before and after 6 months' treatment with quetiapine. *Int J Neuropsychopharmacol,* 13, No. 10, pp. 1383-1395, 1469-5111

APA (2000). *Diagnostic and statistical manual of mental disorders, DSM-IV-TR* (4th ed), American Psychiatric Association, Washington, D.C.

Ashdown H., Dumont Y., Ng M., Poole S., Boksa P., & Luheshi G.N. (2006). The role of cytokines in mediating effects of prenatal infection on the fetus: implications for schizophrenia. *Mol Psychiatry,* 11, No. 1, pp. 47-55, 1359-4184

Bakshi V.P., Alsene K.M., Roseboom P.H., & Connors E.E. (2011). Enduring sensorimotor gating abnormalities following predator exposure or corticotropin-releasing factor in rats: A model for PTSD-like information-processing deficits? *Neuropharmacology,* 1873-7064

Bakshi V.P., Geyer M.A. (1999). Ontogeny of isolation rearing-induced deficits in sensorimotor gating in rats. *Physiol Behav,* 67, No. 3, pp. 385-392, 0031-9384

Belforte J.E., Zsiros V., Sklar E.R., et al. (2010). Postnatal NMDA receptor ablation in corticolimbic interneurons confers schizophrenia-like phenotypes. *Nat Neurosci,* 13, No. 1, pp. 76-83, 1546-1726

Bijlsma E.Y., Oosting R.S., Olivier B., & Groenink L. (2010). Disrupted startle modulation in animal models for affective disorders. *Behav Brain Res,* 208, No. 2, pp. 383-390, 1872-7549

Borrell J., Vela J.M., Arevalo-Martin A., Molina-Holgado E., & Guaza C. (2002). Prenatal immune challenge disrupts sensorimotor gating in adult rats. Implications for the etiopathogenesis of schizophrenia. *Neuropsychopharmacology,* 26, No. 2, pp. 204-215

Bortolato M., Aru G.N., Frau R., et al. (2005). Kappa opioid receptor activation disrupts prepulse inhibition of the acoustic startle in rats. *Biol Psychiatry,* 57, No. 12, pp. 1550-1558, 0006-3223

Braff D., Stone C., Callaway E., Geyer M., Glick I., & Bali L. (1978). Prestimulus effects on human startle reflex in normals and schizophrenics. *Psychophysiology,* 15, No. 4, pp. 339-343, 0048-5772

Braff D.L., Greenwood T.A., Swerdlow N.R., Light G.A., Schork N.J., & The Investigators of the Consortium on the Genetics of Schizophrenia (2008). Advances in endophenotyping schizophrenia. *World Psychiatry,* 7, No. 1, pp. 11-18, 1723-8617

Braff D.L., Geyer M.A., & Swerdlow N.R. (2001a). Human studies of prepulse inhibition of startle: normal subjects, patient groups, and pharmacological studies. *Psychopharmacology (Berl),* 156, No. 2-3, pp. 234-258, 0033-3158

Braff D.L., Geyer M.A., & Swerdlow N.R. (2001b). Human studies of prepulse inhibition of startle: normal subjects, patient groups, and pharmacological studies. *Psychopharmacology (Berl),* 156, No. 2-3, pp. 234-258, 0033-3158

Brenner K., Liu A., Laplante D.P., et al. (2009). Cortisol response to a psychosocial stressor in schizophrenia: blunted, delayed, or normal? *Psychoneuroendocrinology,* 34, No. 6, pp. 859-868, 1873-3360

Brown A.S., Derkits E.J. (2010). Prenatal infection and schizophrenia: a review of epidemiologic and translational studies. *Am J Psychiatry,* 167, No. 3, pp. 261-280, 1535-7228

Brzozka M.M., Fischer A., Falkai P., & Havemann-Reinecke U. (2011). Acute treatment with cannabinoid receptor agonist WIN55212.2 improves prepulse inhibition in psychosocially stressed mice. *Behav Brain Res,* 218, No. 2, pp. 280-287, 1872-7549

Charney D.S., Deutch A.Y., Krystal J.H., Southwick S.M., & Davis M. (1993). Psychobiologic mechanisms of posttraumatic stress disorder. *Arch Gen Psychiatry,* 50, No. 4, pp. 295-305, 0003-990X

Choy K.H., de Visser Y.P., & van den Buuse M. (2009). The effect of 'two hit' neonatal and young-adult stress on dopaminergic modulation of prepulse inhibition and dopamine receptor density. *Br J Pharmacol,* 156, No. 2, pp. 388-396, 1476-5381

Choy K.H., van den Buuse M. (2008). Attenuated disruption of prepulse inhibition by dopaminergic stimulation after maternal deprivation and adolescent corticosterone treatment in rats. *Eur Neuropsychopharmacol,* 18, No. 1, pp. 1-13, 0924-977X

Conti L.H. (2005). Characterization of the effects of corticotropin-releasing factor on prepulse inhibition of the acoustic startle response in Brown Norway and Wistar-Kyoto rats. *Eur J Pharmacol,* 507, No. 1-3, pp. 125-134, 0014-2999

Conti L.H., Murry J.D., Ruiz M.A., & Printz M.P. (2002). Effects of corticotropin-releasing factor on prepulse inhibition of the acoustic startle response in two rat strains. *Psychopharmacology (Berl),* 161, No. 3, pp. 296-303, 0033-3158

Cornwell B.R., Echiverri A.M., Covington M.F., & Grillon C. (2008). Modality-specific attention under imminent but not remote threat of shock: evidence from differential prepulse inhibition of startle. *Psychol Sci,* 19, No. 6, pp. 615-622, 0956-7976

Czyrak A., Mackowiak M., Chocyk A., Fijal K., Gadek-Michalska A., & Wedzony K. (2003). 8-OHDPAT-induced disruption of prepulse inhibition in rats is attenuated by prolonged corticosterone treatment. *Neuropsychopharmacology,* 28, No. 7, pp. 1300-1310 de Jongh R., Groenink L., van Der Gugten J., & Olivier B. (2002). The light-enhanced startle paradigm as a putative animal model for anxiety: effects of chlordiazepoxide, flesinoxan and fluvoxamine. *Psychopharmacology (Berl),* 159, No. 2, pp. 176-180, 0033-3158

Dirks A., Groenink L., Bouwknecht J.A., et al. (2002). Overexpression of corticotropin-releasing hormone in transgenic mice and chronic stress-like autonomic and physiological alterations. *Eur J Neurosci,* 16, No. 9, pp. 1751-1760, 0953-816X

Duncan G.E., Moy S.S., Perez A., et al. (2004). Deficits in sensorimotor gating and tests of social behavior in a genetic model of reduced NMDA receptor function. *Behav Brain Res,* 153, No. 2, pp. 507-519

Eells J.B., Misler J.A., & Nikodem V.M. (2006). Early postnatal isolation reduces dopamine levels, elevates dopamine turnover and specifically disrupts prepulse inhibition in Nurr1-null heterozygous mice. *Neuroscience,* 140, No. 4, pp. 1117-1126, 0306-4522

Einon D.F., Morgan M.J. (1977). A critical period for social isolation in the rat. *Dev Psychobiol,* 10, No. 2, pp. 123-132, 0012-1630

Ellenbroek B.A., Cools A.R. (2002). Early maternal deprivation and prepulse inhibition: the role of the postdeprivation environment. *Pharmacol Biochem Behav,* 73, No. 1, pp. 177-184, 0091-3057

Ellenbroek B.A., Cools A.R. (2000). The long-term effects of maternal deprivation depend on the genetic background. *Neuropsychopharmacology,* 23, No. 1, pp. 99-106, 0893-133X

Ellenbroek B.A., van den Kroonenberg P.T., & Cools A.R. (1998). The effects of an early stressful life event on sensorimotor gating in adult rats. *Schizophr Res,* 30, No. 3, pp. 251-260, 0920-9964

Ermutlu M.N., Karamursel S., Ugur E.H., Senturk L., & Gokhan N. (2005). Effects of cold stress on early and late stimulus gating. *Psychiatry Res,* 136, No. 2-3, pp. 201-209, 0165-1781

Esslinger C., Walter H., Kirsch P., et al. (2009). Neural mechanisms of a genome-wide supported psychosis variant. *Science,* 324, No. 5927, pp. 605, 1095-9203

Faraday M.M. (2002). Rat sex and strain differences in responses to stress. *Physiol Behav,* 75, No. 4, pp. 507-522, 0031-9384

Faraday M.M., O'Donoghue V.A., & Grunberg N.E. (1999). Effects of nicotine and stress on startle amplitude and sensory gating depend on rat strain and sex. *Pharmacol Biochem Behav,* 62, No. 2, pp. 273-284, 0091-3057

Fatemi S.H., Folsom T.D. (2009). The neurodevelopmental hypothesis of schizophrenia, revisited. *Schizophr Bull,* 35, No. 3, pp. 528-548, 0586-7614

Fatemi S.H., Emamian E.S., Kist D., et al. (1999). Defective corticogenesis and reduction in Reelin immunoreactivity in cortex and hippocampus of prenatally infected neonatal mice. *Mol Psychiatry,* 4, No. 2, pp. 145-154, 1359-4184

Fortier M.E., Luheshi G.N., & Boksa P. (2007). Effects of prenatal infection on prepulse inhibition in the rat depend on the nature of the infectious agent and the stage of pregnancy. *Behav Brain Res,* 181, No. 2, pp. 270-277, 0166-4328

Geyer M.A., Krebs-Thomson K., Braff D.L., & Swerdlow N.R. (2001). Pharmacological studies of prepulse inhibition models of sensorimotor gating deficits in schizophrenia: a decade in review. *Psychopharmacology (Berl),* 156, No. 2-3, pp. 117-154, 0033-3158

Goldberg T.E., Kotov R., Lee A.T., et al. (2009). The serotonin transporter gene and disease modification in psychosis: evidence for systematic differences in allelic directionality at the 5-HTTLPR locus. *Schizophr Res,* 111, No. 1-3, pp. 103-108

Grillon C., Davis M. (1997). Effects of stress and shock anticipation on prepulse inhibition of the startle reflex. *Psychophysiology,* 34, No. 5, pp. 511-517, 0048-5772

Groenink L., Bijlsma E.Y., van Bogaert M.J., Oosting R.S., & Olivier B. (2011). Serotonin1A receptor deletion does not interact with maternal separation-induced increases in startle reactivity and prepulse inhibition deficits. *Psychopharmacology (Berl),* 214, No. 1, pp. 353-365, 1432-2072

Guidotti A., Auta J., Davis J.M., et al. (2000). Decrease in reelin and glutamic acid decarboxylase67 (GAD67) expression in schizophrenia and bipolar disorder: a postmortem brain study. *Arch Gen Psychiatry,* 57, No. 11, pp. 1061-1069, 0003-990X

Harrison P.J. (1997). Schizophrenia: a disorder of neurodevelopment? *Curr Opin Neurobiol,* 7, No. 2, pp. 285-289, 0959-4388

Harte M.K., Powell S.B., Swerdlow N.R., Geyer M.A., & Reynolds G.P. (2007). Deficits in parvalbumin and calbindin immunoreactive cells in the hippocampus of isolation reared rats. *J Neural Transm,* 114, No. 7, pp. 893-898, 1435-1463

Herringa R.J., Roseboom P.H., & Kalin N.H. (2006). Decreased amygdala CRF-binding protein mRNA in post-mortem tissue from male but not female bipolar and schizophrenic subjects. *Neuropsychopharmacology,* 31, No. 8, pp. 1822-1831

Jensen K.S., Oranje B., Wienberg M., & Glenthoj B.Y. (2007). The effects of increased central serotonergic activity on prepulse inhibition and habituation of the human startle response. *Neuropsychopharmacology,* 32, No. 10, pp. 2117-2124, 0893-133X

Johnson M.R., Adler L.E. (1993). Transient impairment in P50 auditory sensory gating induced by a cold-pressor test. *Biol Psychiatry,* 33, No. 5, pp. 380-387, 0006-3223

Kaneyuki H., Yokoo H., Tsuda A., et al. (1991). Psychological stress increases dopamine turnover selectively in mesoprefrontal dopamine neurons of rats: reversal by diazepam. *Brain Res,* 557, No. 1-2, pp. 154-161, 0006-8993

Kendler K.S., Kuhn J.W., Vittum J., Prescott C.A., & Riley B. (2005). The interaction of stressful life events and a serotonin transporter polymorphism in the prediction of episodes of major depression: a replication. *Arch Gen Psychiatry,* 62, No. 5, pp. 529-535, 0003-990X

Keshavan M.S. (1999). Development, disease and degeneration in schizophrenia: a unitary pathophysiological model. *J Psychiatr Res,* 33, No. 6, pp. 513-521, 0022-3956

Keshavan M.S., Hogarty G.E. (1999). Brain maturational processes and delayed onset in schizophrenia. *Dev Psychopathol,* 11, No. 3, pp. 525-543, 0954-5794

Krebs-Thomson K., Giracello D., Solis A., & Geyer M.A. (2001). Post-weaning handling attenuates isolation-rearing induced disruptions of prepulse inhibition in rats. *Behav Brain Res,* 120, No. 2, pp. 221-224, 0166-4328

Leitner D.S. (1989). Multisensory deficits in rats produced by acute exposure to cold swim stress. *Behav Neurosci,* 103, No. 1, pp. 151-157, 0735-7044

Leitner D.S. (1986). Alterations in other sensory modalities accompanying stress analgesia as measured by startle reflex modification. *Ann N Y Acad Sci,* 467, pp. 82-92, 0077-8923

Li L., Du Y., Li N., Wu X., & Wu Y. (2009a). Top-down modulation of prepulse inhibition of the startle reflex in humans and rats. *Neurosci Biobehav Rev,* 33, No. 8, pp. 1157-1167, 1873-7528

Li Q., Cheung C., Wei R., et al. (2009b). Prenatal immune challenge is an environmental risk factor for brain and behavior change relevant to schizophrenia: evidence from MRI in a mouse model. *PLoS One,* 4, No. 7, pp. e6354, 1932-6203

Madden J.,4th, Akil H., Patrick R.L., & Barchas J.D. (1977). Stress-induced parallel changes in central opioid levels and pain responsiveness in the rat. *Nature,* 265, No. 5592, pp. 358-360, 0028-0836

Marinelli M., Rudick C.N., Hu X.T., & White F.J. (2006). Excitability of dopamine neurons: modulation and physiological consequences. *CNS Neurol Disord Drug Targets,* 5, No. 1, pp. 79-97, 1871-5273

Markham J.A., Koenig J.I. (2011). Prenatal stress: role in psychotic and depressive diseases. *Psychopharmacology (Berl),* 214, No. 1, pp. 89-106, 1432-2072

Maynard T.M., Sikich L., Lieberman J.A., & LaMantia A.S. (2001). Neural development, cell-cell signaling, and the "two-hit" hypothesis of schizophrenia. *Schizophr Bull,* 27, No. 3, pp. 457-476, 0586-7614

Meyer U., Feldon J. (2009). Neural basis of psychosis-related behaviour in the infection model of schizophrenia. *Behav Brain Res,* 204, No. 2, pp. 322-334, 1872-7549

Millstein R.A., Holmes A. (2007). Effects of repeated maternal separation on anxiety- and depression-related phenotypes in different mouse strains. *Neurosci Biobehav Rev,* 31, No. 1, pp. 3-17, 0149-7634

Naert A., Callaerts-Vegh Z., & D'Hooge R. (2011). Nocturnal hyperactivity, increased social novelty preference and delayed extinction of fear responses in post-weaning socially isolated mice. *Brain Res Bull,* 1873-2747

Nemeroff C.B., Widerlov E., Bissette G., et al. (1984). Elevated concentrations of CSF corticotropin-releasing factor-like immunoreactivity in depressed patients. *Science,* 226, No. 4680, pp. 1342-1344, 0036-8075

Oliver P.L., Davies K.E. (2009). Interaction between environmental and genetic factors modulates schizophrenic endophenotypes in the Snap-25 mouse mutant blind-drunk. *Hum Mol Genet,* 18, No. 23, pp. 4576-4589, 1460-2083

Oranje B., Wienberg M., & Glenthoj B.Y. (2011). A single high dose of escitalopram disrupts sensory gating and habituation, but not sensorimotor gating in healthy volunteers. *Psychiatry Res,* 186, No. 2-3, pp. 431-436, 0165-1781

Oranje B., Kahn R.S., Kemner C., & Verbaten M.N. (2004). Modulating sensorimotor gating in healthy volunteers: the effects of desipramine and haloperidol. *Psychiatry Res,* 127, No. 3, pp. 195-205, 0165-1781

Ozawa K., Hashimoto K., Kishimoto T., Shimizu E., Ishikura H., & Iyo M. (2006). Immune activation during pregnancy in mice leads to dopaminergic hyperfunction and cognitive impairment in the offspring: a neurodevelopmental animal model of schizophrenia. *Biol Psychiatry,* 59, No. 6, pp. 546-554, 0006-3223

Palmer A.A., Dulawa S.C., Mottiwala A.A., Conti L.H., Geyer M.A., & Printz M.P. (2000). Prepulse startle deficit in the Brown Norway rat: a potential genetic model. *Behav Neurosci,* 114, No. 2, pp. 374-388, 0735-7044

Pappas G.D., Kriho V., & Pesold C. (2001). Reelin in the extracellular matrix and dendritic spines of the cortex and hippocampus: a comparison between wild type and heterozygous reeler mice by immunoelectron microscopy. *J Neurocytol,* 30, No. 5, pp. 413-425, 0300-4864

Phillips L.J., Francey S.M., Edwards J., & McMurray N. (2007). Stress and psychosis: towards the development of new models of investigation. *Clin Psychol Rev,* 27, No. 3, pp. 307-317, 0272-7358

Phillips L.J., McGorry P.D., Garner B., et al. (2006). Stress, the hippocampus and the hypothalamic-pituitary-adrenal axis: implications for the development of psychotic disorders. *Aust N Z J Psychiatry,* 40, No. 9, pp. 725-741, 0004-8674

Piacentini M.F., Meeusen R., Buyse L., De Schutter G., & De Meirleir K. (2004). Hormonal responses during prolonged exercise are influenced by a selective DA/NA reuptake inhibitor. *Br J Sports Med,* 38, No. 2, pp. 129-133, 0306-3674

Pietropaolo S., Crusio W.E. (2009). Strain-Dependent Changes in Acoustic Startle Response and its Plasticity Across Adolescence in Mice. *Behav Genet,* 1573-3297

Pietropaolo S., Singer P., Feldon J., & Yee B.K. (2008). The postweaning social isolation in C57BL/6 mice: preferential vulnerability in the male sex. *Psychopharmacology (Berl),* 197, No. 4, pp. 613-628, 0033-3158

Pijlman F.T., Herremans A.H., van de Kieft J., Kruse C.G., & van Ree J.M. (2003). Behavioural changes after different stress paradigms: prepulse inhibition increased after physical, but not emotional stress. *Eur Neuropsychopharmacol,* 13, No. 5, pp. 369-380, 0924-977X

Piontkewitz Y., Assaf Y., & Weiner I. (2009). Clozapine administration in adolescence prevents postpubertal emergence of brain structural pathology in an animal model of schizophrenia. *Biol Psychiatry,* 66, No. 11, pp. 1038-1046, 1873-2402

Powell S.B., Geyer M.A., Preece M.A., Pitcher L.K., Reynolds G.P., & Swerdlow N.R. (2003). Dopamine depletion of the nucleus accumbens reverses isolation-induced deficits in prepulse inhibition in rats. *Neuroscience,* 119, No. 1, pp. 233-240, 0306-4522

Pruessner J.C., Champagne F., Meaney M.J., & Dagher A. (2004). Dopamine release in response to a psychological stress in humans and its relationship to early life maternal care: a positron emission tomography study using [11C]raclopride. *J Neurosci,* 24, No. 11, pp. 2825-2831, 1529-2401

Rehn A.E., Rees S.M. (2005). Investigating the neurodevelopmental hypothesis of schizophrenia. *Clin Exp Pharmacol Physiol,* 32, No. 9, pp. 687-696, 0305-1870

Richter S., Schulz A., Zech C.M., et al. (2010). Cortisol rapidly disrupts prepulse inhibition in healthy men. *Psychoneuroendocrinology,* 1873-3360

Risbrough V.B., Hauger R.L., Roberts A.L., Vale W.W., & Geyer M.A. (2004). Corticotropin-releasing factor receptors CRF1 and CRF2 exert both additive and opposing influences on defensive startle behavior. *J Neurosci,* 24, No. 29, pp. 6545-6552, 1529-2401

Romero E., Guaza C., Castellano B., & Borrell J. (2010). Ontogeny of sensorimotor gating and immune impairment induced by prenatal immune challenge in rats: implications for the etiopathology of schizophrenia. *Mol Psychiatry,* 15, No. 4, pp. 372-383, 1476-5578

Romero E., Ali C., Molina-Holgado E., Castellano B., Guaza C., & Borrell J. (2007). Neurobehavioral and immunological consequences of prenatal immune activation in rats. Influence of antipsychotics. *Neuropsychopharmacology,* 32, No. 8, pp. 1791-1804

Sautter F.J., Bissette G., Wiley J., et al. (2003). Corticotropin-releasing factor in posttraumatic stress disorder (PTSD) with secondary psychotic symptoms, nonpsychotic PTSD, and healthy control subjects. *Biol Psychiatry,* 54, No. 12, pp. 1382-1388, 0006-3223

Schmajuk N.A., Larrauri J.A., De la Casa L.G., & Levin E.D. (2009). Attenuation of auditory startle and prepulse inhibition by unexpected changes in ambient illumination through dopaminergic mechanisms. *Behav Brain Res,* 197, No. 2, pp. 251-261, 1872-7549

Selten J.P., Cantor-Graae E. (2007). Hypothesis: social defeat is a risk factor for schizophrenia? *Br J Psychiatry Suppl,* 51, pp. s9-12, 0960-5371

Shi L., Fatemi S.H., Sidwell R.W., & Patterson P.H. (2003). Maternal influenza infection causes marked behavioral and pharmacological changes in the offspring. *J Neurosci,* 23, No. 1, pp. 297-302, 1529-2401

St Clair D., Xu M., Wang P., et al. (2005). Rates of adult schizophrenia following prenatal exposure to the Chinese famine of 1959-1961. *JAMA,* 294, No. 5, pp. 557-562, 1538-3598

Stahl S.M. (2008). *Stahl's essential psychopharmacology: neuroscientific basis and practical applications* (3rd ed), Cambridge University Press, 978-0-521-85702-4, New York

Stefansson H., Ophoff R.A., Steinberg S., et al. (2009). Common variants conferring risk of schizophrenia. *Nature,* 460, No. 7256, pp. 744-747, 1476-4687

Susser E., Hoek H.W., & Brown A. (1998). Neurodevelopmental disorders after prenatal famine: The story of the Dutch Famine Study. *Am J Epidemiol,* 147, No. 3, pp. 213-216, 0002-9262

Susser E., Neugebauer R., Hoek H.W., et al. (1996). Schizophrenia after prenatal famine. Further evidence. *Arch Gen Psychiatry,* 53, No. 1, pp. 25-31, 0003-990X

Susser E.S., Lin S.P. (1992). Schizophrenia after prenatal exposure to the Dutch Hunger Winter of 1944-1945. *Arch Gen Psychiatry,* 49, No. 12, pp. 983-988, 0003-990X

Sutherland J.E., Conti L.H. (2011). Restraint stress-induced reduction in prepulse inhibition in Brown Norway rats: role of the CRF2 receptor. *Neuropharmacology,* 60, No. 4, pp. 561-571, 1873-7064

Swerdlow N.R., Weber M., Qu Y., Light G.A., & Braff D.L. (2008). Realistic expectations of prepulse inhibition in translational models for schizophrenia research. *Psychopharmacology (Berl),* 199, No. 3, pp. 331-388, 0033-3158

Swerdlow N.R., Talledo J., Sutherland A.N., Nagy D., & Shoemaker J.M. (2006). Antipsychotic effects on prepulse inhibition in normal 'low gating' humans and rats. *Neuropsychopharmacology,* 31, No. 9, pp. 2011-2021

Swerdlow N.R., Geyer M.A., & Braff D.L. (2001). Neural circuit regulation of prepulse inhibition of startle in the rat: current knowledge and future challenges. *Psychopharmacology (Berl),* 156, No. 2-3, pp. 194-215, 0033-3158

van den Buuse M., Morris M., Chavez C., Martin S., & Wang J. (2004). Effect of adrenalectomy and corticosterone replacement on prepulse inhibition and locomotor activity in mice. *Br J Pharmacol,* 142, No. 3, pp. 543-550, 0007-1188

Van den Buuse M., Garner B., & Koch M. (2003). Neurodevelopmental animal models of schizophrenia: effects on prepulse inhibition. *Curr Mol Med,* 3, No. 5, pp. 459-471, 1566-5240

Van Pett K., Viau V., Bittencourt J.C., et al. (2000). Distribution of mRNAs encoding CRF receptors in brain and pituitary of rat and mouse. *J Comp Neurol,* 428, No. 2, pp. 191-212, 0021-9967

van Venrooij J.A., Fluitman S.B., Lijmer J.G., et al. (2010). Impaired Neuroendocrine and Immune Response to Acute Stress in Medication-Naive Patients With a First Episode of Psychosis. *Schizophr Bull,* 1745-1701

Varty G.B., Powell S.B., Lehmann-Masten V., Buell M.R., & Geyer M.A. (2006). Isolation rearing of mice induces deficits in prepulse inhibition of the startle response. *Behav Brain Res,* 169, No. 1, pp. 162-167, 0166-4328

Varty G.B., Braff D.L., & Geyer M.A. (1999). Is there a critical developmental 'window' for isolation rearing-induced changes in prepulse inhibition of the acoustic startle response? *Behav Brain Res,* 100, No. 1-2, pp. 177-183, 0166-4328

Varty G.B., Geyer M.A. (1998). Effects of isolation rearing on startle reactivity, habituation, and prepulse inhibition in male Lewis, Sprague-Dawley, and Fischer F344 rats. *Behav Neurosci,* 112, No. 6, pp. 1450-1457, 0735-7044

Varty G.B., Higgins G.A. (1995). Examination of drug-induced and isolation-induced disruptions of prepulse inhibition as models to screen antipsychotic drugs. *Psychopharmacology (Berl),* 122, No. 1, pp. 15-26, 0033-3158

Vuillermot S., Weber L., Feldon J., & Meyer U. (2010). A longitudinal examination of the neurodevelopmental impact of prenatal immune activation in mice reveals primary defects in dopaminergic development relevant to schizophrenia. *J Neurosci,* 30, No. 4, pp. 1270-1287, 1529-2401

Walker E., Mittal V., & Tessner K. (2008). Stress and the hypothalamic pituitary adrenal axis in the developmental course of schizophrenia. *Annu Rev Clin Psychol,* 4, pp. 189-216

Walker E.F., Diforio D. (1997). Schizophrenia: a neural diathesis-stress model. *Psychol Rev,* 104, No. 4, pp. 667-685, 0033-295X

Wan F.J., Swerdlow N.R. (1993). Intra-accumbens infusion of quinpirole impairs sensorimotor gating of acoustic startle in rats. *Psychopharmacology (Berl),* 113, No. 1, pp. 103-109, 0033-3158

Weiss I.C., Di Iorio L., Feldon J., & Domeney A.M. (2000). Strain differences in the isolation-induced effects on prepulse inhibition of the acoustic startle response and on locomotor activity. *Behav Neurosci,* 114, No. 2, pp. 364-373, 0735-7044

Weiss I.C., Feldon J., & Domeney A.M. (1999). Isolation rearing-induced disruption of prepulse inhibition: further evidence for fragility of the response. *Behav Pharmacol,* 10, No. 2, pp. 139-149, 0955-8810

White P.M., Yee C.M. (1997). Effects of attentional and stressor manipulations on the P50 gating response. *Psychophysiology,* 34, No. 6, pp. 703-711, 0048-5772

Wilkinson L.S., Killcross S.S., Humby T., Hall F.S., Geyer M.A., & Robbins T.W. (1994). Social isolation in the rat produces developmentally specific deficits in prepulse inhibition of the acoustic startle response without disrupting latent inhibition. *Neuropsychopharmacology,* 10, No. 1, pp. 61-72, 0893-133X

Willer J.C., Ernst M. (1986). Somatovegetative changes in stress-induced analgesia in man: an electrophysiological and pharmacological study. *Ann N Y Acad Sci,* 467, pp. 256-272, 0077-8923

Yeap S., Thakore J.H. (2005). Stress axis dysfunction in schizophrenia. *Eur Psychiatry,* 20 Suppl 3, pp. S307-12, 0924-9338

Zubin J., Spring B. (1977). Vulnerability--a new view of schizophrenia. *J Abnorm Psychol,* 86, No. 2, pp. 103-126, 0021-843X

6

Childhood and Adolescent Schizophrenia and Other Early-Onset Psychoses

Hojka Gregoric Kumperscak
Child and Adolescent Psychiatry Unit, Paediatrics Clinic
University Clinical Center Maribor
Slovenia

1. Introduction

Children and adolescents can have a variety of psychotic disorders from acute and transitory psychoses to chronic ones, such as schizophrenia. Their psychotic symptomatology, however, can also be the consequence of an organic cause or drug-inducted. Comparing to adolescence and adulthood, psychotic disorders in childhood seem to occur more rarely, which can be explained by lower incidence and diagnostic problems - hallucinations and delusions in children are quite difficult to recognise (Turk et al., 2007).

While schizophrenia is a very rare disorder in childhood, it becomes increasingly common during adolescence. It is actually the most frequent psychotic disorder in the age group of more than 12 years. This is the reason why this chapter will discuss schizophrenia in greater detail, highlighting possible difficulties a therapist can face during a diagnostic process. Some of these diagnostic difficulties will also be emphasized by the case report describing a metabolic disease which can mimic schizophrenia symptoms.

Even though childhood and adolescent schizophrenia lie on a continuum with schizophrenia in adults and the same diagnostic criteria are valid no matter the age group, there are special difficulties in applying the adult criteria to children. Symptoms at an early stage are less specific and in addition show remarkable overlap with a number of developmental disorders. So, diagnosing schizophrenia in children or adolescents could be a much harder task than diagnosing adults.

In childhood and adolescence, schizophrenia most often has a slow and insidious onset with many precursors in the shape of developmental, cognitive and emotional symptoms or retardation. None of these precursors is schizophrenia-specific, therefore it is striking to see the number of children and adolescents with schizophrenia that seem to be multidimensionally impaired.

The fact is that schizophrenic psychoses are a very heterogeneous group of disorders. Consequently, it is difficult to find a unique etiology. Studies in recent years have focused on the neurobiological and neurodevelopmental approaches, including genetics, and have produced interesting results which have not been yet integrated into conclusive and convincing theory of schizophrenia (Remschmidt, 2001).

The prognosis of early-onset schizophrenia is worse than schizophrenia that starts in adulthood, hence early recognition and treatment is crucial. Children and adolescents with any psychotic disorder, especially with schizophrenia, thus require a broad,

multidimensional treatment approach, very often including hospital treatment, with the focus on the socialization and rehabilitation. Pharmacotherapy does not differ a lot from adult patients.
As it will be seen in a case report and afterwards discussion the importance of excluding possible organic causes, whose clinical manifestation can mimic a psychotic disorder, can not be overestimated. Thus careful clinical, laboratory and imaging diagnostic evaluation must always be performed.

2. History of psychotic disorders in childhood and adolescence

The term psychosis was used very broadly in children and adolescents. It also covered the children with behavioural and autistic spectrum symptoms. The clinical distinction between autism and other psychotic disorders was first established by Kolvin in 1971 (Kolvin, 1971), but there is still confusion and misdiagnosis between the two disorders. The presence of fleeting hallucinations and delusions in nonpsychotic children can also be often misleading in a variety of other diagnoses, such as acute or reactive psychosis. But the onset of schizophrenia during adolescence and childhood has been accepted already in the twentieth century, and it is even more today. The child, adolescent and adult forms of schizophrenia could be regarded as a qualitatively similar and continuous, while allowing for developmental variation (Remschmidt, 2001).

3. Classification of psychotic disorders

Psychotic disorders can be classified into (modified after Turk et al., Turk, 2007):
- acute and transitory psychotic disorders
- schizophrenia
- organic psychotic disorders or psychotic disorders due to general medical condition
- substance-induced psychotic disorders
- schizoaffective disorders.

In schizoaffective disorders, symptoms of schizophrenia and affective symptoms are present at the same time. Since they are very rare in children and adolescents, they will not be considered in detail here. Psychotic symptoms, on the other hand, can be found in 58% of patients with bipolar disorder (see the subchapter 5.6 Differential Diagnosis of schizophrenia for more detail), which is classified under affective disorders.

4. Developmental aspects of psychotic disorders

Main characteristic for any psychotic disorder is loosing the reality control. Understanding the reality and sharing the same view on reality with other members of the same culture has a strong developmental basis. Young children cannot distinguish between fantasy and reality (Remschmidt, 2001). Therefore, it is extremely difficult to demonstrate psychotic processes until children develop reasonably cognitive and linguistic abilities. Beliefs in fantasy figures, imaginary friends are common in preschool children. Transient psychotic-like symptoms, such as hallucinations, can be thus observed in preschool children in relation to stress and anxiety (Rothstein, 1981). Children under 4 years cannot develop typical psychotic symptoms (delusions of persecution or influence) because they lack a fully formed perception of social relations (Remschmidt, 2004).

In school children, psychotic phenomena are not common, but if they are present, they show the tendency to persist and are frequently associated with schizophrenia (Carlson & Kashani, 1988; Del Beccaro et al., 1988; Russel et al., 1989; Volkmar et al., 1988). In adolescents, the levels of psychotic disorders increase markedly and clinical pictures are similar to those seen in the adulthood. Also, the differential diagnosis becomes difficult in the adolescence because of frequent substance abuse in this age range and also because of increased frequency of brief psychotic episodes associated with other conditions such as borderline personality and others (McKenna, 1994).

5. Childhood and adolescent schizophrenia

5.1 Epidemiology

Early-onset schizophrenia can be divided into a very early-onset or childhood-onset schizophrenia (major symptoms of schizophrenia are present at or under the age of 12) and adolescent-onset schizophrenia (with major symptoms in the 13-19 year age range) (Martin & Volkmar, 2007; Remschmidt, 2001).

The lifetime prevalence of schizophrenia is around 1%. It is very rare before the age of 12 and it peaks between the age of 13 and 17 (Remschmidt, 1994). The prevalence of early-onset schizophrenia (childhood and adolescent schizophrenia) is 0.23%. Only 0.1-1% of schizophrenic disorders start before the age of 10, 4% start before the age of 15 and 10% start between the age of 16 and 20. According to one population study, adolescent onset schizophrenia affects 0.23% of the general population and according to another population study, it affects 1.34% of the general population of teenagers with mental retardation (Remschmidt, 2001). Before the age of 15, there is a higher proportion of boys (male:female ratio is 3:1), but soon after the age of 15 the male:female ratio reaches 1:1 (Remschmidt, 2004).

In Europe, childhood-onset schizophrenia is only occasionally diagnosed. An outcome study in Germany covering a 30-year period reported only 40 cases, many of which had onset after the age of 10, but before the age of 13 (Eggers,1978). The NIHM childhood-onset schizophrenia study, which has been ongoing since 1990 in USA has found 89 cases of childhood schizophrenia (Martin &Volkmar, 2007).

In general, mean IQ in children with schizophrenia seems to be lower than in the general population. About 10-20% score about 70 or under. This fact is considered a premorbid feature and not a consequence of schizophrenia (Aylward, 1984). The same seems to be true for adolescents with schizophrenia. Altogether, 1.34% of them have an IQ under 70, a percentage that is much higher than in the general population where it is just 0.23% (Remschmidt, 2001).

5.2 Etiology

Schizophrenia is a complex multifactor disorder, where genetics is an important vulnerability factor. The actual occurrence of the disease and its form, however, depend upon many other familiar and unfamiliar internal and external – environment factors (Sadock & Sadock, 2007). Schizophrenia can thus be seen as a syndrome at the end of dynamic processes, which can be explained with neurodevelopment and neurodegenerative models.

Neurodevelopmental model proposes that the biological origins of schizophrenia lie in the fetal neurodevelopment, and this early developmental lesion can be traced in premorbid developmental, behavioural and cognitive impairments. This neuropathology is finally expressed as classical psychotic symptoms (Purves &Lichtmen, 1980). There is still a lively debate about the value of neurodevelopmental model, since not all patients with schizophrenia show premorbid abnormalietis.

In the last 50 years, neurotransmitter (dopaminergic, serotonergic and glutaminergic) hypotheses have prevailed in an etiology of schizophrenia. However, neurobiological in-vivo and post-mortem studies of neurotransmitter system have yielded inconsistent and contradictory results rather than providing more precise knowledge of schizophrenia etiology. But on the other hand, they were crucial in pharmacotherapy improvement for schizophrenia (Haroutunian, 2007).

Also, in the last decades, it is the genetic studies that have come to the forefront of schizophrenia research. Linkage analysis of microsatellite regions in schizophrenic families has shown that regions associated with schizophrenia can be found on many chromosomes. The impact of one single gene on the disease is very small, probably less than 1% (Gill, 1996; Riley, 2006). The second frequently used genetic method is searching for candidate genes for schizophrenia (Riley, 2006). Among those that are researched in relation to schizophrenia are also the genes that encode dopamine and serotonin receptors and promoters.

As evidenced by the research, there are no genes that would significantly impact the onset of schizophrenia. Instead, schizophrenia seems to be a product of various risk factors in people that are genetically sensitive. This sensitivity is complex and it is most likely represented by a changing combination of various genes with small impact (Sadock & Sadock, 2007). Genetic sensitivity alone, however, is not sufficient for the development of the clinical picture of schizophrenia. Other risk factors must be present too (Riley, 2006; Prathikanti & Weinberger, 2005).

It is possible that childhood schizophrenia has a higher genetic loading, since the outcome of childhood schizophrenia is very poor and probably much worse than for adolescent- and adult-onset schizophrenia (Remschmidt, 2001).

It seems that multiple gene influences result in continuous dimensions rather than in categorical disorders. Thus the dimensional model for schizophrenia seems to be more appropriate than the categorical one (dimensional model will be explained in the subchapter on Diagnosis).

Unfortunately, genetic studies too have failed to fully explain schizophrenia etiology. It remains vaguely and phenotypically broadly defined disorder that represents a complex disease due to the incomplete penetrance and heterogenic genetics (Kendler, 1993; Prathikanti & Weinberger, 2005).

There is, however, a new concept emerging in schizophrenia research, namely endophenotypes. Endophenotypes are particularly useful for understanding the etiology of complex disorders - such as schizophrenia - in which several genes and environmental factors influence the phenotype. Synonyms for endophenotypes are biological markers, biological phenotypes, latent phenotypes or intermediate phenotypes (Gottesman, 2003; Gould, 2006; Holden, 2003; Preston & Weinberger, 2005; Weinberger, 2002). The endophenotype is less genetically complex than the disorder it underlies (Castellanos & Tannock, 2002). It is assumed that it is more closely related to one or more pathophysiological genes for the nosological category, compared with the entire spectrum of disorders included in the nosological category. It is not necessary for an endophenotype to belong to a specific nosological category because nosological categories usually do not have biological background. It is, however, necessary for it to be heritable and to segregate with illness within families (Berrettini, 2005). Cognitive and

biochemical features of psychiatric patients are more associated with genetic factors than the behavioural phenotypes. The idea of endophenotypes is basically to relate some features of schizophrenic patients to the genes (Gottesman & Gould, 2003; Berrettini, 2005). Endophenotypes are stable, state-independent characteristics in contras to behavioural symptoms (Berrettini, 2005). The most studied endophenotypes today are cognitive deficits, an abnormality of the P50 auditory evoked potential and imagining phenotypes (Berrettini, 2005; Burdick et al., 2006; Turner et al., 2006).
Schizophrenia peaks at the age of 15 and this is one of the reasons why many authors see the puberty as a risk factor for schizophrenia (Remschmidt, 2004; Hyde, 1992). Neurobiological changes that occur during the puberty and adolescence can influence more frequent occurrence of schizophrenia during this period of life. These neurobiological changes are: myelinisation of the associative cortex and hippocampus, maturation of the prefrontal cortex, diminishing of the cerebral plasticity, effect of sex hormones on synapses development and changes in dopaminergic innervations (the last two proved only in animals) and changes in neurotransmission (Remschmidt, 2004).

5.3 Diagnosis

No symptom or sign is pathognomonic for schizophrenia. Moreover, patient symptoms change with time. During the last decade, schizophrenic symptoms have been linked to the underlying neurocognitive processes and further to the genetic substrate (for detail please see subchapter on Eetiology - Endophenotypes). It seems that multiple gene influences result in continuous dimensions rather than in categorical disorders. For schizophrenia, five symptom dimensions can be described (positive, negative, disorganized, cognitive and affective symptoms).

Positive symptoms

- Hallucinations, which can be auditory, visual, somatic-tactile, and olfactory. Typical for schizophrenia are voices commenting and/or conversing patient's behaviour or commending him or her what to do (imperative hallucinations).
- Delusions, which can be persecutory, jealousy, guilt and sin, grandiose, religious, and somatic. Typical for patients with schizophrenia are delusions of reference, of being controlled, of mind reading, though broadcasting and thought withdrawal.
- Positive formal thought disorder like distractible speech, pressure of speech, illogicality, and derailment. Some authors classified some of these symptoms among disorganized symptoms.

Negative symptoms

- Affective flattening, which can be seen as unchanged facial expression no matter the circumstances, decreased spontaneous movements, paucity of expressive gestures, and poor eye contact etc.
- Alogia (poverty of speech, poverty of content of speech, blocking, and increased response latency).
- Avolition-apathy (grooming and hygiene, impersistence at work or school, physical anergia).
- Attention (social inattentiveness and inattentiveness during testing).

Disorganized symptoms

- Bizarre behaviour, including bizarre clothing and appearance, social and sexual behaviour, giggling for no reason, aggressive or agitated behaviour and repetitive or stereotyped behaviour.

- Disorganized thinking with illogical, nonsensical thought patterns jumping from one unrelated idea to another, so that it is impossible to understand what the person is trying to say. Making up words is common.

Cognitive symptoms refer to the difficulties with concentration and memory. Thy may include:

- slow thinking
- difficulty understanding
- poor concentration
- poor memory
- difficulty expressing thoughts
- difficulty integrating thoughts, feelings and behaviour.

5.3.1 DSM-IV diagnostic criteria (Diagnostic and Statistical Manual of mental disorders)

DSM-IV (American Psychiatric Association, 1994) contains the American Psychiatric Association's official diagnostic criteria for schizophrenia, which describes several types of schizophrenia. The presence of hallucinations or delusions is not necessary for the diagnosis of schizophrenia. A patient's disorder is diagnosed as schizophrenia also when the two of the symptoms listed as symptoms 3-5 in criterion A are present.

Criterion A characteristic symptoms: two or more of the following, each present for a significant portion of time during a 1-month period (or less if successfully treated):

1. delusions
2. hallucinations
3. disorganized speech
4. grossly disorganized or catatonic behaviour
5. negative symptoms.

For a significant portion of the time since the onset of the disturbance, one or more major areas of functioning such as school or work must be markedly below the level achieved prior to the onset of the disturbance to fulfil the diagnostic criteria for schizophrenia. Continuous symptoms of the disturbance have to persist for at least 6 months. Prodromal symptoms are included in this 6-month period. At least 1 month of acute symptoms (or less if successfully treated) has to be present for the diagnosis of schizophrenia. Schizoaffective disorder, mood disorder with psychotic features, pervasive developmental disorder, direct physiological effects of a substance (a drug abuse, a medication) or a general medical condition have to be ruled out.

DSM-IV advocates the application of the same diagnostic criteria in early-onset schizophrenia as for adult-type disorders with some allowance for different manifestations. It recognises several different types of schizophrenia.

5.3.1.1. *Paranoid type* is the most common type of schizophrenia, typically beginning in adult life. It is the prototype of positive symptoms. The course of disease usually does not lead to personality and cognitive changes (Sadock & Sadock, 2007; Remschmidt, 2005).

5.3.1.2 *Disorganized type* (also cold hebephrenic type) begins most often in puberty with an insidious, slow and unspecific onset. It can often be mistaken for an adolescent crisis. This type is characterized by a marked regression to a primitive, disinhibited and disorganized behaviour. Depersonalization phenomena can be present. The contact with reality is poor, the emotional responses are inappropriate. They can burst into laughter without any apparent reason. Incongruous grinning and grimacing is also common. The behaviour can be described as silly or fatuous (Sadock & Sadock, 2007; Remschmidt, 2005). These patients are usually intelligent with the premorbid personality characteristics such as shyness, passiveness, introverted, with few/no friends. This type can be diagnosed after a few months of observations. Patients with disorganized type show negative symptomatics early in the course of disease. This is also the reason why this type is a prototype for negative symptoms (Remschmidt, 2005).

5.3.1.3 *Catatonic type* was common several decades ago. In Europe and North America, it is quite rare today, most likely because of the antipsychotic treatment. The classic feature is a marked disturbance in motor function which can involve stupor, negativism, rigidity, excitement or posturing. Rapid alternations from one extreme (stupor) to another (excitement) are also possible (Sandock & Sandock, 2007).

5.3.1.4 *Residual type* is a chronic state characterized by the presence of continuing evidence of the schizophrenic disturbance in the absence of a complete set of active symptoms or sufficient symptoms to meet the diagnosis of another type of schizophrenia. Emotional blunting, social withdrawal, eccentric behaviour, illogical thinking and mild loosing of associations commonly appear. Hallucinations or delusions can be present from time to time but are neither prominent nor accompanied with a strong affect (Sandock & Sandock, 2007).

5.3.1.5 Undifferentiated type is a type characterized by the presence of symptoms for schizophrenia, but does not meet criteria for any other type.

5.3.1.6 *Simple schizophrenia* is a type of schizophrenia according to ICD-10 classification (International Statistical Classification of Diseases and Related Health Problems, 1993) with particular insidious onset of withdrawal and social deterioration associated with very poor outcome. It usually starts slowly and untypically in adolescence. In the absence of prominent delusions, hallucinations or disorganized speech, it leads to a profound personal and social destruction. Patients are depressed, anhedonic, without energy and/or motivation. They can leave a school or a job and many of them can be found in marginal populations (homeless etc.). The diagnosing of this type can be quite difficult, since it is not clearly demarcated neither from the schizoid nor from the schizotypal personality disorder (Remschmidt, 2005).

In early-onset schizophrenia there are typically fewer well-formed systematized types when compared to adult schizophrenia. It appears that there is a relative predominance of disorganised and undifferentiated cases and fewer paranoid cases in early-onset schizophrenia, when compared with adult schizophrenia (Remschmidt, 2001).

The definition of schizophrenia is symptom based, so the diagnostic criteria using the adult manifestation of the disorder could miss some of the developmental variability in symptoms seen in children and adolescents. This could result in missed diagnoses, especially in presentation with a slow onset and negative symptoms, which are more commonly seen in children and adolescents (Remschmidt, 2001).

Another factor that has to be taken into consideration is the patient's age, which has a strong impact on the schizophrenic symptom types. Positive symptoms increase linearly with age, while the negative ones occur most frequently in the early childhood and late adolescence (Remschmidt, 2004). Bettes and Walker found a correlation between symptoms and IQ: children with high IQ showed more positive and fewer negative symptoms than low-IQ children (Bettes & Walker, 1987). In the course of schizophrenic symptomatology, there is a clear shift from positive and mixed symptoms to negative ones, which correlates with disease chronicity (Remschmidt, 2005).

Slow and insidious onset of childhood and adolescent schizophrenia is a rule rather than an exception. This is the reason why cases of early-onset schizophrenia are diagnosed with up to two-year delay (Schefer & Ross, 2002). Such delays worsen the course and prognosis of the disease, so early diagnosis and treatment is crucial. Early-onset schizophrenia with acute onset, on the other hand, poses less problems, mostly due to easily recognisable positive symptoms.

5.3.2 Other possible diagnostic aspects

An interesting feature of early-onset schizophrenia compared to adult one seems to be the higher rates of early language, social and motor developmental abnormalities, which are possibly reflecting greater impairment in early brain development (Martin & Volkmar, 2007). This is the reason why Werry suggests at least two clinical phenotypes of schizophrenia. The first one is associated with a long-standing developmental abnormality where the acute psychotic episode develops after some years of pre-existing abnormality. The second phenotype develops in children and adolescents who have had previously normal development (Werry, 1996).

Schizophrenic symptomatic in children and adolescents as well as in adults can also be described using another distinction which differentiates between two type of schizophrenia differing in psychopathological symptoms and premorbid functioning of the patient (Remschmidt, 2005). Type I is characterized by positive symptoms - hallucinations and illusions. Patients are aggressive, restless and excited, they can talk a lot and can make up new words (neologisms). The CAT scan usually reveals a normal brain structure and the response to the pharmacological treatment is usually good. Type II, on the other hand, is characterized by negative symptoms - affective flattening, social withdrawal, loss of interests and cognitive slowness. Here, the CAT scan shows brain structural changes and the response to pharmacotherapy is worse than in type I (Kaplan & Sadock, 1998).

5.4 Preclinical symptoms and associated features

5.4.1 Prodromal states

Before full symptoms of schizophrenia are manifested in a clinical picture, disease pre-stage - prodromal state can be present in 75% of patients with schizophrenia. Prodromal state can last a few days or some years (Remschmidt, 2005). The symptoms are unspecific, ranging from problems with concentration, changes in motivation and sleep disturbances, unspecific fears, irritability and suspiciousness. Family and friends may notice that the person has changed and is no longer functioning well in social, school and/or occupational activities. A patient may develop an interest in abstract ideas, philosophy and in the occult and religious questions. Peculiar behaviour, abnormal affects, unusual speech, bizarre ideas and strange perceptual experiences can be present too. Somatic complains such as headache, back and muscle pain, weakness and digestive problems can also be seen in prodromal state (Sadock & Sadock, 2007). Unspecific prodromal state could be misdiagnosed as adolescent crises or same other psychiatric diagnosis.

Negative symptoms are usually the first schizophrenic symptoms present in a prodromal state, while positive ones usually appear later during the acute state of schizophrenia (Remschmidt, 2005).

5.4.2 Premorbid personality characteristics

Typical, but not invariable, for some children and adolescents with schizophrenia are their premorbid personality characteristics. They are usually quite passive, introverted with few or no friends. They may avoid sport and social activities such as dating and watch TV or listen to the music instead. As children they are often described as special, perpetually unsatisfied and sensitive. Described characteristics may be detected in half of the children and adolescents with schizophrenia (Remschmidt, 2005).

5.4.3 Unspecific developmental abnormalities

In addition to prodromal state and premorbid personality characteristics, patients with early-onset schizophrenia can also show many unspecific developmental abnormalities such as soft neurological signs, unspecific sensory and motoric neurological abnormalities, aggravated autonomic reactions, different perinatal complications and symptoms of hyperkinetic syndrome (Remschmidt, 2004). Prevalent findings in a personal history of children and adolescents with schizophrenia are also cognitive impairments, lower IQ, transient symptoms of pervasive disorder and social withdrawal. A study of Alaghband-Rad et al. found that 36% of patients with childhood schizophrenia had a premorbid history of at least one pervasive developmental disorder feature and 13% had full autism (Alaghband-Rad et al., 1995). In all, 60-70% of children with childhood onset schizophrenia had language and/or motor impairments in infancy (Jacobsen & Rapoport, 1998; Watkins et al., 1988). All described features and impairments are not specific for early-onset schizophrenia, they can also be found in other psychiatric disorders, so they have no diagnostic value.

There is a vivid debate on primary prevention for subjects at high risk for schizophrenia. In short, our knowledge today is not sufficient enough to reliably diagnose pre-schizophrenic states, which is why preventive pharmacological treatment cannot be recommended as yet.

5.5 Course and prognosis

Early-onset schizophrenia has worse prognosis compared to schizophrenia occurring in adulthood. Only 23% of patients with early-onset schizophrenia reach full remission (compared to 25% of adult patients), while 25% of them reach partial remission (compared to 50% of adult patients). Chronic course will have 52% of patients with early-onset schizophrenia (compared to 25% of adult patients) (Remschmidt, 2005). After the hospitalization, 40% of patients with early-onset schizophrenia cannot go back to the same educational/professional level as before the hospitalization. Besides the chronicification of the disease, disfunctional family environment may also be the reason (Remschmidt, 2005).

Moreover, a total of 10% of people with adult schizophrenia die by suicide (Kaplan & Sadock, 1998). There are not many studies on this topic in children and adolescents, but one provides interesting results. Eggers points to the risk of suicide in the prodromal state and growing suicidal risk with onset of schizophrenia; where 65% of adolescents were preoccupied by death thoughts, 20% attempted suicide and 5% committed suicide. Compared to adults, suicide was relatively late phenomena, with the average time of 8.5 years between the onset of schizophrenia and the attempted suicide, and the average time between 6 and 14 years for the committed suicide (Eggers, 1978).

In general, the prognosis for the early-onset schizophrenia is as follows: the earlier the onset, the greater the disability (Remschmidt, 2001). Regarding the gender, girls seem to have somewhat better prognosis, both because they seem to be less vulnerable to the early-onset

than boys, and because they seem to be less affected by the illness. This, however, does not mean that their chance of full recovery is any better than in boys.
Studies show that children with prodromal state that lasted over one year have worse prognosis for clinical improvement during hospitalization (Amminger et al., 1997).

5.6 Differential diagnosis

5.6.1 Conduct and emotional disorders

Hallucination can be present in conduct and emotional disorders, particularly at the times of stress. When focusing on persecutory ideas and ideas of reference, which are often present in conduct and emotional disorders, the misdiagnosis can be the problem (Remschmidt, 2001).

5.6.2 Affective psychosis

In a follow-up study of Werry, over 50% of the bipolar disorder cases had initial diagnosis of schizophrenia (Werry, 1991), which makes a valid distinction between schizophrenia and bipolar disorder in children and adolescents questionable. In affective psychosis, however, the onset of psychotic symptoms is often rapid with relatively good premorbid social and school functioning.

5.6.3 Autistic spectrum disorders

Positive symptoms may develop in autistic spectrum disorders in adolescence, however, they are usually transitory. Children and adolescents with autistic spectrum disorders have more long-standing and progressive deterioration in social and cognitive fields prior to the onset of psychotic symptoms.

5.6.4 Organic brain conditions

At first episode of schizophrenia, one must exclude all other possible organic causes for psychotic symptomatology (drug-inducted psychosis, epilepsy, neuro-degenerative disorders etc.) described in special subchapters.

5.7 Treatment of schizophrenia

5.7.1 Pharmacological treatment

Antipsychotics are the first choice drugs in a pharmacological treatment of schizophrenia. They act suppressively on the symptomatology of the disease, but do not cure the disease. They calm, reduce and eliminate psychotic symptoms in an acute state of schizophrenia. When the acute state has settled down, they act prophylactic against psychotic recidives. Pharmacological treatment in schizophrenia can be divided into three phases:

- Acute phase, in which antipsychotics act suppressively on major schizophrenic symptoms.
- Maintenance phase, which starts in full remission and should last at least six months with the same doses of antiphsychotics as in acute phase. The purpose is to prevent possible relapse, to improve patient's social skills and further relief of symptoms.
- Prophylaxis phase prevents recidive and helps maintaining and/or exceeding the achieved level of patient's functioning and quality of life. This phase should last at least one year after the first episode of schizophrenia and several years after the second episode of schizophrenia. As schizophrenia is a chronic disease, the pharmacological

treatment can be lifelong. The doses of antipsychotics should be lower than in the first two phases (Sandock & Sandock, 2007).

5.7.2 Psychotherapeutic measures

It is crucial that schizophrenic patients and their families are educated about the disease, its etiology, its course and the treatment. Patients and their families have to have the knowledge about the disorder in order to recognise a relapse on time, to prevent preterm drug reduction or cessation, and to strengthen the compliance. Among psychotherapeutic measures, only the most used/applied will be mentioned, i.e. cognitive and other behavioural approaches, emotion management therapy, group programs, family-oriented measures, supportive and structural family therapy and extended development-oriented family therapy.

5.7.3 Rehabilitation

Since nearly half of the patients suffering from schizophrenia cannot return immediately after the hospitalization to their school/occupational and family environment, they are usually directed to rehabilitation centres. On average, the rehabilitation lasts two years and is crucial to the treatment of schizophrenia.

The rehabilitation can be divided into two phases, aiming at growing stepwise independence. During the first phase, much effort should be assigned to the areas of schooling, working skills, social skills training and interpersonal problem solving. It usually lasts one year. The patient is living together with other patients in a rehabilitation centre in a family-like structured program. The second rehabilitation phase, however, should bring major change to the patient in order to gain more independence, self-sufficiency, psychosocial reintegration and the continuation of school and professional work without the significant support from the rehabilitation centre (Remschmidt, 2001).

6. Acute and transient psychotic disorders

There are no reliable data on incidence and prevalence, gender ratio and the mean age at the onset for this psychotic disorder. It seems, however, that it is more frequent in a younger population. The disorder is characterized by a sudden onset (less than in a two-week time) of psychotic symptoms, which may include delusions, hallucinations, disorganized speech or behavior, or catatonic behavior. Also, the symptoms can change frequently during an episode. The duration of an acute and transient psychosis is generally short, non re-occurring, and not better accounted for by another condition. Symptoms generally do not last long, usually just a few days or weeks, but 2-3 months at most. There is a possibility of an eventual return to full baseline functioning (Kaplan & Sadock, 1998). The prognosis is good – 50-80% of patients do not have any psychiatric problems after the acute psychosis has ended. Occasionally, a relation to a stressor can be found. In such cases, the diagnosis of a reactive disorder is appropriate (Sandock & Sandock, 2007).

6.1 Reactive psychoses

Reactive psychosis occurs shortly after (maximum 2 weeks after) and in response to a significant stressor in a person's life (death in the family, war, divorce, abuse, etc.). Psychotic symptoms can be thematically closely related to the trauma. The reactive psychoses are short. Their duration is usually not longer than 2-3 months.

7. Substance-induced psychotic disorder

There are 3 facts that are important when dealing with psychoactive substances associated with psychotic disorders (Kaplan & Sadock, 1998; Remschmidt, 2004).

- Psychoactive substances can cause psychotic symptoms in anyone (typical hallucinogens are LSD, phencyclidine –"*angel dust*", cocaine and amphetamine – "*speed*" and "*ecstasy*").
- In a person who is genetically predisposed to developing a psychosis, psychoactive substances can accelerate the onset of the psychosis and worsen its clinical picture, course and treatment.
- Patients with psychotic disorder (most often schizophrenia) can use psychoactive substances as self-medication because of their effect on symptomatic recovery. Heroin, for instance, can reduce hallucinations, while cannabis, on the other hand, calms the psychotic excitement.

Psychotic symptoms in substance-induced psychotic disorders develop during the intake of a substance or not later than 48 hours after it. Partial remission occurs within one month, while full remission is achieved in 6 months (Remschmidt, 2004). Prominent hallucinations (they typically appear on more than one sensorial level, even though acoustic hallucinations are the most frequent ones), delusions, psychomotor abnormalities (excitment or stupor) and a variety of affective symptoms are typical for a substance-induced psychotic disorder. It is worth mentioning that canabis can cause chronic psychotic state too (Sandock & Sandock, 2007).

In an acute psychotic state, it is difficult to make a distinction between substance-induced psychotic disorders, brief and acute psychotic disorders and schizophrenia. The main facts that militate against the substance-induced psychotic disorders are (Remschmidt, 2005):

- The presence of psychotic symptoms prior to the drug consummation.
- The presence of psychotic episodes prior to the drug consummation.
- Drug-induced psychotic symptoms persist longer than expected.

8. Psychotic disorders due to general medical condition

The evaluation of a psychotic patient requires also a consideration of the possibility that the psychotic symptoms are the result of a general medical condition (brain tumour, head injury, poisoning, infection, metabolic diseases, epilepsy, etc.). These conditions can represent a real diagnostic problem if the psychotic symptoms are the only symptoms in the clinical picture. In such a case, there is a danger to overlook the organic/somatic cause of the symptomatology and to treat the patient incorrectly. When dealing with a case of first psychotic/schizophrenic episode there is a need to preform laboratory tests and imaging investigations in order to exclude the most possible causes of psychotic symptomatology (Sandock & Sandock, 2007).

8.1 Case report

An 18-year-old girl was admitted to the Child and Adolescent Psychiatry Unit of the Maribor University Clinical Centre in Slovenia for suspected disorganized (formerly called hebephrenic) schizophrenia. A year before that, at the age of 17, she had begun to laugh without reason, and her behaviour had become silly and disorganized. Her emotional responses were inappropriate. She started grimacing and became paramimic and parathymic. She withdrew socially and began to shut herself in her room. She had auditory hallucinations, consisting of a running commentary on her behaviour. At that time, there were no changes in her school performance, which was already consistently below average; however, her school performance deteriorated 3 months before admission to hospital, when she became unable to do any schoolwork. She also became disoriented as to her whereabouts and got lost several times.

There had been no aberrations in her developmental milestones. Until recently, she had not had any diseases or needed any medical attention.

Her family history was interesting. She had a 24-year-old brother with moderate mental retardation according to the DSM-IV criteria. He had delayed developmental milestones and difficulties in walking and speaking. She also had a 25-year-old sister who, 4 years before, had had an episode of postpartum depression (according to DSM-IV criteria) that started a few days after she had delivered a baby. She had depressed mood and no interest in her baby or in any other activities. She was motor retarded, complained about loss of energy and diminished ability to think and concentrate, and she reported feelings of worthlessness and guilt about being ill and not being able to take care of her baby. She cried constantly, had no appetite and suffered from insomnia. She recovered in a month without any antidepressants. Her school performance had been below average throughout all 10 years of her education, and she had been unable to find a job either before or after the episode of postpartum depression. She attended night school to become a cook and had achieved average success at the time of writing. There was no history of psychiatric disturbance before or after the episode of postpartum depression. The patient's mother had 7 half-siblings. Two had died, probably of pneumonia, at the age of 6 months. The third sibling was mentally retarded and probably had poliomyelitis at the age of 2 years. Otherwise, there was no family history of psychiatric disorders.

At admission, our patient was disoriented in terms of time, place and person. Her thought process was disorganized, and her behaviour was disorganized and uninhibited. She was paramimic and parathymic with blunted affect. Her rapport with others was poor and her speech monotonous, and her understanding of questions was poor. She had a poor attention span and reported auditory hallucinations, consisting of a running commentary on her behaviour, which she found pleasant. She described the hallucinations as a single young male voice, which was talking to her using short sentences, mostly encouraging her to do everyday tasks and commenting on her behaviour. She revealed a lack of initiative, had poor contact with reality and had no insight into her illness. She was incontinent of urine and had dyspraxia. Psychological tests (Rorschach projective test and Bender Visual-Motor Gestalt test) revealed psychotic disturbance. The results of routine laboratory tests including thyroid-stimulating hormone, vitamin B12 and folic acid were normal. The findings of syphilis and HIV-1 serology were negative, as was serology for Borrelia burgdorferi. Levels of proteins in the cerebrospinal fluid were elevated (0.77 g/L). Electroencephalography (EEG) showed abnormal bilateral synchronous, mainly theta activity, which was most prominent temporally.

According to DSM-IV diagnostic criteria, the patient's disease presented like disorganized schizophrenia (disorganized thought process and behaviour, flattening of the affect, auditory hallucinations and social dysfunction). These symptoms persisted for about 9 months without any marked signs of cognitive impairment, apart from poor attention and slowing in thought process. Therefore, treatment with small doses of an atypical antipsychotic, risperidone (1 mL twice a day) was initiated.

After 1 week of treatment, the patient stopped reporting auditory hallucinations. Although her behaviour was still disorganized, she was more willing to cooperate during the required medical examinations. Neurologic examination revealed positive pyramidal signs in the upper extremities. Tendon-stretch reflexes in the lower extremities were absent distally. Computed tomography revealed signs of advanced cortical atrophy, symmetrical ventricular enlargement and periventricular white-matter hypodensity. Magnetic resonance imaging of the brain showed diffuse signal hyperintensity of the white matter, especially in the periventricular area, as well as in the corpus callosum, cerebral atrophic changes and symmetrical ventricular enlargement. Electromyography showed a slowing of the nerve conduction velocities (NCV) (NCV of the peroneal nerve was 23 m/s [reference range 44–57 m/s]) and marked prolongation of the F-wave latency. Visual evoked potentials showed a normal retinogram, but cortical responses had prolonged latencies with a normal response distribution. Somatosensory and acoustic evoked potentials were within normal limits. Abdominal ultrasonography revealed polyposis of the gall bladder.

Four weeks later, the disorganized and psychotic clinical picture diminished and the patient's cognitive impairment became increasingly obvious. Apart from poor attention and slowing of the thought process, memory (recollection and recent past) was disturbed the most. Therefore neuropsychological tests (Wechsler Intelligence Scale, Wechsler Memory Scale, Trail-making Test, Stroop Test, Hooper Visual Organization Test, Rivermead Behavioural Memory Test and the Controlled Oral Word Association Test) were carried out. The patients' full-scale IQ fell to within the range of severe mental retardation (according to DSM-IV criteria). There was a minor difference between the patient's verbal and performance IQ, favouring the former. The impairments were severe over the whole range of mental functioning. Attention processes, perception, executive functions, communication and motor skills were impaired. Her processing speed was very slow. Memory for verbally presented information and visual memory were found to be severely impaired. She could not independently perform any simple or routine operations. Therefore, an acetylcholinesterase (AChE) inhibitor was added to the therapy (galantamine, 4 mg, twice a day for 1 month, then galantamine, 8 mg, twice a day).

Taking into account the diagnostic findings of neurologic examinations, neuropsychological tests, urinary incontinence and imaging, it was clear that there was most probably an organic disorder underlying the disorganized schizophrenia-like symptoms, which also later caused symptoms of dementia. Therefore, further tests were performed, focusing especially on inherited metabolic disorders.

The results of urine screening tests and screening for very long chain fatty acids in the serum were normal, excluding adrenoleukodystrophy and several disorders of peroxisomal function. Arylsulfatase A activity in leukocytes was markedly reduced (0.047 nmol/h per milligram; normal values in controls 2.82 ± 1.24 nmol/h per milligram). Measurement of urinary sulfatides by electrospray ionization–tandem mass spectrometry showed a 10-fold elevation of 609 nmol/L (values in healthy controls 51.5 ± 33.45 nmol/L), thus confirming the diagnosis of metachrometic leukodystrophia (MLD).

In the patient's sister, who remained clinically asymptomatic apart from the single episode described earlier, biochemical tests also showed clear arylsulfatase, a deficiency in leukocytes (0.155 nmol/h per milligram) and markedly elevated sulfatides in urine (436 nmol/L), thus proving the presence of a metabolic disease metachrometic leukodystrophy (MLD). In accordance with their obligate heterozygosity, intermediate arylsulfatase A activity was found in both of our patients' parents. Our patients' mentally retarded older brother had normal arylsulfatase A activity and normal values of sulfatides in the urine.

8.2 Discussion

Metachromatic leukodystrophy is one of the most serious genetic demyelination disorders (Tylki-Szymanska et al., 1996). It is an autosomal recessive lysosomal disease characterized by demyelination of the white matter in the central nervous system and the peripheral nerves. The relevant gene is located on chromosome 22q13. The disease is caused by a deficiency of the enzyme arylsulfatase A, which hydrolyzes various sulfatides, including the major sulfate-containing lipids of the nervous system. Sulfatide accumulation can be found in the brain and peripheral nerves and nonneural organs (kidney and gallbladder) (Hageman et al., 1995). The incidence of MLD is estimated between 1 and 5 cases per 100 000 newborns (Rentrop et al., 1999)

There are 3 types of MLD: late infantile, juvenile and adult. The late-infantile form, which has its onset at the age of 1–2 years, is characterized by gait and behavioural disturbances. The course of the disease is rapid and the outcome fatal. The juvenile form, which has its onset between the ages of 3 and 15 years, displays a less distinct phenotype, varying from peripheral nerve involvement in younger children to learning problems and behavioural difficulties in older children (Kaye, 2001). It has a more protracted course. The symptoms of adult MLD include dementia, psychosis, behavioural abnormalities, ataxia, polyneuropathy and epileptic seizures. Other psychiatric disorders can present with the following MLD symptoms: personality changes, depressive disorders, alcohol addiction, and worsening of school and/or work performance. Adult MLD has a slowly progressive course. Compared with the late-infantile and juvenile forms, the adult variant of MLD appears to be quite rare. The mean survival for adult MLD is at least 12 years, which is longer than the survival in late-infantile MLD (3–4 years) and juvenile MLD (7–9 years) (Kaye, 2001).

The diagnosis of MLD is based on arylsulfatase A activity in leukocytes or fibroblasts and on sulfatide excretion in the urine.

There is much disagreement in the literature regarding the incidence of psychosis in adult MLD. Hyde et al. (Hyde et al., 1992) suggested that in 53% of patients with adult MLD psychosis is present and is often the initial manifestation. Cengiz et al. (Cengiz et al., 2002) reported the cases of 3 sisters with adult type MLD, 2 of whom were initially diagnosed as having schizophrenia. Hageman et al state that psychosis is a less common symptom than previously suggested. In their group of 13 patients with confirmed adult MLD, the most common symptoms were ataxia and behavioural abnormalities with only 1 patient suffering from psychosis. The findings were similar in the group of 24 patients with confirmed MLD described in the literature, among whom only 4 were psychotic (Hageman et al., 1995).

Disorganized schizophrenia-like symptoms were the initial manifestation of MLD in our patient, and they persisted without any marked signs of cognitive impairment for at least 9 months. Then she got lost several times, and her school performance deteriorated. It is open to discussion whether her school performance deteriorated because of the disorganized schizophrenia-like symptoms or whether this was the first symptom of dementia. The differential diagnosis of dementia became problematic when disorganized and psychotic symptoms diminished after treatment with antipsychotics. We wondered whether disorganized schizophrenia-like symptoms just masked dementia? The first symptoms of disease were disorganized and silly behaviour, disorganized thought process, inappropriate affect, social withdrawal, incongruous grimacing, outbursts of laughter without any apparent reason, paramimia, parathymia, auditory hallucinations, poor contact with reality and no prominent signs of cognitive impairment. All these symptoms can also be found with dementia; however, they usually occur later, have a gradual onset and are rarely all present at the same time. At some point, as MLD progressed, disorganized schizophrenia-like symptoms most probably masked dementia, but dementia was not the initial manifestation of MLD in our patient.

The patient's older sister, in whom the diagnosis of MLD was confirmed biochemically, had had an episode of postpartum depression 4 years before. The literature describes some cases of adult MLD manifesting as major depression, but to our knowledge none of postpartum depression (Ricketts et al., 1996; Vella et al., 1998).

Little is known about the symptomatic treatment of psychotic symptoms and dementia in MLD. Our patient responded well to treatment with small doses of an atypical antipsychotic, showing no side effects. More questionable is the treatment with AChE inhibitors, which is only indicated in Alzheimer's disease.

This report underlines the importance of metabolic or any other somatic disease as a cause of what appears to be a psychosis or schizophrenia. It is crucial to always bear in mind that a full clinical, biochemical and imaging diagnostic evaluations must be performed in any patient with psychotic symptoms (Seidl et al., 1981).

9. Treatment of psychotic disorders

In diagnosing psychosis or any other psychiatric disorder it is important to know how to talk to a child or an adolescent. The communication has to be age appropriate, clear and without any questions that could be misunderstood or confusing. To create a positive transfer it can be helpful to know the topics, films, toys and plays that are popular in a specific age group. Children and adolescents usually like to talk openly without any reservations. They are frank in their answers and compared to adults they minimalize or deny their problems and fears less frequently.

It is equally important that the therapist is calm and relaxed, using short and understandable questions, talking slowly and understandably. Unclear question formulations and irony, must be avoided because they can additionally confuse and excite the patient. Furthermore, the therapist should also clearly explain the patient that he or she is here to help and that in order to do so some questions need to be answered. Discussion about the (un)reality of patient's symptoms and feelings when dealing with an acute psychotic patient should be postponed until the remission phase. It is possible that patient's state of disease will not allow interviewing the patient what have to be recognised soon enough in order not to excite the patients further. But general are psychotic children and adolescents willing to talk about themselves and their symptomatic.

When meeting an acute psychotic patient for a first time, it is difficult to know if the psychotic symptomatics is substance-induced, if it is a result of a general medical condition or whether it is a case of schizophrenia. If the patient's condition allows taking auto- and hetero- anamnestic data, these could be very helpful in further differential diagnostic considerations. For instance, any information on the febrile state or a head injury is very probably associated with a possible organic background. Information on drug consumption is needed to exclude or include a substance-induced psychotic disorders in the diagnosis. Also, schizophrenia positive family history, a symptomatic that is typical for prodromal state or premorbid personal characteristic can be frequently found in the first schizophrenic episode.

Recommended investigations in any first psychotic episode are (Sandock & Sandock, 2007):

- blood biochemical tests (including liver functional tests), thyroid hormones
- drug and alcohol tests
- EEG, ECG, brain imagining investigations (CAT scan or MRI).

If metabolic diseases are suspicious further diagnostic testing should be performed: lactate, pyruvate, ammonia test, aminoacids in serum and urine, organic acids in urine; copper, ceruloplasmine (Mb Wilson); encime arylsulphatase A activity in leukocytes and sulphatides in urine (metachrometic leukodystrophia) (Gregoric Kumperscak, 2005).

Roughly speaking, psychotic patients can clinically present as two different types. Firstly, as acute psychotic, excited and/or physically aggressive patients with vivid hallucinations and illusions without any reality or impulse control and without disease insight. Secondly, as socially withdrawn adolescents with peculiar ideas and interests, diminished school achievements, in whom psychotic symptoms are present but hardly fulfil the needed diagnostic criteria for any psychotic disorder. The first type of patients should be hospitalized and treated with antipsychotics and other medicaments described in following chapter. The second type with a slowly developing clinical picture of psychosis just needs to be carefully followed in order to establish a proper diagnosis. Special care should be taken as prodromal state can be easily misdiagnosed or overlooked. Therefore, it is of outmost importance for the therapist to be familiar with all variations of development and growing up. Sometimes the search of adolescents for their identity can be mistakenly considered as a prodromal state. Only when there is a big difference between premorbid functioning and actual functioning (lower school achievements and social interests), there is a strong likelihood of prodromal state. Adolescents in general feel and describe psychotic symptoms before they can actually be seen in their behaviour and be objectivised. Thus, children and adolescents in a pre-psychotic state often talk about their inner changing, about a strong feeling that there is something happening to them, often stating that they are losing control and their mind. They are very upset and tense without any genuine reason.

9.1 Medication in an acute psychotic and/or excited patient

Acute psychotic and/or excited patients need medication prior to their admission to the hospital. Atypical antipsychotics (AA) and/or benzodiazepines (BD) can be used. The recommendations for acute psychotic and excited child or adolescent treatment follow the recommendations for adult patients. All doses have to be age-adjusted.

AAs and BDs are broadly equally effective in sedation, however the effect of BDs can be quicker. Sometimes the combination of AAs and BDs is necessary and also more effective (Tayler et al., 2009). If the patient is already on AA, then BDs are recommended. If substance-induced psychosis is suspicious, then AAs are appropriate (Tayler et al., 2009).

Before resorting to intramuscular medication (im.), oral medications are always first choice. Clinicians have a good experience with risperidone in suspension, which can be given with water or tea. Oral risperidone suspension 0.5 to 2ml can be first administrated and if no effect is achieved after 2 hours, another dose of risperidone can be given. Olanzepine 5-10mg or haloperidol 0.05-0.15mg per kg per day can also be administrated. Among BDs, lorazepan 1-2 mg or diazepam 5-10mg can be used and the same dose can be repeatedly given after 1-2 hours if no effect is noted. The combination of AAs and BDs could also be administrated.

If there is no possibility for oral medication, im. medication must be used. Among AAs, olazepine 2.5-10mg im. can be administrated or a first generation antipsychotic haloperidol 0.025-0.075mg im. per kg per dose. Among BDs, lorazepam 0.05-0.1 mg im. per kg per dose or diazepam 0.1mg per kg per dose by slow iv. injection can be administrated.

10. Conclusion

To summarize, there are several traps when dealing with children and adolescents who present with symptoms suspicious of being psychosis. The above-described case report clearly shows that it is possible for an organic disease to present with psychotic symptoms only. This, of course, causes problems in accurately diagnosing the disease. Therefore, in order not to overlook a possible organic cause in a psychotic clinical picture, a biochemical, neurological and imagining tests and procedures must always be performed first.

Developmental period with its own special characteristics is another factor that needs to be considered when establishing the diagnosis. Each developmental state can colour the clinical picture differently. It can either overlap or aggravate the psychotic symptoms. For instance, it is completely normal for a 5-years old child to have an imaginary friend, but at age of 15 such friend may indicate pathology.

Also, adolescence is associated with many developmental tasks such as identity formation, independence and autonomy, and development of one's own view of life. All this, of course, brings along at a certain stage of development a detachment from parents, a retreat into their own world, as well as changes in the way of thinking and one's own philosophy, which however should not be confused with the schizophrenia prodromes. On the other hand, due to their key neurodevelopmental changes, puberty and adolescence represent an important risk factor for the development of schizophrenia. Therefore, this should be taken into consideration when establishing the correct diagnosis.

To conclude, though infrequent in childhood, schizophrenia is a major psychiatric disorder of adolescence (Remschmidt, 2001). Bearing in mind that early-onset schizophrenia has worse prognosis than the adult-onset one, early diagnosis followed by treatment is essential. However, in order to diagnose schizophrenia properly, a thorough knowledge of the negative and positive symptoms, prodromal state symptom varieties as well of the full range of normal developmental changes is indispensable. Early-onset schizophrenia frequently starts with negative symptoms, but schizophrenia is usually recognised only when positive symptoms appear in the clinical picture. It also is noteworthy to mention that children and adolescents feel the symptoms and describe them much earlier than their effect on their behaviour can be objectivised and diagnosed.

11. References

Alaghband-Rad, J.; McKenna, K.; Gordon, C.T. et al. (1995). Childhood-onset schizophrenia: the severity of premorbid course. *J Am Child Adolesc Psychiatry*, Vol. 34, pp.1273-83

American Psychiatric Association. (1994). *Diagnostic and statistical manual of mental disorders*, ISBN 0890420254, Washington, USA

Amminger, G.P.; Resch, F.; Mutschlechner, R. et al. (1997). Premorbid adjustment and remission of positive symptoms in first-episode psychosis. *Eur Child Adolesc Psychitry*, Vol. 6, pp. 212-8

Aylward, E.; Walker, E. et al. (1984). Intelligence in schizophrenia: meta-analysis of the research. *Schizophr Bull*, Vol. 10, pp. 430-459

Berrettini, WH. (2005). Genetic bases for endophenotypes in psychiatric disorders. *Dialogues Clin Neurosci*, Vol. 7, pp. 95-101

Bettes, B. A. & Walker, E. (1987). Positive and negative symptoms in psychotic and other psychiatrically disturbed children. *J Child Psychol Psychiatry*, Vol. 28, pp. 555-68

Burdick, K.E.; Goldberg, J.F.; Harrow, M.; Faull, R.N. & Malhotra, A.K. (2006). Neurocognition as a stable endophenotype in bipolar disorder and schizophrenia. *J Nerv Ment Dis*, Vol. 194, pp. 255-60

Carlson, G.A. & Kashani, J.H. (1988). Phenomenology of major depression from childhood through adulthood: analysis of three studies. *Am J of Psychiatry*, Vol. 145, pp. 1222-5

Castellanos, F.X. & Tannock, R. (2002). Neuroscience of attention-deficit/hyperactivity disorder: the search for endophenotypes. *Nat Rev Neurosci*, Vol. 3, pp. 617-28

Cengiz, N.; Ozbenli, T.; Onar, M.; Yildiz, L. & Ertas, B. (2002). Adult metachromatic leukodystrophy: three cases with normal nerve conduction velocities in a family. *Acta Neurol Scand*, Vol. 105, pp. 454-7

Classification of mental and behavioural disorders (ICD-10). (1993). World Health Organization, ISBN-10: 9241544554, Geneva

Del Beccaro, M.A.; Burke, P. & McCaouley, E. (1988). Hallucinations in children: a follow-up study. *J of Am Acad Child Adolesc Psychiatry*, Vol. 27, pp. 462-5

Eggers, C. (1978). Course and prognosis of childhood schizophrenia. *J Autism Child Schizophr*, Vol. 8, pp. 21-36. ISSN 0021-9185

Gill, M.; Vallada, H.; Collier, D.; Sham, P.; Holmans, P.; Murray, R. et al. (1996). A combined analysis of D22S278 marker alleles in affected sib-pairs: support for a susceptibility locus for schizophrenia at chromosome 22q12. Schizophrenia Collaborative Linkage Group (Chromosome 22). *Am J Med Genet*, Vol. 67, pp. 40-5

Gottesman, I.I. & Gould, T.D. (2003). The endophenotype concept in psychiatry: etymology and strategic intentions. *Am J Psychiatry*, Vol. 160, pp. 636-45

Gould, T.D. & Gottesman, I.I. (2006). Psychiatric endophenotypes and the development of valid animal models. *Genes Brain Behav*, Vol.5, pp. 113-9

Gregoric Kumperscak, H.; Paschke, E.; Gradisnik, P.; Vidmar, J. & Umek Bradac, S. (2005). Adult metachromatic leukodystrophy: disorganized schizophrenia-like symptoms and post-partum depression in 2 sisters. *J Psychiatry Neurosci*, Vol. 30, No.1, pp. 33-6

Hageman, A.T.; Gabreels, F.J.; de Jong J,G; Gabreels-Festen, A.A.; van den Berg, C.J.; van Oost, B.A. et al. (1995). Clinical symptoms of adult metachromatic leukodystrophy and arylsulfatase A pseudodeficiency. *Arch Neurol*, Vol. 52, pp. 408-13

Haroutunian, V.; Katsel, P.; Dracheva, S.; Stewart, D.G. & Davis, K.L. (2007). Variations in oligodendrocyte-related gene expression across multiple cortical regions: implications for the pathophysiology of schizophrenia. *Int J Neuropsychopharmacol*, Vol. 10, pp. 565-73

Holden, C. (2003). Neuroscience. Deconstructing schizophrenia. *Science*, Vol. 299, pp. 333-5

Hyde, T.M.; Ziegler, J.C. & Weinberger, D.R. (1992). Psychiatric disturbances in metachromatic leukodystrophy. *Arch Neurol*, Vol. 49, pp. 401-6

Jacobsen, L.K. & Rapoport, J.L. (1998). Research update: childhood-onset schizophrenia: impications of clinical and neurobiological research. *J Child Psychol Psychiatry*, Vol. 39, pp. 101-13

Kaplan, H.I. & Sadock, B.J. (Eds.) (1998). *Kaplan and Sadock's Synopsis of Psychiatry: Behavioral Sciences, Clinical Psychiatry*, Williams & Wilkins, ISBN-10: 0683303309, Baltimore, USA

Kaye, E.M. (2001). Update on genetic disorders affecting white matter. *Pediatr Neurol*, Vol. 24, pp. 11-24

Kendler, K.S. (1993). The genetics of schizophrenia: a current, genetic-epidemiologic perspective. *Schizophrenia Bulletin*, Vol. 19, pp. 2-10

Kolvin, I., Humphrey M. et al. (1971). Studies in the childhood psychoses: cognitive factors in childhood psychoses. *Br J Psychiatry*, Vol. 118, pp. 415-9

Martin, A. & Volkmar, F.R. (Eds.) (2007). *Lewis's child and adolescent psychiatry* (fourth edition) Lippincott, Wiliams&Wilkins. ISBN 13: 978-0-7817-6214-4, London, UK

McKenna, K.; Gordon, C.T. et al. (1994). Looking for childhood-onset schizophrenia: the first 71 cases screened. *J Am Acad Child Adolesc Psychiatry*, Vol. 33, pp. 636-44

Prathikanti, S. & Weinberger, D.R. (2005). Psychiatric genetics--the new era: genetic research and some clinical implications. *Br Med Bull*, Vol. 73-74, pp. 107-22

Preston, G.A. & Weinberger, D.R. (2005). Intermediate phenotypes in schizophrenia: a selective review. *Dialogues Clin Neurosci*, Vol. 7, pp. 165-79

Purves, D. & Lichtman, J.W. (1980). Elimination of synapses in the developing nervous system. *Science*, Vol. 210, pp. 153-7

Remschmidt, H. (1994). Psychosocial milestones in normal puberty and adolescence. *Hor Res*, Vol. 19, pp.19-29

Remschmidt, H. (Ed.) (2001). *Schizophrenia in children and adolescents*. Cambrige University Press, ISBN 0-521-79428-5, Cambrige, UK

Remschmidt, H. (Ed.) (2004). *Schizophrene Erkrankungen im Kindes- und Jugendalter*, Schattauer, ISBN 3-794523288, Stuttgart, Germany

Remschmidt, H. (Ed.) (2005). *Kinder- und Jugendpsychiatry*, Geirg Thieme Verlag, ISBN 3-13-5766047, Stuttgart, Germany

Rentrop, M.; Hakk, K.; Freisleder, F.J.; Kissling, W. & Kockott, G. (1999). Homicide and hebephrenia-like syndrome in metachromatic leukodystrophy. *Nervenarzt*, Vol. 70, pp. 276-80.

Ricketts, M.H.; Amsterdam, J.D.; Park, D.S.; Yang, R.S.; Portez, R.D.; Zhang, X. et al. (1996). A novel arylsulphatase A protein variant and genotype in two patients with major depression. *J Affect Disord*, Vol. 40, pp. 137-47

Riley, B. & Kendler, K.S. (2006). Molecular genetic studies of schizophrenia. *Eur J Hum Genet*, Vol. 14, pp. 669-80

Rothstein, A. (1981). Hallucinatory phenomena in childhood. A critique of the literature. *J Am Acad Child Psychiatry*, Vol. 20, pp. 623-35

Russel, A.T.; Bott, L. & Sammons, C. (1989). The phenomenology of schizophrenia occurring in childhood. *J of Am Acad Child Adolesc Psychiatry*, Vol. 28, pp. 399-407

Sadock, B.J. & Sadock, V.A. (Eds.) (2007). *Kaplan and Sadock's Synopsis of Psychiatry: Behavioral Sciences, Clinical Psychiatry*, Williams & Wilkins, ISBN 9780781773270, Baltimore, USA

Schefer, J.L. & Ross, R.G. (2002). Childhood-onset schizophrenia:premorbid and prodromal diagnostic and treatment histories. *J Am Acad Child Adolesc Psychiatry*, Vol. 41, pp. 538-45

Seidl, D.; Goebel, H.H. & Scholz, W. (1981). Late-onset metachromatic leukodystrophy: diagnostic problems elucidated by case report. *J Neurol*, Vol. 226, pp. 119-24

Tayler, D.; Paton, C. & Kerwin, R. (Eds.) (2009). *Prescribing guidelines*, Martin Dunitz, ISBN-13: 9781841846996, London, UK

Turk, J.; Graham, P. & Verhurst, F. (Eds). (2007). *Child Psychiatry – A Developmental Approach*. Oxford: Oxford University Press, ISBN-13: 9780198526124, Oxford, United Kindom

Turner, J.A.; Smyth, P.; Macciardi, F.; Fallon, J.H.; Kennedy, J.L. & Potkin, S.G. (2006). Imaging phenotypes and genotypes in schizophrenia. *Neuroinformatics*, Vol. 4, pp. 21-49

Tylki-Szymanska, A.; Berger, J.; Loschl, B.; Lugowska, A. & Molzer, B. (1996). Late juvenile metachromatic leukodystrophy (MLD) in three patients with a similar clinical course and identical mutation on one allele. *Clin Genet*, Vol. 50, pp. 287-92

Vella, G.; Loriedo, C.; Raccah, R.; Baldassare, P. & Paolillo, A. (1998). Successful paroxetine treatment of major depression in an adult form of metachromatic leukodystrophy with cognitive disturbance. *Can J Psych*, Vol. 43, pp. 748-9

Volkmar, F.R.; Cohen, D.J.; Hoshino, Y.; Rende, R.D. & Paul, R. (1988). Phenomenology and classification of the childhood psychoses. *Psychol Med*, Vol. 18, pp. 191-201

Watkins, J. M.; Asarnow, R.F. et al. (1988). Symptom development in childhood onset schizophrenia. *J Child Psychol Psychiatry*, Vol. 29, pp. 865-78

Weinberger, D.R. (2002). Biological phenotypes and genetic research on schizophrenia. *World Psychiatry*, Vol. 1, pp. 2-6

Werry, J. S.; McClellan, J.M. et al. (1991). Childhood and adolescent schizophrenic, bipolar, and schizoaffective disorders: a clinical and outcome study. *J Am Acad Child Adolesc Psychiatry* , Vol. 30, pp. 457-65

Werry, J.S. (1996). Childhood schizophrenia. In: *Psychoses and pervasive developmental disorders in childhood and adolescence*. Volkmar, F.R. (Ed.), Amercan Psychiatric Press, ISBN-10: 1882103017, Washington, DC, USA

7

Verbal Behavior Analysis as a Diagnostic and Psychopharmacological Strategy for Differentiating Paranoid and Disorganized Schizophrenics

Frederic Verhaegen and Michel Musiol
Nancy Université (Université Nancy 2)
Laboratoire de Psychologie de l'Interaction et des Relations Intersubjectives,
MSH Lorraine
France

1. Introduction

Schizophrenia is no doubt one of the most controversial psychotic disorders when it comes to describing the symptomatological characteristics (or syndrome groups) that define it. It has no syndrome-specific pathognomonic sign, and its etiology remains poorly understood (Andreasen & Carpenter, 1993; Tsuang, 2000). A century of inquiries supported by considerable progress, especially recent advancements in electrophysiology, imaging, molecular biology, and even cognitive psychology (evolutionary psychology among others), have not yet supplied the needed answers, in such a way that coming up with a single definition of "schizophrenia" is still impossible. Even today, then, this pathology remains an ill-defined reality. Many studies have suggested that one problem with schizophrenia is its heterogeneity (Heinrichs, 1993), an idea supported not only by the discovery of its multiple clinical manifestations but also and especially because it is difficult to find characteristics or features that are shared by all individuals diagnosed with this disease (Chapman & Chapman, 1989; Goldstein, 1990; Heinrichs, 1993).

In this chapter, we will not address the issue of the potential cognitive or neuropsychological processes underlying the symptoms of schizophrenia. Whatever they may be, we believe that the pathology will necessarily be manifest in interactive and discursive settings, whether experimental or clinical; and we hypothesize accordingly that under certain conditions - at least in the natural conditions of language use - the verbal behavior of schizophrenics is likely to reflect the specificities of the disease (Musiol & Trognon, 2000). Locating and analyzing these specificities, if there are any, should therefore improve diagnosis strategies in the middle term.

Based on our view that verbal interaction is the "natural locus of symptom expression" (Trognon & Musiol, 1996), we propose a methodology for analyzing verbal interaction that is inspired by both pragmatics and cognitive psychology. Our aim is, firstly, to detect discourse and dialogue discontinuities as objectively and "decisively" as possible (by "decisively", we mean that there is a high probability of finding pathological dysfunctioning behind the pathological behavior). Then we look at the potential relationship between these discontinuities and the syndrome's specificities, and at a more general level, we discuss how they relate to the question of incoherence. Finally, we show that our pragmatic, cognitive, and formal methodology for dialogue analysis (Musiol, 2002; Musiol & Rebuschi, 2011) enables us to better specify and better differentiate between the various schizophrenic syndromes.

2. Grasping the symptomatological characteristics of schizophrenia

Clinical research on schizophrenia has been making significant progress for nearly thirty years now. In the 1970's and 80's, inquiries into the well-foundedness of the classification into subtypes (paranoid, disorganized, catatonic, etc.) proposed in clinical psychiatry gave way to other models for describing the disease (Andreasen, 1979a; 1984; Andreasen & Olsen, 1982; Crow, 1980; Liddle, 1987). The results of these studies, although growing in number, were contradictory, however, so their heuristic relevance was discredited to some extent. The heterogeneity of the findings led investigators to steer their research towards trying to establish more accurate criteria in view of obtaining greater homogeneity in the populations under study. The development of a number of clinical-information gathering methods, all aimed at producing more global symptom-assessment scales, is an example of this latter approach. New tools like Kay et al.'s (1987) PANSS (Positive and Negative Syndrome Scale), and Andreasen's (1983, 1984) SANS (Scale for the Assessment of Negative Symptoms) and SAPS (Scale for the Assessment of Positive Symptoms) became the first methods used and designed for the specific purpose of evaluating the negative and positive symptoms of schizophrenia. All of these early scales are still widely used today.

The work that produced these tools was thus based on psychometric analyses (mostly factor analyses). Schizophrenia was described first in terms of two dimensions (Andreasen, 1983; 1984; Andreasen & Olsen, 1982; Crow, 1980) and then in terms of three (Liddle, 1987): positive (or productive), negative (or deficient), and disorganized, characterized by formal thought disorders (impoverished and incoherent discourse). In addition, schizophrenics frequently suffer from cognitive deficits affecting attention, memory, and executive functions. The impairment is sometimes massive and is relatively well correlated not only with negative-symptom severity, but also, although to a lesser extent, to positive-symptom severity (Berman et al., 1997; Harvey et al., 1996). These new orientations proved promising and sparked considerable interest, partly due to their satisfactory degree of diagnostic and statistic validity, grounded in particular on their good inter-judge reliability rates. Another advantage of this type of clinical scale for assessing schizophrenic symptomatology is that these psychometric instruments have generally been deemed very useful in evaluating the effectiveness of neuroleptic medication.

2.1 Psychometric approach to communication disorders in schizophrenia

The idea that language abnormalities pervade the discourse of schizophrenic patients is now largely acknowledged by the scientific community. However, although language and communication disorders are among the most widely studied, they are hardly ever examined in an interaction context. Taking a classical clinical approach, Andreasen (1979a, 1979b) drew up an extensive inventory of these disorders based on the symptom-assessment scales she developed for describing the language-related anomalies specific to schizophrenic discourse. Moreover, her work is still valid today (Bazin et al., 2002; Bazin et al., 2005; Docherty et al., 2003; Liddle et al., 2002; Olivier et al., 1997).

Moreover, clinical observation has made a substantial contribution to describing these impairments. Right from the very first descriptions of schizophrenic symptoms, a preponderant concern was language, or even thought disorders (Bleuler, 1911; Chaslin, 1912; Kraepelin, 1971). In fact, it was in a Bleulerian perspective centered on language and communication that Andreasen designed a scale for assessing dissociation (Scale for Assessment of Thought, Language and Communication or TLC) in an attempt to make the concept of "formal thought disorder" fully operational. A such disorder is indeed a key symptom for researchers and clinicians interested in the potential complex thought disorders associated with this pathology. Note that Andreasen's TLC was recently translated into French and validated by Bazin (Bazin et al., 2002).

Studies attempting to gain finer insight into the symptomatology of schizophrenia via a clinical approach continue to grow in number. It has become clear, however, that although these concepts - "formal thought disorder", "incoherence", "disorganized thought" - have been addressed in terms of their relationship to language problems, little research has been conducted to look into how they are related to verbal interaction, that is, interaction in the "natural context" where these phenomena occur (Trognon & Musiol, 1996). In our minds, analyzing this context is a prerequisite for relating these language behaviors to the specific communication, language, and thought abnormalities of these individuals, and in the end, for relating the "incoherent" behaviors rooted in these problems to potential dysfunctions of the underlying cognitive processes, themselves based on the language faculty (Hauser et al., 2002), mental logic (Rips, 1995), reasoning (Politzer, 2002), dialogue (Musiol & Rebuschi, 2011), and the interleaved processes required to manage several of these subcomponents. This brings us directly back to the question of what unit should be used to analyze these phenomena. We will address this question in the next section.

2.2 Features of discontinuity in schizophrenic verbal interaction (pragmatic, cognitive, and dialogical approach)

Instruments based on "quantification", including psychometric scales, do not paint an accurate picture of the cognitive specificities of schizophrenic language and communication disorders. Such instruments are developed using a static type of methodology that is hardly compatible with the naturally dynamic character of communication. In addition, concepts like "incoherence" and "formal thought disorders" are only defined in terms of the items included in the scales (Andreasen & Grove, 1986; Bazin et al., 2002), i.e., solely in terms of the overt behaviors assumed to be associated with the concepts, without reference to the utterance and discourse contexts from which the behaviors arise, nor to the psycholinguistic and/or inferential types of cognitive processes upon which the behaviors rest.

In parallel with the clinical and psychometric approach to schizophrenic communication disorders, a pragmatic and linguistic type of approach began to develop in the 1970's. Unlike the preceding approach, this approach studies the language and communication "disorder" *in situ*, while putting as much emphasis on the speech act as on the syntactic-semantic structure of the utterance and the contextual dimension of the uttering process, grasped in context (Chaïka, 1974; Fromkin, 1975). This means that nearly 20 years before the emergence of the dynamic and resolutely conversational and dialogical approach (Trognon, 1992), the goal had already become to grasp more than just the schizophrenic language disorder itself, but also and especially the impaired way in which these individuals use language in a communication setting (whether in a clinical interview, a therapy session, or an ordinary conversation). Within the past two or three decades, few researchers have challenged the idea that the greatest, if not one of the most important, difficulties of schizophrenic patients lies at the pragmatic level (making use of signs in communication contexts) (Andreasen et al., 1985; Chaïka, 1974, 1990; Frith, 1992; Fromkin, 1975; McKenna & Oh, 2005; Rochester & Martin, 1979; Widlöcher & Hardy-Baylé, 1989). Yet few investigators have attempted to develop tools suited to the ways these disorders are expressed during verbal interaction, i.e., tools that take the process-based, dynamic nature of interaction into account.

By focusing on the properties of conversations involving a psychiatric patient, we propose to develop descriptive, objective, and increasingly "decisive" models of the signs of schizophrenia, and thereby rise to the challenge presented by Chaïka and other linguists in the early seventies. We will do this by considering not only the utterance context of potentially incoherent speech acts, but also the dialogical context that surrounds the interview in which those acts are accomplished. Research on such conversations has provided support for the hypothesis that schizophrenic patients exhibit syndrome-specific impairments at the discourse and communication levels, and more specifically, alterations that affect the psychocognitive principles governing language use (Grice, 1975; 1987; Musiol, 2004; Sperber & Wilson, 1995).

Studies conducted in the pragmatic research trend of cognitive psychopathology since the early 1990's (Musiol, 1992; Trognon, 1992) have shown in this vein that the expression modes of a disorder -- here, schizophrenia -- are largely dependent upon the characteristics of the interaction, particularly the possibility conditions of verbal communication. We thus propose to grasp discourse and dialogue disorders' using a discontinuity-analysis model designed to account for schizophrenic language use and its interrelationships both with the patients' discourse and with their conversational behavior as it is manifested in particular in the turn-taking process. The many properties of verbal interaction -- turn-taking, reciprocity, the hierarchical and dynamic organization of its constituents, and the interlocutionary roles the communicating subjects occupy in the turn-taking process (initiator/speaker versus reacting-partner/listener) -- should all be seen as factors likely to have an impact on our understanding of the significance of a symptom (Musiol, 2002), in such a way that the interlocution can be regarded as the natural locus of expression of psychopathological phenomena (Trognon & Musiol, 1996). Because of its specific properties and the constraints it imposes on the interlocutors' behavior, then, the conversational transaction is the perfect place, methodologically speaking, for observing certain interpretive and inferential processes and their potential dysfunctioning.

Below we present the premises of our investigation strategy, based for the time being on a dialogical and pragmatic type of analysis and aimed at bringing any such dysfunctions and incongruities to the fore. Our task here is to build a predictive model describing the properties of the inferential processes underlying certain forms of incoherence in dialogue, which in our case, should show up in the behaviors that schizophrenic and "normal" interlocutors are led to adopt.

2.2.1 Discontinuity and verbal Interaction

The idea, then, is to build a dialogical and pragmatic model capable of accounting for the dynamic properties of verbal-interaction sequences in which a discontinuity[1] appears. The skills examined -- which belong more specifically to the field we investigate using our pragmatic, dialogical, and cognitive approach to psychopathology -- are thus related to the characteristics of the inferential processes interlocutors are led to act out in a verbal exchange, and more specifically, in a clinical interview. They are also related, among other things, to the cognitive processes used to manage the properties extracted from the various different components of the primary communication units that generate the verbal interaction. These units are elementary illocutionary acts, also called speech acts or discourse acts. On the empirical level, our research in this area over the past fifteen or so years (Musiol & Trognon, 2000; Musiol & Verhaegen, 2009) has enabled us to hypothesize that conversations involving a schizophrenic patient will exhibit many incongruities and discontinuities. Our studies have also led to the hypothesis that the discontinuities formally detected and delineated within a verbal interaction with a schizophrenic fall into two main categories, defined by the so-called hierarchical and functional properties of the discourse structure. Relative to this "hierarchical and functional" structure of discourse (Roulet et al., 1985), we will call the first category "non-decisive" and the second, "decisive".

The idea that discourse must be approached as a verbal interaction, at least in linguistics, dates back to the 1930's and Bakhtine (Bakhtine, 1930), but the concept of hierarchical structure itself was introduced by Pike in the late 1960's (Pike, 1967). This author incorporated the study of language (both languages and discourse) into a unified theory of the structure of human behavior. In his theory, as the author explains, any event involving human behavior (a religious service, for example) can be broken down at the first level into a certain number of constituents linked by specific functions; each constituent can in turn be broken down into lower-level constituents, and so on down until we obtain units of behavior like the utterance or the word.

In this view - and similarly to what is expressed in certain conceptions developed in the linguistics of argumentation (Roulet et al., 1985) or in the psychology of communication (Trognon, 1995; Trognon et al., 1999) - discourse (that is to say, the conversational transaction) can be seen as a "negotiation" process, which makes its structure and functioning easier to grasp, and the conversational transaction can be seen as the relevant unit of analysis. We will define conversational transactions as follows: the most elementary component is the simple or complex speech act (the illocution). Illocutions are defined as acts that apply forces to propositional content (Searle & Vanderveken, 1985); the force defines the type of action (assertive, commissive, directive, declarative, expressive) that the speech act accomplishes, and can be described in terms of a number of properties, of which the illocutionary goal and its direction of fit are among the most important. At a more global level, conversational transactions are regular groups of structures, and structures are regular groups of exchanges and interventions. Accordingly, an exchange is the basic unit of an interlocution, where "basic" means that it is the smallest "dialogical" unit of the interaction (Goffman, 1974; Roulet et al., 1985).

From a microscopic point of view, an exchange is made up of interventions, and the minimal intervention is made up of speech acts (or illocutions). From the macroscopic point of view, exchanges and interventions are organized into structures. Some of these structures

---

[1] Here, we interpret the notion of incoherence in terms of discontinuity

exhibit a typical organization and can be functionally interpreted as if they realized a collective intentionality. Some examples are communicating information, debating, discussing, negotiating, leading a group, making a group decision, as is conducting or participating in a clinical interview or a psychotherapy session.

2.2.2 Properties of non-decisive discontinuity

Earlier studies (see below) have shown that schizophrenic interlocutions (i.e., ones involving a person diagnosed as schizophrenic) exhibit many discontinuities between adjacent segments of discourse, whether at the exchange or intervention level. These discontinuities occur either when the schizophrenic patient is the second speaker and is attempting to adjust his/her reply to the interlocutor's previous intervention, or when the patient is expressing his/her train of thought as he/she accomplishes several speech acts within the same discursive intervention. We will use the term "between-intervention breaks" to refer to coherence problems or discontinuities resulting from a violation of the chaining constraints that guarantee continuity between the speaking turns of two separate interlocutors in an exchange, and "within-intervention breaks" to refer to coherence problems or discontinuities resulting from violation of between-act chaining constraints within the same intervention. Note that in discourse, there exist complex interventions that contain subparts made up of one or more embedded interaction exchanges (Roulet et al., 1985). Failure to satisfy any of these constraints, no matter what kind, suffices to produce a discontinuity. Note in addition that chaining constraints apply locally first, between adjacent speaking turns, but the possibility of embedded exchange sequences authorizes deferred constraint satisfaction (until after this type of sequence is over), which takes place farther along in the unfolding of the discourse. It is also possible to double up embedded sequences recursively (one can always make a parenthetical remark within another parenthetical remark), which means that the interlocutors must be capable of managing a recursive exchange structure (and that the formal analyst of the exchange must be able to take its hierarchical structure into account). To be exact, one must make the distinction between "proximal" breaks, which occur between adjacent interventions, and "distal" breaks, which also result from the violation of a chaining constraint, but this time between non-adjacent interventions. Although distal, these non-adjacent interventions structure the discourse, insofar as the intervention called the speaker's initiative contains the directing utterance that conveys the speaker's intended meaning, and the intervention called the listener's reactive-initiative intervention contains the directing utterance that carries the linguistic trace of the addressee's interpretation of the initial directing utterance. Failure to satisfy these distal constraints in a deferred manner -- no doubt because there is no representation of them -- constitutes failure in a complex task. As such, it reflects severe disorganization of the interlocutive ability (Musiol & Pachoud, 1999).
Below we present a non-decisive discontinuity exemplifying a between-intervention break.
Example 1 (X is the schizophrenic interlocutor) [2]

---

[2] Transcription conventions: (...) stands for the beginning and end of a conversational sequence; (→) stands for prolonged pronunciation of a sound of the language; (↑) stands for a rising intonation; (↓) stands for a falling intonation; (inaudible) means that the passage was inaudible (sometimes its duration is indicated); words in capitals mean that the speaker stressed the word; +5+ stands for a silence of five seconds. Information likely to be important for understanding and analyzing the transcription is shown in parentheses. Ambiguous passages are shown in brackets. For ethical reasons,

V51: (...) and how do you spend your time otherwise (↑) +5+
X52: I watch TV
V53: You watch TV and you watch TV where (↑)
X54: In this room
V55: In this room here and what about when you're not here (↑) when you're somewhere else
X56: I was born in S (city)
V57: Yeah
X58: On September 20th 19xx (...)

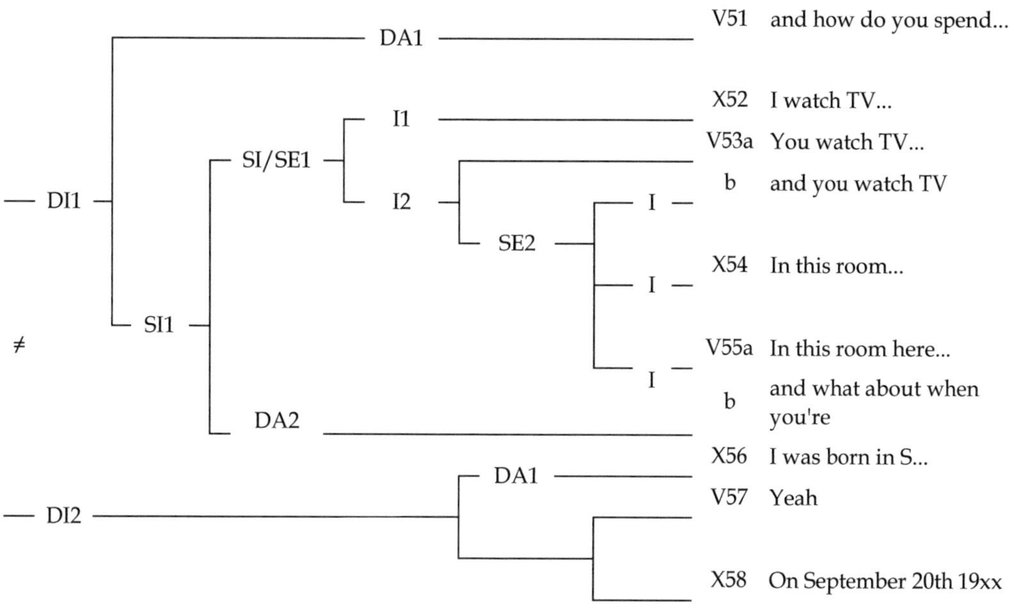

Legend. SE: subordinate exchange. I: intervention. DI: directing intervention. DA: directing act. SI: subordinate intervention. V: interlocutor V. X: interlocutor X. #: discontinuity.

Fig. 1. Commented hierarchical diagram of Example 1.

This exchange consists of two directing interventions (I1 and I2), corresponding to two conversational contributions of two different speakers, the first by the "normal" interlocutor (hetero-initiated from the patient's point of view). This first intervention, I1, can be considered complex. It contains five speaking turns (V51 to V55), and is made up of a directing intervention (a substructure represented by intervention V51/DA1, a first-level directing act), and a subordinate structure, SI1, which takes place between X52 and V55. This subordinate intervention will be called complex too; it consists of a directing substructure V55b/DA2 (second-level directing act) and a subordinate exchange, SE1, which constitutes its subordinate part (SI) insofar as V55b retroactively subordinates this

---

the names of persons, places, and dates have been changed to guarantee the anonymity of all participants.

substructure. Because the schizophrenic interlocutor's reactive-initiative intervention (I2) unfolds between X56 and X58 (with a directing constituent conveyed by X56[3]), one can make the assumption that I1's directing component is carried by the utterance acts performed in DA1 and DA2, as a directive type of complex speech act like [DA1-DA2] would do, here, "*How do you spend your time when you're not here?*"

The hierarchical and functional analysis of this sequence thus ascribes X56 the status of act serving as the "initiative-interpretive reaction" to the initiating directing component, but a discontinuity appears. The break is the result of the lack of continuity here between V51/V55b (I1/DA1-DA2) and X56 (I2/DA1). By definition, we will consider discontinuities that have an effect on the exchange to consist, discursively, of a pair of adjacent interventions (Ii, Ij) whose second element, Ij, is not in a continuity relation with the intervention that precedes it (Ii) in the conversation. The first element, Ii, is seen as a source variable that imposes constraints on the second element, Ij. In Roulet et al.'s (1985) sense, the source variable, Ii, thus defines the set of all between-intervention constraints linked to a question that has a closed set of possible responses. These constraints are:

- Thematic condition: obligation to reply on the theme addressed in the question.
- Propositional-content condition: obligation to give a reply whose content is related to the question's content in an implicative, antonymic, or paraphrastic way.
- Illocutionary condition: obligation to express the content of one's reply in the corresponding illocutionary mode.
- Argumentative-orientation condition: obligation to reply in the expected way, i.e., to confirm the content of the question or its argumentative orientation.

We posit that discontinuity exists as soon as the second element in the pair does not totally or partially satisfy the constraints imposed by the first element (Trognon & Musiol, 1996; Musiol et al., 1998). In line with this definition, V51/V55b (I1/DA1-DA2) is the first element in the pair, Ii, and X56 (I2/DA1) is the second element in the pair, Ij. The discontinuity was generated here by the violation of three out of four conditions: thematic (the patient introduced a new topic), propositional content and argumentative orientation (the new topic in fact introduced a new discourse universe). The second element in the pair, Ij, was an unexpected response to the first element, Ii, in the framework of the general theme of the conversational transaction introduced more globally by the "normal" interlocutor.

Among the different types of constraints described in discourse analysis, within-intervention chaining constraints pertain to the subject's coordination of his/her own discourse; they are discourse planning constraints. Planning operates at various levels, depending on the complexity of the discourse. The following example exhibits a within-intervention discontinuity (non-decisive). By that token, it reveals a disorganized discursive production and thus, impaired discourse planning.

Example 2 (A is the schizophrenic interlocutor)[4]

A25: my mother Sophie
M26: yes
A27: my adopted mother uh (→)
M28: she's not your adopted mother

[3] The utterance act performed in X56, "*I was born in S*" is the constituent which, given the argumentative structure of I2, should satisfy the discursive constraints imposed by I1's directing component

[4] Sequence taken from a corpus of Bernard Pachoud (1996).

A29: I treat her as an adopted mother, don't know why
M30: who who might your mother be (↑)
A31: when I say adopted mother it was to reassure myself it's to (→) uh how can I say this (→) uh I'm (→) uh I'm happy [to see her / to have her] [5] (laughs) I'm taking my glasses off I can't see clearly Mister P (name) +2+

This is a within-intervention discontinuity occurring during a monologue. The patient unexpectedly changes focus in A31, "*uh I'm, uh, I'm happy [to see her/ to have her]*" since he is embarrassed to reply to the request for further information regarding his doubts about his ancestry. Failing to justify his self-doubts, it seems as if he switches to something else. The thing that makes this switch into a discontinuity, i.e., the thing that goes against the listener's expectations, and distinguishes this mode of chaining from a simple avoidance strategy, is that the speaker gives no sign of changing subjects and does not mark his abandonment of his initial plan (Musiol & Pachoud, 1999). Notice also that a syntactic-semantic ambiguity is conveyed by this speech act. Due to the lexical ambiguity of the segment "*to see her/ to have her*", it has at least two potential meanings, endowed with distinct inferential potentials -- the logical form[6] can be instantiated by proposition p1, whose syntactic-semantic structure is "*I'm happy to see her*", or by proposition p2, whose syntactic-semantic structure is "*I'm happy to have her*".

From the pragmatic standpoint, the patient is insufficiently cooperative (Grice, 1975), which shows up in his discourse as a violation of the coordination constraints: the patient changes focus not only without negotiating the change, but also without even marking it (even though a conjunction like "in any case" would have sufficed). This is why we can speak of discontinuity here, a discontinuity that can be interpreted as a violation of the thematic-chaining constraint or the topic-negotiation constraint. Within the intervention structure, the thematic constraint requires "the next constituent to be about a thematic element accessible from the first constituent, or, in the 'strong version' of that constraint, to be about the object of discourse (the intended theme of that constituent)" (Auchlin, 1988).

Note that this discontinuity is followed almost immediately by another one, as if, after violating a coordination constraint, the patient were unable to "get his discourse plan back" and started stringing utterances together in a random fashion, or rather in a one-by-one fashion based on mere contiguity, i.e., by hooking up to one of the last words pronounced, here the word "see", as in the following sequence: "*when I say adopted mother it was to reassure myself* / break 1 ⇒ / *I'm happy [to see her / to have her]* / break 2 ⇒ / *I'm taking my glasses off I can't see clearly*".

Such discontinuities in a speaker's discourse, which can be interpreted as violations of the constraints of coordination, in fact correspond to discontinuities in the speaker's intention (which the "normal" listener was trying to grasp) discontinuities that accentuate the meaning's indeterminate nature and prevent its confirmation later on in the discourse.

---

[5] The patient said /lavwaR/, which has two possible meanings in French: to see her ("*la voir*") and to have her ("*l'avoir*")

[6] For Pollock (1997), "The logical form is an interface between the mental language and the other cognitive systems involved in the intention and the reference [...] Representations of the logical form contain only terms that are semantically interpretable in a universal vocabulary (quantified referential expressions, variables, chains, etc.)."

At the very first level of theoretical interpretation, violation of the coordination constraints underlying the different types of non-decisive discursive discontinuity can be explained in terms of deficits. In the light of the assumptions of cognitive neuropsychology (Frith, 1992), these difficulties could be the expression of an impaired ability to represent actions in the form of "intentions"; such a deficit would have an impact on the ability to plan one's actions. In this view, discourse planning during an interlocution can only be distinguished from more atomic action-planning processes by the greater complexity of the planning strategies it requires. Indeed, planning one's discourse during a conversation is an extremely subtle task that requires not only planning the discourse itself (the linearity of the language imposes a sequential rendition of what one is trying to say), but also, with every new speaking turn, adapting it to what was just said; this means improvising one's next remark to fit the situation, which itself must be reassessed in an ongoing manner (Musiol & Pachoud, 1999; Pachoud, 1996).

2.2.3 Properties of decisive discontinuity

In our model's current state of development, there are two types of decisive discontinuity. We call the first type "conversational gear shifting" (Trognon, 1992; Trognon & Musiol, 1996). Discontinuities of this type disrupt the turn-taking process while sequentially satisfying the chaining constraints of two directing interventions. They are characterized by a surreptitious change in the course of action by the speaker (here, the schizophrenic patient), despite the fact that he/she was the initiator. Consequently, the referential context changes without any indication of that change on the part of the speaker.

This sequence is made up of a ternary exchange, E, so it contains three directing interventions, I1, I2, and I3. The first intervention (the initiating one), I1, is supported by speaking turn G42 and is qualified as complex insofar as it is comprised of several speech acts. The directing act of this intervention is the act "*I was supposed to have a wedding with 3000 guests*". The reactive-initiative intervention (I2) is also complex; it is comprised of three speaking turns (A43-A44). The directing act of this intervention, labelled DA2, is supported by the speech act proffered in A44b "*and a marriage to whom (↑)*" and two subordinate exchanges (SE), each of which consists of two interventions, A43-G43a, and G43b-A44a. Finally, the third intervention (called the reactive intervention), I3 -- also complex because it contains several speech acts (G44a-G44e) -- is supported in particular by the utterance act performed in G44a "*whoever'll want me*", which subordinates the rest of the speech acts in that intervention.

Example 3 (G is a female schizophrenic interlocutor)

G42: (...) so you you has no idea (→) it's a big deal you know (→) having a daughter and being (→) being (stammers) a virgin then being deflowered and all that (→) abandoned you know (→) I'm like you (→) I'm [no longer her / a virgin][7] now (→) I'm a virgin (→) I've got a little girl (→) I have (→) like you (→) but like you (→) but I should have (→) never have (→) gone out with (→) I still would've been a virgin (→) I would've be[8] married in white (→) in a

[7] Due to a language impairment typical of schizophrenics, it was not clear whether the patient said "*pucelle*" /pysel/, a French slang word for "virgin", or "*plus celle*" /plysel/, meaning "I'm no longer her"

[8] Note that the patient's exact words were "*je m'aurais marié*" (use of the auxiliary "*avoir*" instead of "*être*"). This grammatical error is commonly made by native French speakers with poor mastery of the language

big ceremony (→) I was supposed to have a wedding with 3000 guests (→) how does that sound to you (↑)

A43: 3000 (↑)

G43: 3000 guests (→) so you can see that I've got enough

A44: my God I see (→) and a marriage to whom (↑)

G44: whoever'll want me (→) if it's Luke it's Luke (→) if it's not Luke (→) it'll be another (→) another American (→) hey I'm not worrying about it anymore (...)

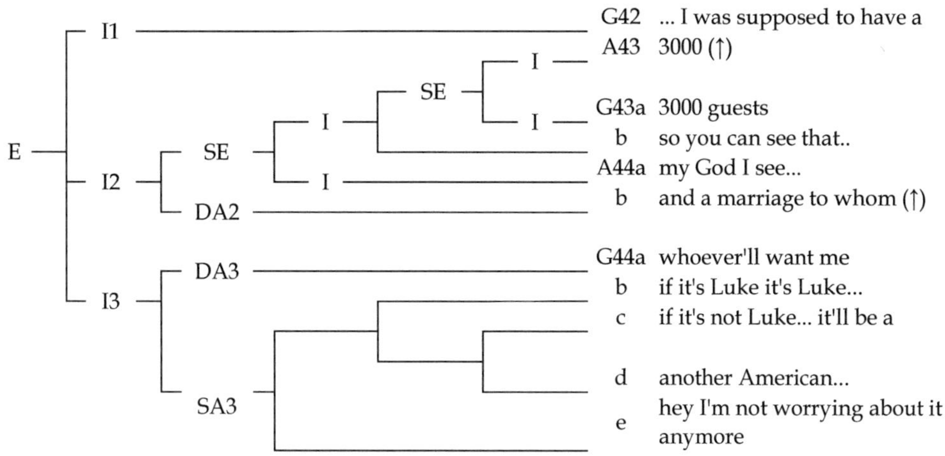

Legend. E: exchange. SE: subordinate exchange. I: intervention. DA: directing act. SA: subordinate act. G: interlocutor G. A: interlocutor A.

Fig. 2. Commented hierarchical diagram of Example 3.

In this sequence, then, it is schizophrenic patient G who, in G42, initiates a narration (in which her interlocutor agrees to participate) of the wedding she was supposed to have (first intervention, labelled the initiating intervention). The directing constituent "*and a marriage to whom (↑)*" (second intervention: A44b) also contributes to this narration. The reference universe of this question corresponds to an "imaginary" wedding related by G. This second intervention can also be interpreted as a question about G's future marriage plans, and this is the interpretation that G links into, via a third directing intervention in G44a. But her remarks are unexpected, to say the least. We will say here that G "shifts gears" during this third phase of the interaction. Now, although a conversational discontinuity like failing to answer a question or not replying to the point being made can be interpreted as a refusal to communicate, a conversational shift of gears cannot be interpreted as such. Indeed, on the third speaking turn, the initial speaker (here the schizophrenic patient) satisfies the between-intervention constraints of the interlocutionary pair at the very same time as she "shifts gears".

Conversational sequences in which the patient shifted gears were in fact quite typical here. They consisted of three interventions that were not necessarily consecutive. The first intervention, made by the patient, initiated a course of action whose realization required the interlocutors to perform a series of subactions, usually involving several speaking turns. The second intervention, by way of which the interlocutor pursued the conversation, had the particularity of being interpretable as an action which both accomplished part of the course of action initiated by the preceding intervention, and initiated a new course of action. The schizophrenic patient linked into this via a third intervention, which in most cases, satisfied the between-intervention constraints (also called "interactional" constraints); however, in cases of gear shifting, the patient pursued the new course of action (Trognon & Musiol, 1996).

Conversational gear shifting can in fact be formally described in the following manner. Let I1, I2, and I3 be three interventions that follow each other in a conversation, although not necessarily consecutively. Of the three component pairs in this sequence, (I1, I2), (I1, I3), (I2, I3), two exhibit continuity and one exhibits discontinuity. The continuous pairs are (I1, I2) and (I2, I3). Intuitively, these pairs exhibit continuity because their components -- for example, I1 and I2 for the pair (I1, I2) -- belong to the same discourse universe. However, the thematic universes of (I1, I2) and (I2, I3) are disjoint, albeit non-contradictory. Furthermore, abstractly speaking, the meaning of I2 is the union of the meanings at play in (I1, I2) and (I2, I3). It all seems as if this three-intervention sequence formed two parallel thematic series, with I2 serving to switch from one series to the other. This is precisely what makes the pair (I1, I3) discontinuous. In switching from the first series to the second series, I2 loses some of its properties. Indeed, two sets of properties characterize a conversational component. The first includes the semantic-pragmatic properties attached to the components' literal meaning, so the illocutionary force belongs to this set. The second includes the properties that describe how the component fits into the organization of the conversation, such as whether the component is directing or subordinate (Trognon & Musiol, 1996). So, the

Example 4 (J is the schizophrenic interlocutor)

J142: Well I where I really suffered it's when I had my concussion

V143: It was due to an accident (↑)

J144: Yes well somebody practically knocked me over (↓) it's really a (→) it's a (→) who threw me (→) who was in front and me behind and who (→) but well I don't care because (→) well I was loaded I actually had 5 liters of wine of (→) of Pineau[9] 5 liters of beer plus 1 or 2 (inaudible)

V145: That you had drunk (↑)

J146: We were going to the farm in S (place) (↓) an abandoned farm (↓) that Henry lives in (→) that belongs to Henry (inaudible) uh (→) a house that what was it what was it (→) that somebody got (↓) + me I liked I like Frank (↓) Frank L (name) (↓) he saved me (→) with his brother (inaudible)

V147: He saved you how (↑)

J148: What (↑)V149: How did he save you (↑)

J150: Ah but uh (→) who uh (→) well he saved me uh because I was with him because he (→) was DRINKing I mean (↓) he wanted to (→) hit me + and besides his brother kidnapped me (↓) +2+ well what helps me here is a good guy it's Damien (↓) um luckily he did that to me because (→) he was doing like this he was making himself disappear +1+ and I can do it myself disappear +1+

V151: So you could disappear and reappear (↑)

J152: Yes (↓)

[9] Pineau is a sweet wine that is slightly stronger than a standard dinner wine.

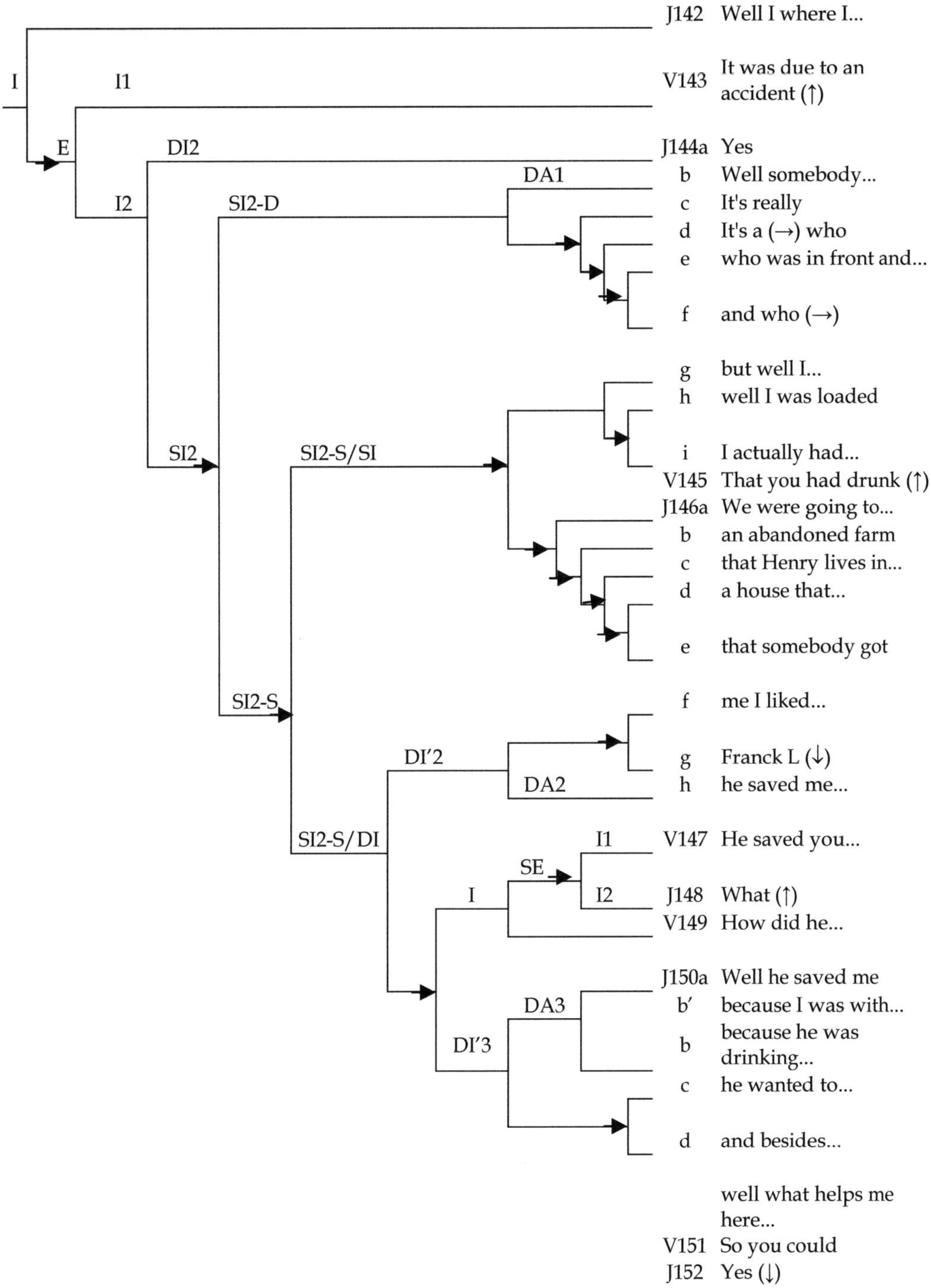

Legend. E: exchange. SE: subordinate exchange. I: intervention. DI: directing intervention. SI: subordinate intervention. DA: directing act. V: interlocutor V. J: interlocutor J.

Fig. 3. Commented hierarchical diagram of Example 4.

meaning of I2 in the second series now only retains the semantic-pragmatic properties of this element, as if I2 could somehow be withdrawn from the conversational structure to which it belongs in order to be treated abstractly and literally.

Our model involves a second type of decisive discontinuity qualified as a "defective conversational initiative". Granted, this type of within-intervention discontinuity consists of chaining that sequentially satisfy the interactional constraints governing the organization of the exchange-level subcomponents of the complex transaction unit. Yet it consists specifically of discontinuities that are inherent in the hierarchical and functional relations governing the sequentialization of speech acts of different levels (in the sense that an act can impose interactive constraints on the constituent that follows it or even precedes it, while still being dependent upon it at the hierarchical and functional level), which subsume or support the argumentation of the interlocutor who initiated the conversational transaction, e.g., the schizophrenic patient.

This hierarchical and functional diagram brings out a complex intervention structure. This intervention will be called self-initiated -- in the present case, initiated by the schizophrenic patient. It can be subdivided into two parts. The first has a single constituent, J142, which is the transaction's directing constituent at the intervention level. The second is a complex exchange-level constituent that progresses through eight other speaking turns in the transaction; it is the subordinate component of the exchange-level transaction that extends from V143 to J150.

The two directing constituents of this exchange are V143, a simple intervention (I1) performed by the "normal" interlocutor, and a complex intervention (I2) which runs from J144 to J150 and is itself made up of two complex parts, DI2 conveyed by speech act J144a -- which is an act of confirmation and is the directing element of this intervention -- and SI2, a subordinate intervention that progresses across J144b and J150d. The second part of this intervention will also be called complex. Its dynamic progression from J144b to J150d unfolds at the first analysis level by way of two subcomponents, themselves endowed with a complex structure: SI2-D (J144b to J144f) and SI2-S (J144g to J150d). The first-level directing act of this constituent is accomplished in J144b, i.e., "*well somebody practically knocked me over*". It is only as the discursive segments of this complex intervention (SI2) progress and are articulated each in turn that we gradually uncover the main characteristics of the defectiveness of the patient's conversational initiative. Statement 144b will be called the "directing act" (DA1) of the first-level directing constituent of this complex intervention-level component. Likewise, 144b is the directing constituent of directing intervention SI2-D, which itself forms the directing part of this complex component (SI2). The substructure SI2-D thus dominates SI2-S, itself highly complex, and as such, dominates the key act of this substructure, here again called "directing". We are speaking of the act accomplished in J146h, i.e., "*he saved me with his brother*". This subordinate part, SI2-S, runs across J144g and J150d. In turn, SI2-S includes a subordinate part going from J144g to J146e (SI2-S/SI) and a directing part going from J146f to J150d (SI2-S/DI). At the hierarchical and functional level, SI2-S/DI is comprised of two complex intervention-level constituents in a subordination relation: DI'2, which extends from J146f to J146h with J146h as its directing act (DA2), and DI'3, which spans from J150a to J150d. The directing act of this intervention is complex; it is composed of two segments, 150a and 150b, articulated around the connective "*because*", which has a causal function. Moreover, directing act DA3 is associated interactively to subordinate act J150b' (preparatory function), which is incorporated into the directing act's structure and into subordinate acts J150c and J150d, both of which fulfill a justifying function. Insofar as we are describing the structure of a complex intervention-level component, namely SI2-S-DI, we will acknowledge -- while drawing from Roulet's (Roulet et al., 1985) model -- that DA2 imposes constraints of the interactive type on DA3. Likewise, insofar as component SI2-S-DI is itself an integral part of complex intervention SI2, of which SI2-D is the directing element, we will acknowledge that DA1 imposes interactive constraints on both DA2 and DA3. Indeed, DA1 is the directing constituent of complex intervention SI2-D, which subordinates SI2-S globally, i.e., dominates both DA2 and DA3.

We can see here that, at the dialogical level, the discontinuity is generated by a multi-layered process, in the sense that DA3, namely utterance J150a-b "*he saved me because he was DRINKing I mean*", satisfies neither the argumentative-relation constraint imposed by DA2, that is, utterance J146h "*he saved me with his brother*", nor the argumentative-relation constraint imposed more distally by DA1, that is, utterance J144b "*well somebody practically knocked me over*". Clearly, the utterance act performed in DA3 "*he saved me because he was DRINKing I mean*" (just like the acts that contribute more globally to the coherence of the subcomponent dominated by DA2, such as "*he saved me with his brother*") can in no way be seen as a discursive constituent of the rhetorical "argument-conclusion" relations imposed on it by discursive constituent DA2, which plays the role of argument here. Moreover, we can also see that this same constituent, DA2, does not satisfy the constraints imposed on it by hierarchical constituent DA1, which dominates it hierarchically. Hence, "*he saved me with his brother*" (DA2) does not satisfy the interactive constraints -- which once again are argumentative-relation constraints -- theoretically imposed on it by DA1, that is, "*well somebody practically knocked me over*". We will agree in addition, based on the hierarchical analysis of this sequence, that DA3 is no better at satisfying the interactive constraints imposed on it by DA1. The rest of the sequence conveys other artefacts and incongruities, but we will stop our commentary at this point since the elements of analysis presented so far suffice for our demonstration.

More generally, J150 is made up of another series of speech acts that introduce a new topic to which the interlocutor will contribute. We are thus in the presence of two distinct conversational transactions: the first (analyzed above) stops precisely at the end of J150d; the second begins with the dialogue-resumption segment "*well what helps me here*".

At the hierarchical and functional level, within-intervention constraints pertain to the proper formulation of interventions. Roulet's (Roulet et al., 1985) book defines them as follows:

- Thematic condition: obligation in the intervention to pursue the object of discourse presented in the intervention's first constituent, whether implicitly or explicitly.
- Argumentative-relation condition: obligation to pursue the intervention using a constituent capable of entering into an argumentative relation (be an argument or conclusion) with the intervention's first constituent.
- Argumentative-orientation condition: obligation, within the intervention, to continue with a constituent that does not contradict the argumentative orientation of the intervention's first constituent.

A complex intervention exhibiting discontinuity is theoretically composed of various act-level components, exchange-level components, and intervention-level components. These various components may be nested (e.g., an intervention can contain an exchange as a subpart of itself) and be combined into more complex units (interrelated hierarchically and functionally). We will call these units the subcomponents of the complex intervention. Being deemed relevant to analyzing this type of conversational transaction, these units are related to each other via domination relations at the rhetorical level; a given subcomponent of the complex intervention always either directs or is subordinate to one or more associated units. In addition, each potential subcomponent has its own internal coherence (if it consists of more than one speech act) and is functionally dependent on the subcomponents that surround it both upstream and downstream, but here again, in a more or less distal way. The functions operating inside a subcomponent are necessarily of the interactional and interactive type (they must satisfy both between- and within-intervention constraints), but the functions that associate the subcomponents to each other are solely of the interactive type.

Sequences exhibiting conversational initiative defectiveness contain at least three directing acts, e1, e2, e3, in a hierarchical and functional relation of domination derived from simple or complex intervention-level constituents. The domination relation defines three pairs [e1, e2], [e2, e3], and [e1, e3] whose dialogical rationality is such that the first element of the pair, e (the source element) puts the second element, e' (the target element) in a strategic interactive relationship with itself that is based on three conditions: the thematic condition, whereby e' must implicitly or explicitly continue with the object of discourse presented in e, the argumentative-relation condition, whereby e' must be an argument or a conclusion of e, and the argumentative-orientation condition, whereby e' must not contradict e in any way. Conversational initiative defectiveness is considered to exist if e3 does not satisfy one or more of the three interactive conditions imposed on it by e2 in the pair [e2, e3] or by e1 in the pair [e1, e3], or if e3 does not satisfy one of more of the three interactive conditions imposed on it by e2 in the pair [e2, e3] and e2 does not satisfy one or more of the three interactive conditions imposed on it by e1 in the pair [e1, e2].

2.2.4 Heuristic aspect of the analysis method

By analyzing numerous sequences from pathological verbal interactions, we were able to bring out several characteristics of the type of discontinuity called manifest or decisive (Musiol, 2002).

Although a patient's utterance discontinuity or discourse incongruity can be counteracted in a conversation by the interlocutor's verbal behavior, it is clear that conversational discontinuities of the within- or between-intervention type retain some degree of non-decisiveness. Only "conversational gear shifting" and sequences containing "conversational initiative defectiveness" can currently be seen as transactions where the patient's behavior might be "incoherent". Furthermore, the mere fact of detecting incoherence does not imply that there is a thought disorder, and therefore does not itself authorize an interpretation of this deficient interlocutionary behavior in terms of dysfunctional thought. What we do hypothesize, however, is that detecting *decisive* incoherence is an intermediate stage -- i.e., *a sufficient but non-necessary condition*[10] for any attempted interpretation in terms of psychopathology. We are also working on articulating the pragmatic-dialogical analysis of decisive sequences with the help of a formal semantic model, in view of "accessing" the properties and rationality of the semantic representations (Musiol & Rebuschi, 2011) of

---

[10] Under this hypothesis, the occurrence of a discontinuity of the decisive type is the sign of a dysfunction in the cognitive system, affecting, for example, cognitive-linguistic processes, cognitive-inferential processes, or their interface. The absence of this type of discontinuity in a corpus is not equivalent to the absence of pathology (the model may simply be insensitive to it).

subjects with a psychiatric disorder, i.e., their intentional, interpretive, or inferential thought processes.

Through the pragmatic-dialogical formalization of the sequences analyzed above (conversational gear shifting and conversational initiative defectiveness), we were able to paint a more precise picture of the form and basic properties of decisive discontinuity. This kind of discontinuity is not sustained by the simple proposition, the speech act, or even the exchange, but by conversational transactions whose structure is based on rhetorical and semantic relations between at least three discursive segments. The conversational transaction is the relevant unit, not the act, the utterance, or the two-or-three turn exchange.

Thus, the decisive nature of incoherence shows up at the transaction level in two types of structures:

- in an exchange, understood *a priori* as a balanced dialogue unit opposing a speaker (e.g., a patient) to his/her interlocutor (e.g., a therapist); the conversational transaction is structured on the basis of at least three symmetrical directing moves.
- in a complex intervention, understood as an asymmetrical dialogue unit where the argumentation of one of the interlocutors (e.g., the patient) overrides that of his/her addressee; the conversational transaction is analyzed on the basis of hierarchical and functional relations between at least three discursive segments detected in the main discourse -- the hierarchical and functional relations between these three or more constituents subsume and support the unfolding of the interlocutor's argumentation.

3. Study

The purpose of this study was to use a pragmatic-dialogical model to link any verbal-behavior discontinuities detected in a patient to that patient's clinical manifestations (or syndromes) as diagnosed on the basis of DSM-IV criteria. The merits of using this model are clear: it provides a more accurate description of the symptomatic manifestations of schizophrenia -- as they are expressed in verbal interaction in the form of syndrome-specific discontinuities -- and thereby allows us to show how these discontinuities co-occur with the clinical manifestations generally described in disease classification systems. From this, we should be able to set forth some specific hypotheses about the potentially distinct properties of the underlying cognitive processes. The models that account for non-decisive discontinuity in verbal interaction are congruent with a potential dysfunction in psychophysiological or neurocognitive processes like the ones involved in planning, for example. The models that account for decisive discontinuity in verbal interaction are congruent with potential impairment of representational or meta-representational cognitive processes (complex thought processes like intentional or inferential processes).

The characteristics of our empirical-investigation corpus (Table 1) also make it possible to control for the potential impact of antipsychotic medication on the expression of symptoms as they show up in verbal interaction. As stated at the beginning of this article, psychometric scales have traditionally been used to measure the effectiveness of neuroleptic treatment, and research in this area has mainly focused on the ability of these scales to assess the comparative effects of conventional (first generation) and atypical (second generation) neuroleptics on schizophrenic symptoms. While few studies contest the effectiveness of neuroleptics on schizophrenic symptoms (especially positive ones), the question of their mechanisms of action and their repercussions on cognition are still widely debated. Some studies have shown that the cognitive performance of schizophrenic patients improves more with atypical than with conventional neuroleptic medication (Goldberg & Weinberger, 1995; Harvey et al., 2003; Meltzer & McGurk, 1999), but their effectiveness is still being questioned.

4. Method

4.1 Participants

Thirty native French-speaking adults (18 men and 12 women, age 41.5±16) participated in the study. Twenty-two of the participants (14 men and 8 women, age 45.0 ±15.4) were assigned to the schizophrenic group (SCH) and eight (4 men and 4 women, age 32.1±14.3) were assigned to the control group (CTR). Two group of schizophrenic patients were formed on the basis of their TLC scores (Thought, Language and Communication Scale, Andreasen, 1979) by two experienced psychologists. Patients without thought disorder (non-thought-disorder patients (NTD), n=11) obtained a TLC score < 7 (mean 3.5 ± 1.7), and patients with thought disorder (thought-disorder patients (TD), n=11) obtained a TLC score > or = 7 (13.6 ± 3.0). The biographical characteristics of the sample are given in Table 1.

Among the 22 schizophrenic participants included fulfilling the Diagnostic and Statistical Manual of Mental Disorders IV (DSM-IV, American Psychiatric Association, 1994), 15 were being treated with antipsychotic drugs ((N)TD-A: mean dose equivalent to 281±118 mg/day of chlorpromazine) and 7 were taking no medication ((N)TD-N). The clinical types of the schizophrenics were as follows: there were 14 paranoid schizophrenics (5 of whom were taking antipsychotic drugs) and 8 disorganized schizophrenics (2 of whom were not taking any antipsychotic medication). The antipsychotic medication taken by the 15 schizophrenic patients was atypical (second generation), conventional (first generation), or a combination of the two. The patients had no neurological disorders and had not suffered from alcoholic intoxication or used any toxic substances for at least three months before the study. The diagnosis of schizophrenia was made by experienced psychiatrists who were not taking part in the study.

The schizophrenic patients were encountered in two different clinical institutions. Seven of them were in the psychiatric emergency ward (Temporary Psychiatric Hospitalization Unit in Troyes, France). They were apparently experiencing their first encounter with the psychiatric world and were not taking antipsychotic drugs. For these participants, no data indicating prior hospitalization in a psychiatric ward could be found. Given that a diagnosis of schizophrenia cannot be pronounced unless the signs of the disorder persist for at least six months (APA, 1994), we had to verify the diagnosis six months later. The diagnosis was indeed confirmed in all cases, although once again, the data was collected at the time of hospitalization. The other 15 patients had been under treatment in a psychiatric ward for at least three years (at the Specialized Hospital of La Rochelle, France). They benefited from daily antipsychotic treatment. Among these 15 patients, 5 were encountered in the specialized hospital where they were inpatients; the other 10, who were hospitalized only intermittently.

Like the schizophrenic patients, the control participants had no neurological disorders and had not suffered from alcoholic intoxication or used toxic substances for at least three months before the study. They had no diagnosed psychiatric disorders and were not taking any psychotropic medication. The controls were encountered in public places.

	SCH (n=22)		CTR (n=8) M±SD	Total
	NTD (n=11) (NTD-A / NTD- N) M±SD	TD (n=11) (TD-A / TD-N) M±SD		
Sex (M-F)	(7-4)	(7-4)	(4-4)	-
Clinical subtypes Paranoid schizophrenics - Disorganized schizophrenics	(7-4)	(7-4)	-	
Age in years	40,2 ± 15,3	49,7 ± 14,7	32.1±14.3	-
Education (in no. of years of schooling from first grade on)	9,6 ± 1,7	7,4 ± 3,2	9.1±1.4	-
Chlorpromazine equivalent in mg per day	200 ± 144 (276 ± 75 / 0)	182 ± 183 (286 ± 146 / 0)	-	-
Time since onset	5,8 ± 4,8	11,2 ± 13,5	-	-
TLC score	3,5 ± 1,7 (3,2 ± 1,9 / 4,3 ± 0,6)	13,6 ± 3 (14,1 ± 3,7 / 12,8 ± 1,3)	-	-
Number of interviews	11 (8 / 3)	11 (7 / 4)	8	30
Number of conversational transactions	124 (105 / 19)	234 (149 / 85)	45	403

Legend. NTD: schizophrenics without thought disorder. TD: schizophrenics with thought disorder. (N)TD-N: schizophrenics with no treatment. (N)TD-A: schizophrenics under antipsychotic treatment. CTR: participants with no diagnosed psychiatric disorders. n: number of patients. M: mean. SD: standard deviation.

Table 1. Characteristics of the Investigation Corpus

Concerning the sociodemographic variables, pairwise comparisons (Student's *t*-test for independent samples) of our groups (NTD vs. TD, NTD vs. CTR, TD vs. CTR) did not yield any significant differences in education ($t[1,20] = 1.694$, $p = .114$; $t[1,17] = 0.654$, $p = .524$; $t[1,17] = -1.368$, $p = .194$) or sex (corrected Chi2: $p = .803$). There was no significant differences for age ($t[1,20] = -1.492$, $p = .151$; $t[1,17] = 1.164$, $p = 0.260$) excepted between group TD and the control group ($t[1,17] = 2.604$, $p = .019$). A comparison of the two schizophrenic groups (NTD and TD) on time-since-onset indicated no significant difference ($t[1,20] = -1.244$, $p = .236$). Regarding the neuroleptic treatment of these two groups (mean chlorpromazine-equivalent dose in mg/day), no significant difference was found

(t[1,20] = .272, p = .789). Given that both patient groups contained neuroleptic-treated and untreated individuals, we also compared the treated schizophrenics with no formal thought disorders (NTD-A) and the treated schizophrenics with formal thought disorders (TD-A): no significant difference was found here either (t[1,13] = -0.154, p = .881). The medication factor should therefore not interfere with the results. The TLC scores of the two schizophrenic groups (NTD and TD) were highly significantly different (t[1,20] = -9.691, $p < .001$). There was a highly significant difference too between group NTD and the control group (t[1,17] = 6.938, $p < .001$) and between group TD and the control group (t[1,17] = 15.030, $p < .001$).

4.2 Procedure

The study was based on a pragmatic and dialogical analysis of verbal transactions taken from a corpus composed of 30 interviews. In all cases, the interviewer was a research psychologist and the interviewee was either a schizophrenic patient or an individual with no psychiatric disorders. All of the interviewees agreed to have the conversation tape recorded so that we could compile our corpus. They were told why they were being recorded, and we did not conceal the fact that they were participating in a study. The instructions were simply to talk to the interviewer. If the interviewee said he/she was having trouble expressing him/herself at the beginning, the interviewer started with a relatively general topic of conversation (everyday activities and/or concerns).
The breakdown of the entire interview corpus gave us 403 conversational sequences (or transactions). Table 1 gives additional information about the interviews.

5. Results

5.1 Classification of conversational sequences, by type of Interlocutor

Our first step was to label the sequences as to whether they contained or did not contain a discontinuity, for each group of interlocutors. Again, the interlocutors were schizophrenics without thought disorder (NTD) or with thought disorder (TD), or individuals with no diagnosed psychiatric disorders (CTR).
Comparisons of the sequences with and without a discontinuity (whether decisive or non-decisive) across participant groups showed that the schizophrenics' conversational sequences (SCH) contained more discontinuities than the "normal" participants' sequences. These two groups were significantly different (Chi2 = 21.175, $p < .001$). There were also more discontinuous sequences in the Thought Disorder schizophrenic subcorpus than in the control-participant subcorpus (Chi2 = 35.300, $p < .001$) and more discontinuous sequences in the Thought Disorder schizophrenic subcorpus than Non-Thought-Disorder schizophrenic subcorpus (Chi2 = 54.726, $p < .001$). These results thus suggest that the models we devised to account for discourse discontinuity are good at differentiating between "pathological conversations" and "normal conversations" in terms of coherence. This is hold true for comparing the two groups of schizophrenics defined on the basis of presence or absence thought disorder. We note a marginally significant between Non-Thought-Disorder group and the control group (Chi2 = 2,966, p = .085).
Now, when the interlocutors were schizophrenics of the paranoid (SCH-P) or disorganized type (SCH-D), or individuals with no diagnosed psychiatric disorders (CTR), comparisons of the sequences with and without a discontinuity (whether decisive or non-decisive) showed that the disorganized-schizophrenics' conversational sequences (SCH) contained

more discontinuities than in the control-participant subcorpus (Chi2 = 17.347, $p < .001$) and there were also discontinuous sequences in the paranoid-schizophrenic subcorpus than in the control subcorpus (Chi2 = 22.323, $p < .001$). These results thus suggest that the models we devised to account for discourse discontinuity are good at differentiating between "pathological conversations" and "normal conversations" in terms of coherence. This does not seem to hold true, however, for comparing the two groups of schizophrenics defined on the basis of clinical type. The sequences in the paranoid-schizophrenic subcorpus did not have more discontinuities than those in the disorganized-schizophrenic subcorpus. These two subgroups did not differ significantly (Chi2 = 0.991, $p = .319$). Thus, irrespective of the medication variable and the type of discontinuity at play, the model failed to detect the specificities of each clinical type of schizophrenia. Our next step, then, will be to look at other variables in order to determine the specificities of each schizophrenic subtype.
Our next step, then, will be to look at other variables in order to determine the specificities of each type of discontinuity.

	NTD	TD	CTR	p-value			
				SCH vs CTR	NTD vs CTR	TD vs CTR	NTD vs TD
Sequences with discontinuity	13 (11%)	117 (50%)	1 (2%)	<.001	p=.085	<.001	<.001
Sequences without discontinuity	111 (89%)	117 (50%)	44 (98%)				
Total	124	234	45				

Legend. SCH: schizophrenics. NTD: schizophrenics without thought disorder. TD: schizophrenics with thought disorder. CTR: individuals with no diagnosed psychiatric disorder.

Table 2. Presence or Absence of Discontinuity, by Participant Group

5.2 Conversational sequences with or without a non-decisive discontinuity, by group of interlocutors

Now let us look at the number of sequences with or without the type of discontinuity we call "non-decisive", for each group of interlocutors. The distribution of these sequences across groups is shown in Table 3, which also gives the significance level in each case. Sequences containing a decisive discontinuity (nine in all) were not included in the table, so the comparison shown here is between non-decisive discontinuous sequences and sequences with no discontinuities.
These results are very similar to those presented above, in that non-decisive discontinuities were more frequent in the schizophrenic subcorpus. When we compare the sequences with a non-decisive discontinuity to ones with no discontinuity across participant groups, we can see that the schizophrenics' conversational sequences contained more such discontinuities than those of the "normal" individuals. These two groups differed significantly (Chi2 = 19.633, $p < .001$). We also found more non-decisive discontinuous sequences in the Thought Disorder schizophrenic subcorpus than in the control-participant subcorpus

(Chi2 = 33. 827, p < .001), and more non-decisive discontinuous sequences in the Thought Disorder schizophrenic subcorpus than Non-Thought-Disorder schizophrenic subcorpus (Chi2 = 59.607, p < .001). Comparing the sequences with or without a non-decisive discontinuity between Non-Thought-Disorder group and the control group, we can see that these two groups were not significantly different (Chi2 = 1.601, p = .206): the Non-Thought-Disorder schizophrenic sequences did not contain more non-decisive discontinuities than the control ones.

	NTD	TD	CTR	p-value			
				SCH vs CTR	NTD vs CTR	TD vs CTR	NTD vs TD
Sequences with non-decisive discontinuity	9 (8%)	112 (49%)	1 (2%)	<.001	=.206	<.001	<.001
Sequences without discontinuity	111 (92%)	117 (51%)	44 (98%)				
Total	120	229	45				

Legend. SCH: schizophrenics. NTD: schizophrenics without thought disorder. TD: schizophrenics with thought disorder. CTR: individuals with no diagnosed psychiatric disorder.

Table 3. Presence or Absence of Non-Decisive Discontinuity, by Participant Group

Now, when we compare the sequences with a non-decisive discontinuity to ones with no discontinuity across participant groups based on the clinical subtypes of schizophrenia (DSM-IV), we also found more non-decisive discontinuous sequences in the disorganized-schizophrenic subcorpus than in the control-participant subcorpus (Chi2 = 17.347, p < .001), and more non-decisive discontinuous sequences in the paranoid-schizophrenic subcorpus than in the control-participant subcorpus (Chi2 = 19.749, p < .001). Comparing the sequences with or without a non-decisive discontinuity across clinical types of schizophrenia, we can see that these two patient groups were not significantly different (Chi2 = 0.208, p = .649): the paranoid-schizophrenic sequences did not contain more non-decisive discontinuities than the disorganized-schizophrenic ones (see Table 4).

However, as suggested above and called for by our experimental design (see Table 1), additional information is needed regarding the potential interaction between our variables "clinical type of schizophrenia" and "medication" (Verhaegen & Musiol, 2009). So we attempted to find out, firstly, whether SCH-P-N conversational sequences had fewer, as many, or more non-decisive discontinuities than other sequences, as compared to SCH-D-N conversational sequences, and secondly, whether SCH-P-A conversational sequences had fewer, as many, or more non-decisive discontinuities than other sequences, as compared to SCH-D-A conversational sequences (see Table 5).

For the schizophrenics who were not under treatment (SCH-N), there were more non-decisive discontinuities among the SCH-D than among the SCH-P (Chi2 = 22.015, p < .001). By contrast, for the patients taking antipsychotic medication (SCH-A), the SCH-P's non-decisive discontinuities outnumbered the SCH-D's (Chi2 = 13.141, p < .001).

	SCH-P	SCH-D	CTR	p-value			
				SCH vs CTR	SCH-P vs CTR	SCH-D vs CTR	SCH-P vs SCH-D
Sequences with non-decisive discontinuity	71 (36%)	50 (33%)	1 (2%)	<.001	<.001	<.001	0.649
Sequences without discontinuity	128 (64%)	100 (67%)	44 (98%)				
Total	199	150	45				

Legend. SCH-P: paranoid schizophrenics. SCH-D: disorganized schizophrenics. SCH: schizophrenics. CTR: individuals with no diagnosed psychiatric disorder.

Table 4. Presence or Absence of Non-Decisive Discontinuity, by Participant Group

		SCH-P	SCH-D
SCH-N	Sequences with non-decisive discontinuity	12 (20%)	28 (67%)
	Sequences with no discontinuity	47 (80%)	(33%)
	Total	59	42
SCH-A	Sequences with non-decisive discontinuity	59 (42%)	22 (20%)
	Sequences with no discontinuity	81 (58%)	86 (80%)
	Total	140	108

Legend. SCH-P: paranoid schizophrenics. SCH-D: disorganized schizophrenics. SCH-N: schizophrenics with no treatment. SCH-A: schizophrenics under treatment.

Table 5. Conversational Sequences With or Without a Non-Decisive Discontinuity, by Presence/Absence of Antipsychotic Medication and Clinical Type of Schizophrenia

5.3 Conversational sequences with or without a decisive discontinuity, by group of interlocutors

Lastly, we looked at the sequences with and without decisive discontinuities for each patient group. Nine sequences were compatible with our decisive-discontinuity model. The Non-thought-Disorder schizophrenic group contains four decisive discontinuity and the Thought-Disorder schizophrenic group contain five ones. The two groups were not significantly different. However, all nine sequences occurred in the paranoid-schizophrenic subcorpus. This subgroup differed significantly from both the disorganized-schizophrenic group (binomial test p = .002) and the "normal" group (binomial test p = .002). Among these nine paranoid schizophrenics, three were from the no-medication group (SCH-P-N) and six were from the antispsychotic-medication group (SCH-P-A).

6. Discussion

These results indicate that the pragmatic and dialogical discontinuity models we developed (decisive and non-decisive models) turned out to be good at discriminating schizophrenic patients from individuals with no psychiatric disorders in terms of conversational coherence. In addition, they accounted for certain coherence-related specificities of the discursive and dialogical productions of patients with each of the subtypes of schizophrenia we studied (paranoid and disorganized). We were able to point out a strong correlation between the paranoid clinical type and a particular kind of "discontinuous" verbal behavior, namely, decisive discontinuity, both for paranoid schizophrenics with and without antipsychotic treatment.

Our decisive-discontinuity model thus allows us to propose some possible explanations for the dysfunctional interpretive and inferential thought processes of schizophrenics of the paranoid type, with the help of an additional model based on formal semantics (Musiol & Rebuschi, 2011). On the other hand, it does not allow us to draw any conclusions about possible similar dysfunctions among schizophrenics of the disorganized type. We are therefore forced to acknowledge that, in the present state of our research, it is impossible to decide which of the following possibilities is correct: either the specific characteristics of verbal interactions between a disorganized schizophrenic patient and a "normal" interlocutor are not captured by the discontinuity model we developed, or these disorganized patients do not exhibit significant incoherency in their dialogue.

The question of what kind of process supports this sort of incoherence arises as soon as we compare the specificities of these incongruous or even incoherent behaviors with theoretical and interpretive models of congruent discourse, such as models of dialogical and pragmatic analysis. We hypothesize that the processes at stake are those underlying the comprehension and calculation of communicative intentions, in Sperber's sense of the term: "Comprehension (or its pragmatic layer) is an inferential process, using as input the output of linguistic decoding and aiming at discovering the speaker's meaning. Comprehension consists, therefore, in inferring a mental state (an intention of a specific kind) from behavior (an utterance)" (Sperber, 2000, p. 129).

Furthermore, we know that decisive verbal-interaction discontinuities have some highly specific proprieties (Musiol, 2002). They appeared here solely in the course of self-initiated conversational sequences (i.e., initiated by the patient). From this standpoint, our model is not only capable of accounting for defective processes that can be grasped in terms of action-planning deficits, as in experimental cognitive neuropsychology for example, but is also and especially very effective for capturing dysfunctions affecting certain cognitive-inferential processes related to spared rationality. This capability is not offered by experimentation, questionnaires, or structured and semi-structured interviews, where the subject (here, the patient) is always in the "reactor's" position and is therefore led to react and adapt to the presentation of a "stimulus" present in the discourse of another person (e.g., in the task instructions given by an experimenter).

While no link was found here between the occurrence of non-decisive discontinuous transaction sequences and the clinical form of the schizophrenic interlocutor's pathology when the medication variable was not controlled, this was no longer true when we did control for this factor. For the schizophrenics who were not under any kind of antipsychotic treatment, we found more non-decisive discontinuities among patients of the disorganized type than among the paranoid ones. For those taking antipsychotic drugs, we found more non-decisive discontinuities among the paranoid schizophrenics than among the disorganized ones.

These results once again stress the merits of taking the medication variable into account in research into this disorder. Although we are not the first to make this recommendation, there are still few studies that look at the impact of medication on dialogue behavior (and not just verbal behavior) or on cognitive-inferential processes. Taking this type of variable into account has another advantage. It brings up the issue of the specificities of the cognitive processes underlying these disorders. Indeed, the present statistical results suggest that only the model of non-decisive discontinuity was able to bring out a significant effect of medication on the type of incoherence (Verhaegen & Musiol, 2009), firstly in terms of a decrease in discontinuity, i.e., the reestablishment of certain forms of coherence solely for patients suffering from the disorganized type of schizophrenia, and secondly, in terms of an increase in discontinuity for the paranoid type of patient.

7. Conclusion

The present findings enable us to define communication disorders in a more precise way than was possible until the late 1980's when the term "pragmatic impairment" was used to mean the same thing as impaired language use. Today, the pragmatic approach in cognitive psychopathology addresses various theoretical and practical dimensions of cognitive psychology and neurocognition. From an empirical point of view, however, descriptions of certain characteristics of severe disorders (psychoses and neuropathologies) remain inadequate. For example, we still do not have a precise symptom-classification system for describing the interpretive and inferential thought disorders of patients.

Psychology studies that take a pragmatic approach attempt to grasp and formalize this type of cognitive activity, thereby putting this approach in a position to supply new knowledge, not only for defining "incoherence" but also for capturing it by relating data obtained in a pragmatic perspective to neurocognitive conceptions of schizophrenia (Musiol & Verhaegen, 2009). The formal semantic approach should then allow us to gain new and better-informed insight into the psychocognitive processes associated with thought disorders (Musiol & Rebuschi, 2011).

Our investigation strategy sheds light on the question of the extent to which clinicians can make valid intuitive judgments about a patient's language and/or communication deficiencies when faced with the patient's behaviors. An apparent communication deficiency of a schizophrenic patient may not imply a thought disorder (even if a thought disorder most likely means impaired communication). From the diagnosis standpoint, the pragmatic approach to cognitive psychopathology allows us to contemplate the possibility of clarifying or even operationalizing the notion of "formal thought disorder". In a general way, our investigation strategy contributes to advancing our understanding of language and communication in relation to schizophrenia (Crow, 2010; Titone, 2010).

8. Acknowledgment

We wish to thank Dr. Jean-Michel Durand (CHS Marius Lacroix, La Rochelle, France) and Dr. Philippe Brun (CH des Hauts-Clos, Troyes, France) for their help with data collection. Thanks are also extended to Vivian Waltz for her translation of this paper.

9. References

Andreasen, N. C. (1979a). Thought, language and communication disorders. I-Clinical assessments definition of terms, and evaluation of their reliability. *Archives of General Psychiatry,* Vol. 36, pp. 1315-1324, ISSN 1538-3636

Andreasen, N. C. (1979b). Thought, language and communication disorders. II-Diagnostic significance. *Archives of General Psychiatry,* Vol. 36, 1325-1330, ISSN 1538-3636

Andreasen, N. C. (1982). Negative symptoms in schizophrenia. *Archives of General Psychiatry,* Vol. 39, 784-788, ISSN 1538-3636

Andreasen, N. C. (1983). *Scale for the Assessment of Negative Symptoms (SANS),* Iowa city, University of Iowa

Andreasen, N. C. (1984). *Scale for the Assessment of Positive Symptoms (SAPS),* Iowa city, University of Iowa

Andreasen, N. C., & Carpenter, W. T. Jr. (1993). Diagnosis and classification of schizophrenia. *Schizophrenia Bulletin,* Vol. 19, pp. 199-214, ISSN 0586-7614

Andreasen, N. C., & Grove, W. M. (1986). Thought, language, and communication in schizophrenia: Diagnosis and prognosis. *Schizophrenia Bulletin,* Vol. 12, 348-359, ISSN 0586-7614

Andreasen, N. C., & Olsen, S. (1982). Negative versus positive Schizophrenia. *Archives of General Psychiatry,* Vol. 39, pp. 789-794, ISSN 1538-3636

Andreasen, N. C., Hoffman, R. E., & Grove, W. M. (1985). Mapping abnormalities in Language and Cognition, In *Controversies in schizophrenia: changes and constancies,* A. Alpert (Ed.), pp. 199-226, Guilford Press, 978-089-8623-75-8, New York

American Psychiatric Association (1994). *Diagnostic and statistical manual of mental disorders. Fourth Edition (DSM IV).* American Psychiatric Association, ISBN 978-089-0420-62-1, Washington DC

Auchlin, A. (1988). Dialogue et stratégies: propositions pour une analyse dynamique de la conversation, In *Echanges sur la conversation,* J. Cosnier, N. Gelas, & C. Kerbrat-Orecchioni (Eds.), pp.33-45), Edition du CNRS, ISBN 978-222-2041-03-0, Paris

Bakhtine, M. (1930/1981). [V.N. Volochinov]. La structure de l'énoncé. In *Mikhaïl Bakhtine, le principe dialogique,* T. Todorov T (Ed.), pp. 287-316, Éditions du Seuil, 978-202-0058-30-8, Paris

Bazin, N., Lefrere, F., Passerieux, C., Sarfati, Y., & Hardy-Bayle, M. C. (2002). Troubles formels de la pensée: traduction française de l'échelle d'évaluation de la pensée, du langage et de la communication (Scale for the Assessment of Thought, Language and Communication: TLC). *L'Encéphale,* Vol. 28, pp. 109-119, ISSN 0013-7006

Bazin, N., Sarfati, Y., Lefrere, F., Passerieux, C., & Hardy-Bayle, M.C. (2005). Scale for the evaluation of communication disorders in patients with schizophrenia: A validation study. *Schizophrenia Research,* Vol. 77, N°1, pp. 75-84, ISSN 0920-9964

Berman, I., Viegner, B., Merson, A., Allan, E., Pappas, D., & Green, A. I. (1997). Relationships between positive and negative symptoms and neuropsychological deficits in schizophrenia. *Schizophrenia Research,* Vol. 25, N°1, pp. 1-10, ISSN 0920-9964

Bleuler, E. (1911). *Dementia praecox ou groupe des schizophrénies.* E.P.E.L., G.R.E.C. French translation of 1993 ISBN 978-290-8855-11-1

Chaïka, E. O. (1974). A linguist looks at 'schizophrenic' language. *Brain and Language,* Vol. 1, pp. 257-276, ISSN 0093-934X

Chaïka, E. O. (1990). *Understanding psychotic speech: Beyond Freud and Chomsky,* Charles C Thomas Pub Ltd, ISBN 978-039-8056-48-3, Illinois, USA.

Chapman, L. J., & Chapman, J. P. (1989). Strategies for resolving the heterogeneity of schizophrenics and their relatives using cognitive measures. *Journal of Abnormal Psychology,* Vol. 98, N°4, pp. 357-366, ISSN 0021-843X

Chaslin, P. (1912). Groupe provisoire des folies discordantes. In *Eléments de sémiologie et clinique mentales.* Asselin et Houzeau, Paris

Crow, T. J. (1980). Molecular Pathology of schizophrenia: More than one disease process? *British Medical Journal,* Vol. 280, pp. 66-68, ISSN 0959-8138

Crow, T. J. (2010). The nuclear symptoms of schizophrenia reveal the four quadrant structure of language and its deficit frame. *Journal of Neurolinguistics,* Vol. 23, N°1, pp. 1-9, ISSN 0911-6044

Docherty, N.M., Cohen, A.S., Nienow, T.M., Dinzeo, T.J., & Dangemaier, R.E. (2003). Stability of formal thought disorder and referential communication disturbances in schizophrenia. *Journal of Abnormal Psychology,* Vol. 112, pp. 469-475, ISSN 0021-843X

Frith, C. D. (1992). *The cognitive Neuropsychology of Schizophrenia.* LEA, ISBN 978-0863773341, Hove

Fromkin, V. A. (1975). A linguist looks at "a linguist looks at schizophrenic language". *Brain and Language,* Vol.2, pp. 498-503, ISSN 0093-934X

Goffman, E. (1974). *Les rites d'interaction.* Minuit, ISBN 2707300225, Paris

Goldberg, T. E. & Weinberger, D. R. (1995). Thought disorder, working memory and attention: interrelationships and the effects of neuroleptic medications. *International Clinical Psychopharmacology,* Vol. 10, N°3, pp. 99-104, ISSN 0268-1315

Goldstein, G. (1990). Neuropsychological heterogeneity in schizophrenia: A consideration of abstraction and problem solving abilities. *Archives of Clinical Neuropsychology,* Vol. 5, pp. 251-264, ISSN 0887-6177

Grice, H. P. (1975). Logic and conversation, In *Syntax and Semantics 3: Speech Acts,* P. Cole, & J. L. Morgan (Eds.), pp.41-58, New York: Academic Press.

Grice, H. P. (1987). Conceptual analysis and the province of philosophy, In *Studies in the way of words,* H.P. Grice (Ed.), pp. 181-185, Harvard University Press, ISBN 978-0674852716, Cambridge (MA), London.

Hardy-Bayle, M. C., Sarfati, Y., & Passerieux, C. (2003). The cognitive basis of disorganization in schizophrenia and its clinical correlates: toward a pathogenetic disorganization scale. *Schizophrenia Bulletin,* Vol. 29, N°3, pp. 459-471, ISSN 0586-7614

Harvey, P. D., Green, M. F., Mc Gurk, S. R., & Meltzer, H. Y. (2003). Changes in cognitive functioning with risperidone and olanzapine treatment: a large-scale, double-blind, randomized study. *Psychopharmacology,* Vol. 69, pp. 404-11, ISSN 0033-3158

Harvey, P. D., Lombardi, J., Leibman, M., White, L., Parrella, M., Powchik, P., & Davidson, M. (1996). Cognitive impairment and negative symptoms in geriatric chronic schizophrenic patients: a follow-up study. *Schizophrenia Research,* Vol. 22, N°3, pp. 223-231, ISSN 0920-9964

Hauser, M. D., Chomsky, N., & Fitch, W. T. (2002). The Faculty of Language: What Is It, Who Has It, and How Did It Evolve?. *Science*, Vol. 298, pp. 1569-1579, ISSN 0036-8075

Heinrichs, R. W. (1993). Schizophrenia and the brain: conditions for a neuropsychology of madness. *American Psychologist*, Vol. 48, N°3, pp. 221-233, ISSN 0003-066X

Kay, S. R., Fiszbein, A., & Opler, L. A. (1987). The Positive and Negative Syndrome Scale (PANSS) for schizophrenia. *Schizophrenia Bulletin*, Vol. 13, pp. 261-276, ISSN 0586-7614

Kraepelin, E. (1919). *Dementia Praecox and Paraphrenia*. Trans. R. M. Barclay, & G. M. Robertson (Eds.). Krieger RE, 1971, ASIN: B000OKQ154, New York.

Liddle, P. F. (1987). The symptoms of chronic schizophrenia. A re-examination of the positive-negative dichotomy. *British Journal of Psychiatry*, Vol. 151, pp. 145-151, ISSN 0007-1250

Liddle, P. F., Ngan, E. T. C., Caissie, S. L., Anderson, C. M., Bates, A. T., Quested, D. J., White, R., & Weg, R. (2002). Thought and Language Index: an instrument for assessing thought and language in schizophrenia. *British Journal of Psychiatry*, Vol. 181, pp. 326-330, ISSN 0007-1250

McKenna, P. & Oh, T. (2005). Schizophrenic speech. Making sense of Bathroots and Ponds that fall in doorways. Cambridge University Press. ISBN 978-052-1810-75-2, Cambridge

Meltzer, H. Y. & McGurk, S. (1999). The effects of clozapine, ripseridone and olanzapine on cognitive function in schizophrenia. *Schizophrenia Bulletin*, Vol. 25, pp. 233-55, ISSN 0586-7614

Musiol, M. (1992). De l'incohérence du discours au désordre de la pensée chez le schizophrène. *Psychologie Française*, Vol. 37, pp. 221-233, ISSN 0033-2984

Musiol, M. (2002). *Les conditions de l'analyse des troubles de la pensée dans l'interaction verbale (Contribution au programme pragmatique et cognitif en psychopathologie)* [HDR]. Université Paris 8, Paris

Musiol, M. (2004). Les contrats de communication au risque des pathologies de la communication, In *Psychologie sociale et communication,* M. Bromberg, & A. Trognon (Eds.), pp. 77-94, Dunod, ISBN 210007166, Paris

Musiol, M. & Pachoud, B. (1999). Les conditions de l'interprétation psychopathologique des troubles du langage chez le schizophrène. *Psychologie Française*, Vol. 44, N°4, pp. 319-332, ISSN 0033-2984

Musiol, M. & Rebuschi, M. (2011). From conversational analysis to a model of conceptual and referential thought. In *Formal Approaches of dialog,* A. Trognon (Ed.), PUN, ISBN 978-281-4300-42-2, Nancy, France

Musiol, M. & Trognon, A. (2000). *Eléments de Psychopathologie Cognitive. Le discours schizophrène*, Armand Colin, ISBN 978-220-0015-69-5, Paris, France

Musiol, M. & Verhaegen, F. (2002). Vers une stratégie de formalisation de la rupture dans l'interaction verbale. *Philosophia Scientiae*, Vol. 6, N°1, pp.125-161, ISSN 1281-2463

Musiol, M. Verhaegen, F. (2009). Appréhension et catégorisation de l'expression de la symptomatologie schizophrénique dans l'interaction verbale. *Annales Medico-Psychologiques*, Vol. 167, 717-727, ISSN 0003-4487

Olivier, V., Hardy-Bayle, M. C., Lancrenon, S., Fermanian, J., Sarfati, Y., Passerieux, C., & Chevalier, J. F. (1997). Rating scale for the assessment of communication disorders in schizophrenics. *European Psychiatry*, Vol. 12, pp. 356-361, ISSN 0924-9338

Pachoud, B. (1996). Les troubles de la compétence interactionnelle dans la schizophrénie. In *Raisons Pratiques (La folie dans la place),* I. Joseph, & J. Proust (Eds.), pp.211-230, Editions de l'Ecole des Hautes Etudes en Sciences Sociales, ISBN EHESS 2-7132-1218-9, Paris

Pike, K. (1967). *Language in relation to unified theory of the structure of human behavior*. Mouton, ISBN 978-902-7918-69-7, The Hague.

Politzer, G. (2002). *Le raisonnement humain*, Hermès, ISBN 2-7462-0501-7, Paris

Pollock, J. Y. (1997). *Langage et cognition*, PUF, ISBN 978-213-0480-90-7, Paris

Rips, L. J. (1995). Deduction and cognition. In *An invitation to cognitive science: Thinking*, E. E. Smith, & D. N. Osherson (Eds.), pp. 297-343, MIT Press, ISBN 978-026-2650-43-4, Cambridge (Ma), London

Rochester, S. & Martin, J. R. (1979). *Crazy Talk. A Study of the Discourse of Schizophrenic Speakers*, Plenum Press, ISBN 978-030-6402-36-4, London

Roulet, E., Auchlin, A., Moeschler, J., Rubattel, C. & Schelling, M. (1985). *L'articulation du discours en français contemporain*, Peter Lang, ISBN, 978-326-1037-94-7, Berne

Searle, J. R. & Vanderveken, D. (1985). *Foundations of illocutionary logic*, Cambridge University Press, ISBN 978-052-1108-85-0, Cambridge.

Sperber, D. (2000). Metarepresentations in an evolutionary perspective. In D *Metarepresentations: An multidisciplinarity perspective*, Sperber (Ed.), pp. 117-137, Oxford University Press, ISBN 978-019-5141-15-3, Oxford.

Sperber, D. & Wilson, D. (1995). *Relevance* (2nd edition), Blackwell, ISBN 978-063-1198-78-9, Oxford/Cambridge.

Titone, D. (2010). Language, communication, & schizophrenia. *Journal of Neurolinguistics*, Vol. 23, pp. 173-175, ISSN 0911-6044

Trognon, A. (1987). Débrayages conversationnels. *DRLAV*, Vol. 36-37, pp.105-122, ISSN 07549296

Trognon, A. (1992). L'approche pragmatique en psychopathologie cognitive. *Psychologie Française*, Vol. 37, pp.189-202, ISSN 0033-2984

Trognon, A. (1995). Structures interlocutoires. *Cahiers de linguistique française*, Vol. 17, pp. 79-98, ISSN 0259-6199

Trognon, A. & Musiol, M. (1996). L'accomplissement interactionnel du trouble schizophrénique. In *Raisons Pratiques (La folie dans la place),* I. Joseph, & J. Proust (Eds.), pp.179-209, Editions de l'Ecole des Hautes Etudes en Sciences Sociales, ISBN EHESS 2-7132-1218-9, Paris

Trognon, A.; Musiol, M. & Kostulski, K. (1999). Une théorie de la conversation est-elle possible? *Verbum*, Vol. XXI, N°2, pp. 133-146, ISSN 0182-5887

Tsuang, M. (2000). Schizophrenia: genes and environment. *Biological Psychiatry*, Vol. 47, pp. 210-220, ISSN 0006-3223

Verhaegen, F. & Musiol, M. (2008). Impact des médicaments antipsychotiques sur les discontinuités du comportement verbal en conversation schizophrénique. *Psychologie de l'interaction*, Vol. 25-26, pp. 164-94, ISSN 1291-0600

Verhaegen, F. & Musiol, M. (2009). Symptomatologie schizophrénique et processus psychopharmacologiques: contribution empirique. *Annales Medico-Psychologiques*, Vol. 167, pp. 728-735, ISSN 0003-4487

Widlocher, D. & Hardy-Bayle, M. C. (1989). Cognition and control of action in psychopathology. *Cahiers de Psychologie Cognitive*, Vol. 9, N°6, 583-616, ISSN 0249-9185

Part 2

Depression

8

Mouse Models of Depression

Nina Dedic, Sandra M. Walser and Jan M. Deussing
Max Planck Institute of Psychiatry
Germany

1. Introduction

Mood disorders such as depression are the most prevalent diseases amongst psychiatric disorders and a leading cause for disability worldwide. Modelling mood disorders in animals is a major challenge considering the complex nature of the diseases. Nevertheless, existing models and paradigms have proven extremely useful not only with respect to the identification and improvement of therapeutic substances, but also regarding the validation of neurobiological underpinnings.

In this chapter we introduce some basic concepts with respect to the questions what and how animal models are able to contribute to our understanding of mood disorders. The chapter centers on the mouse as the key model organism in neuropsychiatric research and gives an overview on the most popular behavioural tests and models with a particular focus on major depression. This chapter is not meant to be fully exhaustive considering the comprehensive literature on this topic, but rather intends to point out general concepts and controversies in the field, for instance to clarify the differences between animal models, behavioural tests and antidepressant screening paradigms. Moreover, the chapter will call the attention to some novel strategies and technologies that are envisioned to significantly impact the future development and application of animal models of mood disorders. Finally, the chapter will introduce latest views on the importance of introducing gene × environment interactions into animal models of etiologic relevance.

1.1 Epidemiology of depression

Depression, officially termed major depressive disorder (MDD) ranks among the most prevalent diseases worldwide. According to the estimations of the World Health Organization, depression will be the second leading cause of disability in 2020 (Murray and Lopez, 1997). Recent epidemiological studies indicate that severe forms of depression affect 2-5% of the population worldwide, and up to 20% are affected by milder forms of the disease (Kessler et al., 2003). Moreover, depressive patients have a 2-4 fold increased risk of developing cardiovascular diseases and 10-15% of individuals with major depression commit suicide (Keck, 2006).

Up to now, depression is diagnosed according to criteria in the Diagnostic Manual of Mental Disorders (DSM-IV), which characterizes a major depressive episode by at least five of the following symptoms: (1) depressed or irritable mood, (2) decreased interest or loss of pleasure, (3) weight gain or loss, (4) insomnia or hypersomnia, (5) psychomotor retardation or agitation, (6) fatigue or loss of energy, (7) feelings of worthlessness or inappropriate guilt,

(8) diminished ability to think or concentrate, (9) recurrent thoughts of death and suicide. The symptoms must be evident almost daily for at least 2 weeks. Additionally, symptoms of anxiety are also often seen in depressed individuals (Berton and Nestler, 2006).

The genetic risk to develop depression is 40–50% (Levinson, 2006), but there are also several environmental risk factors for MDD. These include gender, stressful life events, adverse childhood experiences and certain personality traits (Fava and Kendler, 2000). Many recent studies support the hypothesis that stressful events correlate with an increased vulnerability for depression in a way that stressful situations often precede the onset of illness and are also associated with the severity of depression (Brown et al., 1987;Dunner et al., 1979;Holsboer, 2001;Nemeroff, 1988). Such stressors can lead to a transient hyperactivation of the hypothalamic-pituitary-adrenocortical (HPA) axis, resulting in increased glucocorticoid secretion. In this regard, depression is often associated with a dysregulation of the HPA axis under chronic stress conditions (Holsboer and Barden, 1996). Additionally, treatment of depressed patients with antidepressants can restore the homeostasis of the HPA axis and thereby contributes to clinical improvement (Holsboer, 2000;Holsboer and Barden, 1996).

In contrast to the epidemiological magnitude of the disease, the progress of pharmacological therapy for depression is still limited (Nestler et al., 2002). All available antidepressants act via monoamine neurotransmitter systems, but only 50-70% of the patients exhibit acceptable responses to treatment (Morilak and Frazer, 2004). Additionally, slow onset of clinical effects as well as severe side effects associated with antidepressant therapy frequently lead to discontinuation of treatment. Although the latest generation of drugs has fewer side effects, they still exhibit similar effectiveness rates and show a substantial delay of 4-6 weeks between onset of treatment and clinical improvement. Beside that, 25-35% of the patients remain resistant to the treatment even after 6 weeks of therapy (Berton and Nestler, 2006;Holsboer, 2005). Apart from monoamines, many other targets have been analyzed, including glucocorticoid receptor and corticotropin-releasing hormone receptor antagonists (Berton and Nestler, 2006;Grigoriadis, 2005) as well as histone deacetylase inhibitors (Covington, et al., 2009). However, so far none of these studies has resulted in a new adequate treatment of the disease. Besides these aspects, the molecular mechanisms underlying depression still remain largely unknown.

All these arguments raise the necessity of finding novel approaches to discover different targets for antidepressant treatment and of developing new mouse models to study the effects of monoamine and non-monoamine-related molecules.

1.2 The endophenotype concept – modelling symptoms of depression in mice

1.2.1 The endophenotype concept

The highly variable composition of symptoms, course of illness and response to treatment renders it very difficult to accurately define and consequently diagnose depression. The so-called psychopathological endophenotypes represent key symptoms of major depression. An endophenotype represents a trait that is intermediate between genotype and disease, not necessarily beholden to the diagnostic criteria for single illness, but in many cases useful to simplify our understanding of complex or heterogeneous disorders (Shyn and Hamilton, 2010). An endophenotype is associated with illness in the population, is heritable and is primarily state-independent. Furthermore, endophenotype and illness co-segregate within families and the endophenotype found in affected family members is found in nonaffected family members at a higher rate than in the general population (Gottesman and Gould,

2003;Gould and Gottesman, 2006). The methods available to identify endophenotypes include neuropsychological, cognitive, neurophysiological, neuroanatomical, and biochemical measures (Hasler et al., 2004).

1.2.2 Depression-associated endophenotypes in mice

Mimicking any human behavioural trait in a mouse is extremely difficult, which makes the undertaking to try and model a multifactorial disease such as depression nearly impossible. How do we recapitulate all aspects of depression in an animal, when the criteria used to classify a major depression are of extreme heterogeneous and sometimes even of opposite nature (e.g., substantial weight gain or loss, insomnia or hypersomnia)? On top of that, animals not only lack consciousness of self, self-reflection and consideration of others but also aspects of the disorder such as depressed mood, low self-esteem or suicidality (Deussing JM, 2006). This does not mean that it is impossible to develop useful animal models, but rather highlights the unlikelihood of generating a model that will mirror the full extent of a given human neuropsychiatric disorder (Nestler and Hyman, 2010). Nonetheless, in depression, as well as other mood disorders, certain endophenotypes can be reproduced independently and evaluated in animals (Table 1). As mentioned above, these include physiological, endocrinological, neuroanatomical and behavioural alterations, many of which can be measured in mice.

So far a variety of different mouse models have been established to improve our understanding of the pathophysiology of a wide spectrum of psychiatric diseases. However, a full consensus regarding the prerequisites of a valid animal model is still lacking in the scientific community. Up to now, the three criteria set up by McKinney and Bunney (McKinney and Bunney, 1969) are still widely accepted; they include construct validity, face validity, and predictive validity.

Construct (or etiologic) validity, the most complex of the three terms, requires that the symptoms produced in the animal model are based on the same underlying neurobiological mechanisms as in humans. Thus, one tries to recreate mechanisms/processes in the animal which would also initiate the disease in humans (Nestler and Hyman, 2010). The ideal way would be to introduce a known human disease-causing gene variant into a mouse and thereby alter intracellular mechanisms, which in the end lead to the disease (Chadman et al., 2009). Unfortunately this is currently far from being realistic, since most disease-causing genetic alterations have not been established with certainty and the probability that a single gene is solely responsible for the disease is highly unlikely. In addition, an animal model does not have to be based on a genetic change, but can also be subject to an environmental challenge or a combination of both.

Face validity is achieved when the animal exhibits specific symptoms of the disease which are similar in the human condition. These can be of biochemical, anatomical, neuropathological or behavioural nature. Thus the concept of face validity can also be regarded as the attempt to reproduce certain endophenotypes which can be accurately measured in the animal.

Finally, *predictive validity* refers to the ability of the animal to correctly respond to pharmacological treatment, which should correlate with results from clinical trials.

In this context, it is important to note that the more criteria the proposed model meets, the more compelling it will be (Malkesman et al., 2010). Simply put, researchers are faced with the challenge of 1) constructing a model with similarity in disease progression and symptomatology to humans, 2) detecting these phenotypes with the appropriate behavioural tests and 3) reverting them with treatment modalities that are also effective in humans.

DSM-IV symptoms	Endopenotypes in mice	Appropriate test/analysis
Depressed or irritable mood	Cannot be modeled	
Decreased interest or loss of pleasure	Anhedonia	Sucrose preference Intracranial self-stimulation Conditioned place-preferance Female urine sniffing
Weight gain or loss	Can easily be measured	Abnormal loss or gain of weight after stress
Insomnia or hypersomnia	Abnormal sleep architecture	Assessed by electroencephalogram recordings
Psychomotor retardation or agitation	Alterations in locomotion	open field alterations of homecage activity treadmill running Gate analysis
Fatigue or loss of energy	Alterations in locomotion	Reduced homecage activity Treadmill running Nest building
Feelings of worthlessness or inappropriate guilt	Cannot be modeled	
Diminished ability to think or concentrate	Deficits in working and spatial memory	Morris water maze Y-maze fear conditioning Attentional set-shifting
Recurrent thoughts of death and suicide	Cannot be modeled	
	Additional endophenotypes	
	Anxiety-related behavior	Open field Elevated plus maze Dark-light box Novelty-induced hypophagia Novel object exploration Modified hole board Marble burying
	Changes in social behavior	Social interaction/avoidance Sociability
	Behavioral despair	Forced swim test Tail suspension test Learned helplessness
	Neuroendocrine disturbances	Alterations in corticosterone secretion Dexamethasone suppression Combined dexamethasone/CRH challenge
	Changes in neuroanatomy	Analysis of hippocampal volume by resonance imaging (often reduced in depressed patients)

Table 1. Depression-associated endophenotypes that can be modelled in mice.

Although progress has been made to identify the underlying molecular mechanism of depression, the lack of specific markers and biomarkers still represents a major drawback. In contrast to many other illnesses such as cancer, infectious diseases, cardiovascular arrest, diabetes, stroke, etc., depression cannot simply be diagnosed by making use of the usual methods, such as assessing blood pressure, glucose levels, inflammatory agents, heart rate and others. Clinicians still fully rely on observations and verbal communication. Therefore, behavioural tests that are used to assess phenotypic alterations relevant to depression in mice are of extreme importance and will be discussed in more detail.

2. Behavioural tests – tools used to assess phenotypic alterations in animal models

First, we want to point out the importance of discriminating between an animal model, a behavioural test and an antidepressant screening paradigm. Animal models, as discussed above, are expected to show sufficient construct, face and predictive validity. Behavioural tests on the other hand are used to assess phenotypic alterations relevant to the disease and should be regarded as a technical tool and not a model (Table 1). Likewise, antidepressant screening paradigms, such as the forced swim test, also do not represent a model of depression but should rather be regarded as drug-screening assays.

Nowadays researchers are discordant when it comes to the term "depression-related test". Given the fact that there is no consensus as to what can be regarded as "depression-like" behaviour in animals it has become increasingly popular to look at, and talk of behavioural endophenotypes or sub-categories, which in some cases may, and in others may not represent aspects of depression. These include anxiety-, reward-, social and despair-based behaviour as well as alterations in general locomotion, sleep, food and liquid intake.

2.1 Tests assessing despair-based / stress-coping behaviour

In earlier days, the Porsolt forced swim test (FST) and the tail suspension test (TST) were regarded as typical depression-like paradigms, given the fact that both were developed to screen monoamine-based antidepressant drugs. This is currently a matter of debate, since both assess the response to an acute inescapable stressor, provoking despair-based behaviour/immobility or stress-coping behaviour rather than depression-like behaviour. The FST makes use of the fact that rodents eventually develop immobility when being placed in a cylinder of water after they have stopped active escape behaviours, such as climbing or swimming (Cryan and Holmes, 2005) A related task is the TST, which relies on similar assumptions and interpretations as the FST. Here the mice are hung upside down by their tails and the time spent immobile is assessed. One major advantage of the TST is that it is not confounded by stressful hypothermia as is the case in the FST. However, the TST is restricted to strains that do not tend to climb their tail which otherwise confuses the interpretation of behavioural measures (Mayorga and Lucki, 2001). In either case the underlying principles measuring the lack of active coping behaviour are identical. However, the question whether immobility should be interpreted as passive stress-coping, behavioural despair or even depression-like behaviour remains controversial. One aspect favouring the stress-coping rather than depression-like aspect of the FST are the outcomes when manipulating the corticotropin-releasing hormone (CRH) system. CRH overexpressing animals as well as central application of CRH result in decreased immobility (Butler et al., 1990;van Gaalen et al., 2002;Lu et al., 2008). However, it is widely believed that high levels of CRH are rather pro-depressive (Holsboer and Ising, 2008) and it was shown that CRHR1 antagonists have an effect similar to paroxetine and other antidepressants (Holsboer and Ising, 2008). Thus it is likely that the CRH/CRHR1 stress system also accounts for regulating and/or triggering responses to the test (Refojo and Deussing, 2011). In that regard, Gardier already pointed out that the FST assesses stress-induced anxiety rather than depression (Gardier and Bourin, 2001). In addition, it is very unlikely that such a short period of inescapable stress is able to induce a depression-like state in a wild-type animal. Nevertheless, the FST and TST have proved reliable across many laboratories by demonstrating their ability to detect a broad spectrum of substances with antidepressant efficacy, all of which reduce immobility. However, most effects are already observed after acute treatment, which contrasts the human situation, where chronic application of antidepressants is necessary to achieve clinical responses (Nestler and Hyman, 2010). For this reason, we believe that the FST and TST should rather be viewed as paradigms designed to assess strategies of stress-coping behaviour and monoamine-based antidepressant action (Lucki, 1997), and not as models of depression (Refojo and Deussing, 2011).

In addition to the FST and TST, the learned helplessness paradigm also makes use of stressor uncontrollability and passive vs. active coping responses (Cryan and Holmes, 2005). The paradigm is based on the observation that animals exposed to uncontrolled or unpredictable aversive events (e.g. electrical shocks) for a sufficient period of time will develop long-lasting deficits in escape performance (Seligman and Maier, 1967). Short-term treatment with antidepressants as well as anxiolytics has shown to reverse the enforced behavioural phenotype, which doesn't make the paradigm particularly selective (Cryan and Mombereau, 2004). In addition, only some of the animals develop signs of helplessness and those are usually short-lived. Similar to the FST and TST, the learned helplessness paradigm does not parallel clinical settings with regard to the slow onset of antidepressant action, but remains a good tool for the assessment of stress-coping behaviour (Deussing, 2006).

2.2 Anxiety-based tests

The lack of clear a distinction between depression and anxiety amongst researchers poses a major issue in the interpretation of behavioural tests. Depression, by definition, is considered a pathological mental condition. Anxiety, however, is a normal state of cognitive and behavioural preparedness that an organism mobilizes in response to a future or distant potential threat (Leonardo and Hen, 2008). Although anxiety is often necessary and even protective, excessive anxiety can trigger disabling responses that, in time, lead to anxiety disorders (e.g., generalized anxiety disorder, social phobia, simple phobia, panic disorder, posttraumatic stress disorder (PTSD), and obsessive compulsive disorder) (Bienvenu et al., 2009). Anxiety can often emerge as part of a depressive syndrome, but this does not hold true for all patients and certainly not for all animal models (Krishnan et al., 2007;Wallace et al., 2009). It is also important to note that the underlying neural circuitries are believed to be different in depression and anxiety (Nestler and Hyman, 2010). However, in animal models anxiety is considered a core endophenotype of depression, which is mainly due to the availability of a wide range of standardized tests, all of which assess anxiety-like behaviour. Most of these assays are based on approach-avoidance conflicts and were developed and validated using classical benzodiazepine-like anxiolytic compounds. Mice generally display high levels of exploration of a novel environment but also have an innate aversion to enter exposed, well-lit areas. The elevated plus-maze (EPM) and elevated zero-maze present the subject mouse with the choice of spending time exploring the open areas of a plus-shaped or circular runway, versus spending time exploring the enclosed arms and arcs (Handley and Mithani, 1984;Chadman et al., 2009). Other exploration-based tasks, founded on similar conflicting tendencies to approach versus avoid a potentially dangerous area are the dark-light box (DaLi) and open field (OF) test. In the latter the aversive area is represented by the central zone of a brightly lit open field. In the dark-light box test averseness is achieved by a highly illuminated compartment (Lister, 1990;Belzung and Griebel, 2001). The novel object exploration test makes use of similar principles, the only difference being that mice are first habituated to an environment and then exposed to novelty (novel object). Explorative paradigms such as the EPM, DaLi and brightly lit OF have been suggested to measure state anxiety (Belzung and Le, 1994;van Gaalen and Steckler, 2000). In contrast, exploration of novelty in an area known to be safe has been suggested to fundamentally differ from the exploration of a totally new environment and thus claimed to reflect trait rather than state anxiety (Griebel et al., 1993;van Gaalen and Steckler, 2000). Other tests are the modified hole board the mirrored chamber test, the staircase test and the marble burying test (Broekkamp et al., 1986;Holmes, 2001;Belzung and Griebel, 2001;Ohl et al., 2003). Another emerging paradigm is the novelty-induced suppression of feeding test, which measures the latency until food consumption in a novel environment. Here, rodents have shown to respond to chronic but not acute antidepressant treatment, resulting in decreased latency to feed (Dulawa and Hen, 2005). This goes along with the fact that anxiety in humans can in many cases be treated with chronic antidepressant administration (Nestler and Hyman, 2010).

Even though approach-avoidance tests are critical in the assessment of anxiety-related behaviour in mice, they still have to be interpreted with caution. In most of the tests it is not possible to distinguish between an anxiety response and other phenotypes such as motivation, novelty-seeking, impulsivity or arousal. Thus increased time spent in an aversive area can be interpreted as both, decreased anxiety or increased motivation or arousal. Different exploratory and even coping strategies can also be misinterpreted as alterations in anxiety-like behaviour. Additionally, tests based on exploration can be strongly influenced by differences in basal locomotion and cognition (Refojo and Deussing, 2011). As is the case with the FST and TST, the above mentioned anxiety-based assays represent useful initial screens, but should never be used as definite evidence of a depression-like phenotype. This emphasizes the importance of parallel use of several slightly different anxiety tests, as well as the utilization of internal controls with respect to locomotion. Most importantly, additional non-anxiety based tests should be considered (see below).

2.3 Reward-related and anhedonic behaviour

Anhedonia, a hallmark of depression is defined as the inability to experience pleasure from activities formally found enjoyable. Dopamine neuronal functioning is essential in sustaining a wide variety of pleasurable and rewarding experiences (Wise and Bozarth, 1985;Wise, 2002). Especially dopaminergic neurons, projecting from the ventral tegmental area to the prefrontal cortex, basolateral amygdala, and nucleus accumbens are essential in reward processes (Wise, 2002). The most widely accepted approach to assess reward-seeking behaviour is via the sucrose consumption and preference tests. Decreased intake of palatable solutions, such as sucrose is regarded as a behavioural measure of hedonic deficit/depressive-like state (Willner, 2005). One drawback, however, is that one cannot rule out appetitive, metabolic or sensorial influences, which may be altered in genetically modified animals. In addition, enhanced hedonic drive and motivation, which are hallmarks of manic symptoms in bipolar disorder, may often be misinterpreted as decreased depression-like behaviour (Hasler et al., 2004). Operant paradigms, such as the conditioned place-preference (CPP), are also widely applied to assess anhedonic behaviour. Although mainly used to determine the addiction potential of drugs, CPP can also be employed to test animals in a drug-free state. Even though methodological details differ among laboratories, a typical CPP experiment includes differential pairing of two distinct sets of environmental (contextual) cues with a stimulus (e.g., drug, food, copulatory opportunity) (Bardo and Bevins, 2000). When tested later on in the absence of the stimulus, the approaches and the amount of time spent in the compartments previously associated with the positive stimulus serve as an indicator of preference and a measure of reward learning. Obvious drawbacks include the rather elaborate testing procedure as well as the fact that the paradigm is heavily dependent on learning, memory and motor activity. Operant self-administration, using the so-called operant box (or Skinner box), represent additional methods in anhedonic research (Sanchis-Segura and Spanagel, 2006). In contrast, intracranial self-stimulation-based procedures make use of the phenomenon that direct stimulation of distinct brain regions through electrical or chemical means can activate the reward system and serve as an operant reinforcer (Sanchis-Segura and Spanagel, 2006). However, the use of brain stimulation reward techniques requires surgery and sometimes extensive periods of training that often exceed the recovery time from the surgery (Malkesman et al., 2010). Alternatives are for instance the recently developed female urine sniffing test (FUST). The FUST is a nonoperant test, designed to measure reward-seeking behaviour in rodents based on the interest in pheromonal odors from the opposite sex (Malkesman et al., 2010). The duration of female urine sniffing was significantly decreased after foot-shock stress and could be reverted upon antidepressant treatment (Malkesman et al., 2010). As with other tests, the FUST faces limitations when working with transgenic animals, which in some cases may suffer from olfactory system dysfunction (Hull and Dominguez, 2007). Furthermore, the preference for estrus female odour might also be related to social and not just sexual behaviour (Wersinger et al., 2004). As with anxiety tests, multiple tasks that evaluate different aspects of reward sensitivity should be considered, and are likely to provide more insights into the behavioural and neurobiological processes of mood disorders such as depression.

2.4 Cognition-based tests

A majority of depressed patients, especially older adults, show pronounced cognitive deficits typically consisting of memory impairments, poor attention, and executive dysfunction (Butters et al., 2004;Crocco et al., 2010). Hence, it is of great interest to model altered cognitive behaviours in mice. However, this undertaking faces many challenges, given the fact that the rodent cortex is much more primitive than the human, which makes it extremely difficult to address many aspects of cognitive processing in mice (Cryan and Holmes, 2005). Therefore, many of the applied cognition tasks, such as the Morris water maze (MWM) and Y-maze test, focus on general cognitive function mediated by the hippocampal region. Developed by Morris in 1984, the MWM test assesses spatial learning in mice and rats and is strongly reflective of hippocampal synaptic plasticity and NMDA receptor function. The test relies on distal, visual cues that can help the animal to locate and navigate to a submerged escape platform from different starting locations within an open swimming arena. Spatial learning is evaluated across repeated trials and reference memory is assessed by preference for the platform area once the platform is absent (Morris, 1984;D'Hooge and De Deyn, 2001). Similarly, the Y-maze also assesses spatial memory and hippocampal integrity. It is based on the animal's natural curiosity to discover novel environments (Conrad et al., 1996;Dellu et al., 2000), but is not confounded by possible effects of hypothermia. Incidents of chronic social stress, a precondition of many depressed patients, have shown to alter cognitive performance in a battery of tests including the MWM and Y-maze task (McEwen and Sapolsky, 1995;Song et al., 2006;Wang et al., 2011).

It is important to note that many cognitive deficits, such as misappraisal and over-attention to threatening stimuli, are also observed in panic disorder, generalized anxiety disorders and phobias (Cryan and Holmes, 2005). Thus, researchers often speak of emotional cognition, which can be analysed in rodents with certain well established concepts such as Pavlovian fear-conditioning (Davis, 1990;Fendt and Fanselow, 1999;Maren, 2001). Such contextual and cued fear conditioning tasks represent additional methodologies to investigate memory, as they require that the animals learn the association of a non-aversive context or cue with an aversive stimulus. The ability to learn this association is measured by the amount of freezing exhibited in response to the cue or context alone (Amann et al., 2010). Many variations of the paradigm exist, including altering the type of cue and stimulus, and, once learned, testing the rate at which learning is extinguished (Fanselow, 1980). The failure to extinguish learned fear responses is one key feature of post-traumatic stress disorder, phobias and other anxiety disorders (El-Ghundi et al., 2001).

Another recently validated test in rats is the attentional set-shifting test (Birrell and Brown, 2000;Bondi et al., 2008). The animals are trained to dig for food in bowls which are presented in pairs, only one being baited. The rat has to select the bowl to dig in based on the texture that covers the bowl's surface or the odor of the medium with which it is filled. Once the training procedure is completed, the animals perform a series of discrimination tasks, including reversal, an intradimensional shift, and an extradimensional shift. The number of trials required to perform six consecutive correct responses in different stages is scored. Rats subjected to chronic unpredictable stress exhibited impairments in the attentional set-shifting test, which were prevented by desipramine or escitalopram treatment (Bondi et al., 2008). In addition, lesions of the medial prefrontal cortex selectively disrupted extradimensional set shifting (Birrell and Brown, 2000). Although this paradigm is quite labour intensive and not yet validated for the mouse, it represents a very interesting means to evaluate prefrontal cortex function as a cognitive trait relevant for depression.

Although cognitive tests are not used as standard tools when assessing depression-like behaviour, they certainly provide insights into the cognitive aspects of the emotional state. Thus, it is strongly recommended to include cognitive tasks in schedules for testing emotional behaviour especially in combination with some of the well-established anxiety tests described above.

2.5 Assessing behaviour via social tests

Social behaviour can be defined as any behaviour that influences, or is influenced by, other members of the same species. A variety of neuropsychiatric disorders, including depression, are characterized by disruptions of social behaviour (Nestler and Hyman, 2010). Many of the social test paradigms were originally developed to study schizophrenia and autism-like behaviour, in which alterations in social behaviour represent core symptoms of the disease. However, social withdrawal also represents a common symptom in psychiatric conditions such as depression, social phobia, and PTSD (Berton and Nestler, 2006). Exposure to chronic social stress, after which rodents show signs of anhedonia and increased anxiety-like behaviour, is also effective in inducing social withdrawal (Krishnan et al., 2007). Although most social tasks in mice are employed after repeated exposure to a stressor, it should be considered to employ these tests also under basal conditions especially when evaluating transgenic mouse lines.

The classical social interaction paradigm encompasses the free exploration of an unfamiliar congener by the experimental mouse. Social interaction is measured by the time spent in close proximity to the unfamiliar mouse as well as the amount and duration of additional behaviour including sniffing, following, grooming, biting, mounting etc. In many cases, social avoidance behaviour is associated with anxiety- and depression-like behaviour.

The social avoidance paradigm represents a similar but faster and more systematic approach to assess social avoidance. In contrast to the standard tests, social approach towards an unfamiliar mouse enclosed in a wire mesh cage is measured (Berton et al., 2006). This excludes subject bias from the observer, since only the time spent in close proximity to the target is assessed. In addition, aggressive behaviours such as biting and fighting can be excluded. Other paradigms, including the sociability test can be used to assess the social preference between a stranger/conspecific and an object (Moy et al., 2004). In addition, social novelty can be evaluated by introducing a second unfamiliar mouse. In rats, it was shown that social behaviour is individually stable and that sociability is related to 5-HT metabolism in the prefrontal cortex (Tonissaar et al., 2004;Tonissaar et al., 2008b). Additionally, sociability and anxiety were shown to be closely related domains (Tonissaar et al., 2004;Tonissaar et al., 2008a). Even though preclinical research has clearly favoured the rat for the assessment of social behaviour, the propagation of transgenic and gene targeting technologies in the mouse has established it as a unique model in psychiatric research. Thus, an ever increasing number of social tasks is established in mice and should definitely be considered when assessing animal models of depression.

3. Outline of existing mouse models of depression

Most animal models of depression are either based on environmental challenges or on manipulation of sensory and integrative functions of the brain. By means of a variety of stressful conditions, certain symptoms that are inferred to be "depression-like" can be evoked in animals. In contrast, molecular and cellular tools, which allow the development of targeted genetic manipulation strategies in embryonic stem cells, are also widely applied to generate so called "depression models". Below, the most prominent and widely used animal models of depression will be considered. In addition, innovative strategies and state-of-the-art technologies used to construct novel genetic mouse models of depression will be discussed.

3.1 Lesion models

Patients exhibiting depression or other psychiatric syndromes often show alterations in structures related to olfactory function. Olfactory performance was shown to be reduced in depressed patients (Pause et al., 2001) together with morphological differences in olfactory projection areas, noticeably in the amygdala (Nestler et al., 2002). Thus, the bulbectomized rat or mouse has been considered a model of agitated depression (Leonard and Tuite, 1981;Kelly et al., 1997). After ablation of the olfactory bulb, mice demonstrate typical loss of smell but also disruptions of the limbic-hypothalamic axis with the consequence of behavioural, neurochemical, neuroendocrine and neuroimmune alterations, all of which may resemble changes in depressed patients (Song and Leonard, 2005). The behavioural outcome of olfactory bulbectomy is largely thought to result from compensatory mechanisms of neuronal reorganisation. Thus, most of the literature indicates that the olfactory bulb is not a mere sensory area, suggesting that it could have non-olfactory functions relevant for modulation of behaviour (Edwards et al., 1972;Cain and Paxinos, 1974;Mucignat-Caretta et al., 2004). In addition, peripheral anosmia fails to produce the observed behavioural changes in mice, indicating once more that loss of smell alone is not the sole cause for the observed syndromes (Mar et al., 2000). Underlying changes are thought to involve alterations in synaptic strength and/or loss of spine density in various limbic regions including the amygdala and hippocampus (Kelly and Leonard, 1999). Marked changes in major neurotransmitter systems have also been observed in bulbectomized rodents (Kelly, 1999). However, the most consistent behavioural phenotype of bulbectomized animals is a hyperactive response in the open field paradigm, which is reversible upon antidepressant treatment (Cryan et al., 1999). This model of depression shows high face validity as it mimics the slow onset of antidepressant action reported in clinical studies (Willner and Mitchell, 2002). However, high construct validity is not achieved as the model fails to recapitulate the etiology of disease progression.

3.2 Pharmacological models

Pharmacological models in the ideal sense should induce behavioural changes and treatment responses partly similar to depression. Reserpine, a sympatholytic drug that depletes catecholamines in the brain (Eranco and Hopsu, 1958;Mascorro and Yates, 1971), is believed to chemically evoke a depression-like phenotype in animals. The drug was shown to induce a syndrome of locomotor hypomotility and reduced body temperature in rodents. In addition, reserpine exhibits effects on the adrenal glands which resemble those of physiological stress (Joh et al., 1973). This model is based on the capability of antidepressants to reverse the inhibitory effects caused by reserpine on motility in rats and mice (Nutt, 2006). The psychostimulant withdrawal paradigm, another widely applied pharmacological model, displays both, responsiveness to antidepressants and induces characteristic symptoms of depression. In humans, withdrawal from chronic psychostimulants generates symptoms that have strong behavioural and psychological parallels to depression including diminished interest in pleasure. Withdrawal from chronic amphetamine treatment results in behavioural changes that were shown to be analogous to some aspects of depression. These included reward deficits and increased immobility in the FST (Kokkinidis et al., 1986;Cryan et al., 2003). Therefore, examination of the behavioural effects of drug withdrawal may provide insights into the underlying neurobiological mechanisms and aid in the development of animal models of depression that are sensitive to antidepressant agents. Although many of these models show robust predictive and even face validity, most of them fail to mimic disease etiology. In that regard, pharmacological models such as those mentioned above, significantly contributed to the strengthening of the monoamine theory of depression, which assumes that an elevation of serotonin and norepinephrine levels will improve depressive symptomatology. However, they are limited in their value as effective models of depression given the ever expanding impact of genetic and environmental models.

3.3 Genetic mouse models

Genetically engineered mice represent a powerful tool to study candidate genes thought to participate in a particular disease. In general, scientists discriminate between forward and reverse genetics. Forward genetics allows the identification of relevant genes without any prior knowledge of genetic or mechanistic underpinnings of a phenotype of interest. Classically, forward genetics involves larger scale random mutagenesis screens such as ENU-(N-ethyl-N-nitrosourea) or gene-trap-based approaches which have resulted in a great number of mutants displaying aspects of depression-like behaviour. On the other hand, reverse genetics involves genetic manipulations that result in loss- or gain-of-function mutants. These include classical transgenic mice that have additional copies of certain genes in their genome, which results in a gain-of-function. Similarly, knock-in techniques are frequently applied to generate gain-of-function animals. However, transgenes can also be used to induce a loss-of-function if the inserted transgene produces an antisense mRNA of the target gene. Similarly, short hairpin RNAs directed against the gene of interest have also been widely used (Kleinhammer et al., 2010). However, disruption of specific target genes is most commonly achieved via generation of knockout mice. Embryonic stem (ES) cell technology has been widely used to produce null mutants or 'conventional' knockouts (Capecchi, 2005). In that case, the targeting vector is constructed to allow the precise disruption of a gene resulting in the complete ablation of protein and/or mRNA production within every cell. Such conventional knockout mice were of immense importance in identifying candidate genes involved in depression and other mood disorders (see below). However, they were limited in their ability to further uncover specific brain regions and neural circuitries involved in disease etiology. In many cases, homozygous knockouts were not viable or induced developmental and peripheral changes such as reduced weight or organ dysfunction. Since then, technologies in this field have expanded rapidly, introducing sophisticated conditional strategies (Branda and Dymecki, 2004). This progress has allowed an increasingly refined control of spatial and temporal gene expression. In particular, the propagation of site-specific recombinases makes it possible to address gene function in a spatially and temporally restricted manner. For example, mouse lines expressing Cre recombinases selectively in neurons of a specific neurotransmitter type allow for gene targeting of specific populations of neurons. Moreover, increasing availability of mouse lines expressing the tamoxifen-inducible Cre recombinase variant CreERT2 (Branda and Dymecki, 2004) offers additional temporal control and avoids obscurities due to developmental functions of targeted genes. In addition, conditional strategies such as RNAi technology or virus-mediated genetic manipulation also enable the control over spatial and temporal gene expression, and are thus becoming increasingly important.

Currently, three main theories try to conceptualize the molecular mechanisms underlying depression. These include the monoamine and neurotrophic hypothesis, and the HPA system. Thus, most genetic approaches aim at altering the expression of genes that are involved in these systems and thereby analyse their respective role in animal behaviour, neuroendocrine and molecular parameters (Urani et al., 2005). The monoamine hypothesis postulates that depression is caused by an impairment of serotonergic, noradrenergic or dopaminergic neurotransmission. The monoaminergic deficiency can be due to several factors including decreased synthesis or early degradation of neurotransmitters, altered expression or function of neurotransmitter receptors and impairment of signal transduction systems activated by post-synaptic neurotransmitter receptors (Berton and Nestler, 2006).

The neurotrophic hypothesis of depression assumes that the cAMP responsive element-binding protein (CREB) - brain derived neurotrophic factor (BDNF) - tyrosine kinase B receptor (TRKB) pathway is involved in the pathophysiology of depression and action of antidepressants. Originally the theory was based on findings in rodents, demonstrating that acute or chronic stress decreases BDNF expression in the hippocampus and that diverse classes of antidepressants produce the opposite effect and can prevent the actions of stress (Berton and Nestler, 2006).

A dysregulation of the HPA axis, the major neuroendocrine stress system in mammals, has also been postulated to play a role in human depression. Hyperactivity of the HPA axis is observed in the majority of patients with depression, as manifested by increased expression of CRH in the hypothalamus, increased levels of CRH in the cerebrospinal fluid (CSF) and reduced feedback inhibition of the axis by CRH and glucocorticoids (Sapolsky, 2000;Barden, 2004;de Kloet et al., 2005;Deussing and Wurst, 2005;Muller and Holsboer, 2006).

Although the above mentioned systems are commonly accepted, other neuromodulatory systems have also been implicated in depression, e.g. substance P, neuropeptide Y, aquaporines, and the immune system, in particular the activation of cytokines (Rosenkranz, 2007;Kong et al., 2009;Morales-Medina et al., 2010;Blume et al., 2011). Most likely, neither of the theories will ever hold true on its own in explaining all underlying mechanisms of depression. An interaction of these systems, combining dysregulations of more than one neuronal circuit with environmental factors, is probably more likely to explain the etiology of depression. Nevertheless, these theories represented initial starting points for the generation of possibly valid "depression-models". Among many of the generated mouse mutants based on the mentioned hypothesis, only very few, if any, can be considered valid genetic depression models, but rather represent models of predisposition to depression (Cryan and Mombereau, 2004). Some of the seminal genetic models will be discussed in more detail below.

3.3.1 Models based on the monoamine hypothesis of depression

Several knockout mice of candidate genes related to the monoamine hypothesis were generated in the past. The main ones included the serotonin-(SERT), noradrenaline (NAT)-, and dopamine (DAT) transporters, which represent major targets of antidepressants and psychostimulants such as cocaine and 3,4-methylendioxy-N-methylamphetamine (MDMA/ecstasy). The monoamine transporters (MATs) are localized at the presynaptic mebranes of monoaminergic neurons where they modulate the fate and restrict the lifetime of the released monoamines (Haenisch and Bonisch, 2011). Most classical antidepressants act via MAT inhibition thereby increasing the availability of monoamines in the synaptic cleft. Thus one would speculate that MAT knockouts would show a similar phenotype to that observed after antidepressant treatment. Interestingly, SERT knockout mice show a strong anxiety-like phenotype and are not resistant to depression. Although they display an excess of extracellular 5HT during embryonic development, marked depletion of 5HT was shown in several regions of the adult mouse brain (Bengel et al., 1998). This favoured the assumption that life-long absence of SERT can lead to chronic serotonin depletion resulting in depression-like behaviour (Gross et al., 2000;Gross et al., 2002).

In order to study the endophenotypes of dopaminergic dysregulation Caron and co-workers (Giros et al., 1996) developed conventional DAT knockout (DAT-KO) mice. These animals show persistent hyperdopaminergia, resulting in a downregulation of pre- and postsynaptic dopamine receptors (Gainetdinov et al., 1999;Jones et al., 1999). Concerning the behavioural phenotype, DAT-KO mice show very pronounced hyperlocomotion (Giros et al., 1996;Gainetdinov et al., 1999;Pogorelov et al., 2005), decreased immobility in the FST (Spielewoy et al., 2000), increased sucrose preference (Perona et al., 2008), impairments in cognitive function (Gainetdinov et al., 1999) and deficits in reversal learning (Morice et al., 2007). These observations support a certain role of the dopamine transporter in mediating an antidepressant-like phenotype.

In contrast, the phenotype of conventional NAT knockouts fits the profile of antidepressant efficacy of drugs that antagonize the noradrenalin transporter (Xu et al., 2000). These mice behave like antidepressant-treated animals, exhibiting decreased immobility in the FST and TST (Xu et al., 2000) as well as increased sucrose consumption (Haenisch et al., 2009). In addition, NAT knockout mice show less susceptibility towards acute and chronic stress (Haenisch et al., 2009). Thus, NAT knockout animals seem to be a good model to obtain more in-depth knowledge on the pathophysiology of depression and antidepressant action.

MAT deficient mice represent interesting tools to study human genetic conditions in which these transporters are downregulated, but render them less useful for investigating their normal role in the adult brain. It should also be noted that monoamine transporters can often compensate for each other if they are completely knocked out (Haenisch and Bonisch, 2011). For example, noradrenaline can be taken up and stored in striatal dopaminergic neurons (Gobert et al., 2004). These compensatory processes represent an additional difficulty in understanding the transporter role in the adult brain. In this regard, the conventional SERT and DAT knockout mice rendered insights into the brain serotonergic and dopaminergic systems, but could not fully address the involvement of these monoamines in a depression-like state. A conditional knockout of SERT and DAT within the CNS serotonergic and dopaminergic neurons, respectively, would greatly aid in this undertaking. Unfortunately, until now, no tissue-specific conditional knockouts of the SERT and DAT have been generated. However, SERT knockdown via siRNA led to a reduction of SERT mRNA levels in the dorsal and medial raphe nuclei as well as immobility in the FST, which was identical to the response obtained from wildtype mice treated with the antidepressant citalopram (Hoyer et al., 2006). Knockdown of the dopamine transporter within the ventral tegmental area led to behavioural alterations also found in patients with bipolar disorder (Young et al., 2010;Young et al., 2011). These models represent interesting and valuable pharmacological tools and stress the importance of developing conditional monoamine-transporter knockouts in the future.

In addition to MATs, conventional monoamine receptor mutant mice also mimic some aspects of depression-like behaviour. Fourteen subtypes of 5HT receptors have been identified so far (Hoyer and Martin, 1997) many of which have been targeted genetically

(Holmes, 2001). However, it is far from clear which receptors are mediating specific aspects of emotional behaviour. So far, the $5HT_{1A}$ receptor ($5HT_{1A}$-R) has been investigated in greater detail. $5HT_{1A}$-R knockouts display increased anxiety-related behaviour (Heisler et al., 1998;Ramboz et al., 1998;Sibille et al., 2000) and HPA axis dysregulation (Gross et al., 2000). Most of the other serotonin receptor knockout mice show no behavioural alterations. Although the behavioural effects in $5HT_{1A}$-R knockout mice were rather small, they still represent a valuable pharmacological model to study pharmacodynamical, biochemical and behavioural characteristics of serotonergic antidepressants (Urani et al., 2005). Similarly, there are hardly any pharmacological tools available that are selective enough to discriminate between the different subtypes of α_2 adrenergic receptors. Thus, mice carrying deletions for these receptors could help to better understand receptor function and improve drug specificity. Mutant α_{2A} adrenergic receptor mice show an increase in anxiety-like behaviour (Lahdesmaki et al., 2002), increased immobility in the FST and have a disrupted circadian rhythm (Schramm et al., 2001), a symptom often observed in human depression.
Although monoamine receptor KOs represent valuable pharmacological tools, they are limited in their value as an animal model of depression. This is mostly due to the fact that deletion of a signal receptor is probably not sufficient to induce reliable depression-like phenotypes. In addition, compensatory mechanisms in early embryogenesis can lead to misinterpretations of receptor function pointing out once more the importance of conditional KOs.

3.3.2 Models based on the neurotrophic factor-related hypothesis of depression

The neurotrophin hypothesis of depression has also been addressed in the mouse by targeting neurotrophic factors such as BDNF and the respective TRKB receptors. However, conventional BDNF and TRKB receptor KOs are not viable (Conover et al., 1995). Thus, most of the earlier studies were conducted with heterozygous knockout mice. These were behaviourally indistinguishable from control littermates, consequently not representing a genetic model of depression (MacQueen et al., 2001). In contrast, forebrain-specific BDNF deletion leads to hyperactivity, obesity and increased anxiety-like behaviour (Rios et al., 2001). In addition, inducible knockout of BDNF from the hippocampus and other forebrain regions prevented the antidepressant effects of certain reuptake inhibitors (Monteggia et al., 2004). These animal models were of great value in linking the role of BDNF in the adult brain with antidepressant-like activity of certain drugs. However, complications arise from the fact that BDNF seems to exert quite opposite effects in different neural circuits. Although it shows antidepressant-like effects at the level of the hippocampus, BDNF infusion into the ventral tegmental area induces a prodepression-like effect (Eisch et al., 2003;Berton and Nestler, 2006). Conversely, conditional forebrain deletion of the BDNF receptor TRKB induced only a few behavioural changes, many of which are inconsistent (Zorner et al., 2003). Nevertheless, the conditional BDNF knockouts significantly contributed to the dissection of the role of BDNF in depression-related behaviours and responses to antidepressant drugs.

3.3.3 Models based on alterations of the HPA axis

3.3.3.1 The CRH/CRHR1 System

The generation and analysis of numerous constitutive mouse mutants affecting different parts of the HPA axis is another example where genetically modified mice have demonstrated their enormous potential. The genetic dissection of the organism's major stress-integrating system in the mouse has confirmed a major role of corticosteroid receptors and of the CRH system in the pathogenesis of affective disorders including depression (Deussing and Wurst, 2005). Therefore it seemed obvious to target the major player of the system, CRH. However, homozygous CRH knockout mice are viable and show no behavioural abnormalities compared to control littermates (Muglia et al., 1995). Basal pituitary ACTH secretion is compensated by an increased expression of the co-secretagogue neuropeptide vasopressin (AVP), thus CRH deficiency impairs but does not fully block pituitary-adrenal responses to diverse stressors (Venihaki and Majzoub, 1999). In contrast, conventional CRH receptor 1 knockouts display a severe impairment of stress-induced HPA axis activation and marked glucocorticoid deficiency (Muller and Holsboer, 2006). In addition, they demonstrate increased locomotor activity and decreased anxiety-like behaviour, both under basal conditions and after ethanol withdrawal (Timpl et al., 1998;Sillaber et al., 2002). As a result, conventional CRHR1 deletion was shown to affect behaviour as well as neuroendocrine regulation, which obstructs the analyses of the role of CRH as a neuromodulator independent of HPA axis activation. By generating forebrain-specific CRHR1 knockouts, this problem was overcome (Muller et al., 2003). These animals demonstrated a marked decrease in anxiety-related behaviour, which was not influenced by central nervous system effects of circulating stress hormones. In addition, forebrain CRHR1 deficiency has been shown to attenuate chronic stress-induced cognitive deficits and dendritic remodelling (Wang et al., 2011). However, it remains a matter of debate which brain structures and circuits are mediating anxiety-like behaviour in mice. So far, most of the results provide evidence that amygdalar CRHR1 is responsible for the observed phenotypes (Liebsch et al., 1995;Sztainberg et al., 2010). Thus it would be of great importance to further dissect the origin of these effects by generating mice with deletions of CRHR1 in certain neuronal subpopulations and/or specific brain regions.

Taking into account that depression is often accompanied with excessive glucocorticoids and elevated CRH levels in the cerebrospinal fluid, the generation of mice overexpressing CRH was of utter importance. Different lines of CRH-overexpressing mice consistently display an increase in anxiety-related behaviour (Stenzel-Poore et al., 1996;Kolber et al., 2010). However, in all cases unrestricted CRH overexpression resulted in elevated corticosterone levels accompanied by symptoms of Cushing-like syndrome, complicating the interpretation of stress-related behavioural results. This problem was circumvented by designing mutants overexpressing CRH under the CNS-specific Nestin and the forebrain-specific Camk2a promotors (Lu et al., 2008). In both lines, the basal HPA axis activity remained unaltered. CRH overexpression in the whole CNS, but not when expressed in specific forebrain regions, resulted in stress-induced hypersecretion of corticosterone and decreased immobility in the FST and TST (Lu et al., 2008). These changes were probably due to acute effects of overexpressed CRH as they were normalized by CRH-R1 antagonist treatment. However, forebrain-specific CRH overexpression during postnatal development was shown to cause long-lasting anxiogenic and despair-like phenotypes (Kolber et al., 2010). This supports the hypothesis that CRH in limbic regions such as the amygdala, hippocampus and prefrontal cortex can induce anxiety-like changes. This further coincides with results obtained from conditional forebrain-specific CRHR1 knockout animals, which demonstrate decreased anxiety-like behaviour. However, the problems concerning ectopic expression cannot be neglected and thus it remains unclear whether CRH overexpressing mouse mutants show sufficient, if any, construct validity. The best way to address this issue would be to generate a CRH overexpressing mouse under the control of its endogenous promoter, thereby restricting the overexpression to its actual expression sites.

3.3.3.2 Glucocorticoids and glucocorticoid receptors

Excessive stimulation of the HPA axis, implicated in depression, is mostly reflected by excessive glucocorticoids. Conventional glucocorticoid receptor knockouts have thus been developed in order to address the function of the GR in depression. Initially, a GR-antisense transgenic mouse was developed (Pepin et al., 1992), which demonstrated behavioural and neuroendocrine signs and symptoms common among depressed patients. These included reduced negative feedback sensitivity to dexamethasone (Stec et al., 1994) and enhanced stress hormone response (Pepin et al., 1992). Most importantly, this model showed good predictive validity evident in an antidepressant response which induced numerous changes including increased GR mRNA, reduced HPA axis activity (Montkowski et al., 1995) and enhanced hippocampal LTP (Steckler et al., 2001). A few years later, conventional GR knockouts were developed (Cole et al., 1995). These showed a similar phenotype to that observed in GR-antisense transgenic mice. In addition, they exhibited increased helplessness after stress exposure and reduced hippocampal BDNF content (Ridder et al., 2005). Forebrain-specific GR deletion produces non-suppression of corticosterone following dexamethasone administration, altered circadian HPA axis activity, and increased hypothalamic vasopressin expression, which are all hallmarks of depression. Interestingly, they also exhibited a robust despair-like phenotype, which was reverted by antidepressant treatment (Boyle et al., 2005). Taking into account the observations from the conventional GR knockouts, it does not seem surprising that GR antagonists are being considered and currently tested as possible non-monoamine-based antidepressants.

Conditional, forebrain-restricted overexpressing GR mutants were also developed in order to address the function of the receptor in the pathophysiology of depression. However, increased GR expression specifically in the forebrain is unlikely to occur under normal circumstances (Muller and Holsboer, 2006). Nevertheless, some important insights into how the GR modulates emotional responsiveness have been obtained (Wei et al., 2004). Increased anxiety-related behaviour was observed in conditional GR overexpressing mice, which was reverted by desipramine treatment. However, the HPA axis remained unchanged, rendering this line a model of "increased emotional lability". In contrast, when GR overexpression was achieved by means of inserting two additional copies of the gene using a yeast artificial chromosome, the animals demonstrated a stress-resistant HPA system and showed reduced helplessness after stress exposure (Reichardt et al., 2000). However, it should be noted that in this case the GR overexpression was not restricted to the central nervous system. In this regard, both transgenic lines provided some insights concerning stress responsiveness, but are not very suitable as a model for depression.

It becomes quite clear that no single model fulfils all the criteria necessary to be coined "depression-model". Future technologies, such as constitutive and conditional RNAi transgenesis, zinc-finger and optogenetic approaches will have a great impact on the development of more suitable models for depression and other psychiatric disorders.

4. Next generation of genetic models – new techniques and strategies

4.1 Models based on Genome-Wide Association Studies (GWAS)

In a genome-wide association study (GWAS) a large number of genetic polymorphisms across the whole genome is examined to identify genetic associations with an observable trait or disease. The power of a GWAS is restricted by the sample size and the technical properties of the genotyping platform used with regard to the coverage of genomic locations. GWASs can be used to detect case-control- or family-based associations (Craddock et al., 2008). The great advantage of this method compared to classical candidate gene studies is that it allows genetic investigation of a disease in a non-hypothesis-driven manner. Using this unbiased approach increases the possibility to find new and even unexpected genes associated with a certain disease. A key factor for this kind of study is a preferably large sample size in order to detect even small effect sizes. There is evidence that for psychiatric disorders most of the heritable risk is due to interactions of combinations of genetic risk variants each with a relatively small effect on the general outcome (Cichon et al., 2009). An obvious challenge concerning the genetic investigation of psychiatric disorders in comparison to non-psychiatric diseases is that the phenotype and the clinical picture of mood disorders are more difficult to define. Therefore, the patient samples used for a GWAS are often rather heterogeneous with regard to sex, age, symptoms, environmental factors and other issues. To increase the statistical power of GWAS studies a so-called meta-analysis can be performed by pooling all GWAS data available for a certain disease and subsequent statistical evaluation in order to increase the sample size. Associations for several candidate genes have been identified in a meta-analysis of genetic studies on major depression, including apolipoprotein E (*APOE)*, dopamine receptor D4 (*DRD4)*, guanine nucleotide-binding protein (*GNB3)*, methylenetetrahydrofolate reductase (*MTHFR)*, dopamine transporter (*SLC6A3)* and serotonin transporter (*SLC6A4)* (Lopez-Leon et al., 2008). Additionally, several associations with immune-related genes have been reported, for instance *P2RX7* which is a purinergic ATP-gated calcium channel that modulates macrophage-induced inflammatory responses and is also expressed in neurons and glia cells in the brain. A non-synonymous coding SNP in the *P2RX7* gene (rs2230912) leading to an amino acid substitution (Gln460Arg) has been found to be associated with major depression and bipolar disorder in several independent studies (Barden et al., 2006;Lucae et al., 2006;McQuillin et al., 2009;Hejjas et al., 2009;Soronen et al., 2011). These data highlight *P2RX7* as a new interesting candidate gene for mood disorders even though these findings need further investigation. The proper way to validate the biological significance of such implicated risk variations is the generation of an appropriate *in vivo* model. Using knock-in mouse models, human association data can be validated and pharmacological compounds can be tested *in vivo*. In a study of Chen et al (Chen et al., 2006) a common single-nucleotide polymorphism (SNP) in the brain-derived neurotrophic factor (BDNF) gene, leading to a substitution of methionine for valine at codon 66 (Val66Met) was investigated in a mouse model carrying the BDNF variant. This SNP was shown to be associated with alterations in brain anatomy and memory, but its relevance for psychiatric disorders has been unclear. In response to stress these mutant mice exhibited increased anxiety-related behaviour suggesting that this genetic predisposition combined with an environmental challenge may increase the risk to develop anxiety and depressive disorders (Chen et al., 2006).

4.2 Generating models using optogenetics

The use of traditional electrophysiological, pharmacological and genetic methods goes along with considerable deficits, which make them partly unsuitable to study neural circuits with fine spatial and temporal resolution *in vivo* (Carter and de, 2011). To overcome these limitations, a new technology termed optogenetics (Deisseroth et al., 2006) has been developed to precisely stimulate, inhibit or alter the activity of specific cells and their processes with high temporal accuracy and rapid reversibility. The special feature of this approach are effectors which can be activated by light and are genetically encoded allowing direct control of specific cell populations *in vitro* and *in vivo*. The most commonly used optogenetic effectors are genetically engineered variants of natural opsins, light-sensitive ion channels that can be stimulated in response to specific wavelengths of light leading either to membrane depolarisation, hyperpolarisation or change in intracellular signalling (Carter and de, 2011). The first class includes channelrhodopsin-2 (ChR2), isolated from the green algae *Chlamydomonas reinhardtii* which is sensitive to blue light and has already successfully been used in transgenic mice (Arenkiel et al., 2007;Tsai et al., 2009;Huber et al., 2008). Photons are absorbed by the all-*trans*-retinal cofactor of ChR2 that is endogenously expressed at sufficient levels in the central nervous system of vertebrates (Li et al., 2005;Bi et al., 2006;Ishizuka et al., 2006;Zhang et al., 2006). ChR2 can be activated and closed very rapidly upon light on- and offset, respectively, allowing stimulation of neurons within milliseconds (Boyden et al., 2005;Li et al., 2005). The inhibitory counterpart of ChR2, the chloride pump halorhodopsin (NpHR), was isolated from the bacteria *Natronomonas pharaoni* and possesses an activation spectrum in the yellow range, complementary to that of channelrhodopsin. Similarly to ChR2, NpHR uses all-*trans* retinal as chromophore and can therefore be applied in vertebrate organisms without exogenous cofactors. By expressing both proteins in the same cell, one can either activate or silence it by illumination with different wavelengths (Fiala et al., 2010). A third strategy is to design artificial rhodopsin-GPCR chimeras that combine the light responsive elements of rhodopsin with the biochemical signalling functionality of specific GPCRs termed Opto-XRs (Kramer et al., 2009;Airan et al., 2009). Recently, this method was used to develop an Opto-XR that controls serotonin signalling via the 5-HT(1A) receptor (Oh et al., 2010).

Several studies have used optogenetic techniques to investigate the neural circuitries and molecular mechanisms underlying mammalian behaviour and the etiology of neurological disorders (Carter and de, 2011). For instance, recent studies used optogenetics to dissect the neural circuitry within basal ganglia underlying Parkinson´s disease (Gradinaru et al., 2009;Kravitz et al., 2010). It was also shown that optogenetic stimulation of the *locus coeruleus* (LC) leads to an immediate shift from sleep to wakefulness whereas optogenetic inhibiton causes a decrease in wakefulness (Carter and de, 2011). However, sustained stimulation of the LC produces a behavioural state resembling cataplexy, a transient loss of muscle tone which is a hallmark of narcolepsy. These results suggest that overstimulation can cause behavioural arrests similar to those seen in neuropsychiatric disorders. In addition, using optogenetics, selective phasic photostimulation of dopaminergic neurons in the ventral tegmental area (VTA) was able to trigger behavioural conditioning whereas tonic activity was not (Tsai et al., 2009). Stimulation of dopaminergic neurons in the VTA led to secretion of glutamate into the nucleus accumbens in addition to dopamine, suggesting that mesolimbic reward signalling may involve glutamatergic transmission (Tecuapetla et al., 2010;Stuber et al., 2010). Many other studies using optogenetic probes have been performed, including associative fear memory (Ciocchi et al., 2010;Johansen et al., 2010;Haubensak et al., 2010), epilepsy (Tonnesen et al., 2009) and others. Thus, optogenetics represents an uprising and promising technique in molecular brain research, which will certainly aid in the development and analysis of new mouse models of depression.

4.3 Mouse engineering by means of zinc finger nucleases

Another new promising technique called genome editing enables efficient and precise genetic modification by induction of a double-strand break in a specific target sequence in the genome using zinc finger nucleases (ZFN), followed by the generation of genetic modifications during subsequent DNA repair. These zinc finger nucleases are sequence-specific endonucleases that can be modified to cleave a desired DNA target. This method was initially applied to *Drosophila melanogaster* (Bibikova et al., 2002) and has already been used to disrupt endogenous loci in rats (Geurts and Moreno, 2010), by using this technique, basically any eukaryote can be genetically modified.

Genetic disruption using this technology is achieved by taking advantage of errors introduced during DNA repair to destroy the function of a gene or genomic region in a single step without selection for the desired event (Urnov et al., 2010). This process is called non-homologous end-joining, a template-independent and therefore imperfect repair mechanism resulting in deletions or insertions. For gene disruption in rats, engineered zinc finger nucleases with extended recognition sites were used to produce knockout animals for two different endogenous genes, and transmission of the disrupted alleles occurred at a frequency of 10–100% (Geurts and Moreno, 2010). The great advantage of this ZFN-driven knockout approach is that only one generation is needed, and compares favourably with others strategies such as classical gene targeting in mouse embryonic stem cells considering duration and screening effort.

A second, more complex approach using a ZFN-induced double-strand break which is recombinogenic in higher eukaryotes is called homology-based genome editing. This technique requires the simultaneous provision of an appropriately designed, homology-containing donor DNA molecule along with the locus-specific ZFNs. This enables the study of gene function and modelling of disease-causing mutations through the creation of a point mutation that is characteristic of a known disease-predisposing allele or that disables a motif that is thought to be crucial for function (Urnov et al., 2010). This method was applied to three different genes in *D. melanogaster*, and in up to 90% the offspring of treated animals carried the donor-specific alleles of the target gene (Beumer et al., 2006).

Meyer and colleagues have recently explored whether gene targeting can be directly performed in murine zygotes by the use of zinc-finger nucleases. They reported that gene targeting could be successfully achieved in murine one-cell embryos upon the coinjection of targeting vectors with zinc-finger nucleases, without preselection (Meyer et al., 2010).

Using the ZFN technology will enable to identify and validate genes involved in complex diseases such as depression. Especially for the validation of candidate genes for disease susceptibility identified in linkage and association studies this method could provide a powerful tool in the future (Geurts and Moreno, 2010).

Furthermore, other types of nucleases based on engineered transcription activator-like effectors (TALEs) are currently under development (Christian et al., 2010). TAL effector nucleases have the advantage that they are very simple to engineer and have already been used to target endogenous loci in human cells (Miller et al., 2011). Up to now, no transgenic organisms based on TALE nuclease technology have been reported yet, but this certainly is just a matter of time.

5. Mouse models based on environmental challenges

Besides genetic risk factors, many studies have implicated environmental alterations including stressful life events with the development of affective disorders (Pezawas et al., 2005;Ising and Holsboer, 2006). Exposure to stress or to traumatic life experiences has a strong impact on the manifestation of depression, suggesting an impairment of proper stress-coping strategies in depressed patients (Kessler, 1997;de Kloet et al., 2005). Therefore, depression is also regarded as a stress-related disorder, and, accordingly, many of the animal models of depression are based on the exposure to various types of acute or chronic stressors. However, up to now little consensus exists on the definition of stress. Many studies interpret the presence of a stress response, evident in a sudden increase of corticosterone, as an indicator of stress exposure. However, appetitive and rewarding situations such as sexual behaviour and winning a social interaction elicit HPA axis responses that are similar in magnitude as highly aversive situations like social defeat (Koolhaas et al., 2011). This points out that the physiological response per se does not necessarily indicate a state of stress. In other words, when is a stimulus a stressor and what makes a response a stress response? Koolhaas and colleagues agreed on the view that stress should be considered as a cognitive perception of uncontrollability and/or unpredictability that is expressed in a physiological and behavioural response. Hence, an unpredictable situation should be characterized by the absence of an anticipatory response, whereas uncontrollability can be defined as a reduced recovery of the neuroendocrine reaction (Koolhaas et al., 2011). In that regard the most prominent models will be explained below.

5.1 Chronic stress models

The chronic character of stressors is generally considered an important factor in the development of various forms of stress-related pathologies. Several chronic stress procedures have been employed in the past, trying to achieve a measure of construct and face validity. Chronic mild or chronic unpredictable stress involves exposing rodents to a series of repeated physical stressors, including foot shock, restraint, low temperatures, loud music etc, over a period of weeks or longer (Willner, 2005;Nestler and Hyman, 2010). Towards the end of the stress procedure the animals develop signs of anhedonia, which can be reverted by chronic, but not acute, administration of antidepressants. Although this model shows aspects of construct and face validity, it is not easily reproduced across laboratories. This is probably caused by repeated exposure to a certain stimulus, which eventually renders it predictable. Thus, stimuli which have been perceived as stressors at the beginning cease to be perceived as such after a while. This holds especially true for repeated restraint (immobilization) stress in view of the strong decline of the physiological response upon its repetition (Grissom et al., 2008). In this regard, some commonly used animal models of chronic stress may represent models of adaptation rather than models of stress-related pathology (Koolhaas et al., 2011). A means of circumventing this problem is to use stressors with a certain degree of ecological validity. These stressors should be unpredictable, uncontrollable and challenge the natural defence mechanisms of the animal. So far only a few models seem to meet these criteria including chronic social defeat stress. Here, an animal is repeatedly exposed to an aggressive dominant animal, leading to social subordination, after which the mice show a range of depression-like symptoms, including anhedonia, social withdrawal and cognitive impairments (Berton et al., 2006;Wang et al., 2011). Most of these are reversible by chronic, but not acute, antidepressant treatment (Berton et al., 2006). In addition, chronic social defeat was shown to induce a metabolic syndrome in mice characterized by weight gain, insulin and leptin resistance (Chuang et al., 2010), consistent with homeostatic abnormalities observed in depressed patients. In addition, experience of social defeat leads to changes in the state of the serotonergic and noradrenergic systems of various parts of the brain (Berton et al., 1998). A further advantage of chronic social defeat is the potential to segregate defeated subjects into susceptible and unsusceptible populations on the basis of considerable individual variance to social defeat behavioural outcomes (Krishnan et al., 2007). Thus, the social defeat procedure exhibits features of construct, face and predictive validity, although the intensity of the stress used is more severe than that seen in humans. The main drawback of chronic stress paradigms is that the evoked phenotypes often "resemble social anxiety" and not depression. It is difficult to identify the required stress duration which induces depression-like symptoms rather than sole anxiety responses. Kudryavtseva and colleagues propose that longer sessions of social stress (at least 20 days) are required to induce depression-like phenotypes, whereas Nestler and colleagues claim to observe such behavioural alterations already after 10 days (Berton et al., 2006). Additional studies will help to further elaborate on this aspect and possibly pave the road for improved strategies in modelling depression.

5.2 Early life stress models

Similar validity compared to the chronic social defeat model was achieved for early life stress, including prenatal stress, early postnatal handling, and most of all maternal separation (Francis et al., 1996;Ladd et al., 2000;Caldji et al., 2000;Meaney, 2001). Traumatic life events in childhood have been shown to result in an increased sensitivity to the effects of stress later in life and alter the individual's vulnerability to stress-related psychiatric disorders such as depression (Graham et al., 1999;Heim and Nemeroff, 2001). Early life stress in mice produces neuroendocrine and behavioural changes that persist into adulthood, some of which can be reverted by antidepressants (Meaney, 2001). The most widely used model is the maternal separation paradigm of early life deprivation, in which pups are separated from the dam for 1-24 h per day during the first two postnatal weeks. This results in increased anxiety-like and despair-based behaviour as well as increased HPA axis response, all of which can be observed in adulthood (de Kloet et al., 2005). It is important to mention that shorter periods of separation tend to produce opposite effects. Thus early life challenges may conversely induce changes that prepare an individual for life in a more hostile environment and therefore be predominantly beneficial. Hence, it has be proposed that adult diseases such as depression might not be promoted by early life adversity per se, but by a mismatch of the programmed and the later actual environment in combination with a more vulnerable or resilient genetic predisposition (Schmidt, 2011). Although the exact physiological nature of the effects of postnatal maternal separation is not fully understood, the paradigm demonstrated its value for studying the neurobiological basis of the impact of early life stress on emotional behaviour (Cryan and Holmes, 2005). More recently, a new early life stress model based on similar principles has been developed. The main difference is that the new model omits the separation from the mother and thereby avoids metabolic disturbances, exhaustion, or hypothermia of the pups. This is evoked by means of fragmented maternal care, generated by reducing the amount of nesting and bedding material available to the dam (Rice et al., 2008).

6. Gene-environment interactions

Although chronic stress has been implicated in the onset of psychiatric disorders, it has to be kept in mind that not all individuals exposed to severe stress will progress to disease. In that sense, it is also quite unlikely that a single genetic variant is responsible for a specific disorder. Therefore, it is of great necessity to understand the cause of individual differences and the consequences of variation in vulnerability, with regard to disease progression. It is clear that major efforts should be directed towards the combination of genetic modifications and environmental challenges in the same subject. Such stimulation of gene-environment interactions is more likely to reflect the pathophysiological mechanisms of depression. Many studies have already applied this concept by subjecting transgenic lines to chronic social stress procedures (Berton et al., 2006;Wagner et al., 2010;Wang et al., 2011). These studies provide further evidence that disease-associated genetic alterations do not have to be pathological/beneficial under normal conditions, but in combination with chronic stress can either cause vulnerability or resilience towards the development of depression-like phenotypes.

7. Classical antidepressants – limitations and future prospects

The majority of antidepressant drug discovery efforts during the past decades have focused on finding more selective serotonin- or noradrenaline-based agonists or antagonists having modes of action similar to already available drugs, only with the ability to act more quickly and safely. However, until now this approach has not lead to improved treatment. There are some novel drugs known as atypical antidepressants which have ascribed monoamine-based mechanisms, but there is only weak evidence that their implied mechanisms actually account for their clinical efficacy. In parallel, non-monoamine systems that might contribute to the pathophysiology of depression have been analyzed in the past, revealing potential biomarkers for depression, such as CRH, P2RX7, BDNF, etc. (see above). However, none of these discoveries has been translated into a new bona fide treatment for depression so far. Ironically, the search for non-monoamine-based antidepressants has often relied on the actions of monoamine-based drugs. This highlights the necessity to develop improved animal models of depression. Applying the techniques and approaches mentioned above should aid in this undertaking and hopefully translate into the development of new treatment modalities apart from classical antidepressants.

8. Conclusion

The major problem in the establishment of a suitable animal model of depression is that the development of such a model requires a better understanding of the etiology of the disorders. The current state of clinical knowledge lacks objective diagnostic tests and validated biomarkers of such a highly heterogeneous illness. However, such models are of great necessity for understanding disease pathophysiology and for hastening the development of treatments based on new molecular targets. We have given a general overview of the current mouse models of depression and outlined some of the difficulties in the generation and validation of such models. In addition, new strategies and technologies have been discussed, which will greatly contribute to our understanding of disease pathology. Nevertheless, it is very unlikely that mice will ever recapitulate all of the salient features of a human mental illness. Above all, models are meant to serve as investigative tools. In that regard, researchers should critically judge construct, face and predictive validity and not simply assume that behavioural alterations in one or more tests are sufficient to render a model of depression. In addition, differences between males and females are often not addressed in preclinical research. Extensive literature reports that mood disorders are more frequent in women than in men, but the great majority of basic research has focussed on male rodents as animal models (Palanza, 2001). This emphasizes the need for reliable depression models in females. In addition other endophenotypes of depression, such as alterations in sleep, should also be addressed more consistently in mice. To accomplish the goal of creating more appropriate animal models of depression, it will be necessary to implement and combine all recent advances in genetics, pharmacology and electrical stimulation with environmental challenges (Fig. 1). This will hopefully initiate the development of new treatment modalities which are based on knowledge and not serendipity.

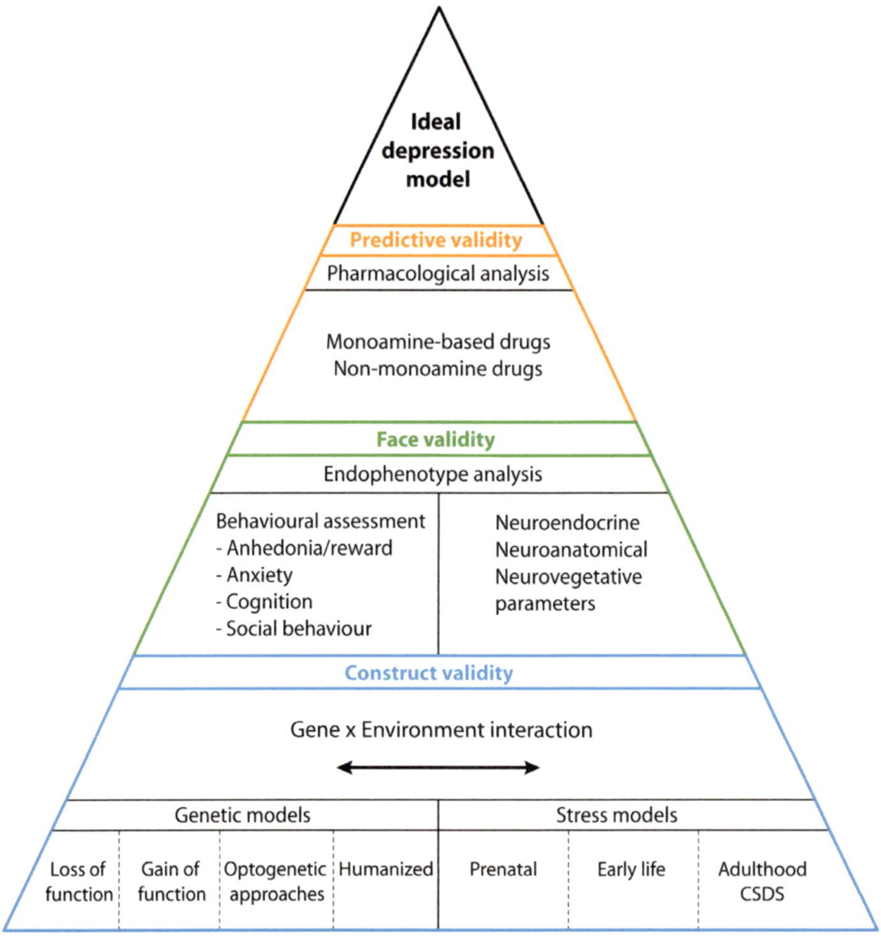

Fig. 1. Towards an ideal mouse model of depression.

In order to generate more suitable depression models with strong construct validity, major efforts should be directed towards the combination of genetic modification and environmental challenges in the same subject. This would simulate gene-environment interactions that more plausibly reflect the pathophysiological mechanisms of depression. Such models should show sufficient face validity, as assessed by behavioural and/or physiological parameters and respond to classical and/or novel drugs (predictive validity).

9. References

Airan RD, Thompson KR, Fenno LE, Bernstein H, Deisseroth K (2009) Temporally precise in vivo control of intracellular signalling. Nature 458:1025-1029.

Amann LC, Gandal MJ, Halene TB, Ehrlichman RS, White SL, McCarren HS, Siegel SJ (2010) Mouse behavioral endophenotypes for schizophrenia. Brain Res Bull 83:147-161.

Arenkiel BR, Peca J, Davison IG, Feliciano C, Deisseroth K, Augustine GJ, Ehlers MD, Feng G (2007) In vivo light-induced activation of neural circuitry in transgenic mice expressing channelrhodopsin-2. Neuron 54:205-218.

Barden N (2004) Implication of the hypothalamic-pituitary-adrenal axis in the physiopathology of depression. J Psychiatry Neurosci 29:185-193.

Barden N, Harvey M, Gagne B, Shink E, Tremblay M, Raymond C, Labbe M, Villeneuve A, Rochette D, Bordeleau L, Stadler H, Holsboer F, Muller-Myhsok B (2006) Analysis of single nucleotide polymorphisms in genes in the chromosome 12Q24.31 region points to P2RX7 as a susceptibility gene to bipolar affective disorder. Am J Med Genet B Neuropsychiatr Genet 141B:374-382.

Bardo MT, Bevins RA (2000) Conditioned place preference: what does it add to our preclinical understanding of drug reward? Psychopharmacology (Berl) 153:31-43.

Belzung C, Griebel G (2001) Measuring normal and pathological anxiety-like behaviour in mice: a review. Behav Brain Res 125:141-149.

Belzung C, Le PG (1994) Comparison of different behavioral test situations used in psychopharmacology for measurement of anxiety. Physiol Behav 56:623-628.

Bengel D, Murphy DL, Andrews AM, Wichems CH, Feltner D, Heils A, Mossner R, Westphal H, Lesch KP (1998) Altered brain serotonin homeostasis and locomotor insensitivity to 3, 4-methylenedioxymethamphetamine ("Ecstasy") in serotonin transporter-deficient mice. Mol Pharmacol 53:649-655.

Berton O, Aguerre S, Sarrieau A, Mormede P, Chaouloff F (1998) Differential effects of social stress on central serotonergic activity and emotional reactivity in Lewis and spontaneously hypertensive rats. Neuroscience 82:147-159.

Berton O, McClung CA, Dileone RJ, Krishnan V, Renthal W, Russo SJ, Graham D, Tsankova NM, Bolanos CA, Rios M, Monteggia LM, Self DW, Nestler EJ (2006) Essential role of BDNF in the mesolimbic dopamine pathway in social defeat stress. Science 311:864-868.

Berton O, Nestler EJ (2006) New approaches to antidepressant drug discovery: beyond monoamines. Nat Rev Neurosci 7:137-151.

Beumer K, Bhattacharyya G, Bibikova M, Trautman JK, Carroll D (2006) Efficient gene targeting in Drosophila with zinc-finger nucleases. Genetics 172:2391-2403.

Bi A, Cui J, Ma YP, Olshevskaya E, Pu M, Dizhoor AM, Pan ZH (2006) Ectopic expression of a microbial-type rhodopsin restores visual responses in mice with photoreceptor degeneration. Neuron 50:23-33.

Bibikova M, Golic M, Golic KG, Carroll D (2002) Targeted chromosomal cleavage and mutagenesis in Drosophila using zinc-finger nucleases. Genetics 161:1169-1175.

Bienvenu OJ, Stein MB, Samuels JF, Onyike CU, Eaton WW, Nestadt G (2009) Personality disorder traits as predictors of subsequent first-onset panic disorder or agoraphobia. Compr Psychiatry 50:209-214.

Birrell JM, Brown VJ (2000) Medial frontal cortex mediates perceptual attentional set shifting in the rat. J Neurosci 20:4320-4324.

Blume J, Douglas SD, Evans DL (2011) Immune suppression and immune activation in depression. Brain Behav Immun 25:221-229.

Bondi CO, Rodriguez G, Gould GG, Frazer A, Morilak DA (2008) Chronic unpredictable stress induces a cognitive deficit and anxiety-like behavior in rats that is prevented by chronic antidepressant drug treatment. Neuropsychopharmacology 33:320-331.

Boyden ES, Zhang F, Bamberg E, Nagel G, Deisseroth K (2005) Millisecond-timescale, genetically targeted optical control of neural activity. Nat Neurosci 8:1263-1268.

Boyle MP, Brewer JA, Funatsu M, Wozniak DF, Tsien JZ, Izumi Y, Muglia LJ (2005) Acquired deficit of forebrain glucocorticoid receptor produces depression-like changes in adrenal axis regulation and behavior. Proc Natl Acad Sci U S A 102:473-478.

Branda CS, Dymecki SM (2004) Talking about a revolution: The impact of site-specific recombinases on genetic analyses in mice. Dev Cell 6:7-28.

Broekkamp CL, Rijk HW, Joly-Gelouin D, Lloyd KL (1986) Major tranquillizers can be distinguished from minor tranquillizers on the basis of effects on marble burying and swim-induced grooming in mice. Eur J Pharmacol 126:223-229.

Brown GW, Bifulco A, Harris TO (1987) Life events, vulnerability and onset of depression: some refinements. Br J Psychiatry 150:30-42.

Butler PD, Weiss JM, Stout JC, Nemeroff CB (1990) Corticotropin-releasing factor produces fear-enhancing and behavioral activating effects following infusion into the locus coeruleus. J Neurosci 10:176-183.

Butters MA, Bhalla RK, Mulsant BH, Mazumdar S, Houck PR, Begley AE, Dew MA, Pollock BG, Nebes RD, Becker JT, Reynolds CF, III (2004) Executive functioning, illness course, and relapse/recurrence in continuation and maintenance treatment of late-life depression: is there a relationship? Am J Geriatr Psychiatry 12:387-394.

Cain DP, Paxinos G (1974) Olfactory bulbectomy and mucosal damage: effects on copulation, irritability, and interspecific aggression in male rats. J Comp Physiol Psychol 86:202-212.

Caldji C, Diorio J, Meaney MJ (2000) Variations in maternal care in infancy regulate the development of stress reactivity. Biol Psychiatry 48:1164-1174.

Capecchi MR (2005) Gene targeting in mice: functional analysis of the mammalian genome for the twenty-first century. Nat Rev Genet 6:507-512.

Carter ME, de LL (2011) Optogenetic investigation of neural circuits in vivo. Trends Mol Med 17:197-206.

Chadman KK, Yang M, Crawley JN (2009) Criteria for validating mouse models of psychiatric diseases. Am J Med Genet B Neuropsychiatr Genet 150B:1-11.

Chen ZY, Jing D, Bath KG, Ieraci A, Khan T, Siao CJ, Herrera DG, Toth M, Yang C, McEwen BS, Hempstead BL, Lee FS (2006) Genetic variant BDNF (Val66Met) polymorphism alters anxiety-related behavior. Science 314:140-143.

Christian M, Cermak T, Doyle EL, Schmidt C, Zhang F, Hummel A, Bogdanove AJ, Voytas DF (2010) Targeting DNA double-strand breaks with TAL effector nucleases. Genetics 186:757-761.

Chuang JC, Cui H, Mason BL, Mahgoub M, Bookout AL, Yu HG, Perello M, Elmquist JK, Repa JJ, Zigman JM, Lutter M (2010) Chronic social defeat stress disrupts regulation of lipid synthesis. J Lipid Res 51:1344-1353.

Cichon S, Craddock N, Daly M, Faraone SV, Gejman PV, Kelsoe J, Lehner T, Levinson DF, Moran A, Sklar P, Sullivan PF (2009) Genomewide association studies: history, rationale, and prospects for psychiatric disorders. Am J Psychiatry 166:540-556.

Ciocchi S, Herry C, Grenier F, Wolff SB, Letzkus JJ, Vlachos I, Ehrlich I, Sprengel R, Deisseroth K, Stadler MB, Muller C, Luthi A (2010) Encoding of conditioned fear in central amygdala inhibitory circuits. Nature 468:277-282.

Cole TJ, Blendy JA, Monaghan AP, Krieglstein K, Schmid W, Aguzzi A, Fantuzzi G, Hummler E, Unsicker K, Schutz G (1995) Targeted disruption of the glucocorticoid receptor gene blocks adrenergic chromaffin cell development and severely retards lung maturation. Genes Dev 9:1608-1621.

Conover JC, Erickson JT, Katz DM, Bianchi LM, Poueymirou WT, McClain J, Pan L, Helgren M, Ip NY, Boland P, . (1995) Neuronal deficits, not involving motor neurons, in mice lacking BDNF and/or NT4. Nature 375:235-238.

Conrad CD, Galea LA, Kuroda Y, McEwen BS (1996) Chronic stress impairs rat spatial memory on the Y maze, and this effect is blocked by tianeptine pretreatment. Behav Neurosci 110:1321-1334.

Covington HE, III, Maze I, LaPlant QC, Vialou VF, Ohnishi YN, Berton O, Fass DM, Renthal W, Rush AJ, III, Wu EY, Ghose S, Krishnan V, Russo SJ, Tamminga C, Haggarty SJ, Nestler EJ (2009) Antidepressant actions of histone deacetylase inhibitors. J Neurosci 29:11451-11460.

Craddock N, O'Donovan MC, Owen MJ (2008) Genome-wide association studies in psychiatry: lessons from early studies of non-psychiatric and psychiatric phenotypes. Mol Psychiatry 13:649-653.

Crocco EA, Castro K, Loewenstein DA (2010) How late-life depression affects cognition: neural mechanisms. Curr Psychiatry Rep 12:34-38.

Cryan JF, Holmes A (2005) The ascent of mouse: advances in modelling human depression and anxiety. Nat Rev Drug Discov 4:775-790.

Cryan JF, Hoyer D, Markou A (2003) Withdrawal from chronic amphetamine induces depressive-like behavioral effects in rodents. Biol Psychiatry 54:49-58.

Cryan JF, McGrath C, Leonard BE, Norman TR (1999) Onset of the effects of the 5-HT1A antagonist, WAY-100635, alone, and in combination with paroxetine, on olfactory bulbectomy and 8-OH-DPAT-induced changes in the rat. Pharmacol Biochem Behav 63:333-338.

Cryan JF, Mombereau C (2004) In search of a depressed mouse: utility of models for studying depression-related behavior in genetically modified mice. Mol Psychiatry 9:326-357.

D'Hooge R, De Deyn PP (2001) Applications of the Morris water maze in the study of learning and memory. Brain Res Brain Res Rev 36:60-90.

Davis M (1990) Animal models of anxiety based on classical conditioning: the conditioned emotional response (CER) and the fear-potentiated startle effect. Pharmacol Ther 47:147-165.

de Kloet ER, Joels M, Holsboer F (2005) Stress and the brain: from adaptation to disease. Nat Rev Neurosci 6:463-475.

Deisseroth K, Feng G, Majewska AK, Miesenbock G, Ting A, Schnitzer MJ (2006) Next-generation optical technologies for illuminating genetically targeted brain circuits. J Neurosci 26:10380-10386.

Dellu F, Contarino A, Simon H, Koob GF, Gold LH (2000) Genetic differences in response to novelty and spatial memory using a two-trial recognition task in mice. Neurobiol Learn Mem 73:31-48.

Deussing JM (2006) Animal models of depression. Drug Discovery Today: Disease Models 3.

Deussing J, Wurst W (2005) Dissecting the genetic effect of the CRH system on anxiety and stress-related behaviour. Elsevier.

Dulawa SC, Hen R (2005) Recent advances in animal models of chronic antidepressant effects: the novelty-induced hypophagia test. Neurosci Biobehav Rev 29:771-783.

Dunner DL, Patrick V, Fieve RR (1979) Life events at the onset of bipolar affective illness. Am J Psychiatry 136:508-511.

Edwards DA, Thompson ML, Burge KG (1972) Olfactory bulb removal vs peripherally induced anosmia: differential effects on the aggressive behavior of male mice. Behav Biol 7:823-828.

Eisch AJ, Bolanos CA, de WJ, Simonak RD, Pudiak CM, Barrot M, Verhaagen J, Nestler EJ (2003) Brain-derived neurotrophic factor in the ventral midbrain-nucleus accumbens pathway: a role in depression. Biol Psychiatry 54:994-1005.

El-Ghundi M, O'Dowd BF, George SR (2001) Prolonged fear responses in mice lacking dopamine D1 receptor. Brain Res 892:86-93.

Eranco O, Hopsu V (1958) Effect of reserpine on the histochemistry and content of adrenaline and noradrenaline in the adrenal medulla of the rat and the mouse. Endocrinology 62:15-23.

Fanselow MS (1980) Conditioned and unconditional components of post-shock freezing. Pavlov J Biol Sci 15:177-182.

Fava M, Kendler KS (2000) Major depressive disorder. Neuron 28:335-341.

Fendt M, Fanselow MS (1999) The neuroanatomical and neurochemical basis of conditioned fear. Neurosci Biobehav Rev 23:743-760.

Fiala A, Suska A, Schluter OM (2010) Optogenetic approaches in neuroscience. Curr Biol 20:R897-R903.

Francis D, Diorio J, LaPlante P, Weaver S, Seckl JR, Meaney MJ (1996) The role of early environmental events in regulating neuroendocrine development. Moms, pups, stress, and glucocorticoid receptors. Ann N Y Acad Sci 794:136-152.

Gainetdinov RR, Jones SR, Caron MG (1999) Functional hyperdopaminergia in dopamine transporter knock-out mice. Biol Psychiatry 46:303-311.

Gardier AM, Bourin M (2001) Appropriate use of "knockout" mice as models of depression or models of testing the efficacy of antidepressants. Psychopharmacology (Berl) 153:393-394.

Geurts AM, Moreno C (2010) Zinc-finger nucleases: new strategies to target the rat genome. Clin Sci (Lond) 119:303-311.

Giros B, Jaber M, Jones SR, Wightman RM, Caron MG (1996) Hyperlocomotion and indifference to cocaine and amphetamine in mice lacking the dopamine transporter. Nature 379:606-612.

Gobert A, Billiras R, Cistarelli L, Millan MJ (2004) Quantification and pharmacological characterization of dialysate levels of noradrenaline in the striatum of freely-moving rats: release from adrenergic terminals and modulation by alpha2-autoreceptors. J Neurosci Methods 140:141-152.

Gottesman II, Gould TD (2003) The endophenotype concept in psychiatry: etymology and strategic intentions. Am J Psychiatry 160:636-645.

Gould TD, Gottesman II (2006) Psychiatric endophenotypes and the development of valid animal models. Genes Brain Behav 5:113-119.

Gradinaru V, Mogri M, Thompson KR, Henderson JM, Deisseroth K (2009) Optical deconstruction of parkinsonian neural circuitry. Science 324:354-359.

Graham YP, Heim C, Goodman SH, Miller AH, Nemeroff CB (1999) The effects of neonatal stress on brain development: implications for psychopathology. Dev Psychopathol 11:545-565.

Griebel G, Belzung C, Misslin R, Vogel E (1993) The free-exploratory paradigm: an effective method for measuring neophobic behaviour in mice and testing potential neophobia-reducing drugs. Behav Pharmacol 4:637-644.

Grigoriadis DE (2005) The corticotropin-releasing factor receptor: a novel target for the treatment of depression and anxiety-related disorders. Expert Opin Ther Targets 9:651-684.

Grissom N, Kerr W, Bhatnagar S (2008) Struggling behavior during restraint is regulated by stress experience. Behav Brain Res 191:219-226.

Gross C, Santarelli L, Brunner D, Zhuang X, Hen R (2000) Altered fear circuits in 5-HT(1A) receptor KO mice. Biol Psychiatry 48:1157-1163.

Gross C, Zhuang X, Stark K, Ramboz S, Oosting R, Kirby L, Santarelli L, Beck S, Hen R (2002) Serotonin1A receptor acts during development to establish normal anxiety-like behaviour in the adult. Nature 416:396-400.

Haenisch B, Bilkei-Gorzo A, Caron MG, Bonisch H (2009) Knockout of the norepinephrine transporter and pharmacologically diverse antidepressants prevent behavioral and brain neurotrophin alterations in two chronic stress models of depression. J Neurochem 111:403-416.

Haenisch B, Bonisch H (2011) Depression and antidepressants: insights from knockout of dopamine, serotonin or noradrenaline re-uptake transporters. Pharmacol Ther 129:352-368.

Handley SL, Mithani S (1984) Effects of alpha-adrenoceptor agonists and antagonists in a maze-exploration model of 'fear'-motivated behaviour. Naunyn Schmiedebergs Arch Pharmacol 327:1-5.

Hasler G, Drevets WC, Manji HK, Charney DS (2004) Discovering endophenotypes for major depression. Neuropsychopharmacology 29:1765-1781.

Haubensak W, Kunwar PS, Cai H, Ciocchi S, Wall NR, Ponnusamy R, Biag J, Dong HW, Deisseroth K, Callaway EM, Fanselow MS, Luthi A, Anderson DJ (2010) Genetic dissection of an amygdala microcircuit that gates conditioned fear. Nature 468:270-276.

Heim C, Nemeroff CB (2001) The role of childhood trauma in the neurobiology of mood and anxiety disorders: preclinical and clinical studies. Biol Psychiatry 49:1023-1039.

Heisler LK, Chu HM, Brennan TJ, Danao JA, Bajwa P, Parsons LH, Tecott LH (1998) Elevated anxiety and antidepressant-like responses in serotonin 5-HT1A receptor mutant mice. Proc Natl Acad Sci U S A 95:15049-15054.

Hejjas K, Szekely A, Domotor E, Halmai Z, Balogh G, Schilling B, Sarosi A, Faludi G, Sasvari-Szekely M, Nemoda Z (2009) Association between depression and the Gln460Arg polymorphism of P2RX7 gene: a dimensional approach. Am J Med Genet B Neuropsychiatr Genet 150B:295-299.

Holmes A (2001) Targeted gene mutation approaches to the study of anxiety-like behavior in mice. Neurosci Biobehav Rev 25:261-273.

Holsboer F (2000) The corticosteroid receptor hypothesis of depression. Neuropsychopharmacology 23:477-501.

Holsboer F (2001) Stress, hypercortisolism and corticosteroid receptors in depression: implications for therapy. J Affect Disord 62:77-91.

Holsboer F (2005) The future of antidepressant pharmacogenetics is arriving. Introduction. Prog Neuropsychopharmacol Biol Psychiatry 29:996-998.

Holsboer F, Barden N (1996) Antidepressants and hypothalamic-pituitary-adrenocortical regulation. Endocr Rev 17:187-205.

Holsboer F, Ising M (2008) Central CRH system in depression and anxiety--evidence from clinical studies with CRH1 receptor antagonists. Eur J Pharmacol 583:350-357.

Hoyer D, Martin G (1997) 5-HT receptor classification and nomenclature: towards a harmonization with the human genome. Neuropharmacology 36:419-428.

Hoyer D, Thakker DR, Natt F, Maier R, Huesken D, Muller M, Flor P, VAN DER PH, Schmutz M, Bilbe G, Cryan JF (2006) Global down-regulation of gene expression in the brain using RNA interference, with emphasis on monoamine transporters and GPCRs: implications for target characterization in psychiatric and neurological disorders. J Recept Signal Transduct Res 26:527-547.

Huber D, Petreanu L, Ghitani N, Ranade S, Hromadka T, Mainen Z, Svoboda K (2008) Sparse optical microstimulation in barrel cortex drives learned behaviour in freely moving mice. Nature 451:61-64.

Hull EM, Dominguez JM (2007) Sexual behavior in male rodents. Horm Behav 52:45-55.

Ishizuka T, Kakuda M, Araki R, Yawo H (2006) Kinetic evaluation of photosensitivity in genetically engineered neurons expressing green algae light-gated channels. Neurosci Res 54:85-94.

Ising M, Holsboer F (2006) Genetics of stress response and stress-related disorders. Dialogues Clin Neurosci 8:433-444.

Joh TH, Geghman C, Reis D (1973) Immunochemical demonstration of increased accumulation of tyrosine hydroxylase protein in sympathetic ganglia and adrenal medulla elicited by reserpine. Proc Natl Acad Sci U S A 70:2767-2771.

Johansen JP, Hamanaka H, Monfils MH, Behnia R, Deisseroth K, Blair HT, LeDoux JE (2010) Optical activation of lateral amygdala pyramidal cells instructs associative fear learning. Proc Natl Acad Sci U S A 107:12692-12697.

Jones SR, Gainetdinov RR, Caron MG (1999) Application of microdialysis and voltammetry to assess dopamine functions in genetically altered mice: correlation with locomotor activity. Psychopharmacology (Berl) 147:30-32.

Keck ME (2006) Corticotropin-releasing factor, vasopressin and receptor systems in depression and anxiety. Amino Acids 31:241-250.

Kelly JP, Leonard BE (1999) An investigation of the antidepressant properties of lofepramine and its desmethylated metabolites in the forced swim and olfactory bulbectomized rat models of depression. Eur Neuropsychopharmacol 9:101-105.

Kelly JP, Wrynn AS, Leonard BE (1997) The olfactory bulbectomized rat as a model of depression: an update. Pharmacol Ther 74:299-316.

Kessler RC (1997) The effects of stressful life events on depression. Annu Rev Psychol 48:191-214.

Kessler RC, Berglund P, Demler O, Jin R, Koretz D, Merikangas KR, Rush AJ, Walters EE, Wang PS (2003) The epidemiology of major depressive disorder: results from the National Comorbidity Survey Replication (NCS-R). JAMA 289:3095-3105.

Kleinhammer A, Wurst W, Kuhn R (2010) Gene knockdown in the mouse through RNAi. Methods Enzymol 477:387-414.

Kokkinidis L, Zacharko RM, Anisman H (1986) Amphetamine withdrawal: a behavioral evaluation. Life Sci 38:1617-1623.

Kolber BJ, Boyle MP, Wieczorek L, Kelley CL, Onwuzurike CC, Nettles SA, Vogt SK, Muglia LJ (2010) Transient early-life forebrain corticotropin-releasing hormone elevation causes long-lasting anxiogenic and despair-like changes in mice. J Neurosci 30:2571-2581.

Kong H, Sha LL, Fan Y, Xiao M, Ding JH, Wu J, Hu G (2009) Requirement of AQP4 for antidepressive efficiency of fluoxetine: implication in adult hippocampal neurogenesis. Neuropsychopharmacology 34:1263-1276.

Koolhaas JM, Bartolomucci A, Buwalda B, de Boer SF, Flugge G, Korte SM, Meerlo P, Murison R, Olivier B, Palanza P, Richter-Levin G, Sgoifo A, Steimer T, Stiedl O, van DG, Wohr M, Fuchs E (2011) Stress revisited: a critical evaluation of the stress concept. Neurosci Biobehav Rev 35:1291-1301.

Kramer RH, Fortin DL, Trauner D (2009) New photochemical tools for controlling neuronal activity. Curr Opin Neurobiol 19:544-552.

Kravitz AV, Freeze BS, Parker PR, Kay K, Thwin MT, Deisseroth K, Kreitzer AC (2010) Regulation of parkinsonian motor behaviours by optogenetic control of basal ganglia circuitry. Nature 466:622-626.

Krishnan V, et al. (2007) Molecular adaptations underlying susceptibility and resistance to social defeat in brain reward regions. Cell 131:391-404.

Ladd CO, Huot RL, Thrivikraman KV, Nemeroff CB, Meaney MJ, Plotsky PM (2000) Long-term behavioral and neuroendocrine adaptations to adverse early experience. Prog Brain Res 122:81-103.

Lahdesmaki J, Sallinen J, MacDonald E, Kobilka BK, Fagerholm V, Scheinin M (2002) Behavioral and neurochemical characterization of alpha(2A)-adrenergic receptor knockout mice. Neuroscience 113:289-299.

Leonard BE, Tuite M (1981) Anatomical, physiological, and behavioral aspects of olfactory bulbectomy in the rat. Int Rev Neurobiol 22:251-286.

Leonardo ED, Hen R (2008) Anxiety as a developmental disorder. Neuropsychopharmacology 33:134-140.

Levinson DF (2006) The genetics of depression: a review. Biol Psychiatry 60:84-92.

Li X, Gutierrez DV, Hanson MG, Han J, Mark MD, Chiel H, Hegemann P, Landmesser LT, Herlitze S (2005) Fast noninvasive activation and inhibition of neural and network activity by vertebrate rhodopsin and green algae channelrhodopsin. Proc Natl Acad Sci U S A 102:17816-17821.

Liebsch G, Landgraf R, Gerstberger R, Probst JC, Wotjak CT, Engelmann M, Holsboer F, Montkowski A (1995) Chronic infusion of a CRH1 receptor antisense oligodeoxynucleotide into the central nucleus of the amygdala reduced anxiety-related behavior in socially defeated rats. Regul Pept 59:229-239.

Lister RG (1990) Ethologically-based animal models of anxiety disorders. Pharmacol Ther 46:321-340.

Lopez-Leon S, Janssens AC, Gonzalez-Zuloeta Ladd AM, Del-Favero J, Claes SJ, Oostra BA, van Duijn CM (2008) Meta-analyses of genetic studies on major depressive disorder. Mol Psychiatry 13:772-785.

Lu A, Steiner MA, Whittle N, Vogl AM, Walser SM, Ableitner M, Refojo D, Ekker M, Rubenstein JL, Stalla GK, Singewald N, Holsboer F, Wotjak CT, Wurst W, Deussing JM (2008) Conditional mouse mutants highlight mechanisms of corticotropin-releasing hormone effects on stress-coping behavior. Mol Psychiatry 13:1028-1042.

Lucae S, Salyakina D, Barden N, Harvey M, Gagne B, Labbe M, Binder EB, Uhr M, Paez-Pereda M, Sillaber I, Ising M, Bruckl T, Lieb R, Holsboer F, Muller-Myhsok B (2006) P2RX7, a gene coding for a purinergic ligand-gated ion channel, is associated with major depressive disorder. Hum Mol Genet 15:2438-2445.

Lucki I (1997) The forced swimming test as a model for core and component behavioral effects of antidepressant drugs. Behav Pharmacol 8:523-532.

MacQueen GM, Ramakrishnan K, Croll SD, Siuciak JA, Yu G, Young LT, Fahnestock M (2001) Performance of heterozygous brain-derived neurotrophic factor knockout mice on behavioral analogues of anxiety, nociception, and depression. Behav Neurosci 115:1145-1153.

Malkesman O, Scattoni ML, Paredes D, Tragon T, Pearson B, Shaltiel G, Chen G, Crawley JN, Manji HK (2010) The female urine sniffing test: a novel approach for assessing reward-seeking behavior in rodents. Biol Psychiatry 67:864-871.

Mar A, Spreekmeester E, Rochford J (2000) Antidepressants preferentially enhance habituation to novelty in the olfactory bulbectomized rat. Psychopharmacology (Berl) 150:52-60.
Maren S (2001) Neurobiology of Pavlovian fear conditioning. Annu Rev Neurosci 24:897-931.
Mascorro JA, Yates RD (1971) Ultrastructural studies of the effects of reserpine on mouse abdominal sympathetic paraganglia. Anat Rec 170:269-279.
Mayorga AJ, Lucki I (2001) Limitations on the use of the C57BL/6 mouse in the tail suspension test. Psychopharmacology (Berl) 155:110-112.
McEwen BS, Sapolsky RM (1995) Stress and cognitive function. Curr Opin Neurobiol 5:205-216.
McKinney WT, Jr., Bunney WE, Jr. (1969) Animal model of depression. I. Review of evidence: implications for research. Arch Gen Psychiatry 21:240-248.
McQuillin A, Bass NJ, Choudhury K, Puri V, Kosmin M, Lawrence J, Curtis D, Gurling HM (2009) Case-control studies show that a non-conservative amino-acid change from a glutamine to arginine in the P2RX7 purinergic receptor protein is associated with both bipolar- and unipolar-affective disorders. Mol Psychiatry 14:614-620.
Meaney MJ (2001) Maternal care, gene expression, and the transmission of individual differences in stress reactivity across generations. Annu Rev Neurosci 24:1161-1192.
Meyer M, de Angelis MH, Wurst W, Kuhn R (2010) Gene targeting by homologous recombination in mouse zygotes mediated by zinc-finger nucleases. Proc Natl Acad Sci U S A 107:15022-15026.
Miller JC, Tan S, Qiao G, Barlow KA, Wang J, Xia DF, Meng X, Paschon DE, Leung E, Hinkley SJ, Dulay GP, Hua KL, Ankoudinova I, Cost GJ, Urnov FD, Zhang HS, Holmes MC, Zhang L, Gregory PD, Rebar EJ (2011) A TALE nuclease architecture for efficient genome editing. Nat Biotechnol 29:143-148.
Monteggia LM, Barrot M, Powell CM, Berton O, Galanis V, Gemelli T, Meuth S, Nagy A, Greene RW, Nestler EJ (2004) Essential role of brain-derived neurotrophic factor in adult hippocampal function. Proc Natl Acad Sci U S A 101:10827-10832.
Montkowski A, Barden N, Wotjak C, Stec I, Ganster J, Meaney M, Engelmann M, Reul JM, Landgraf R, Holsboer F (1995) Long-term antidepressant treatment reduces behavioural deficits in transgenic mice with impaired glucocorticoid receptor function. J Neuroendocrinol 7:841-845.
Morales-Medina JC, Dumont Y, Quirion R (2010) A possible role of neuropeptide Y in depression and stress. Brain Res 1314:194-205.
Morice E, Billard JM, Denis C, Mathieu F, Betancur C, Epelbaum J, Giros B, Nosten-Bertrand M (2007) Parallel loss of hippocampal LTD and cognitive flexibility in a genetic model of hyperdopaminergia. Neuropsychopharmacology 32:2108-2116.
Morilak DA, Frazer A (2004) Antidepressants and brain monoaminergic systems: a dimensional approach to understanding their behavioural effects in depression and anxiety disorders. Int J Neuropsychopharmacol 7:193-218.
Morris R (1984) Developments of a water-maze procedure for studying spatial learning in the rat. J Neurosci Methods 11:47-60.

Moy SS, Nadler JJ, Perez A, Barbaro RP, Johns JM, Magnuson TR, Piven J, Crawley JN (2004) Sociability and preference for social novelty in five inbred strains: an approach to assess autistic-like behavior in mice. Genes Brain Behav 3:287-302.

Mucignat-Caretta C, Bondi' M, Caretta A (2004) Animal models of depression: olfactory lesions affect amygdala, subventricular zone, and aggression. Neurobiol Dis 16:386-395.

Muglia L, Jacobson L, Dikkes P, Majzoub JA (1995) Corticotropin-releasing hormone deficiency reveals major fetal but not adult glucocorticoid need. Nature 373:427-432.

Muller MB, Holsboer F (2006) Mice with mutations in the HPA-system as models for symptoms of depression. Biol Psychiatry 59:1104-1115.

Muller MB, Zimmermann S, Sillaber I, Hagemeyer TP, Deussing JM, Timpl P, Kormann MS, Droste SK, Kuhn R, Reul JM, Holsboer F, Wurst W (2003) Limbic corticotropin-releasing hormone receptor 1 mediates anxiety-related behavior and hormonal adaptation to stress. Nat Neurosci 6:1100-1107.

Murray CJ, Lopez AD (1997) Alternative projections of mortality and disability by cause 1990-2020: Global Burden of Disease Study. Lancet 349:1498-1504.

Nemeroff CB (1988) The role of corticotropin-releasing factor in the pathogenesis of major depression. Pharmacopsychiatry 21:76-82.

Nestler EJ, Gould E, Manji H, Buncan M, Duman RS, Greshenfeld HK, Hen R, Koester S, Lederhendler I, Meaney M, Robbins T, Winsky L, Zalcman S (2002) Preclinical models: status of basic research in depression. Biol Psychiatry 52:503-528.

Nestler EJ, Hyman SE (2010) Animal models of neuropsychiatric disorders. Nat Neurosci 13:1161-1169.

Nutt DJ (2006) The role of dopamine and norepinephrine in depression and antidepressant treatment. J Clin Psychiatry 67 Suppl 6:3-8.

Oh E, Maejima T, Liu C, Deneris E, Herlitze S (2010) Substitution of 5-HT1A receptor signaling by a light-activated G protein-coupled receptor. J Biol Chem 285:30825-30836.

Ohl F, Roedel A, Binder E, Holsboer F (2003) Impact of high and low anxiety on cognitive performance in a modified hole board test in C57BL/6 and DBA/2 mice. Eur J Neurosci 17:128-136.

Palanza P (2001) Animal models of anxiety and depression: how are females different? Neurosci Biobehav Rev 25:219-233.

Pause BM, Miranda A, Goder R, Aldenhoff JB, Ferstl R (2001) Reduced olfactory performance in patients with major depression. J Psychiatr Res 35:271-277.

Pepin MC, Pothier F, Barden N (1992) Impaired type II glucocorticoid-receptor function in mice bearing antisense RNA transgene. Nature 355:725-728.

Perona MT, Waters S, Hall FS, Sora I, Lesch KP, Murphy DL, Caron M, Uhl GR (2008) Animal models of depression in dopamine, serotonin, and norepinephrine transporter knockout mice: prominent effects of dopamine transporter deletions. Behav Pharmacol 19:566-574.

Pezawas L, Angst J, Kasper S (2005) Recurrent brief depression revisited. Int Rev Psychiatry 17:63-70.

Pogorelov VM, Rodriguiz RM, Insco ML, Caron MG, Wetsel WC (2005) Novelty seeking and stereotypic activation of behavior in mice with disruption of the Dat1 gene. Neuropsychopharmacology 30:1818-1831.

Ramboz S, Oosting R, Amara DA, Kung HF, Blier P, Mendelsohn M, Mann JJ, Brunner D, Hen R (1998) Serotonin receptor 1A knockout: an animal model of anxiety-related disorder. Proc Natl Acad Sci U S A 95:14476-14481.

Refojo D, Deussing J (2011) Animal models of depression. In: Neurobiology of Depression (Lopez-Munoz F, Alamon, eds), Taylor & Francis, in press.

Reichardt HM, Tuckermann JP, Bauer A, Schutz G (2000) Molecular genetic dissection of glucocorticoid receptor function in vivo. Z Rheumatol 59 Suppl 2:II/1-II/5.

Rice CJ, Sandman CA, Lenjavi MR, Baram TZ (2008) A novel mouse model for acute and long-lasting consequences of early life stress. Endocrinology 149:4892-4900.

Ridder S, Chourbaji S, Hellweg R, Urani A, Zacher C, Schmid W, Zink M, Hortnagl H, Flor H, Henn FA, Schutz G, Gass P (2005) Mice with genetically altered glucocorticoid receptor expression show altered sensitivity for stress-induced depressive reactions. J Neurosci 25:6243-6250.

Rios M, Fan G, Fekete C, Kelly J, Bates B, Kuehn R, Lechan RM, Jaenisch R (2001) Conditional deletion of brain-derived neurotrophic factor in the postnatal brain leads to obesity and hyperactivity. Mol Endocrinol 15:1748-1757.

Rosenkranz MA (2007) Substance P at the nexus of mind and body in chronic inflammation and affective disorders. Psychol Bull 133:1007-1037.

Sanchis-Segura C, Spanagel R (2006) Behavioural assessment of drug reinforcement and addictive features in rodents: an overview. Addict Biol 11:2-38.

Sapolsky RM (2000) Glucocorticoids and hippocampal atrophy in neuropsychiatric disorders. Arch Gen Psychiatry 57:925-935.

Schmidt MV (2011) Animal models for depression and the mismatch hypothesis of disease. Psychoneuroendocrinology 36:330-338.

Schramm NL, McDonald MP, Limbird LE (2001) The alpha(2a)-adrenergic receptor plays a protective role in mouse behavioral models of depression and anxiety. J Neurosci 21:4875-4882.

Seligman ME, Maier SF (1967) Failure to escape traumatic shock. J Exp Psychol 74:1-9.

Shyn SI, Hamilton SP (2010) The genetics of major depression: moving beyond the monoamine hypothesis. Psychiatr Clin North Am 33:125-140.

Sibille E, Pavlides C, Benke D, Toth M (2000) Genetic inactivation of the Serotonin(1A) receptor in mice results in downregulation of major GABA(A) receptor alpha subunits, reduction of GABA(A) receptor binding, and benzodiazepine-resistant anxiety. J Neurosci 20:2758-2765.

Sillaber I, Rammes G, Zimmermann S, Mahal B, Zieglgansberger W, Wurst W, Holsboer F, Spanagel R (2002) Enhanced and delayed stress-induced alcohol drinking in mice lacking functional CRH1 receptors. Science 296:931-933.

Song C, Leonard BE (2005) The olfactory bulbectomised rat as a model of depression. Neurosci Biobehav Rev 29:627-647.

Song L, Che W, Min-Wei W, Murakami Y, Matsumoto K (2006) Impairment of the spatial learning and memory induced by learned helplessness and chronic mild stress. Pharmacol Biochem Behav 83:186-193.

Soronen P, Mantere O, Melartin T, Suominen K, Vuorilehto M, Rytsala H, Arvilommi P, Holma I, Holma M, Jylha P, Valtonen HM, Haukka J, Isometsa E, Paunio T (2011) P2RX7 gene is associated consistently with mood disorders and predicts clinical outcome in three clinical cohorts. Am J Med Genet B Neuropsychiatr Genet 156B:435-447.

Spielewoy C, Roubert C, Hamon M, Nosten-Bertrand M, Betancur C, Giros B (2000) Behavioural disturbances associated with hyperdopaminergia in dopamine-transporter knockout mice. Behav Pharmacol 11:279-290.

Stec I, Barden N, Reul JM, Holsboer F (1994) Dexamethasone nonsuppression in transgenic mice expressing antisense RNA to the glucocorticoid receptor. J Psychiatr Res 28:1-5.

Steckler T, Rammes G, Sauvage M, van Gaalen MM, Weis C, Zieglgansberger W, Holsboer F (2001) Effects of the monoamine oxidase A inhibitor moclobemide on hippocampal plasticity in GR-impaired transgenic mice. J Psychiatr Res 35:29-42.

Stenzel-Poore MP, Duncan JE, Rittenberg MB, Bakke AC, Heinrichs SC (1996) CRH overproduction in transgenic mice: behavioral and immune system modulation. Ann N Y Acad Sci 780:36-48.

Stuber GD, Hnasko TS, Britt JP, Edwards RH, Bonci A (2010) Dopaminergic terminals in the nucleus accumbens but not the dorsal striatum corelease glutamate. J Neurosci 30:8229-8233.

Sztainberg Y, Kuperman Y, Tsoory M, Lebow M, Chen A (2010) The anxiolytic effect of environmental enrichment is mediated via amygdalar CRF receptor type 1. Mol Psychiatry 15:905-917.

Tecuapetla F, Patel JC, Xenias H, English D, Tadros I, Shah F, Berlin J, Deisseroth K, Rice ME, Tepper JM, Koos T (2010) Glutamatergic signaling by mesolimbic dopamine neurons in the nucleus accumbens. J Neurosci 30:7105-7110.

Timpl P, Spanagel R, Sillaber I, Kresse A, Reul JM, Stalla GK, Blanquet V, Steckler T, Holsboer F, Wurst W (1998) Impaired stress response and reduced anxiety in mice lacking a functional corticotropin-releasing hormone receptor 1. Nat Genet 19:162-166.

Tonissaar M, Herm L, Eller M, Koiv K, Rinken A, Harro J (2008a) Rats with high or low sociability are differently affected by chronic variable stress. Neuroscience 152:867-876.

Tonissaar M, Mallo T, Eller M, Haidkind R, Koiv K, Harro J (2008b) Rat behavior after chronic variable stress and partial lesioning of 5-HT-ergic neurotransmission: effects of citalopram. Prog Neuropsychopharmacol Biol Psychiatry 32:164-177.

Tonissaar M, Philips MA, Eller M, Harro J (2004) Sociability trait and serotonin metabolism in the rat social interaction test. Neurosci Lett 367:309-312.

Tonnesen J, Sorensen AT, Deisseroth K, Lundberg C, Kokaia M (2009) Optogenetic control of epileptiform activity. Proc Natl Acad Sci U S A 106:12162-12167.

Tsai HC, Zhang F, Adamantidis A, Stuber GD, Bonci A, de LL, Deisseroth K (2009) Phasic firing in dopaminergic neurons is sufficient for behavioral conditioning. Science 324:1080-1084.
Urani A, Chourbaji S, Gass P (2005) Mutant mouse models of depression: candidate genes and current mouse lines. Neurosci Biobehav Rev 29:805-828.
Urnov FD, Rebar EJ, Holmes MC, Zhang HS, Gregory PD (2010) Genome editing with engineered zinc finger nucleases. Nat Rev Genet 11:636-646.
van Gaalen MM, Steckler T (2000) Behavioural analysis of four mouse strains in an anxiety test battery. Behav Brain Res 115:95-106.
van Gaalen MM, Stenzel-Poore MP, Holsboer F, Steckler T (2002) Effects of transgenic overproduction of CRH on anxiety-like behaviour. Eur J Neurosci 15:2007-2015.
Venihaki M, Majzoub JA (1999) Animal models of CRH deficiency. Front Neuroendocrinol 20:122-145.
Wagner K, Wang X, Liebl C, Scharf S, Muller M, Schmidt M (2010) Pituitary glucocorticoid receptor deletion reduces vulnerability to chronic stress. Psychoneuroendocrinology 36:579-587.
Wallace DL, Han MH, Graham DL, Green TA, Vialou V, Iniguez SD, Cao JL, Kirk A, Chakravarty S, Kumar A, Krishnan V, Neve RL, Cooper DC, Bolanos CA, Barrot M, McClung CA, Nestler EJ (2009) CREB regulation of nucleus accumbens excitability mediates social isolation-induced behavioral deficits. Nat Neurosci 12:200-209.
Wang XD, Chen Y, Wolf M, Wagner KV, Liebl C, Scharf SH, Harbich D, Mayer B, Wurst W, Holsboer F, Deussing JM, Baram TZ, Muller MB, Schmidt MV (2011) Forebrain CRHR1 deficiency attenuates chronic stress-induced cognitive deficits and dendritic remodeling. Neurobiol Dis 42:300-310.
Wei Q, Lu XY, Liu L, Schafer G, Shieh KR, Burke S, Robinson TE, Watson SJ, Seasholtz AF, Akil H (2004) Glucocorticoid receptor overexpression in forebrain: a mouse model of increased emotional lability. Proc Natl Acad Sci U S A 101:11851-11856.
Wersinger SR, Kelliher KR, Zufall F, Lolait SJ, O'Carroll AM, Young WS, III (2004) Social motivation is reduced in vasopressin 1b receptor null mice despite normal performance in an olfactory discrimination task. Horm Behav 46:638-645.
Willner P (2005) Chronic mild stress (CMS) revisited: consistency and behavioural-neurobiological concordance in the effects of CMS. Neuropsychobiology 52:90-110.
Willner P, Mitchell PJ (2002) The validity of animal models of predisposition to depression. Behav Pharmacol 13:169-188.
Wise RA (2002) Brain reward circuitry: insights from unsensed incentives. Neuron 36:229-240.
Wise RA, Bozarth MA (1985) Brain mechanisms of drug reward and euphoria. Psychiatr Med 3:445-460.
Xu F, Gainetdinov RR, Wetsel WC, Jones SR, Bohn LM, Miller GW, Wang YM, Caron MG (2000) Mice lacking the norepinephrine transporter are supersensitive to psychostimulants. Nat Neurosci 3:465-471.
Young JW, Goey AK, Minassian A, Perry W, Paulus MP, Geyer MA (2010) The mania-like exploratory profile in genetic dopamine transporter mouse models is diminished in

a familiar environment and reinstated by subthreshold psychostimulant administration. Pharmacol Biochem Behav 96:7-15.

Young JW, van EJ, Winstanley CA, Geyer MA (2011) Increased risk-taking behavior in dopamine transporter knockdown mice: further support for a mouse model of mania. J Psychopharmacol 25:934-943.

Zhang F, Wang LP, Boyden ES, Deisseroth K (2006) Channelrhodopsin-2 and optical control of excitable cells. Nat Methods 3:785-792.

Zorner B, Wolfer DP, Brandis D, Kretz O, Zacher C, Madani R, Grunwald I, Lipp HP, Klein R, Henn FA, Gass P (2003) Forebrain-specific trkB-receptor knockout mice: behaviorally more hyperactive than "depressive". Biol Psychiatry 54:972-982.

9

Biological Alterations in Depression

C. Benton and T. Wiltshire
The University of North Carolina at Chapel Hill
United States of America

1. Introduction

According to the World Health Organization, depression is among the leading cause of disability worldwide with approximately 121 million people affected (http://www.who.int). It is estimated that 5% of men and 9% of women will experience depression in a given year (Kessler et al., 2005). Major Depressive Disorder (MDD) is characterized by persistent depressed mood or loss of interest or pleasure from daily activities. Additionally, patients may experience feelings of guilt or worthlessness, as well as psychomotor, physiological, and cognitive disturbances (DSM IV). Given that the etiology of depression is unclear, current antidepressant treatments are ineffective for most patients. Presently, less than 30% of patients achieve response or remission (Trivedi et al., 2006). Depression is a clinically and genetically heterogeneous disorder, which complicates efforts to identify causative factors of disease and replicate findings. In addition, diagnosis and therapeutic assessment are primarily based on subjective measures, making patient selection and outcome measures amenable to inconsistencies and irreproducibility.

Biomarkers that objectively establish diagnosis, prognosis, and antidepressant response can facilitate research and clinical management of patients with depression. Many analytes, including brain-derived neurotrophic factor (BDNF), serotonin transporter, and monoamines, have been linked with depressive symptoms and response to antidepressant therapy (Manji et al., 2001; Nestler et al., 2002; Thase, 2007). Although much progress has been made in identifying neurobiological correlates of depression, it is unclear whether these alterations are causally linked or are due to disease and/or treatment. With the goal of facilitating the search for depression biomarkers, this chapter will discuss several key molecular and neurochemical alterations that have been linked with depressive disorder.

2. Genetic studies

The role of genetics in the development of MDD is supported by findings from family, twin, and adoption studies. Studies that compared the prevalence of depression in monozygotic versus dizygotic twins indicate a heritability estimate of 35-50% (Bierut et al., 1999; Kendler et al., 1993; Sullivan et al., 2000). There is a two-to-threefold increased risk of developing MDD among first degree relatives of depressed individuals (Kelsoe, 2004; Sullivan et al., 2000), indicating that genetic variants can be used as prognostic and diagnostic markers. There are two widely used approaches to determine genetic markers of depression. Candidate gene analysis examines the frequency of genetic alleles between cases and controls. Hypotheses are generated *a priori* based on the likelihood that the gene affects the risk of depression. Alternatively, advances in genotyping capabilities and more recently, gene sequencing, have enabled scientists to look for unbiased genome-wide associations between common single nucleotide polymorphisms (SNPs) and behavior. Genes that confer risk to depression have been primarily identified using candidate gene analysis approaches, while recent efforts to uncover genetic markers of antidepressant response include the Sequenced Treatment Alternatives to Relieve Depression (STAR*D) trial and Genome-Based Therapeutic Drugs for Depression (GENDEP) study, which looked at genome-wide associations of common variants with antidepressant response. Genetic studies of depression (Levinson, 2006; Lohoff, 2010; Shyn & Hamilton, 2010) and antidepressant response (Crisafulli et al., 2011; Kato & Serretti, 2010; Porcelli et al., 2010) are reviewed in this chapter with a focus on several genes.

2.1 Genetic predictors of depression and antidepressant response

Antidepressant medications primarily work on altering neurotransmitters in the brain, thus much attention has been given to genes within the monoaminergic pathway (Kato & Serretti, 2010). An insertion/deletion polymorphism on the 5′ promoter region of the serotonin transporter gene (*5-HTTLPR*) produces a long (*L*) allele or a short (*S*) lower-expressing allele. The *5-HTTLPR* variant alters expression of the serotonin transporter *in vitro* (Lesch et al., 1996) and has been linked with MDD (Caspi et al., 2010; Goldman et al., 2010; Uher & McGuffin, 2010), neuroticism (Lesch et al., 1996), affective disorder (Collier et al., 1996; Lasky-Su et al., 2005), suicidality (Anguelova et al., 2003; P. Y. Lin & Tsai, 2004), and anxiety related personality traits (Schinka et al., 2004; Sen et al., 2004). Patients with the low expressing allele exhibited increased amygdala activation in response to sad faces (Hariri et al., 2002), reduced gray matter volume in amygdala and perigenual cingulate cortex (Pezawas et al., 2005), as well as altered functional coupling in both regions (Pezawas et al., 2005), thus supporting the role of the serotonin transporter in the development of the amygdala-cingulate feedback circuitry. Carriers of the S allele who experienced stressful life events in the past were more vulnerable to depression and suicidality (Caspi et al., 2003; Kendler et al., 2005). However, several groups did not find an association between depression and *5-HTTLPR* alone (Middeldorp et al., 2010; Munafo & Flint, 2009; Risch et al., 2009) or in interaction with stressful life events (Risch et al., 2009). Homozygous carriers of the *L* allele showed higher response and remission rates (Serretti et al., 2005) and more favorable side effect profiles (Kato & Serretti, 2010; Kraft et al., 2007; Murphy et al., 2004), which did not replicate to a recent large clinical trial that did not find a link between *5-HTTLPR* and treatment response (Kraft et al., 2007). Altogether, these findings indicate that environment must be taken into account when evaluating the potential use of *5-HTTLPR* as a genetic marker of depression.

Other genes in the monoamine pathway have been studied for their link with depressive behavior. The serotonin-1A receptor (*HTR1A*) is located in the serotonergic neurons and on their post-synaptic targets. In the pre-synaptic neuron, 5HT1A auto-inhibits raphe firing and 5-HT synthesis. The -1019C/G variant (rs6295) found in the promoter region of *HTR1A* results in higher expression of serotonin-1A auto-receptor (5-HT1A), which leads to reduction in serotonergic neurotransmission (Stahl, 1994). The -1019C/G mutation is correlated with anxiety and depression (Gross et al., 2002; Lemonde et al., 2004; Strobel et al., 2003). In Asians, the G allele is associated with improved treatment outcomes (Hong et al., 2006; Kato et al., 2009). However, this finding was not observed in Caucasians (Lemonde et al., 2004; Serretti et al., 2004), suggesting a confounding effect of race. The relationship between *HTR2A* and antidepressant response is unclear due to conflicting results (reviewed in Kato 2010). A recent meta-analysis did not find any association between *HTR1A* and *HTR2A* and treatment response; however, a polymorphism within *HTR2A* was correlated with tolerability(Kato & Serretti, 2010). No association has been established between *HTR2A* and MDD (Anguelova et al., 2003).

The tryptophan hydroxylases 1 and 2 (TPH1 and TPH2) catalyze the rate-limiting step in 5-HT biosynthesis. A functional variant in *TPH2* (Arg441His) results in 80% reduction of 5-HT in the brain (X. Zhang et al., 2004) and was found to be more frequent in patients with MDD (X. Zhang et al., 2005). However, other studies failed to replicate this finding (Delorme et al., 2006). Furthermore, the *TPH* 218A allele is associated with poor antidepressant response (Serretti et al., 2001a; Serretti et al., 2001b), a finding that was supported by a meta-analysis study (Kato & Serretti, 2010). Patients with the 218 C/C genotype were more likely to respond to antidepressant therapy (Kato & Serretti, 2010). Interestingly, the significant pooled odds ratio score (OR) was primarily influenced by the sum of the three studies that looked at the association between remission rates and the 218 genotype, suggesting that the *TPH* gene may be important in regulating long-term antidepressant response. Of interest is the recent correlation between *TPH2* haplotype markers and suicidality (De Luca et al., 2004; Lopez et al., 2007), suggesting that *TPH2* may mediate a subset of depressive symptoms like suicidal thoughts and feelings of guilt and worthlessness.

Enzymes that mediate clearance of catecholamines including, monoamine oxidase A (MAO-A) and catechol-O-methyl transferase (COMT) have been linked to antidepressant response. Higher transcription efficiency is observed with the variable number tandem repeat (VNTR) sequence located 1.2kb upstream of the *MAO-A* gene (Sabol et al., 1998). Alternatively, the Val to Met substitution at codon 158 for membrane-bound COMT protein (codon 108 for soluble COMT) has been linked to lower enzymatic activity(Mannisto & Kaakkola, 1999) and improved response to citalopram (Arias et al., 2006) and mirtazapine (Szegedi et al., 2005) but not paroxetine (Arias et al., 2006; Szegedi et al., 2005).

A locus on Chr. 12 has been linked with MDD (Abkevich et al., 2003; McGuffin et al., 2005) and anxiety (Erhardt et al., 2007). Within this putative region lies the purinergic ATP-binding calcium channel gene (*P2X7)*. A non-synonymous coding SNP within *P2X7* (Gln460Arg) is associated with MDD risk (Lucae et al., 2006). P2X7 protein is required for IL-1 (interleukin-1) processing and secretion (Ferrari et al., 2006), highlighting the potential role of immune function in depressive behavior. Moreover, the FK506 binding protein 5 (*FKBP5*) in complex with Hsp90 regulates glucocorticoid receptor sensitivity. A functional variant within *FKBP5* that results in increased intracellular concentration of FKBP5 has been linked with recurrence of depressive episodes (Binder et al., 2004) and antidepressant response (Binder et al., 2004; Lekman et al., 2008b). FKBP5 activates glucocorticoid receptors and the hypothalamic-pituitary-adrenal axis, which regulate response to stress (Binder et al., 2004). Additionally, the corticotropin releasing hormone 1 (*CRH1*) variant is correlated with early onset of depressive symptoms (Papiol et al., 2007). CRH activates the HPA axis, thus supporting the role of the HPA axis in mediating depressive behavior.

Small low-powered studies were combined in a meta-analysis to clarify the associations of several genes with depression, which were unclear due to inconsistent or non-replicated findings. Lopez-Leon et al. found a protective effect for the *APOE* ε2 allele (combined OR, 0.51; CI, 0.27-0.97) with no evidence of between-study heterogeneity (Lopez-Leon et al.,

2008). Alternatively, an increased risk were found for the methylenetetrahydrofolate reductase *MTHFR* C677T polymorphism (pooled OR, 1.36), the guanine nucleotide binding protein 3 *GNB3* C825T variant (pooled OR, 1.38; CI, 1.13-1.69), and the dopamine transporter *SLC6A3* 40 bp VNTR (pooled OR, 2.06; CI, 1.25-3.40) (Lopez-Leon et al., 2008).
Pharmacogenetic studies of antidepressants in the STAR*D trial have identified genes associated with treatment response (Hu et al., 2007; Lekman et al., 2008a; McMahon et al., 2006; Paddock, 2008), treatment resistance (Perlis et al., 2008), and treatment-emergent suicidal ideation (Laje et al., 2009; Laje et al., 2007; Perlis et al., 2007). In addition, polymorphisms in genes that encode drug-metabolizing enzymes and transporters have been tested for correlation with treatment response (Peters et al., 2008). Genes that were significantly associated with response to citalopram include *FKBP5* (Lekman et al., 2008a), glutamate receptor, ionotropic kainite 1 (*GRIK1*), N-methyl d-aspartate 2A (*GRIN2A*), 5-hydrxytryptamine receptor 2A (*HTR2A*), potassium channel, subfamily K, member 2 (KCNK2), phosphodiesterase (PDE), and solute carrier family 6 member 4 (*SLC6A4*) (E. Lin & Chen, 2008).
A link between genes and depression exists, however, putative genes identified to date do not significantly account for the phenotypic variance observed (Mann & Currier, 2006). Although these initial results may seem disappointing, they indicate that the genetics of depression is far from simple. It is likely that multiple genes with minor effect sizes interact with environmental factors to affect mood, making identification of genetic biomarkers challenging. Efforts to investigate gene by environmental effects can further delineate the contribution of each gene on disease and treatment outcomes (Lesch, 2004; Wermter et al., 2010).

3. Biochemical alterations

Several mechanisms are altered in depression and these include neurotransmission, neuroendocrine signaling, and neuroimmune functions. It is unclear whether these biochemical alterations are products or causative factors of depression. This section will discuss common biological alterations that have been observed in depression, facilitating identification of candidate biochemical markers for depression and antidepressant response.

3.1 Monoamines

The monoamine theory of depression developed following the observation that iproniazid, a drug that inhibits the metabolism of monoamines by blocking MAO, improved the mood of patients who are taking the drug (Delay et al., 1952). In addition, depletion of monoamines by agents like reserpine was found to induce depression (Goodwin & Bunney, 1971). This theory led to the development of antidepressant drugs that elevate monoamine levels at the synapse by blocking uptake transporters, catabolic enzymes or inhibitory pre-synaptic auto- or hetero-receptors. The monoamines provided a biochemical basis for depression, whereby depression is thought to result from a 'chemical imbalance' of monoamines in the brain (Schildkraut, 1965). However, several observations have cast doubt on the major role of monoamines in MDD. In addition to the untimely manner in which elevation of monoamines occur with respect to symptom resolution (Baldessarini, 1989), treatments that do not elevate monoamine levels like electroconvulsive therapy (ECT) have been effectively shown to treat depression (Pagnin et al., 2004). The monoamine theory of depression was then modified to indicate that elevation of monoamines is the first step in a cascade of molecular events that ultimately leads to symptom improvement (Pineyro & Blier, 1999). Research focus began to shift towards evaluating the long-term adaptive changes that result from increased monoamines in the synapse. It was hypothesized that elevation in monoamines leads to reduction in the sensitivity and/or number of monoamine receptors. Although desensitization and internalization of monoamine receptors have been observed in several animal and post-mortem studies, results were often inconsistent and conflicting (Elhwuegi, 2004). Effective antidepressant agents that do not act by inhibiting monoamine reuptake proteins or metabolizing enzymes can still facilitate receptor internalization despite the absence of pre-synaptic input (Fishman & Finberg, 1987; Kientsch et al., 2001). More recently, it has been shown that monoamine elevation may lead to cellular genesis. Various antidepressant agents including, specific serotonin reuptake inhibitor (fluoxetine), monoamine oxidase inhibitor (tranylcypromine), specific norepinephrine reuptake inhibitor (reboxetine), and serotonin/norepinephrine uptake inhibitor (tricyclic antidepressants) have been shown to induce cell proliferation and neurogenesis (Santarelli et al., 2003), which suggests that monoamine elevation leads to other downstream molecular effects that can alter behavior.

Despite decades of research aimed to evaluate the relationship between depression and monoamine alteration, direct evidence supporting the causative role of monoamines in MDD is lacking (Nestler, 1998), thus prompting efforts to study other pathways that may underlie depressive behavior.

3.2 Hypothalamic Pituitary Adrenal (HPA) axis

Dysregulation in the HPA axis, which is characterized by elevated plasma cortisol and CRH is a common finding in depressed patients (Holsboer, 2000; Raison & Miller, 2003). In response to stress, the parvocellular neurons in the hypothalamus secrete CRH, stimulating the release of adenocorticotropin releasing hormone (ACTH) from the anterior pituitary. ACTH, in turn, activates the synthesis and release of glucocorticoids (cortisol from humans and corticosterone in rodents) from the adrenal cortex. Glucocorticoids negatively regulate the HPA axis by inhibiting the synthesis and release of CRH from the hypothalamus.

Activation of the HPA axis mediates physiologic adaptation to stress, however, persistent stimulation can lead to glucocorticoid receptor (GR) desensitization (de Kloet et al., 2005). Patients with depression typically exhibit high levels of cortisol in plasma, saliva, and urine, as well as an increase in the size and activity of the pituitary and adrenal glands (Nemeroff & Vale, 2005). Impairment of the HPA axis, which is primarily characterized by the inability to suppress cortisol levels following pharmacologic stimulation of GR by dexamethasone, has been observed in depressed patients (Ising et al., 2005; Kunzel et al., 2003; Sher, 2006). HPA alterations normalize with antidepressant therapy (Holsboer, 2000) and this is associated with less relapse (Ising et al., 2007). Glucocorticoids not only exhibit immune and metabolic functions but it also regulates neurogenesis, neuronal survival, hippocampal size and structure, and acquisition of new memories (Herbert et al., 2006). Reduced maternal handling increases CRH signaling (Ladd et al., 1996) and sustains HPA hyperactivity, inducing depressive-like behavior in the pups (Francis et al., 1999; Meaney, 2001). In humans, early stressful life event is associated with dysregulated HPA axis (Heim et al., 2002) and development of depressive symptoms (Chapman et al., 2004; McCauley et al., 1997). One of the mechanisms by which antidepressants induce hippocampal neurogenesis is by activating GR (Anacker et al., 2011), thus implicating a direct relationship between HPA axis and neural brain signaling.

3.3 Other neuroendocrine markers

It was discovered that hypothyroidism elicits depressive behavior and that these symptoms can be reversed by thyroxine therapy (Asher, 1949). Similar symptoms are observed in depression and hypothyroidism, which include dysphoric mood, fatigue, anhedonia, and alteration in weight (Jackson, 1998). Low levels of thyroid hormones (T_3 and T_4) stimulate the release of thyrotropin releasing hormone (TRH) from the hypothalamus to the anterior pituitary. The pituitary, in turn, releases thyrotropin-stimulating hormone (TSH), which leads to the release of triiodothyronine (T_3) and thyroxine (T_4) from the thyroid. Thyroid hormones primarily regulate metabolism but may also be involved in neurotransmission (Dratman & Gordon, 1996). Although not all depressed patients display abnormalities in thyroid function, alterations have been observed including, elevation in T_4 (Baumgartner et al., 1988; Kirkegaard & Faber, 1991), lower TSH levels (Maes et al., 1989), as well as blunted response of TSH to TRH (Hein & Jackson, 1990; Maes et al., 1989). Type-II deiodinase (D-II) catalyzes deiodination of T_4 to T_3. Psychotropic medications like lithium (Baumgartner et al., 1994b), desipramine (Campos-Barros et al., 1994), carbamezapine (Baumgartner et al., 1994a), and fluoxetine (Baumgartner et al., 1994c) stimulate the activity of D-II, indicating that mood regulatory agents indirectly regulate T_3 levels. Others, however, did not find any effects of antidepressant on thyroid function (Brambilla et al., 1982). Interestingly, one study found that morning and nocturnal changes in TSH may predict antidepressant response (Duval et al., 1996).

There is increasing evidence implicating the involvement of stress-responsive neuropeptide systems in depression and anxiety. The involvement of various neuropeptides has been reviewed (Alldredge, 2010; Holmes et al., 2003) and a number of them will be described here. Administration of neuropeptide antagonists/agonists results in altered responses in rodent models of anxiety and depression (Rotzinger et al., 2010). Stress stimulates the release of vasopressin, which in turn enhances the effects of CRH on ACTH (G. Aguilera et al., 2003; Engelmann et al., 2004; J. N. Zhou et al., 2001). Depressed patients display altered levels of vasopressin in the suprachiasmatic nucleus (SCN) (J. N. Zhou et al., 2001), paraventricular nucleus (Purba et al., 1996), and supraoptic nucleus (Meynen et al., 2006). A polymorphism in the vasopressin receptor (V_{1B}) may be protective against MDD (Overstreet & Griebel, 2005; Salome et al., 2006). Antagonism of the V_{1B} receptor reduced depressive-like behavior (Griebel et al., 2002), which was comparable to treatment with antidepressant agents (Salome et al., 2006). This effect was mainly due to inhibition of the V_{1B} receptors in the lateral septum and amygdala (Stremmelin 2005). Similar to vasopressin, neuropeptide Y (NPY) is released under stress. NPY is abundantly expressed in the brain and is co-localized with noradrenaline, somatostatin, and GABA (γ-aminobutyric acid) (Kask et al., 2002). Reduction in NPY is associated with increased sensitivity to depression and stress, indicating that NPY agonists may exhibit antidepressive effects (Redrobe et al., 2002). A variant in the promoter region of *Npy* alters the expression of NPY *in vivo* and is linked with anxiety behavior and neural responses to stress (Z. Zhou et al., 2008). Substance P (SP), a known modulator of pain signaling, has been shown to interact with serotonergic signaling (Schwarz et al., 1999). Substance P binds to neurokinin-1 (NK_1) receptors found in the brain and in the periphery. Genetic ablation or pharmacologic antagonism of NK_1 receptors promotes monoaminergic activity (Froger et al., 2001; Maubach et al., 2002; Santarelli et al., 2001) and reduces anxiety-like behavior (Santarelli et al., 2001). Depressed patients have higher SP levels in the serum (Bondy et al., 2003). Interestingly, NK_1 antagonists activate the serotonergic system similarly to serotonin reuptake inhibitor (escitalopram)(Guiard et al., 2004), indicating that NK1 antagonists may have antidepressive effects. Galanin is a 29-30 amino acid peptide that regulates various physiological responses like metabolism and food intake. Galanin binds to several galanin receptors (GALR), which in turn interacts with different G proteins, activating various signal transduction pathways (K. E. Smith et al., 1998; Wang et al., 1998). Galanin administration in rodents produces a variety of effects including, nerve regeneration, nociception, and alteration in sexual and feeding behavior (Wrenn & Crawley, 2001; Yoshitake et al., 2003). Galanin mediates 5-HT and norepinephrine levels (Ogren et al., 2006) and antagonism of GALR can enhance or reduce depressive-like behavior depending on which GALR subtype is being inhibited (Barr et al., 2006; X. Lu et al., 2005).

Many years of research implicate the role of the neuroendocrine system in depression. Most neuroendocrine regulatory mechanisms occur through the bidirectional communication between the hypothalamus and pituitary. These findings indicate that the neural circuitry, neuronal signaling, and structural plasticity within this region are likely to be critical in behavioral responses.

4. Metabolic alterations

Metabolic syndrome is comprised of several features including, central obesity and insulin resistance, which, in concert, increases risk for developing cardiovascular disease and diabetes. Compared to healthy controls, depressed individuals are more likely to develop obesity, diabetes, and hypertension (Lindley et al., 2009), indicating potential overlap between depressive symptoms and metabolic syndrome. Independent of the criteria used to define metabolic syndrome (Raikkonen et al., 2007), a strong bidirectional association between depression and metabolic syndrome exists in women (Gil et al., 2006; Kinder et al., 2004; Raikkonen et al., 2007). The correlation between depressive symptoms and metabolic syndrome is slightly higher in monozygotic twins than dizygotic twins, suggesting that genetics play a critical role in both disorders (McCaffery et al., 2003). Resistance to insulin, which is a risk factor for developing metabolic syndrome, is a common occurrence in depressed patients (Koslow et al., 1982; Okamura et al., 2000; Winokur et al., 1988), which suggests that insulin links depression with metabolic syndrome. Insulin exerts dose-dependent effects on food intake and energy regulation. Ablation of insulin receptors on neuronal cells leads to an increased in body fat disposition, suggesting that insulin negatively regulates adiposity (Bruning et al., 2000). Additionally, insulin regulates monoamine uptake and metabolism, phosphoinositol turnover, as well as norepinephrine and dopamine transporter mRNA levels (Craft & Watson, 2004). It has been shown that insulin can recruit GABA receptors (Wan et al., 1997) and promote internalization of α-amino-3-hydroxy-5-methylisoxazole-4-propionic acid (AMPA) receptors, which suggests that insulin plays a critical role in neuronal signaling and synaptic plasticity (Huang et al., 1998). Interestingly, brain volume abnormalities and neurocognitive deficits commonly found in MDD patients have been observed in individuals with diabetes mellitus (DM), suggesting overlapping pathophysiology between MDD and DM (McIntyre et al., 2010). Insensitivity to insulin likely develops due to HPA axis hyperactivity (Rizza et al., 1982), impaired immune system (Fernandez-Real et al., 2001; Maes, 1995; Moller, 2000), and altered central serotonergic signaling (Goodnick et al., 1995; Horacek et al., 1999), all of which are common findings in depressed patients (Belmaker, 2008; Krishnan & Nestler, 2008).

Association between depression and obesity has been identified in several cross sectional studies (de Wit et al., 2010; Faith et al., 2002; Scott et al., 2008). A recent meta-analysis looked at the association between obesity and depression in a community-based setting and found that obese patients have an 18% increased risk of developing depressive symptoms (overall OR, 1.18) (de Wit et al., 2010). Subsequent sub-group analyses showed that the association with obesity holds true for depressed women but not for men, which suggests that comorbidity is likely to be affected by sex (de Wit et al., 2010). Similarly, a meta-analysis of longitudinal studies showed that baseline obesity increased the risk of depression (pooled OR, 1.57) and that depression increased the odds for developing obesity (pooled OR, 1.40). Prospective analysis of the cause-effect relationship between obesity and depression indicate reciprocal findings, whereby obesity was found to be a predictor of depression in eight out of the ten studies reviewed, while 53% of the studies found that depression predicts obesity (Faith et al., 2011). Interestingly, the positive association between depression and obesity is only detected in studies conducted in the United States but not in other European countries, indicating a strong contributory effect of environment (Atlantis & Baker, 2008). It is increasingly recognized that similar neural circuitry that regulate memory, reward, mood, and emotion also controls appetite, body weight, and energy homeostasis (Dallman, 2009; Zheng et al., 2009). Food induces olfactory and visual sensory inputs, which stimulate the orbitofrontal cortex, where acquisition, storage, and processing of memory and experiences associated with food is thought to occur (Verhagen, 2007). Stimulation of the mu-opioid receptor in the nucleus accumbens and ventral pallidum results in further intake of pleasurable foods (Will et al., 2003; M. Zhang & Kelley, 2000). The ventral tegmental area and the nucleus accumbens are part of the mesolimbic dopaminergic system, which regulates behavioral response (motivation) towards favorable stimuli (Berridge, 1996, 2007; Pecina et al., 2006), indicating that food intake and motivation are, at least partly, co-regulated by similar circuitry. The hypothalamus regulates homeostatic responses to altered nutrient levels and adiposity levels (Berthoud, 2002; Xue & Kahn, 2006) through various endocrine hormones including, leptin (Farooqi et al., 2002; Friedman, 1999; O'Rahilly, 2002) and NPY (Luquet et al., 2005). Although leptin is primarily known for its role in appetite suppression and energy expenditure, leptin also mediates reproduction and cognition (Chehab, 2000; Farr et al., 2006). Independent of body mass, depressed patients show lower plasma levels of leptin (Jow et al., 2006; Kraus et al., 2001) although other studies did not find similar results (Antonijevic et al., 1998; Deuschle et al., 1996; Rubin et al., 2002). Rodents exposed to chronic unpredictable stress showed reduction in sucrose preference and higher depressive-like behavior, which was reversed by leptin administration, indicating that leptin exhibits antidepressive effects likely through innervations of the limbic brain circuitry (X. Y. Lu et al., 2006). In response to stressful events, leptin suppresses CRH, ACTH, and corticosterone secretion, suggesting a direct impact of leptin on the HPA axis (Ahima et al., 1996; Heiman et al., 1997; Huang et al., 1998). In addition, leptin-deficient *ob/ob* mice display altered *Slc6a4* expression (Collin et al., 2000), decreased neuronal and glial cells, and reduced brain weight and cortical volume (Ahima 1999, Stepan 1999), further supporting the role of leptin in MDD.

A common thread between MDD, DM, and heart disease exists. The co-occurrence and pathophysiologic overlap between metabolic syndrome, obesity, and depression may explain the significant association between depression, diabetes, and cardiovascular disease (Frasure-Smith et al., 1993; Goldney et al., 2004; Paile-Hyvarinen et al., 2007).

5. Neuroimmune

An interaction between behavior and the immune system was first recognized in 200 AD, when Galen observed that melancholic women were more susceptible to cancer (Leonard, 1988). Depressed patients exhibit reduced neutrophil phagocytosis, natural killer cell activity, and mitogen stimulated lymphocyte proliferation (Irwin et al., 1990). Furthermore, patients with MDD show increased cytokine secretion from activated macrophages and elevated acute phase proteins in the liver (Sluzewska et al., 1996), indicating dysregulation in immune response. Antidepressants inhibit the ability of lipopolysaccharide (LPS) to induce the synthesis and the release of pro-inflammatory cytokines, likely through elevation of cyclic adenosine monophosphate (cAMP) levels (Xia et al., 1996). It has been hypothesized that abnormal secretion of macrophage monokines leads to depressive behavior (R. S. Smith, 1991). Macrophages secrete neuroendocrine and immune modulators, including, interleukins (IL), tumor necrosis factors (TNF), ACTH, and endorphins (Nathan, 1987), thus indicating a regulatory role for macrophages in mediating the neuro-endocrine-immune interface.

A bidirectional relationship between the brain, neuroendocrine, and immune systems exists, particularly in response to stress. Overactivity of the HPA axis, which is a common finding in depressed individuals (Holsboer, 2000; Raison & Miller, 2003), results in hypercortisolemia and suppression of the immune system. Conversely, persistent stress can result in fewer B cells, T cells, and lymphocytes (Olff, 1999), which can confer susceptibility to infections and cancer (Garssen & Goodkin, 1999; Kiecolt-Glaser et al., 1995; Reiche et al., 2005). Stressful events like separation or divorce are correlated with increased cancer risk, low proportions of NK and T cells, impairment of DNA repair, and abnormal immune response (Kiecolt-Glaser et al., 1987). The presence of reactive oxygen species has been detected in depressed patients (Irie et al., 2005). Levels of 8-hydroxydeoxyguanosine (8-OH-dG), a biomarker of cancer-related oxidative DNA damage, is positively correlated with depressive symptoms (Irie et al., 2005), which suggests that depression may be associated with cancer.

In 1987, Wagner-Jauregg demonstrated that activation of the immune system can affect various mental states (Raju, 1998). Cytokines regulate growth, differentiation, and function of many cells (Turnbull & Rivier, 1999). They can be broadly classified as pro-inflammatory or anti-inflammatory cytokines. Pro-inflammatory cytokines like interleukin-1 (IL-1), interleukin-6 (IL-6), and TNF-α stimulate immune cell production, activation, and proliferation. On the other hand, anti-inflammatory cytokines including, interleukin-4 (IL-4), interleukin-10 (IL-10), and interleukin-13 (IL-13) dampen the immune response. The role of cytokines in depression was identified following observation that interferon treatment induces 'sickness behavior,' which mimics depressive symptoms such as dysphoric mood, fatigue, anorexia, weight loss, and altered sleep patterns (Papanicolaou et al., 1998; Yirmiya, 2000). Depression is characterized by elevation of pro-inflammatory markers IL-6, c-reactive protein (CRP) (Maes, 1995), IL-1, and IL-2 (Dunn et al., 2005; Song et al., 1994). Treatment with LPS stimulated depressive-like behavior and cytokine secretion, which were reversed by antidepressants or cytokine antagonists (Yirmiya, 2000). Administration of IL-6 and IL-1 results in elevation of vasopressin, cortisol, CRH, and ACTH (Brebner et al., 2000; Harbuz et al., 1992; Xu et al., 1999), which suggests a pivotal role of cytokines in HPA axis activation (Dentino et al., 1999). In rodents, treatment with IL-1 resulted in increased DA, NE, and 5-HT activity in the brain (Dunn & Swiergiel, 1999; Merali et al., 1997; Song et al., 1999).

Cytokines acutely stimulate 5-HT neurotransmission and reduce its production by stimulating indoleamine 2,3-dioxygenase (IDO), an enzyme that converts the precursor of 5-HT (tryptophan) into kynurenine (Wichers & Maes, 2002). Pro-inflammatory cytokines have been shown to up-regulate serotonin transporter (Morikawa et al., 1998; Mossner & Lesch, 1998; Wichers & Maes, 2002), while anti-inflammatory cytokines like IL-4 reduces 5-HT uptake (Mossner et al., 2001). Together, these findings suggest that cytokines affect depressive behavior likely through regulation of monoamines and the HPA axis.

The symptom heterogeneity observed in depressed patients suggests that biological abnormalities are likely to be patient-dependent and disease-specific. Collectively, these results indicate that biochemical mechanisms likely interact to mediate a complex behavior like mood and anhedonia. It is therefore unlikely that a single biological marker will characterize a heterogeneous disorder like depression. Significant benefits can be rendered in evaluating the behavioral effects of a panel of biological markers or biochemical signatures, particularly since reciprocal communication between nervous, endocrine, and immune systems have been noted (Cserr & Knopf, 1992; Felten, 1991; Reichlin, 1993). For most cases, when associations between biochemical alterations and depression are detected, the causal relationship is often poorly understood.

6. Brain and molecular correlates

Direct and indirect evidence from neurostructural, neurofunctional, and molecular studies indicate impairments in neural circuitry, structural plasticity, and cellular resilience. These abnormalities reflect the molecular neurobiological underpinnings of depression as discussed below.

6.1 Neurostructural and neurofunctional studies

The cortical-limbic circuitry is implicated to mediate emotional processing in depressed patients (Davidson et al., 2002; Dougherty & Rauch, 1997; Mayberg, 1997). Results from positron emission tomography (PET) studies indicate that unmedicated patients with MDD exhibit increased activity and cerebral blood flow (CBF) to the amygdala, orbital cortex, and medial thalamus, as well as decreased CBF to the pre-frontal cortex (PFC) and anterior cingulate cortex (ACC) (Drevets, 2000a; Drevets et al., 1999). Meta-analyses of structural neuroimaging studies indicate that MDD is characterized by reduction of gray matter volumes in the ACC (Koolschijn et al., 2009), subgenual cingulate cortex (Hajek et al., 2008), and hippocampus (McKinnon et al., 2009). Post-mortem neuropathological studies have shown that patients with MDD show reduced cortex volume, decreased number of glial cells, and/or reduced neuron sizes (Ongur et al., 1998; Rajkowska, 2000; Rajkowska et al., 1999). Given the functional roles of specific brain regions in emotional processing, neuropathological abnormalities observed in depression suggest that areas that mediate autonomic and neuroendocrine responses (amygdala) is associated with increased activity and cerebral blood flow, while reduction in activity is observed in brain regions that control emotional processing (cortex) (Manji et al., 2001). Antidepressant treatment reduces CBF and metabolism in the amygadala (Drevets, 2000b; Drevets et al., 1999), attenuating hyperresponsiveness to stress (Rosenkranz et al., 2010). Similarly, larger hippocampal volume (Frodl et al., 2008; Kronmuller et al., 2008; MacQueen et al., 2008) and gray matter density in the ACC (Costafreda et al., 2009) were positively correlated with antidepressant response.

Inferences regarding the structural integrity of neural tracts can be made through diffusion tensor imaging (DTI), which measures the diffusion properties of water through brain tissues, *in vivo*. Patients that did not respond to 12 weeks of escitalopram (Alexopoulos et al., 2008) or citalopram (Alexopoulos et al., 2002) treatment showed microstructural abnormalities in white matter pathways connecting the cortex with the limbic and paralimbic areas, which indicates that poor therapeutic outcome is related to impaired cortical-limbic connectivity (Mayberg, 2003). Patients with prior exposure to parental verbal abuse (Choi et al., 2009) or have genetic polymorphisms (*5-HTTLPR*) (Alexopoulos et al., 2009) exhibit microstructural white matter abnormalities, suggesting that neural brain structure is subject to genetic and environmental control. Of note, impairment in brain morphology, neural circuitry, and brain function have been linked with monoaminergic and non-monoaminergic genetic variants (Scharinger et al., 2010). In addition to evaluating the structural integrity of neural brain circuits, functional activity within the limbic-cortical circuitry has been investigated. Brain activity can be evaluated by measuring blood oxygen level-dependent (BOLD) signals while patients are resting (intrinsic activity) or when performing a task (task-related activity). BOLD signaling is associated with changes in blood flow and tissue oxygen concentration, which are markers of brain activity. Depressed individuals have reduced activity in the limbic and cortical regions (Anand et al., 2005), which normalizes as symptoms resolve (Anand et al., 2005). Patients with MDD show hyperactivity in the amygdala (Surguladze et al., 2005) and reduced co-activation of the dorsal ACC (Matthews et al., 2008) when viewing negative facial expressions. These changes in brain activity are ameliorated with chronic antidepressant treatment (Chen et al., 2008; Fu et al., 2004; Sheline et al., 2001).

Similar to the electrocardiogram (ECG), unfiltered electrical activity generated by the brain can be measured by an electroencephalogram (EEG). EEG signals can be converted to show a topographical representation of the distribution of the EEG waveforms across the cortex known as the quantitative electroencephalograph (QEEG) brain map. The QEEG image is used to assess brain activity and metabolism in real-time, providing a global assessment of brain activity. Brain electrical activity can be measured using cordance, low-resolution brain electromagnetic tomography (LORETA), and antidepressant treatment (ATR) index. Cordance, which uses QEEG measurements conducted from a full scalp electrode array, assesses perfusion of cerebral cortex and brain activity on cortical convexities like PFC (Cook et al., 1998; Leuchter et al., 1999). Several groups have demonstrated the usefulness of cordance in characterizing antidepressant response (Bares et al., 2008; Cook et al., 2002). Responders and non-responders differ in QEEG measurements at rest and during task-oriented activities (Bruder et al., 2008). LORETA, which assesses activity of deeper cortical regions like ACC and orbitofrontal cortex (Pizzagalli et al., 2001), identifies cortical alterations in relation to depression and antidepressant response (Anderer et al., 2002; Saletu et al., 2010). Both cordance and LORETA require whole-head electrode montages for data collection, which entails up to 75 minutes of QEEG recording, limiting its clinical utility. On the other hand, the ATR only uses a five-electrode montage placed on the frontal brain regions, which limits QEEG recording to 10 minutes (Leuchter et al., 2009a; Leuchter et al., 2009b). The largest study that evaluated the use of ATR in predicting antidepressant response is the Biomarkers for Rapid Identification of Treatment Effectiveness trial in Major Depression (BRITE-MD) trial. In this study, positive ATR predicted response and remission to escitalopram. Patients with negative ATR values were either switched to bupropion or continued to be treated with escitalopram. In comparison to patients who stayed on escitalopram, patients who switched to bupropion were 1.9 times more likely to respond to treatment (Leuchter et al., 2009a; Leuchter et al., 2009b). These results support the use of ATR as a biomarker for monitoring treatment response and clinical progression.

6.2 Cellular and molecular markers

Lower hippocampal volume (Videbech & Ravnkilde, 2004), which is commonly found in post-mortem brain tissues of depressed individuals (MacQueen et al., 2003), results in reduced hippocampal plasticity. Reduction in neurogenesis, brain volume, and thickness is likely due to decreased neurotrophins and/or changes in neuroplasticity (Geuze et al., 2005). Neurotrophins, including brain-derived neurotrophic factor (BDNF), have been repeatedly implicated in the pathogenesis and treatment of MDD (Duman & Monteggia, 2006). Administration of BDNF induces cell proliferation and neurogenesis (Pencea et al., 2001; Zigova et al., 1998), and leads to lower depressive-like behavior (Shirayama et al., 2002; Siuciak et al., 1997). Neurogenesis, resulting from either antidepressant treatment or cell implantation, attenuates depressive behavior (Tfilin et al., 2009). Depressed patients show reduced BDNF levels (Sen et al., 2008), which can result in lower number of dendrites in the synapse (Manji et al., 2003; Nestler et al., 2002). Antidepressants stimulate BDNF synthesis (Duman, 2004) and normalizes reduced BDNF levels in depressed patients (Brunoni et al., 2008; Sen et al., 2008). A functional variant at codon 66, resulting in a valanine to methionine change (Val66Met), is reported to correspond with drug response. Carriers of the Met allele were reported to have better treatment outcomes (Gratacos et al., 2008; Kato & Serretti, 2010), however, others did not find any correlation between the Val66Met variant and treatment response (Kato & Serretti, 2010; Tsai et al., 2003; Wilkie et al., 2007). Furthermore, genetic susceptibility to depression was not associated with the *BDNF* Val166Met variant (Gratacos et al., 2007; Lopez-Leon et al., 2008). The Met allele is associated with impaired intra-cellular packaging and activity dependent secretion of BDNF, which disrupts hippocampal function (Egan et al., 2003). Impaired suppression of the HPA axis following dexamethasone treatment was also observed in the *BDNF* Met carriers (Schule et al., 2006). Of note, mouse lines that did not express *Bdnf* during fetal development or post-natal development were hyperactive, hyperaggressive, and showed higher depressive-like behavior compared to transgenic mice that were conditioned to express *Bdnf* during post-natal development (Chan et al., 2006), suggesting that the behavioral effects of BDNF are region and time-dependent. Interestingly, an interaction between the *BDNF* G196A variant, the serotonin transporter gene, and stressful life events has been observed (M. Aguilera et al., 2009; Pezawas et al., 2008).

BDNF is activated by cyclic-AMP response element-binding protein (CREB). The cAMP-CREB cascade has been extensively studied for its involvement in cell survival and neural plasticity (D'Sa & Duman, 2002; Duman et al., 1997). The cAMP-CREB pathway is upregulated following chronic antidepressant treatment (Duman et al., 1999). Activation of the CREB pathway is thought to result in neurogenesis. Activated or phosphorylated CREB is found in actively dividing neural progenitor cells in the hippocampal subgranular zone (SGZ) (Nakagawa et al., 2002a). Mice lacking *Creb* show markedly reduced cell proliferation (Nakagawa et al., 2002b) and administration of a phosphodiesterase inhibitor, which activates the cAMP cascade, increases neurogenesis and improve depressive behavior (Takahashi et al., 1999). Although CREB plays a critical role in neurogenesis, CREB is not necessary to elicit antidepressant effects. After antidepressant treatment, no difference in depressive-like responses was observed between *Creb* deficient mice and wild-type controls, indicating that the behavioral effects of antidepressant drugs may occur through other CREB-independent mechanisms.

Given that depressed patients exhibit reduced neuronal and glial cells, molecular mechanisms that stimulate neurogenesis (activation of CREB and BDNF synthesis) are likely to be critical in MDD. Presently, the clinical significance of cellular genesis in depression is largely unknown. It is likely that cellular proliferative and survival processes interact to facilitate remodeling of synaptic connections that can lead to altered mood. It is noteworthy to consider, however, that in the absence of stress, the neural circuitry underlying depression may be different (Krishnan & Nestler, 2008). There is a possibility that reversal of stress-induced neural plasticity changes is not required for antidepressive effects (Nestler et al., 2002).

7. Depression signatures

7.1 Gene expression signatures

Gene expression profiling studies provide an unbiased look at the relationship between gene expression and depressive disorder, which is useful in identifying novel targets for antidepressant therapy (for a detailed review see Sequeira & Turecki, 2006). Bernard and colleagues collected gene expression data from the locus coeruleus of healthy, depressed, and bipolar patients. In this study, they found significant alterations in patients with MDD but not bipolar subjects. Gene expression alterations were detected in the glutamate signaling genes (*SLC1A2, SLC1A3* and *GLUL*), growth factor genes (*FGFR3* and *TrkB*), and several astroglial genes (Bernard et al., 2010). Similarly, dysregulation of fibroblast growth factor genes (*FGF1, FGF2, FGFR2,* and, *FGF3)* were detected in cortical regions of depressed patients, irrespective of previous antidepressant treatment (Evans et al., 2004). Consistent with previous findings, expression of genes involved in signal transmission of glutamate and GABA were found to be dysregulated in depressed patients (Choudary et al., 2005) and in suicide victims with and without depression (Sequeira et al., 2009). Alteration in genes regulating oligodendrocyte function (Sequeira & Turecki, 2006) and cell-cell communication (Sequeira et al., 2009) were altered in MDD, suggesting impairment in brain circuitry. Notably, reduced oligodendrocyte expression and neuronal changes in amygdala were detected in both depressed individuals and in rodents exposed to unpredictable chronic mild stress (Sibille et al., 2009), indicating a connection between stress response and neural circuitry.

For biomarkers to be clinically useful, putative analytes must be detected in easily accessible samples like plasma or serum. Using LPS-stimulated blood samples, Spijker et al. compared gene expression profiles between healthy and unmedicated patients with MDD. A significant difference in gene expression pattern was observed in a subset of genes, all of which have not been previously associated with depression (Spijker et al., 2010). Transcriptome changes in the leukocyte mRNA is correlated with response to antidepressant agents or lithium therapy (Iga et al., 2008). The authors found that normalization in gene expression pattern correlates with antidepressant response (Iga et al., 2008). In addition to analyzing global changes in the brain or plasma transcriptome, genetic regulatory elements of depression or antidepressant response can be identified using quantitative trait loci (QTL) mapping analysis. In this approach, DNA variants that regulate gene expression locally or distally (*cis* or *trans*-regulatory elements) are analyzed for correlation with depressive behavior, thereby facilitating analysis for regulatory genes underlying depressive behavior. This approach has been used to detect regulatory genetic elements for several behaviors (Bryant et al., 2009; Radcliffe et al., 2006).

7.2 Protein signatures

Other efforts to identify depression signatures include protein expression profiling. Plasma samples from control, depressed, and schizophrenic patients were analyzed for 79 plasma protein biomarkers including, cytokines, neurotrophins, and chemokines (Domenici et al., 2010). Interestingly, insulin and matrix metallopeptidase 9 (MMP-9) displayed the biggest difference between control and depressed patients (Domenici et al., 2010). Efforts to expand the panel of protein markers to include peripheral and neuropsychological markers are currently underway (Tadic et al., 2011). The global analysis of protein expression is still in its infancy although several groups have performed proteomic analysis in the cerebrospinal fluid (CSF) (Raedler & Wiedemann, 2006) and in discrete brain regions collected post-mortem (Beasley et al., 2006). In order to characterize the cause-effect relationship between biological alterations, treatment, and behavior, protein profiling studies in human samples should be complemented with proteomic studies in animals, which are more amenable for determination of disease and treatment effects.

8. Other mechanisms

8.1 Epigenetics

Discordance of depression between monozygotic twins suggests other non-genetic factors are involved (Mill & Petronis, 2007). Alteration in gene expression can occur without changes in the DNA sequence through epigenetic mechanisms like histone modification and methylation of DNA CpG islands. Deacytelation of histones results in DNA coiling, which prevents binding of transcription factors to the DNA, suppressing gene transcription. Alternatively, methylation alters DNA chemistry, which blocks gene transcription. Epigenetic mechanisms can explain how genetically weak signals of risk combined with environmental factors predispose patients to depression (Caspi & Moffitt, 2006).

Adverse childhood experiences confer risk to depressive behavior (Heim & Nemeroff, 2001) likely through epigenetic alteration. Offspring who received minimal maternal care had higher DNA methylation at the glucocorticoid receptor (GR) promoter region and were more responsive to stress compared to control animals (Liu et al., 1997; Weaver et al., 2004). Methylation in the GR promoter region leads to reduced binding of the nerve growth factor induced protein-A (NGF-1A), affecting GR regulation (Weaver et al., 2004; Weaver et al., 2007). Notably, low levels of maternal care led to epigenetic repression of the estrogen-alpha receptor that resulted in transmission of maternal behavior to offspring (Champagne et al., 2006; Champagne et al., 2003), thus indicating transgenerational phenotypic transfer through epigenetic alterations.

Mice that are deficient in *Hdac5* display enhanced vulnerability to stress, suggesting that stress reduces histone deacytelase activity leading to down-regulation of gene expression (Renthal et al., 2007). The adverse effect of stress on *Hdac5* activity is reversed by chronic antidepressant treatment (Renthal et al., 2007). Antidepressant treatment increases histone acetylation at the *Bdnf* promoter region, activating *Bdnf* expression (Tsankova et al., 2006). BDNF mediates formation and differentiation of new neurons, facilitating long-term potentiation and memory development.

RNA-mediated modifications through non-coding RNAs (ncRNA) and microRNAs (miRNA) can activate or silence gene transcription. The role of miRNA in regulating serotonergic transmission has been reviewed (Millan, 2011). MicroRNAs are short RNAs (22-24 nucleotides) that bind to complementary sequences on target mRNAs, typically leading to gene silencing (Bartel, 2009; Carthew & Sontheimer, 2009; Winter et al., 2009). A recent study by Baudry et al. shows that miR-16 negatively regulates the expression of serotonin transporter (SERT). Fluoxetine treatment stimulates the release of S100 calcium binding protein B (S100β) in the raphe, leading to elevation of miR-16 and reduction in SERT (Baudry et al., 2010). MiR-16 also represses the expression of anti-apoptotic protein (B-cell lymphoma 2) Bcl-2 (Cimmino et al., 2005), indicating a critical role of miR-16 in neurotransmission as well as cell proliferation. In addition, genetic studies using seahare (*Aplysia*) identified miR-124 as a translational repressor of CREB, which suggests that microRNAs indirectly regulate secondary messenger pathways by modulating CREB expression (Rajasethupathy et al., 2009). Overexpression of ncRNA was found in Alzheimer's patients (Faghihi et al., 2010), however, an association between ncRNA and depression is yet to be established.

Consistent with the notion that genes are interconnected within a network, it is conceivable that an epigenetic regulatory network exists. Efforts to identify epigenomic signatures are underway (Akbarian & Huang, 2009) and this data should be integrated with other data sets like the brain transcriptome and behavior to identify causative pathways in depression. Of great interest is the assessment of epigenetic transgenerational transmission of a trait and genomic imprinting (epigenetic alteration on gene expression is based on whether the gene is inherited from the father or the mother). These epigenetic phenomena facilitate our understanding of how environment and genetics interact to mediate behavior, ultimately providing a comprehensive picture of the molecular mechanisms underlying depression.

8.2 Sleep and circadian rhythm

It was previously thought that insomnia is a risk factor for depression (Breslau et al., 1996; Ford & Kamerow, 1989; Hohagen et al., 1993) and years of research did not clarify the exact relationship between insomnia and depression (Riemann, 2007; Riemann et al., 2001). In an EEG, normal sleep can be partitioned into several stages. The first is progression from light sleep (N1 stage), followed by an "intermediate" level of sleep (stage N2) that leads to the "deep" sleep, which is characterized by slow delta waves on the EEG (stage N3). Stages N1-N3 are part of non-rapid eye movement sleep, which alternates with rapid eye movement (REM) sleep throughout the night (Benca & Peterson, 2008). Depression is characterized by abnormal sleep (difficulty falling asleep, nocturnal awakenings, early-morning awakenings), decreased slow-wave sleep, shortened rapid eye movement (REM) latency, and increased REM density (Thase et al., 1997; Tsuno et al., 2005). Interestingly, total sleep deprivation improves symptoms in 40-60% of depressed patients (Giedke & Schwarzler, 2002; Wirz-Justice & Van den Hoofdakker, 1999), which is thought to be due to activation of the limbic dopaminergic pathways (Ebert et al., 1994; Ebert et al., 1996). Additionally, the slow-wave sleep is marginally affected by antidepressant therapy (Sharpley & Cowen, 1995; Tsuno et al., 2005), indicating partial involvement of monoamines in sleep regulation.

In addition to disruption in sleep pattern, depressed patients also exhibit alteration in biological rhythms, including appetite and hormone levels. Patients with seasonal affective disorders (SAD) have depressive symptoms during the winter months when daylight is shorter. The bright light therapy has been effectively used to treat SAD (Lam, 2006) and non-seasonal depression (Terman & Terman, 2005) and is thought to work by shifting the circadian clock (Wirz-Justice et al., 2005). Similar to 5-HT, melatonin is derived from tryptophan and is a critical regulator of circadian rhythm. Depressed patients display altered melatonin release and abnormal melatonin levels (Rubin et al., 1992; Wetterberg, 1999), particularly in the acute phase of depressive illness (Srinivasan et al., 2006). Antidepressant therapy increases melatonin (Srinivasan et al., 2006; Thompson et al., 1985). Of note, a pilot study that looked at the use of melatonin in addition to cortisol as a prognostic marker for depression found promising results (Buckley & Schatzberg, 2010).

Genetic regulators of the molecular clock (*Clock, Bmal1, Npas2, GSK3β,* and *Timeless*) have been linked with various mood disorders (McClung, 2007). Mutant mouse models exhibiting point mutations on the *Clock* gene display anxiety-like and depressive-like behavior (Roybal et al., 2007) and increased dopamine transmission in the ventral tegmental area (VTA) (McClung et al., 2005; Nestler & Carlezon, 2006), suggesting that the *Clock* gene regulates dopamine signaling. Interestingly, there is circadian rhythm with regards to concentration, release, and synthesis of 5-HT, norepinephrine, and dopamine (Barassin et al., 2002; Shieh et al., 1997; Weiner et al., 1992), as well as in the expression and activity of monoamine receptors (Kafka et al., 1983; Wesemann & Weiner, 1990; Witte & Lemmer, 1991), indicating a link between monoamine signaling and circadian rhythm.

9. Future directions: Moving towards a systems biology approach

Based on these findings, it is unlikely that a single biomarker can describe a multifactorial disorder like depression. Data from the last decades indicate that alterations in MDD are interconnected (**Figure 1**). This figure illustrates that there are neuroanatomical, neurobiochemical, neuroimmune, neuroendocrine, genetic, and metabolic mechanisms underlying MDD. Given the involvement of various biological systems, it is no surprise that depression is characterized by heterogeneous molecular and clinical manifestations, which complicate the search for depressive biomarkers. Therefore, uncovering the etiology and mechanism underlying depression necessitates modification of clinical and pre-clinical study designs and the use of combinatorial approaches to assess multiple phenotypic variances.

To obtain an in-depth clinical and biological assessment of depression, methodological aspects that should be considered when conducting clinical studies include obtaining a detailed family, medical, drug, and experiential history, performing longer patient follow-up (6 months to 1 year), assessing for metabolic, psychosomatic, and behavioral symptoms, and collecting blood samples for biological assessment of disease or changes in symptoms. This information can aid in identifying genetic, environmental, and biological factors that contribute to patient-specific depressive behavior, which can further delineate behavioral and biological alterations that differ or overlap between depressed patients.

Animal studies offer several advantages including lower cost, subject availability, and ease in brain and blood sample accessibility. In addition, the behavioral effects of drugs, genetics, and environment are more feasible to investigate in animal models of depression since the genome and the environment can be easily manipulated. Despite apparent advantages in using animals for depression studies, pre-clinical models of depression suffer from lack of face and construct validity (Nestler & Hyman, 2010). Depressive symptoms are challenging to model in animals given that diagnosis and prognosis are based on empirical clinical observations and patients' phenomenological accounts. In an effort to better assess clinical depressive measures in pre-clinical studies, the National Institute of Mental Health has adopted a set of constructs, known as the Research Domain Criteria (RDoC) (http://www.nimh.nih.gov), that are useful in conducting animal studies. The RDoC provides a framework in which scientific approaches like genomics and neuroscience can be used to interrogate for specific domains including negative affect and cognition. It remains to be seen if the use of RDoC will result in definitive findings that are likely to be replicated and validated.

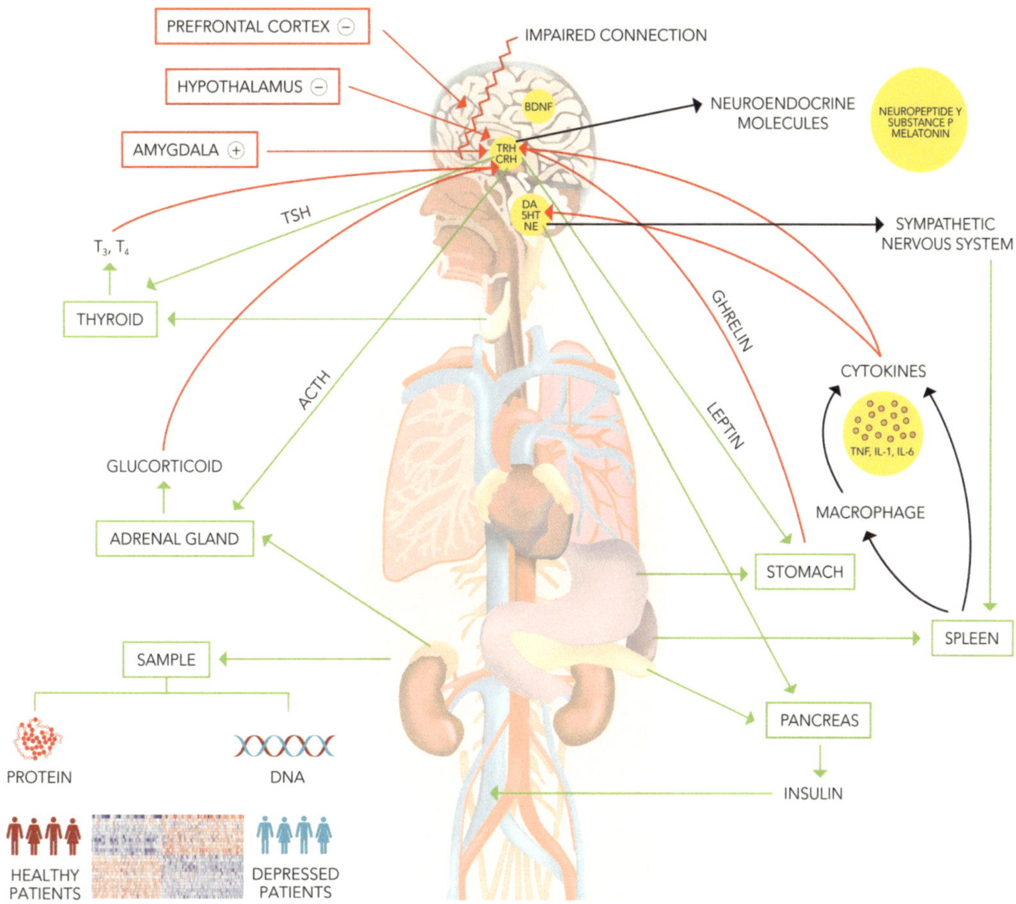

Fig. 1. *Biological Alterations in Depression.* Impairment in the HPA axis, neural circuitry, neuroendocrine, neuroimmune, neuronal signaling, neurogenesis, and metabolic functions have been observed in depressed patients, resulting in symptom heterogeneity. As shown, bidirectional communication among several pathways exists (i.e. crosstalk between sympathetic nervous system and inflammatory markers). Cellular (genetic) and molecular (proteomic) alterations in depression can be identified by performing global gene and protein expression analyses between healthy controls and depressed individuals (bottom left), leading to identification of depression molecular signatures.

Advancements in methodologies and information technology have facilitated identification of molecular and neurochemical correlates of MDD. Optogenetics helps elucidate the inter-relationship between neural circuitry, brain signaling, and biological response. Genomics, proteomics, epigenomics, and metabolomics provide an unbiased way to characterize biological alterations that underlie depressive behavior. In light of the many biological systems that are affected in depression, combinatorial approaches should be used to examine changes in various (cellular, molecular, biochemical, and behavioral) phenotypes, providing us with a comprehensive disease model.

Research studies conducted over the last forty years have not led to a detailed understanding of the mechanisms underlying MDD. Although this may seem disappointing at first, advances in technology and scientific approach indicate that the road to elucidating depression is one filled with hope and excitement.

10. References

Abkevich, V., Camp, N.J., Hensel, C.H., Neff, C.D., Russell, D.L., Hughes, D.C., Plenk, A.M., Lowry, M.R., Richards, R.L., Carter, C., Frech, G.C., Stone, S., Rowe, K., Chau, C.A., Cortado, K., Hunt, A., Luce, K., O'Neil, G., Poarch, J., Potter, J., Poulsen, G.H., Saxton, H., Bernat-Sestak, M., Thompson, V., Gutin, A., Skolnick, M.H., Shattuck, D. & Cannon-Albright, L. (2003). Predisposition locus for major depression at chromosome 12q22-12q23.2. *Am J Hum Genet,* Vol.73, No.6, (Dec 2003), pp. 1271-1281.

Aguilera, G., Volpi, S. & Rabadan-Diehl, C. (2003). Transcriptional and post-transcriptional mechanisms regulating the rat pituitary vasopressin V1b receptor gene. *J Mol Endocrinol,* Vol.30, No.2, (Apr 2003), pp. 99-108.

Aguilera, M., Arias, B., Wichers, M., Barrantes-Vidal, N., Moya, J., Villa, H., van Os, J., Ibanez, M.I., Ruiperez, M.A., Ortet, G. & Fananas, L. (2009). Early adversity and 5-HTT/BDNF genes: new evidence of gene-environment interactions on depressive symptoms in a general population. *Psychol Med,* Vol.39, No.9, (Sep 2009), pp. 1425-1432.

Ahima, R.S., Prabakaran, D., Mantzoros, C., Qu, D., Lowell, B., Maratos-Flier, E. & Flier, J.S. (1996). Role of leptin in the neuroendocrine response to fasting. *Nature,* Vol.382, No.6588, (Jul 18 1996), pp. 250-252.

Akbarian, S. & Huang, H.S. (2009). Epigenetic regulation in human brain-focus on histone lysine methylation. *Biol Psychiatry,* Vol.65, No.3, (Feb 1 2009), pp. 198-203.

Alexopoulos, G.S., Kiosses, D.N., Choi, S.J., Murphy, C.F. & Lim, K.O. (2002). Frontal white matter microstructure and treatment response of late-life depression: a preliminary study. *Am J Psychiatry,* Vol.159, No.11, (Nov 2002), pp. 1929-1932.

Alexopoulos, G.S., Murphy, C.F., Gunning-Dixon, F.M., Glatt, C.E., Latoussakis, V., Kelly, R.E., Jr., Kanellopoulos, D., Klimstra, S., Lim, K.O., Young, R.C. & Hoptman, M.J. (2009). Serotonin transporter polymorphisms, microstructural white matter abnormalities and remission of geriatric depression. *J Affect Disord,* Vol.119, No.1-3, (Dec 2009), pp. 132-141.

Alexopoulos, G.S., Murphy, C.F., Gunning-Dixon, F.M., Latoussakis, V., Kanellopoulos, D., Klimstra, S., Lim, K.O. & Hoptman, M.J. (2008). Microstructural white matter abnormalities and remission of geriatric depression. *Am J Psychiatry,* Vol.165, No.2, (Feb 2008), pp. 238-244.

Alldredge, B. (2010). Pathogenic involvement of neuropeptides in anxiety and depression. *Neuropeptides,* Vol.44, No.3, (Jun 2010), pp. 215-224.

Anacker, C., Zunszain, P.A., Carvalho, L.A. & Pariante, C.M. (2011). The glucocorticoid receptor: pivot of depression and of antidepressant treatment? *Psychoneuroendocrinology,* Vol.36, No.3, (Apr 2011), pp. 415-425.

Anand, A., Li, Y., Wang, Y., Wu, J., Gao, S., Bukhari, L., Mathews, V.P., Kalnin, A. & Lowe, M.J. (2005). Antidepressant effect on connectivity of the mood-regulating circuit: an FMRI study. *Neuropsychopharmacology,* Vol.30, No.7, (Jul 2005), pp. 1334-1344.

Anderer, P., Saletu, B., Semlitsch, H.V. & Pascual-Marqui, R.D. (2002). Structural and energetic processes related to P300: LORETA findings in depression and effects of antidepressant drugs. *Methods Find Exp Clin Pharmacol,* Vol.24 Suppl D, 2002), pp. 85-91.

Anguelova, M., Benkelfat, C. & Turecki, G. (2003). A systematic review of association studies investigating genes coding for serotonin receptors and the serotonin transporter: II. Suicidal behavior. *Mol Psychiatry,* Vol.8, No.7, (Jul 2003), pp. 646-653.

Antonijevic, I.A., Murck, H., Frieboes, R.M., Horn, R., Brabant, G. & Steiger, A. (1998). Elevated nocturnal profiles of serum leptin in patients with depression. *J Psychiatr Res,* Vol.32, No.6, (Nov-Dec 1998), pp. 403-410.

Arias, B., Serretti, A., Lorenzi, C., Gasto, C., Catalan, R. & Fananas, L. (2006). Analysis of COMT gene (Val 158 Met polymorphism) in the clinical response to SSRIs in depressive patients of European origin. *J Affect Disord,* Vol.90, No.2-3, (Feb 2006), pp. 251-256.

Asher, R. (1949). Myxoedematous madness. *Br Med J,* Vol.2, No.4627, (Sep 10 1949), pp. 555-562.

Atlantis, E. & Baker, M. (2008). Obesity effects on depression: systematic review of epidemiological studies. *Int J Obes (Lond),* Vol.32, No.6, (Jun 2008), pp. 881-891.

Baldessarini, R.J. (1989). Current status of antidepressants: clinical pharmacology and therapy. *J Clin Psychiatry,* Vol.50, No.4, (Apr 1989), pp. 117-126.

Barassin, S., Raison, S., Saboureau, M., Bienvenu, C., Maitre, M., Malan, A. & Pevet, P. (2002). Circadian tryptophan hydroxylase levels and serotonin release in the suprachiasmatic nucleus of the rat. *Eur J Neurosci,* Vol.15, No.5, (Mar 2002), pp. 833-840.

Bares, M., Brunovsky, M., Kopecek, M., Novak, T., Stopkova, P., Kozeny, J., Sos, P., Krajca, V. & Hoschl, C. (2008). Early reduction in prefrontal theta QEEG cordance value predicts response to venlafaxine treatment in patients with resistant depressive disorder. *Eur Psychiatry,* Vol.23, No.5, (Aug 2008), pp. 350-355.

Barr, A.M., Kinney, J.W., Hill, M.N., Lu, X., Biros, S., Rebek, J., Jr. & Bartfai, T. (2006). A novel, systemically active, selective galanin receptor type-3 ligand exhibits antidepressant-like activity in preclinical tests. *Neurosci Lett,* Vol.405, No.1-2, (Sep 11 2006), pp. 111-115.

Bartel, D.P. (2009). MicroRNAs: target recognition and regulatory functions. *Cell,* Vol.136, No.2, (Jan 23 2009), pp. 215-233.

Baudry, A., Mouillet-Richard, S., Schneider, B., Launay, J.M. & Kellermann, O. (2010). miR-16 targets the serotonin transporter: a new facet for adaptive responses to antidepressants. *Science,* Vol.329, No.5998, (Sep 17 2010), pp. 1537-1541.

Baumgartner, A., Campos-Barros, A., Gaio, U., Hessenius, C., Flechner, A. & Meinhold, H. (1994a). Carbamazepine affects triiodothyronine production and metabolization in rat hippocampus. *Life Sci,* Vol.54, No.23, 1994a), pp. PL401-407.

Baumgartner, A., Campos-Barros, A., Gaio, U., Hessenius, C., Frege, I. & Meinhold, H. (1994b). Effects of lithium on thyroid hormone metabolism in rat frontal cortex. *Biol Psychiatry,* Vol.36, No.11, (Dec 1 1994b), pp. 771-774.

Baumgartner, A., Dubeyko, M., Campos-Barros, A., Eravci, M. & Meinhold, H. (1994c). Subchronic administration of fluoxetine to rats affects triiodothyronine production and deiodination in regions of the cortex and in the limbic forebrain. *Brain Res,* Vol.635, No.1-2, (Jan 28 1994c), pp. 68-74.

Baumgartner, A., Graf, K.J., Kurten, I. & Meinhold, H. (1988). The hypothalamic-pituitary-thyroid axis in psychiatric patients and healthy subjects: Parts 1-4. *Psychiatry Res,* Vol.24, No.3, (Jun 1988), pp. 271-332.

Beasley, C.L., Pennington, K., Behan, A., Wait, R., Dunn, M.J. & Cotter, D. (2006). Proteomic analysis of the anterior cingulate cortex in the major psychiatric disorders: Evidence for disease-associated changes. *Proteomics,* Vol.6, No.11, (Jun 2006), pp. 3414-3425.

Belmaker, R.H. (2008). The future of depression psychopharmacology. *CNS Spectr,* Vol.13, No.8, (Aug 2008), pp. 682-687.

Benca, R.M. & Peterson, M.J. (2008). Insomnia and depression. *Sleep Med,* Vol.9 Suppl 1, (Sep 2008), pp. S3-9.

Bernard, R., Kerman, I.A., Thompson, R.C., Jones, E.G., Bunney, W.E., Barchas, J.D., Schatzberg, A.F., Myers, R.M., Akil, H. & Watson, S.J. (2010). Altered expression of glutamate signaling, growth factor, and glia genes in the locus coeruleus of patients with major depression. *Mol Psychiatry,* Vol.16, No.6, (Jun 2010), pp. 634-646.

Berridge, K.C. (1996). Food reward: brain substrates of wanting and liking. *Neurosci Biobehav Rev,* Vol.20, No.1, 1996), pp. 1-25.

Berridge, K.C. (2007). The debate over dopamine's role in reward: the case for incentive salience. *Psychopharmacology (Berl),* Vol.191, No.3, (Apr 2007), pp. 391-431.

Berthoud, H.R. (2002). Multiple neural systems controlling food intake and body weight. *Neurosci Biobehav Rev,* Vol.26, No.4, (Jun 2002), pp. 393-428.

Bierut, L.J., Heath, A.C., Bucholz, K.K., Dinwiddie, S.H., Madden, P.A., Statham, D.J., Dunne, M.P. & Martin, N.G. (1999). Major depressive disorder in a community-based twin sample: are there different genetic and environmental contributions for men and women? *Arch Gen Psychiatry,* Vol.56, No.6, (Jun 1999), pp. 557-563.

Binder, E.B., Salyakina, D., Lichtner, P., Wochnik, G.M., Ising, M., Putz, B., Papiol, S., Seaman, S., Lucae, S., Kohli, M.A., Nickel, T., Kunzel, H.E., Fuchs, B., Majer, M., Pfennig, A., Kern, N., Brunner, J., Modell, S., Baghai, T., Deiml, T., Zill, P., Bondy, B., Rupprecht, R., Messer, T., Kohnlein, O., Dabitz, H., Bruckl, T., Muller, N., Pfister, H., Lieb, R., Mueller, J.C., Lohmussaar, E., Strom, T.M., Bettecken, T., Meitinger, T., Uhr, M., Rein, T., Holsboer, F. & Muller-Myhsok, B. (2004). Polymorphisms in FKBP5 are associated with increased recurrence of depressive episodes and rapid response to antidepressant treatment. *Nat Genet,* Vol.36, No.12, (Dec 2004), pp. 1319-1325.

Bondy, B., Baghai, T.C., Minov, C., Schule, C., Schwarz, M.J., Zwanzger, P., Rupprecht, R. & Moller, H.J. (2003). Substance P serum levels are increased in major depression: preliminary results. *Biol Psychiatry,* Vol.53, No.6, (Mar 15 2003), pp. 538-542.

Brambilla, F., Smeraldi, E., Sacchetti, E., Bellodi, L., Genazzani, A.R., Facchinetti, F. & Muller, E.E. (1982). Neuroendocrine abnormalities in depressive illness. *Adv Biochem Psychopharmacol,* Vol.32, 1982), pp. 329-340.

Brebner, K., Hayley, S., Zacharko, R., Merali, Z. & Anisman, H. (2000). Synergistic effects of interleukin-1beta, interleukin-6, and tumor necrosis factor-alpha: central monoamine, corticosterone, and behavioral variations. *Neuropsychopharmacology,* Vol.22, No.6, (Jun 2000), pp. 566-580.

Breslau, N., Roth, T., Rosenthal, L. & Andreski, P. (1996). Sleep disturbance and psychiatric disorders: a longitudinal epidemiological study of young adults. *Biol Psychiatry,* Vol.39, No.6, (Mar 15 1996), pp. 411-418.

Bruder, G.E., Sedoruk, J.P., Stewart, J.W., McGrath, P.J., Quitkin, F.M. & Tenke, C.E. (2008). Electroencephalographic alpha measures predict therapeutic response to a selective serotonin reuptake inhibitor antidepressant: pre- and post-treatment findings. *Biol Psychiatry,* Vol.63, No.12, (Jun 15 2008), pp. 1171-1177.

Bruning, J.C., Gautam, D., Burks, D.J., Gillette, J., Schubert, M., Orban, P.C., Klein, R., Krone, W., Muller-Wieland, D. & Kahn, C.R. (2000). Role of brain insulin receptor in control of body weight and reproduction. *Science,* Vol.289, No.5487, (Sep 22 2000), pp. 2122-2125.

Brunoni, A.R., Lopes, M. & Fregni, F. (2008). A systematic review and meta-analysis of clinical studies on major depression and BDNF levels: implications for the role of neuroplasticity in depression. *Int J Neuropsychopharmacol,* Vol.11, No.8, (Dec 2008), pp. 1169-1180.

Bryant, C.D., Chang, H.P., Zhang, J., Wiltshire, T., Tarantino, L.M. & Palmer, A.A. (2009). A major QTL on chromosome 11 influences psychostimulant and opioid sensitivity in mice. *Genes Brain Behav,* Vol.8, No.8, (Nov 2009), pp. 795-805.

Buckley, T.M. & Schatzberg, A.F. (2010). A pilot study of the phase angle between cortisol and melatonin in major depression - a potential biomarker? *J Psychiatr Res,* Vol.44, No.2, (Jan 2010), pp. 69-74.

Campos-Barros, A., Meinhold, H., Stula, M., Muller, F., Kohler, R., Eravci, M., Putzien, O. & Baumgartner, A. (1994). The influence of desipramine on thyroid hormone metabolism in rat brain. *J Pharmacol Exp Ther,* Vol.268, No.3, (Mar 1994), pp. 1143-1152.

Carthew, R.W. & Sontheimer, E.J. (2009). Origins and Mechanisms of miRNAs and siRNAs. *Cell,* Vol.136, No.4, (Feb 20 2009), pp. 642-655.

Caspi, A., Hariri, A.R., Holmes, A., Uher, R. & Moffitt, T.E. (2010). Genetic sensitivity to the environment: the case of the serotonin transporter gene and its implications for studying complex diseases and traits. *Am J Psychiatry,* Vol.167, No.5, (May 2010), pp. 509-527.

Caspi, A. & Moffitt, T.E. (2006). Gene-environment interactions in psychiatry: joining forces with neuroscience. *Nat Rev Neurosci,* Vol.7, No.7, (Jul 2006), pp. 583-590.

Caspi, A., Sugden, K., Moffitt, T.E., Taylor, A., Craig, I.W., Harrington, H., McClay, J., Mill, J., Martin, J., Braithwaite, A. & Poulton, R. (2003). Influence of life stress on depression: moderation by a polymorphism in the 5-HTT gene. *Science,* Vol.301, No.5631, (Jul 18 2003), pp. 386-389.

Champagne, F.A., Weaver, I.C., Diorio, J., Dymov, S., Szyf, M. & Meaney, M.J. (2006). Maternal care associated with methylation of the estrogen receptor-alpha1b promoter and estrogen receptor-alpha expression in the medial preoptic area of female offspring. *Endocrinology,* Vol.147, No.6, (Jun 2006), pp. 2909-2915.

Champagne, F.A., Weaver, I.C., Diorio, J., Sharma, S. & Meaney, M.J. (2003). Natural variations in maternal care are associated with estrogen receptor alpha expression and estrogen sensitivity in the medial preoptic area. *Endocrinology,* Vol.144, No.11, (Nov 2003), pp. 4720-4724.

Chan, J.P., Unger, T.J., Byrnes, J. & Rios, M. (2006). Examination of behavioral deficits triggered by targeting Bdnf in fetal or postnatal brains of mice. *Neuroscience,* Vol.142, No.1, (Sep 29 2006), pp. 49-58.

Chapman, D.P., Whitfield, C.L., Felitti, V.J., Dube, S.R., Edwards, V.J. & Anda, R.F. (2004). Adverse childhood experiences and the risk of depressive disorders in adulthood. *J Affect Disord,* Vol.82, No.2, (Oct 15 2004), pp. 217-225.

Chehab, F.F. (2000). Leptin as a regulator of adipose mass and reproduction. *Trends Pharmacol Sci,* Vol.21, No.8, (Aug 2000), pp. 309-314.

Chen, C.H., Suckling, J., Ooi, C., Fu, C.H., Williams, S.C., Walsh, N.D., Mitterschiffthaler, M.T., Pich, E.M. & Bullmore, E. (2008). Functional coupling of the amygdala in depressed patients treated with antidepressant medication. *Neuropsychopharmacology,* Vol.33, No.8, (Jul 2008), pp. 1909-1918.

Choi, J., Jeong, B., Rohan, M.L., Polcari, A.M. & Teicher, M.H. (2009). Preliminary evidence for white matter tract abnormalities in young adults exposed to parental verbal abuse. *Biol Psychiatry,* Vol.65, No.3, (Feb 1 2009), pp. 227-234.

Choudary, P.V., Molnar, M., Evans, S.J., Tomita, H., Li, J.Z., Vawter, M.P., Myers, R.M., Bunney, W.E., Jr., Akil, H., Watson, S.J. & Jones, E.G. (2005). Altered cortical glutamatergic and GABAergic signal transmission with glial involvement in depression. *Proc Natl Acad Sci U S A,* Vol.102, No.43, (Oct 25 2005), pp. 15653-15658.

Cimmino, A., Calin, G.A., Fabbri, M., Iorio, M.V., Ferracin, M., Shimizu, M., Wojcik, S.E., Aqeilan, R.I., Zupo, S., Dono, M., Rassenti, L., Alder, H., Volinia, S., Liu, C.G., Kipps, T.J., Negrini, M. & Croce, C.M. (2005). miR-15 and miR-16 induce apoptosis by targeting BCL2. *Proc Natl Acad Sci U S A,* Vol.102, No.39, (Sep 27 2005), pp. 13944-13949.

Collier, D.A., Stober, G., Li, T., Heils, A., Catalano, M., Di Bella, D., Arranz, M.J., Murray, R.M., Vallada, H.P., Bengel, D., Muller, C.R., Roberts, G.W., Smeraldi, E., Kirov, G., Sham, P. & Lesch, K.P. (1996). A novel functional polymorphism within the promoter of the serotonin transporter gene: possible role in susceptibility to affective disorders. *Mol Psychiatry,* Vol.1, No.6, (Dec 1996), pp. 453-460.

Collin, M., Hakansson-Ovesjo, M.L., Misane, I., Ogren, S.O. & Meister, B. (2000). Decreased 5-HT transporter mRNA in neurons of the dorsal raphe nucleus and behavioral depression in the obese leptin-deficient ob/ob mouse. *Brain Res Mol Brain Res,* Vol.81, No.1-2, (Sep 30 2000), pp. 51-61.

Cook, I.A., Leuchter, A.F., Morgan, M., Witte, E., Stubbeman, W.F., Abrams, M., Rosenberg, S. & Uijtdehaage, S.H. (2002). Early changes in prefrontal activity characterize clinical responders to antidepressants. *Neuropsychopharmacology,* Vol.27, No.1, (Jul 2002), pp. 120-131.

Cook, I.A., O'Hara, R., Uijtdehaage, S.H., Mandelkern, M. & Leuchter, A.F. (1998). Assessing the accuracy of topographic EEG mapping for determining local brain function. *Electroencephalogr Clin Neurophysiol,* Vol.107, No.6, (Dec 1998), pp. 408-414.

Costafreda, S.G., Chu, C., Ashburner, J. & Fu, C.H. (2009). Prognostic and diagnostic potential of the structural neuroanatomy of depression. *PLoS One,* Vol.4, No.7, 2009), pp. e6353.

Craft, S. & Watson, G.S. (2004). Insulin and neurodegenerative disease: shared and specific mechanisms. *Lancet Neurol,* Vol.3, No.3, (Mar 2004), pp. 169-178.

Crisafulli, C., Fabbri, C., Porcelli, S., Drago, A., Spina, E., De Ronchi, D. & Serretti, A. (2011). Pharmacogenetics of antidepressants. *Front Pharmacol,* Vol.2, 2011), pp. 6.

Cserr, H.F. & Knopf, P.M. (1992). Cervical lymphatics, the blood-brain barrier and the immunoreactivity of the brain: a new view. *Immunol Today,* Vol.13, No.12, (Dec 1992), pp. 507-512.

D'Sa, C. & Duman, R.S. (2002). Antidepressants and neuroplasticity. *Bipolar Disord,* Vol.4, No.3, (Jun 2002), pp. 183-194.

Dallman, M.F. (2009). Stress-induced obesity and the emotional nervous system. *Trends Endocrinol Metab,* Vol.21, No.3, (Mar 2009), pp. 159-165.

Davidson, R.J., Pizzagalli, D., Nitschke, J.B. & Putnam, K. (2002). Depression: perspectives from affective neuroscience. *Annu Rev Psychol,* Vol.53, 2002), pp. 545-574.

de Kloet, E.R., Joels, M. & Holsboer, F. (2005). Stress and the brain: from adaptation to disease. *Nat Rev Neurosci,* Vol.6, No.6, (Jun 2005), pp. 463-475.

De Luca, V., Mueller, D.J., Tharmalingam, S., King, N. & Kennedy, J.L. (2004). Analysis of the novel TPH2 gene in bipolar disorder and suicidality. *Mol Psychiatry,* Vol.9, No.10, (Oct 2004), pp. 896-897.

de Wit, L., Luppino, F., van Straten, A., Penninx, B., Zitman, F. & Cuijpers, P. (2010). Depression and obesity: a meta-analysis of community-based studies. *Psychiatry Res,* Vol.178, No.2, (Jul 30 2010), pp. 230-235.

Delay, J., Laine, B. & Buisson, J.F. (1952). [The action of isonicotinyl-hydrazide used in the treatment of depressive states]. *Ann Med Psychol (Paris),* Vol.110, No.2:5, (Dec 1952), pp. 689-692.

Delorme, R., Durand, C.M., Betancur, C., Wagner, M., Ruhrmann, S., Grabe, H.-J., Nygren, G., Gillberg, C., Leboyer, M., Bourgeron, T., Courtet, P., Jollant, F., Buresi, C., Aubry, J.-M., Baud, P., Bondolfi, G., Bertschy, G., Perroud, N. & Malafosse, A. (2006). No human tryptophan hydroxylase-2 gene R441H mutation in a large cohort of psychiatric patients and control subjects. *Biological Psychiatry,* Vol.60, No.2, 2006), pp. 202-203 %U http://www.ncbi.nlm.nih.gov/pubmed/16581035.

Dentino, A.N., Pieper, C.F., Rao, M.K., Currie, M.S., Harris, T., Blazer, D.G. & Cohen, H.J. (1999). Association of interleukin-6 and other biologic variables with depression in older people living in the community. *J Am Geriatr Soc,* Vol.47, No.1, (Jan 1999), pp. 6-11.

Deuschle, M., Blum, W.F., Englaro, P., Schweiger, U., Weber, B., Pflaum, C.D. & Heuser, I. (1996). Plasma leptin in depressed patients and healthy controls. *Horm Metab Res,* Vol.28, No.12, (Dec 1996), pp. 714-717.

Domenici, E., Wille, D.R., Tozzi, F., Prokopenko, I., Miller, S., McKeown, A., Brittain, C., Rujescu, D., Giegling, I., Turck, C.W., Holsboer, F., Bullmore, E.T., Middleton, L., Merlo-Pich, E., Alexander, R.C. & Muglia, P. (2010). Plasma protein biomarkers for depression and schizophrenia by multi analyte profiling of case-control collections. *PLoS One,* Vol.5, No.2, 2010), pp. e9166.

Dougherty, D. & Rauch, S.L. (1997). Neuroimaging and neurobiological models of depression. *Harv Rev Psychiatry,* Vol.5, No.3, (Sep-Oct 1997), pp. 138-159.

Dratman, M.B. & Gordon, J.T. (1996). Thyroid hormones as neurotransmitters. *Thyroid,* Vol.6, No.6, (Dec 1996), pp. 639-647.

Drevets, W.C. (2000a). Functional anatomical abnormalities in limbic and prefrontal cortical structures in major depression. *Prog Brain Res,* Vol.126, 2000a), pp. 413-431.

Drevets, W.C. (2000b). Neuroimaging studies of mood disorders. *Biol Psychiatry,* Vol.48, No.8, (Oct 15 2000b), pp. 813-829.

Drevets, W.C., Frank, E., Price, J.C., Kupfer, D.J., Holt, D., Greer, P.J., Huang, Y., Gautier, C. & Mathis, C. (1999). PET imaging of serotonin 1A receptor binding in depression. *Biol Psychiatry,* Vol.46, No.10, (Nov 15 1999), pp. 1375-1387.

Duman, R.S. (2004). Role of neurotrophic factors in the etiology and treatment of mood disorders. *Neuromolecular Med,* Vol.5, No.1, 2004), pp. 11-25.

Duman, R.S., Heninger, G.R. & Nestler, E.J. (1997). A molecular and cellular theory of depression. *Arch Gen Psychiatry,* Vol.54, No.7, (Jul 1997), pp. 597-606.

Duman, R.S., Malberg, J. & Thome, J. (1999). Neural plasticity to stress and antidepressant treatment. *Biol Psychiatry,* Vol.46, No.9, (Nov 1 1999), pp. 1181-1191.

Duman, R.S. & Monteggia, L.M. (2006). A neurotrophic model for stress-related mood disorders. *Biol Psychiatry,* Vol.59, No.12, (Jun 15 2006), pp. 1116-1127.

Dunn, A.J. & Swiergiel, A.H. (1999). Behavioral responses to stress are intact in CRF-deficient mice. *Brain Res,* Vol.845, No.1, (Oct 16 1999), pp. 14-20.

Dunn, A.J., Swiergiel, A.H. & de Beaurepaire, R. (2005). Cytokines as mediators of depression: what can we learn from animal studies? *Neurosci Biobehav Rev,* Vol.29, No.4-5, 2005), pp. 891-909.

Duval, F., Mokrani, M.C., Crocq, M.A., Jautz, M., Bailey, P., Diep, T.S. & Macher, J.P. (1996). Effect of antidepressant medication on morning and evening thyroid function tests during a major depressive episode. *Arch Gen Psychiatry,* Vol.53, No.9, (Sep 1996), pp. 833-840.

Ebert, D., Feistel, H., Barocka, A. & Kaschka, W. (1994). Increased limbic blood flow and total sleep deprivation in major depression with melancholia. *Psychiatry Res,* Vol.55, No.2, (Jun 1994), pp. 101-109.

Ebert, D., Feistel, H., Loew, T. & Pirner, A. (1996). Dopamine and depression--striatal dopamine D2 receptor SPECT before and after antidepressant therapy. *Psychopharmacology (Berl),* Vol.126, No.1, (Jul 1996), pp. 91-94.

Egan, M.F., Kojima, M., Callicott, J.H., Goldberg, T.E., Kolachana, B.S., Bertolino, A., Zaitsev, E., Gold, B., Goldman, D., Dean, M., Lu, B. & Weinberger, D.R. (2003). The BDNF val66met polymorphism affects activity-dependent secretion of BDNF and human memory and hippocampal function. *Cell,* Vol.112, No.2, (Jan 24 2003), pp. 257-269.

Elhwuegi, A.S. (2004). Central monoamines and their role in major depression. *Prog Neuropsychopharmacol Biol Psychiatry,* Vol.28, No.3, (May 2004), pp. 435-451.

Engelmann, M., Landgraf, R. & Wotjak, C.T. (2004). The hypothalamic-neurohypophysial system regulates the hypothalamic-pituitary-adrenal axis under stress: an old concept revisited. *Front Neuroendocrinol,* Vol.25, No.3-4, (Sep-Dec 2004), pp. 132-149.

Erhardt, A., Lucae, S., Unschuld, P.G., Ising, M., Kern, N., Salyakina, D., Lieb, R., Uhr, M., Binder, E.B., Keck, M.E., Muller-Myhsok, B. & Holsboer, F. (2007). Association of polymorphisms in P2RX7 and CaMKKb with anxiety disorders. *J Affect Disord,* Vol.101, No.1-3, (Aug 2007), pp. 159-168.

Evans, S.J., Choudary, P.V., Neal, C.R., Li, J.Z., Vawter, M.P., Tomita, H., Lopez, J.F., Thompson, R.C., Meng, F., Stead, J.D., Walsh, D.M., Myers, R.M., Bunney, W.E., Watson, S.J., Jones, E.G. & Akil, H. (2004). Dysregulation of the fibroblast growth factor system in major depression. *Proc Natl Acad Sci U S A,* Vol.101, No.43, (Oct 26 2004), pp. 15506-15511.

Faghihi, M.A., Zhang, M., Huang, J., Modarresi, F., Van der Brug, M.P., Nalls, M.A., Cookson, M.R., St-Laurent, G., 3rd & Wahlestedt, C. (2010). Evidence for natural antisense transcript-mediated inhibition of microRNA function. *Genome Biol,* Vol.11, No.5, 2010), pp. R56.

Faith, M.S., Butryn, M., Wadden, T.A., Fabricatore, A., Nguyen, A.M. & Heymsfield, S.B. (2011). Evidence for prospective associations among depression and obesity in population-based studies. *Obes Rev,* Vol.12, No.5, (May 2011), pp. e438-453.

Faith, M.S., Matz, P.E. & Jorge, M.A. (2002). Obesity-depression associations in the population. *J Psychosom Res,* Vol.53, No.4, (Oct 2002), pp. 935-942.

Farooqi, I.S., Matarese, G., Lord, G.M., Keogh, J.M., Lawrence, E., Agwu, C., Sanna, V., Jebb, S.A., Perna, F., Fontana, S., Lechler, R.I., DePaoli, A.M. & O'Rahilly, S. (2002). Beneficial effects of leptin on obesity, T cell hyporesponsiveness, and neuroendocrine/metabolic dysfunction of human congenital leptin deficiency. *J Clin Invest,* Vol.110, No.8, (Oct 2002), pp. 1093-1103.

Farr, S.A., Banks, W.A. & Morley, J.E. (2006). Effects of leptin on memory processing. *Peptides,* Vol.27, No.6, (Jun 2006), pp. 1420-1425.

Felten, D.L. (1991). Neurotransmitter signaling of cells of the immune system: important progress, major gaps. *Brain Behav Immun,* Vol.5, No.1, (Mar 1991), pp. 2-8.

Fernandez-Real, J.M., Vayreda, M., Richart, C., Gutierrez, C., Broch, M., Vendrell, J. & Ricart, W. (2001). Circulating interleukin 6 levels, blood pressure, and insulin sensitivity in apparently healthy men and women. *J Clin Endocrinol Metab,* Vol.86, No.3, (Mar 2001), pp. 1154-1159.

Ferrari, D., Pizzirani, C., Adinolfi, E., Lemoli, R.M., Curti, A., Idzko, M., Panther, E. & Di Virgilio, F. (2006). The P2X7 receptor: a key player in IL-1 processing and release. *J Immunol,* Vol.176, No.7, (Apr 1 2006), pp. 3877-3883.

Fishman, P.H. & Finberg, J.P. (1987). Effect of the tricyclic antidepressant desipramine on beta-adrenergic receptors in cultured rat glioma C6 cells. *J Neurochem,* Vol.49, No.1, (Jul 1987), pp. 282-289.

Ford, D.E. & Kamerow, D.B. (1989). Epidemiologic study of sleep disturbances and psychiatric disorders. An opportunity for prevention? *JAMA,* Vol.262, No.11, (Sep 15 1989), pp. 1479-1484.

Francis, D., Diorio, J., Liu, D. & Meaney, M.J. (1999). Nongenomic transmission across generations of maternal behavior and stress responses in the rat. *Science,* Vol.286, No.5442, (Nov 5 1999), pp. 1155-1158.

Frasure-Smith, N., Lesperance, F. & Talajic, M. (1993). Depression following myocardial infarction. Impact on 6-month survival. *JAMA,* Vol.270, No.15, (Oct 20 1993), pp. 1819-1825.

Friedman, J.M. (1999). Leptin and the regulation of body weight. *Harvey Lect,* Vol.95, 1999), pp. 107-136.

Frodl, T., Jager, M., Smajstrlova, I., Born, C., Bottlender, R., Palladino, T., Reiser, M., Moller, H.J. & Meisenzahl, E.M. (2008). Effect of hippocampal and amygdala volumes on clinical outcomes in major depression: a 3-year prospective magnetic resonance imaging study. *J Psychiatry Neurosci,* Vol.33, No.5, (Sep 2008), pp. 423-430.

Froger, N., Gardier, A.M., Moratalla, R., Alberti, I., Lena, I., Boni, C., De Felipe, C., Rupniak, N.M., Hunt, S.P., Jacquot, C., Hamon, M. & Lanfumey, L. (2001). 5-hydroxytryptamine (5-HT)1A autoreceptor adaptive changes in substance P (neurokinin 1) receptor knock-out mice mimic antidepressant-induced desensitization. *J Neurosci,* Vol.21, No.20, (Oct 15 2001), pp. 8188-8197.

Fu, C.H., Williams, S.C., Cleare, A.J., Brammer, M.J., Walsh, N.D., Kim, J., Andrew, C.M., Pich, E.M., Williams, P.M., Reed, L.J., Mitterschiffthaler, M.T., Suckling, J. & Bullmore, E.T. (2004). Attenuation of the neural response to sad faces in major depression by antidepressant treatment: a prospective, event-related functional magnetic resonance imaging study. *Arch Gen Psychiatry,* Vol.61, No.9, (Sep 2004), pp. 877-889.

Garssen, B. & Goodkin, K. (1999). On the role of immunological factors as mediators between psychosocial factors and cancer progression. *Psychiatry Res,* Vol.85, No.1, (Jan 18 1999), pp. 51-61.

Geuze, E., Vermetten, E. & Bremner, J.D. (2005). MR-based in vivo hippocampal volumetrics: 2. Findings in neuropsychiatric disorders. *Mol Psychiatry,* Vol.10, No.2, (Feb 2005), pp. 160-184.

Giedke, H. & Schwarzler, F. (2002). Therapeutic use of sleep deprivation in depression. *Sleep Med Rev,* Vol.6, No.5, (Oct 2002), pp. 361-377.

Gil, K., Radzillowicz, P., Zdrojewski, T., Pakalska-Korcala, A., Chwojnicki, K., Piwonski, J., Ignaszewska-Wyrzykowska, A., Zaluga, L., Mielczarek, M., Landowski, J. & Wyrzykowski, B. (2006). Relationship between the prevalence of depressive symptoms and metabolic syndrome. Results of the SOPKARD Project. *Kardiol Pol,* Vol.64, No.5, (May 2006), pp. 464-469.

Goldman, N., Glei, D.A., Lin, Y.H. & Weinstein, M. (2010). The serotonin transporter polymorphism (5-HTTLPR): allelic variation and links with depressive symptoms. *Depress Anxiety,* Vol.27, No.3, (Mar 2010), pp. 260-269.

Goldney, R.D., Fisher, L.J. & Hawthorne, G. (2004). Depression and the CIDI. *Br J Psychiatry,* Vol.185, (Dec 2004), pp. 518-519.

Goodnick, P.J., Henry, J.H. & Buki, V.M. (1995). Treatment of depression in patients with diabetes mellitus. *J Clin Psychiatry,* Vol.56, No.4, (Apr 1995), pp. 128-136.

Goodwin, F.K. & Bunney, W.E., Jr. (1971). Depressions following reserpine: a reevaluation. *Semin Psychiatry,* Vol.3, No.4, (Nov 1971), pp. 435-448.

Gratacos, M., Gonzalez, J.R., Mercader, J.M., de Cid, R., Urretavizcaya, M. & Estivill, X. (2007). Brain-derived neurotrophic factor Val66Met and psychiatric disorders: meta-analysis of case-control studies confirm association to substance-related disorders, eating disorders, and schizophrenia. *Biol Psychiatry,* Vol.61, No.7, (Apr 1 2007), pp. 911-922.

Gratacos, M., Soria, V., Urretavizcaya, M., Gonzalez, J.R., Crespo, J.M., Bayes, M., de Cid, R., Menchon, J.M., Vallejo, J. & Estivill, X. (2008). A brain-derived neurotrophic factor

(BDNF) haplotype is associated with antidepressant treatment outcome in mood disorders. *Pharmacogenomics J*, Vol.8, No.2, (Apr 2008), pp. 101-112.

Griebel, G., Simiand, J., Serradeil-Le Gal, C., Wagnon, J., Pascal, M., Scatton, B., Maffrand, J.P. & Soubrie, P. (2002). Anxiolytic- and antidepressant-like effects of the non-peptide vasopressin V1b receptor antagonist, SSR149415, suggest an innovative approach for the treatment of stress-related disorders. *Proc Natl Acad Sci U S A*, Vol.99, No.9, (Apr 30 2002), pp. 6370-6375.

Gross, C., Zhuang, X., Stark, K., Ramboz, S., Oosting, R., Kirby, L., Santarelli, L., Beck, S. & Hen, R. (2002). Serotonin1A receptor acts during development to establish normal anxiety-like behaviour in the adult. *Nature*, Vol.416, No.6879, (Mar 28 2002), pp. 396-400.

Guiard, B.P., Przybylski, C., Guilloux, J.P., Seif, I., Froger, N., De Felipe, C., Hunt, S.P., Lanfumey, L. & Gardier, A.M. (2004). Blockade of substance P (neurokinin 1) receptors enhances extracellular serotonin when combined with a selective serotonin reuptake inhibitor: an in vivo microdialysis study in mice. *J Neurochem*, Vol.89, No.1, (Apr 2004), pp. 54-63.

Hajek, T., Kozeny, J., Kopecek, M., Alda, M. & Hoschl, C. (2008). Reduced subgenual cingulate volumes in mood disorders: a meta-analysis. *J Psychiatry Neurosci*, Vol.33, No.2, (Mar 2008), pp. 91-99.

Harbuz, M.S., Stephanou, A., Sarlis, N. & Lightman, S.L. (1992). The effects of recombinant human interleukin (IL)-1 alpha, IL-1 beta or IL-6 on hypothalamo-pituitary-adrenal axis activation. *J Endocrinol*, Vol.133, No.3, (Jun 1992), pp. 349-355.

Hariri, A.R., Mattay, V.S., Tessitore, A., Kolachana, B., Fera, F., Goldman, D., Egan, M.F. & Weinberger, D.R. (2002). Serotonin transporter genetic variation and the response of the human amygdala. *Science*, Vol.297, No.5580, (Jul 19 2002), pp. 400-403.

Heim, C. & Nemeroff, C.B. (2001). The role of childhood trauma in the neurobiology of mood and anxiety disorders: preclinical and clinical studies. *Biol Psychiatry*, Vol.49, No.12, (Jun 15 2001), pp. 1023-1039.

Heim, C., Newport, D.J., Wagner, D., Wilcox, M.M., Miller, A.H. & Nemeroff, C.B. (2002). The role of early adverse experience and adulthood stress in the prediction of neuroendocrine stress reactivity in women: a multiple regression analysis. *Depress Anxiety*, Vol.15, No.3, 2002), pp. 117-125.

Heiman, M.L., Ahima, R.S., Craft, L.S., Schoner, B., Stephens, T.W. & Flier, J.S. (1997). Leptin inhibition of the hypothalamic-pituitary-adrenal axis in response to stress. *Endocrinology*, Vol.138, No.9, (Sep 1997), pp. 3859-3863.

Hein, M.D. & Jackson, I.M. (1990). Review: thyroid function in psychiatric illness. *Gen Hosp Psychiatry*, Vol.12, No.4, (Jul 1990), pp. 232-244.

Herbert, J., Goodyer, I.M., Grossman, A.B., Hastings, M.H., de Kloet, E.R., Lightman, S.L., Lupien, S.J., Roozendaal, B. & Seckl, J.R. (2006). Do corticosteroids damage the brain? *J Neuroendocrinol*, Vol.18, No.6, (Jun 2006), pp. 393-411.

Hohagen, F., Rink, K., Kappler, C., Schramm, E., Riemann, D., Weyerer, S. & Berger, M. (1993). Prevalence and treatment of insomnia in general practice. A longitudinal study. *Eur Arch Psychiatry Clin Neurosci*, Vol.242, No.6, 1993), pp. 329-336.

Holmes, A., Heilig, M., Rupniak, N.M., Steckler, T. & Griebel, G. (2003). Neuropeptide systems as novel therapeutic targets for depression and anxiety disorders. *Trends Pharmacol Sci*, Vol.24, No.11, (Nov 2003), pp. 580-588.

Holsboer, F. (2000). The stress hormone system is back on the map. *Curr Psychiatry Rep,* Vol.2, No.6, (Dec 2000), pp. 454-456.

Hong, C.J., Chen, T.J., Yu, Y.W. & Tsai, S.J. (2006). Response to fluoxetine and serotonin 1A receptor (C-1019G) polymorphism in Taiwan Chinese major depressive disorder. *Pharmacogenomics J,* Vol.6, No.1, (Jan-Feb 2006), pp. 27-33.

Horacek, J., Kuzmiakova, M., Hoschl, C., Andel, M. & Bahbonh, R. (1999). The relationship between central serotonergic activity and insulin sensitivity in healthy volunteers. *Psychoneuroendocrinology,* Vol.24, No.8, (Nov 1999), pp. 785-797.

Hu, X.Z., Rush, A.J., Charney, D., Wilson, A.F., Sorant, A.J., Papanicolaou, G.J., Fava, M., Trivedi, M.H., Wisniewski, S.R., Laje, G., Paddock, S., McMahon, F.J., Manji, H. & Lipsky, R.H. (2007). Association between a functional serotonin transporter promoter polymorphism and citalopram treatment in adult outpatients with major depression. *Arch Gen Psychiatry,* Vol.64, No.7, (Jul 2007), pp. 783-792.

Huang, Q., Rivest, R. & Richard, D. (1998). Effects of leptin on corticotropin-releasing factor (CRF) synthesis and CRF neuron activation in the paraventricular hypothalamic nucleus of obese (ob/ob) mice. *Endocrinology,* Vol.139, No.4, (Apr 1998), pp. 1524-1532.

Iga, J., Ueno, S. & Ohmori, T. (2008). Molecular assessment of depression from mRNAs in the peripheral leukocytes. *Ann Med,* Vol.40, No.5, 2008), pp. 336-342.

Irie, M., Miyata, M. & Kasai, H. (2005). Depression and possible cancer risk due to oxidative DNA damage. *J Psychiatr Res,* Vol.39, No.6, (Nov 2005), pp. 553-560.

Irwin, M., Patterson, T., Smith, T.L., Caldwell, C., Brown, S.A., Gillin, J.C. & Grant, I. (1990). Reduction of immune function in life stress and depression. *Biol Psychiatry,* Vol.27, No.1, (Jan 1 1990), pp. 22-30.

Ising, M., Horstmann, S., Kloiber, S., Lucae, S., Binder, E.B., Kern, N., Kunzel, H.E., Pfennig, A., Uhr, M. & Holsboer, F. (2007). Combined dexamethasone/corticotropin releasing hormone test predicts treatment response in major depression - a potential biomarker? *Biol Psychiatry,* Vol.62, No.1, (Jul 1 2007), pp. 47-54.

Ising, M., Kunzel, H.E., Binder, E.B., Nickel, T., Modell, S. & Holsboer, F. (2005). The combined dexamethasone/CRH test as a potential surrogate marker in depression. *Prog Neuropsychopharmacol Biol Psychiatry,* Vol.29, No.6, (Jul 2005), pp. 1085-1093.

Jackson, I.M. (1998). The thyroid axis and depression. *Thyroid,* Vol.8, No.10, (Oct 1998), pp. 951-956.

Jow, G.M., Yang, T.T. & Chen, C.L. (2006). Leptin and cholesterol levels are low in major depressive disorder, but high in schizophrenia. *J Affect Disord,* Vol.90, No.1, (Jan 2006), pp. 21-27.

Kafka, M.S., Wirz-Justice, A., Naber, D., Moore, R.Y. & Benedito, M.A. (1983). Circadian rhythms in rat brain neurotransmitter receptors. *Fed Proc,* Vol.42, No.11, (Aug 1983), pp. 2796-2801.

Kask, A., Harro, J., von Horsten, S., Redrobe, J.P., Dumont, Y. & Quirion, R. (2002). The neurocircuitry and receptor subtypes mediating anxiolytic-like effects of neuropeptide Y. *Neurosci Biobehav Rev,* Vol.26, No.3, (May 2002), pp. 259-283.

Kato, M., Fukuda, T., Wakeno, M., Okugawa, G., Takekita, Y., Watanabe, S., Yamashita, M., Hosoi, Y., Azuma, J., Kinoshita, T. & Serretti, A. (2009). Effect of 5-HT1A gene polymorphisms on antidepressant response in major depressive disorder. *Am J Med Genet B Neuropsychiatr Genet,* Vol.150B, No.1, (Jan 5 2009), pp. 115-123.

Kato, M. & Serretti, A. (2010). Review and meta-analysis of antidepressant pharmacogenetic findings in major depressive disorder. *Mol Psychiatry,* Vol.15, No.5, (May 2010), pp. 473-500.

Kelsoe, J.R., (2004). Mood disorders: Genetics, in: Sadock, BJ, Sadock, VA (Eds.), *Kaplan and Sadock's Comprehensive Textbook of Psychiatry*. Lippincott Williams & Wilkins, pp. 1582-1594 %@ 0781734347 %0781734347 Eighth.

Kendler, K.S., Kuhn, J.W., Vittum, J., Prescott, C.A. & Riley, B. (2005). The interaction of stressful life events and a serotonin transporter polymorphism in the prediction of episodes of major depression: a replication. *Arch Gen Psychiatry,* Vol.62, No.5, (May 2005), pp. 529-535.

Kendler, K.S., Neale, M.C., Kessler, R.C., Heath, A.C. & Eaves, L.J. (1993). A longitudinal twin study of 1-year prevalence of major depression in women. *Arch Gen Psychiatry,* Vol.50, No.11, (Nov 1993), pp. 843-852.

Kessler, R.C., Chiu, W.T., Demler, O., Merikangas, K.R. & Walters, E.E. (2005). Prevalence, severity, and comorbidity of 12-month DSM-IV disorders in the National Comorbidity Survey Replication. *Arch Gen Psychiatry,* Vol.62, No.6, (Jun 2005), pp. 617-627.

Kiecolt-Glaser, J.K., Fisher, L.D., Ogrocki, P., Stout, J.C., Speicher, C.E. & Glaser, R. (1987). Marital quality, marital disruption, and immune function. *Psychosom Med,* Vol.49, No.1, (Jan-Feb 1987), pp. 13-34.

Kiecolt-Glaser, J.K., Marucha, P.T., Malarkey, W.B., Mercado, A.M. & Glaser, R. (1995). Slowing of wound healing by psychological stress. *Lancet,* Vol.346, No.8984, (Nov 4 1995), pp. 1194-1196.

Kientsch, U., Burgi, S., Ruedeberg, C., Probst, S. & Honegger, U.E. (2001). St. John's wort extract Ze 117 (Hypericum perforatum) inhibits norepinephrine and serotonin uptake into rat brain slices and reduces 3-adrenoceptor numbers on cultured rat brain cells. *Pharmacopsychiatry,* Vol.34 Suppl 1, (Jul 2001), pp. S56-60.

Kinder, L.S., Carnethon, M.R., Palaniappan, L.P., King, A.C. & Fortmann, S.P. (2004). Depression and the metabolic syndrome in young adults: findings from the Third National Health and Nutrition Examination Survey. *Psychosom Med,* Vol.66, No.3, (May-Jun 2004), pp. 316-322.

Kirkegaard, C. & Faber, J. (1991). Free thyroxine and 3,3',5'-triiodothyronine levels in cerebrospinal fluid in patients with endogenous depression. *Acta Endocrinol (Copenh),* Vol.124, No.2, (Feb 1991), pp. 166-172.

Koolschijn, P.C., van Haren, N.E., Lensvelt-Mulders, G.J., Hulshoff Pol, H.E. & Kahn, R.S. (2009). Brain volume abnormalities in major depressive disorder: a meta-analysis of magnetic resonance imaging studies. *Hum Brain Mapp,* Vol.30, No.11, (Nov 2009), pp. 3719-3735.

Koslow, S.H., Stokes, P.E., Mendels, J., Ramsey, A. & Casper, R. (1982). Insulin tolerance test: human growth hormone response and insulin resistance in primary unipolar depressed, bipolar depressed and control subjects. *Psychol Med,* Vol.12, No.1, (Feb 1982), pp. 45-55.

Kraft, J.B., Peters, E.J., Slager, S.L., Jenkins, G.D., Reinalda, M.S., McGrath, P.J. & Hamilton, S.P. (2007). Analysis of association between the serotonin transporter and antidepressant response in a large clinical sample. *Biol Psychiatry,* Vol.61, No.6, (Mar 15 2007), pp. 734-742.

Kraus, T., Haack, M., Schuld, A., Hinze-Selch, D. & Pollmacher, T. (2001). Low leptin levels but normal body mass indices in patients with depression or schizophrenia. *Neuroendocrinology,* Vol.73, No.4, (Apr 2001), pp. 243-247.

Krishnan, V. & Nestler, E.J. (2008). The molecular neurobiology of depression. *Nature,* Vol.455, No.7215, (Oct 16 2008), pp. 894-902.

Kronmuller, K.T., Pantel, J., Kohler, S., Victor, D., Giesel, F., Magnotta, V.A., Mundt, C., Essig, M. & Schroder, J. (2008). Hippocampal volume and 2-year outcome in depression. *Br J Psychiatry,* Vol.192, No.6, (Jun 2008), pp. 472-473.

Kunzel, H.E., Binder, E.B., Nickel, T., Ising, M., Fuchs, B., Majer, M., Pfennig, A., Ernst, G., Kern, N., Schmid, D.A., Uhr, M., Holsboer, F. & Modell, S. (2003). Pharmacological and nonpharmacological factors influencing hypothalamic-pituitary-adrenocortical axis reactivity in acutely depressed psychiatric in-patients, measured by the Dex-CRH test. *Neuropsychopharmacology,* Vol.28, No.12, (Dec 2003), pp. 2169-2178.

Ladd, C.O., Owens, M.J. & Nemeroff, C.B. (1996). Persistent changes in corticotropin-releasing factor neuronal systems induced by maternal deprivation. *Endocrinology,* Vol.137, No.4, (Apr 1996), pp. 1212-1218.

Laje, G., Allen, A.S., Akula, N., Manji, H., John Rush, A. & McMahon, F.J. (2009). Genome-wide association study of suicidal ideation emerging during citalopram treatment of depressed outpatients. *Pharmacogenet Genomics,* Vol.19, No.9, (Sep 2009), pp. 666-674.

Laje, G., Paddock, S., Manji, H., Rush, A.J., Wilson, A.F., Charney, D. & McMahon, F.J. (2007). Genetic markers of suicidal ideation emerging during citalopram treatment of major depression. *Am J Psychiatry,* Vol.164, No.10, (Oct 2007), pp. 1530-1538.

Lam, R.W. (2006). Sleep disturbances and depression: a challenge for antidepressants. *Int Clin Psychopharmacol,* Vol.21 Suppl 1, (Feb 2006), pp. S25-29.

Lasky-Su, J.A., Faraone, S.V., Glatt, S.J. & Tsuang, M.T. (2005). Meta-analysis of the association between two polymorphisms in the serotonin transporter gene and affective disorders. *Am J Med Genet B Neuropsychiatr Genet,* Vol.133B, No.1, (Feb 5 2005), pp. 110-115.

Lekman, M., Laje, G., Charney, D., Rush, A.J., Wilson, A.F., Sorant, A.J., Lipsky, R., Wisniewski, S.R., Manji, H., McMahon, F.J. & Paddock, S. (2008a). The FKBP5-gene in depression and treatment response--an association study in the Sequenced Treatment Alternatives to Relieve Depression (STAR*D) Cohort. *Biol Psychiatry,* Vol.63, No.12, (Jun 15 2008a), pp. 1103-1110.

Lekman, M., Paddock, S. & McMahon, F.J. (2008b). Pharmacogenetics of major depression: insights from level 1 of the Sequenced Treatment Alternatives to Relieve Depression (STAR*D) trial. *Mol Diagn Ther,* Vol.12, No.5, 2008b), pp. 321-330.

Lemonde, S., Du, L., Bakish, D., Hrdina, P. & Albert, P.R. (2004). Association of the C(-1019)G 5-HT1A functional promoter polymorphism with antidepressant response. *Int J Neuropsychopharmacol,* Vol.7, No.4, (Dec 2004), pp. 501-506.

Leonard, B.E. (1988). Stress, the immune system and psychiatric illness. *Stress Medicine,* Vol.4, No.4, 1988), pp. 207-213 %U http://onlinelibrary.wiley.com/doi/210.1002/smi.2460040405/abstract.

Lesch, K.P. (2004). Gene-environment interaction and the genetics of depression. *J Psychiatry Neurosci,* Vol.29, No.3, (May 2004), pp. 174-184.

Lesch, K.P., Bengel, D., Heils, A., Sabol, S.Z., Greenberg, B.D., Petri, S., Benjamin, J., Muller, C.R., Hamer, D.H. & Murphy, D.L. (1996). Association of anxiety-related traits with a polymorphism in the serotonin transporter gene regulatory region. *Science,* Vol.274, No.5292, (Nov 29 1996), pp. 1527-1531.

Leuchter, A.F., Cook, I.A., Gilmer, W.S., Marangell, L.B., Burgoyne, K.S., Howland, R.H., Trivedi, M.H., Zisook, S., Jain, R., Fava, M., Iosifescu, D. & Greenwald, S. (2009a). Effectiveness of a quantitative electroencephalographic biomarker for predicting differential response or remission with escitalopram and bupropion in major depressive disorder. *Psychiatry Res,* Vol.169, No.2, (Sep 30 2009a), pp. 132-138.

Leuchter, A.F., Cook, I.A., Marangell, L.B., Gilmer, W.S., Burgoyne, K.S., Howland, R.H., Trivedi, M.H., Zisook, S., Jain, R., McCracken, J.T., Fava, M., Iosifescu, D. & Greenwald, S. (2009b). Comparative effectiveness of biomarkers and clinical indicators for predicting outcomes of SSRI treatment in Major Depressive Disorder: results of the BRITE-MD study. *Psychiatry Res,* Vol.169, No.2, (Sep 30 2009b), pp. 124-131.

Leuchter, A.F., Uijtdehaage, S.H., Cook, I.A., O'Hara, R. & Mandelkern, M. (1999). Relationship between brain electrical activity and cortical perfusion in normal subjects. *Psychiatry Res,* Vol.90, No.2, (Apr 26 1999), pp. 125-140.

Levinson, D.F. (2006). The genetics of depression: a review. *Biol Psychiatry,* Vol.60, No.2, (Jul 15 2006), pp. 84-92.

Lin, E. & Chen, P.S. (2008). Pharmacogenomics with antidepressants in the STAR*D study. *Pharmacogenomics,* Vol.9, No.7, (Jul 2008), pp. 935-946.

Lin, P.Y. & Tsai, G. (2004). Association between serotonin transporter gene promoter polymorphism and suicide: results of a meta-analysis. *Biol Psychiatry,* Vol.55, No.10, (May 15 2004), pp. 1023-1030.

Lindley, T.E., Infanger, D.W., Rishniw, M., Zhou, Y., Doobay, M.F., Sharma, R.V. & Davisson, R.L. (2009). Scavenging superoxide selectively in mouse forebrain is associated with improved cardiac function and survival following myocardial infarction. *Am J Physiol Regul Integr Comp Physiol,* Vol.296, No.1, (Jan 2009), pp. R1-8.

Liu, D., Diorio, J., Tannenbaum, B., Caldji, C., Francis, D., Freedman, A., Sharma, S., Pearson, D., Plotsky, P.M. & Meaney, M.J. (1997). Maternal care, hippocampal glucocorticoid receptors, and hypothalamic-pituitary-adrenal responses to stress. *Science,* Vol.277, No.5332, (Sep 12 1997), pp. 1659-1662.

Lohoff, F.W. (2010). Overview of the genetics of major depressive disorder. *Curr Psychiatry Rep,* Vol.12, No.6, (Dec 2010), pp. 539-546.

Lopez-Leon, S., Janssens, A.C., Gonzalez-Zuloeta Ladd, A.M., Del-Favero, J., Claes, S.J., Oostra, B.A. & van Duijn, C.M. (2008). Meta-analyses of genetic studies on major depressive disorder. *Mol Psychiatry,* Vol.13, No.8, (Aug 2008), pp. 772-785.

Lopez, V.A., Detera-Wadleigh, S., Cardona, I., Kassem, L. & McMahon, F.J. (2007). Nested association between genetic variation in tryptophan hydroxylase II, bipolar affective disorder, and suicide attempts. *Biol Psychiatry,* Vol.61, No.2, (Jan 15 2007), pp. 181-186.

Lu, X., Lundstrom, L., Langel, U. & Bartfai, T. (2005). Galanin receptor ligands. *Neuropeptides,* Vol.39, No.3, (Jun 2005), pp. 143-146.

Lu, X.Y., Kim, C.S., Frazer, A. & Zhang, W. (2006). Leptin: a potential novel antidepressant. *Proc Natl Acad Sci U S A,* Vol.103, No.5, (Jan 31 2006), pp. 1593-1598.

Lucae, S., Salyakina, D., Barden, N., Harvey, M., Gagne, B., Labbe, M., Binder, E.B., Uhr, M., Paez-Pereda, M., Sillaber, I., Ising, M., Bruckl, T., Lieb, R., Holsboer, F. & Muller-Myhsok, B. (2006). P2RX7, a gene coding for a purinergic ligand-gated ion channel, is associated with major depressive disorder. *Hum Mol Genet,* Vol.15, No.16, (Aug 15 2006), pp. 2438-2445.

Luquet, S., Perez, F.A., Hnasko, T.S. & Palmiter, R.D. (2005). NPY/AgRP neurons are essential for feeding in adult mice but can be ablated in neonates. *Science,* Vol.310, No.5748, (Oct 28 2005), pp. 683-685.

MacQueen, G.M., Campbell, S., McEwen, B.S., Macdonald, K., Amano, S., Joffe, R.T., Nahmias, C. & Young, L.T. (2003). Course of illness, hippocampal function, and hippocampal volume in major depression. *Proc Natl Acad Sci U S A,* Vol.100, No.3, (Feb 4 2003), pp. 1387-1392.

MacQueen, G.M., Yucel, K., Taylor, V.H., Macdonald, K. & Joffe, R. (2008). Posterior hippocampal volumes are associated with remission rates in patients with major depressive disorder. *Biol Psychiatry,* Vol.64, No.10, (Nov 15 2008), pp. 880-883.

Maes, M. (1995). Evidence for an immune response in major depression: a review and hypothesis. *Prog Neuropsychopharmacol Biol Psychiatry,* Vol.19, No.1, (Jan 1995), pp. 11-38.

Maes, M., Vandewoude, M., Schotte, C., Martin, M., Blockx, P., Scharpe, S. & Cosyns, P. (1989). Hypothalamic-pituitary-adrenal and -thyroid axis dysfunctions and decrements in the availability of L-tryptophan as biological markers of suicidal ideation in major depressed females. *Acta Psychiatr Scand,* Vol.80, No.1, (Jul 1989), pp. 13-17.

Manji, H.K., Drevets, W.C. & Charney, D.S. (2001). The cellular neurobiology of depression. *Nat Med,* Vol.7, No.5, (May 2001), pp. 541-547.

Manji, H.K., Quiroz, J.A., Sporn, J., Payne, J.L., Denicoff, K., N, A.G., Zarate, C.A., Jr. & Charney, D.S. (2003). Enhancing neuronal plasticity and cellular resilience to develop novel, improved therapeutics for difficult-to-treat depression. *Biol Psychiatry,* Vol.53, No.8, (Apr 15 2003), pp. 707-742.

Mann, J.J. & Currier, D. (2006). Effects of genes and stress on the neurobiology of depression. *Int Rev Neurobiol,* Vol.73, 2006), pp. 153-189.

Mannisto, P.T. & Kaakkola, S. (1999). Catechol-O-methyltransferase (COMT): biochemistry, molecular biology, pharmacology, and clinical efficacy of the new selective COMT inhibitors. *Pharmacol Rev,* Vol.51, No.4, (Dec 1999), pp. 593-628.

Matthews, S.C., Strigo, I.A., Simmons, A.N., Yang, T.T. & Paulus, M.P. (2008). Decreased functional coupling of the amygdala and supragenual cingulate is related to increased depression in unmedicated individuals with current major depressive disorder. *J Affect Disord,* Vol.111, No.1, (Nov 2008), pp. 13-20.

Maubach, K.A., Martin, K., Chicchi, G., Harrison, T., Wheeldon, A., Swain, C.J., Cumberbatch, M.J., Rupniak, N.M. & Seabrook, G.R. (2002). Chronic substance P (NK1) receptor antagonist and conventional antidepressant treatment increases burst firing of monoamine neurones in the locus coeruleus. *Neuroscience,* Vol.109, No.3, 2002), pp. 609-617.

Mayberg, H.S. (1997). Limbic-cortical dysregulation: a proposed model of depression. *J Neuropsychiatry Clin Neurosci,* Vol.9, No.3, (Summer 1997), pp. 471-481.

Mayberg, H.S. (2003). Modulating dysfunctional limbic-cortical circuits in depression: towards development of brain-based algorithms for diagnosis and optimised treatment. *Br Med Bull,* Vol.65, 2003), pp. 193-207.

McCaffery, J.M., Niaura, R., Todaro, J.F., Swan, G.E. & Carmelli, D. (2003). Depressive symptoms and metabolic risk in adult male twins enrolled in the National Heart, Lung, and Blood Institute twin study. *Psychosom Med,* Vol.65, No.3, (May-Jun 2003), pp. 490-497.

McCauley, J., Kern, D.E., Kolodner, K., Dill, L., Schroeder, A.F., DeChant, H.K., Ryden, J., Derogatis, L.R. & Bass, E.B. (1997). Clinical characteristics of women with a history of childhood abuse: unhealed wounds. *JAMA,* Vol.277, No.17, (May 7 1997), pp. 1362-1368.

McClung, C.A. (2007). Circadian genes, rhythms and the biology of mood disorders. *Pharmacol Ther,* Vol.114, No.2, (May 2007), pp. 222-232.

McClung, C.A., Sidiropoulou, K., Vitaterna, M., Takahashi, J.S., White, F.J., Cooper, D.C. & Nestler, E.J. (2005). Regulation of dopaminergic transmission and cocaine reward by the Clock gene. *Proc Natl Acad Sci U S A,* Vol.102, No.26, (Jun 28 2005), pp. 9377-9381.

McGuffin, P., Knight, J., Breen, G., Brewster, S., Boyd, P.R., Craddock, N., Gill, M., Korszun, A., Maier, W., Middleton, L., Mors, O., Owen, M.J., Perry, J., Preisig, M., Reich, T., Rice, J., Rietschel, M., Jones, L., Sham, P. & Farmer, A.E. (2005). Whole genome linkage scan of recurrent depressive disorder from the depression network study. *Hum Mol Genet,* Vol.14, No.22, (Nov 15 2005), pp. 3337-3345.

McIntyre, R.S., Park, K.Y., Law, C.W., Sultan, F., Adams, A., Lourenco, M.T., Lo, A.K., Soczynska, J.K., Woldeyohannes, H., Alsuwaidan, M., Yoon, J. & Kennedy, S.H. (2010). The association between conventional antidepressants and the metabolic syndrome: a review of the evidence and clinical implications. *CNS Drugs,* Vol.24, No.9, (Sep 1 2010), pp. 741-753.

McKinnon, M.C., Yucel, K., Nazarov, A. & MacQueen, G.M. (2009). A meta-analysis examining clinical predictors of hippocampal volume in patients with major depressive disorder. *J Psychiatry Neurosci,* Vol.34, No.1, (Jan 2009), pp. 41-54.

McMahon, F.J., Buervenich, S., Charney, D., Lipsky, R., Rush, A.J., Wilson, A.F., Sorant, A.J., Papanicolaou, G.J., Laje, G., Fava, M., Trivedi, M.H., Wisniewski, S.R. & Manji, H. (2006). Variation in the gene encoding the serotonin 2A receptor is associated with outcome of antidepressant treatment. *Am J Hum Genet,* Vol.78, No.5, (May 2006), pp. 804-814.

Meaney, M.J. (2001). Maternal care, gene expression, and the transmission of individual differences in stress reactivity across generations. *Annu Rev Neurosci,* Vol.24, 2001), pp. 1161-1192.

Merali, Z., Lacosta, S. & Anisman, H. (1997). Effects of interleukin-1beta and mild stress on alterations of norepinephrine, dopamine and serotonin neurotransmission: a regional microdialysis study. *Brain Res,* Vol.761, No.2, (Jul 4 1997), pp. 225-235.

Meynen, G., Unmehopa, U.A., van Heerikhuize, J.J., Hofman, M.A., Swaab, D.F. & Hoogendijk, W.J. (2006). Increased arginine vasopressin mRNA expression in the

human hypothalamus in depression: A preliminary report. *Biol Psychiatry,* Vol.60, No.8, (Oct 15 2006), pp. 892-895.
Middeldorp, C.M., de Geus, E.J., Willemsen, G., Hottenga, J.J., Slagboom, P.E. & Boomsma, D.I. (2010). The serotonin transporter gene length polymorphism (5-HTTLPR) and life events: no evidence for an interaction effect on neuroticism and anxious depressive symptoms. *Twin Res Hum Genet,* Vol.13, No.6, (Dec 2010), pp. 544-549.
Mill, J. & Petronis, A. (2007). Molecular studies of major depressive disorder: the epigenetic perspective. *Mol Psychiatry,* Vol.12, No.9, (Sep 2007), pp. 799-814.
Millan, M.J. (2011). MicroRNA in the regulation and expression of serotonergic transmission in the brain and other tissues. *Curr Opin Pharmacol,* Vol.11, No.1, (Feb 2011), pp. 11-22.
Moller, D.E. (2000). Potential role of TNF-alpha in the pathogenesis of insulin resistance and type 2 diabetes. *Trends Endocrinol Metab,* Vol.11, No.6, (Aug 2000), pp. 212-217.
Morikawa, O., Sakai, N., Obara, H. & Saito, N. (1998). Effects of interferon-alpha, interferon-gamma and cAMP on the transcriptional regulation of the serotonin transporter. *Eur J Pharmacol,* Vol.349, No.2-3, (May 22 1998), pp. 317-324.
Mossner, R., Daniel, S., Schmitt, A., Albert, D. & Lesch, K.P. (2001). Modulation of serotonin transporter function by interleukin-4. *Life Sci,* Vol.68, No.8, (Jan 12 2001), pp. 873-880.
Mossner, R. & Lesch, K.P. (1998). Role of serotonin in the immune system and in neuroimmune interactions. *Brain Behav Immun,* Vol.12, No.4, (Dec 1998), pp. 249-271.
Munafo, M.R. & Flint, J. (2009). Replication and heterogeneity in gene x environment interaction studies. *Int J Neuropsychopharmacol,* Vol.12, No.6, (Jul 2009), pp. 727-729.
Murphy, G.M., Jr., Hollander, S.B., Rodrigues, H.E., Kremer, C. & Schatzberg, A.F. (2004). Effects of the serotonin transporter gene promoter polymorphism on mirtazapine and paroxetine efficacy and adverse events in geriatric major depression. *Arch Gen Psychiatry,* Vol.61, No.11, (Nov 2004), pp. 1163-1169.
Nakagawa, S., Kim, J.E., Lee, R., Chen, J., Fujioka, T., Malberg, J., Tsuji, S. & Duman, R.S. (2002a). Localization of phosphorylated cAMP response element-binding protein in immature neurons of adult hippocampus. *J Neurosci,* Vol.22, No.22, (Nov 15 2002a), pp. 9868-9876.
Nakagawa, S., Kim, J.E., Lee, R., Malberg, J.E., Chen, J., Steffen, C., Zhang, Y.J., Nestler, E.J. & Duman, R.S. (2002b). Regulation of neurogenesis in adult mouse hippocampus by cAMP and the cAMP response element-binding protein. *J Neurosci,* Vol.22, No.9, (May 1 2002b), pp. 3673-3682.
Nathan, C.F. (1987). Secretory products of macrophages. *J Clin Invest,* Vol.79, No.2, (Feb 1987), pp. 319-326.
Nemeroff, C.B. & Vale, W.W. (2005). The neurobiology of depression: inroads to treatment and new drug discovery. *J Clin Psychiatry,* Vol.66 Suppl 7, 2005), pp. 5-13.
Nestler, E.J. (1998). Antidepressant treatments in the 21st century. *Biol Psychiatry,* Vol.44, No.7, (Oct 1 1998), pp. 526-533.
Nestler, E.J., Barrot, M., DiLeone, R.J., Eisch, A.J., Gold, S.J. & Monteggia, L.M. (2002). Neurobiology of depression. *Neuron,* Vol.34, No.1, (Mar 28 2002), pp. 13-25.
Nestler, E.J. & Carlezon, W.A., Jr. (2006). The mesolimbic dopamine reward circuit in depression. *Biol Psychiatry,* Vol.59, No.12, (Jun 15 2006), pp. 1151-1159.

Nestler, E.J. & Hyman, S.E. (2010). Animal models of neuropsychiatric disorders. *Nat Neurosci*, Vol.13, No.10, (Oct 2010), pp. 1161-1169.

O'Rahilly, S. (2002). Leptin: defining its role in humans by the clinical study of genetic disorders. *Nutr Rev*, Vol.60, No.10 Pt 2, (Oct 2002), pp. S30-34; discussion S68-84, 85-37.

Ogren, S.O., Kuteeva, E., Hokfelt, T. & Kehr, J. (2006). Galanin receptor antagonists : a potential novel pharmacological treatment for mood disorders. *CNS Drugs*, Vol.20, No.8, 2006), pp. 633-654.

Okamura, F., Tashiro, A., Utumi, A., Imai, T., Suchi, T., Tamura, D., Sato, Y., Suzuki, S. & Hongo, M. (2000). Insulin resistance in patients with depression and its changes during the clinical course of depression: minimal model analysis. *Metabolism*, Vol.49, No.10, (Oct 2000), pp. 1255-1260.

Olff, M. (1999). Stress, depression and immunity: the role of defense and coping styles. *Psychiatry Res*, Vol.85, No.1, (Jan 18 1999), pp. 7-15.

Ongur, D., Drevets, W.C. & Price, J.L. (1998). Glial reduction in the subgenual prefrontal cortex in mood disorders. *Proc Natl Acad Sci U S A*, Vol.95, No.22, (Oct 27 1998), pp. 13290-13295.

Overstreet, D.H. & Griebel, G. (2005). Antidepressant-like effects of the vasopressin V1b receptor antagonist SSR149415 in the Flinders Sensitive Line rat. *Pharmacol Biochem Behav*, Vol.82, No.1, (Sep 2005), pp. 223-227.

Paddock, S. (2008). Genetic variation in GRIK4 and the implications for antidepressant treatment. *Pharmacogenomics*, Vol.9, No.2, (Feb 2008), pp. 133-135.

Pagnin, D., de Queiroz, V., Pini, S. & Cassano, G.B. (2004). Efficacy of ECT in depression: a meta-analytic review. *J ECT*, Vol.20, No.1, (Mar 2004), pp. 13-20.

Paile-Hyvarinen, M., Raikkonen, K., Forsen, T., Kajantie, E., Yliharsila, H., Salonen, M.K., Osmond, C. & Eriksson, J.G. (2007). Depression and its association with diabetes, cardiovascular disease, and birth weight. *Ann Med*, Vol.39, No.8, 2007), pp. 634-640.

Papanicolaou, D.A., Wilder, R.L., Manolagas, S.C. & Chrousos, G.P. (1998). The pathophysiologic roles of interleukin-6 in human disease. *Ann Intern Med*, Vol.128, No.2, (Jan 15 1998), pp. 127-137.

Papiol, S., Arias, B., Gasto, C., Gutierrez, B., Catalan, R. & Fananas, L. (2007). Genetic variability at HPA axis in major depression and clinical response to antidepressant treatment. *J Affect Disord*, Vol.104, No.1-3, (Dec 2007), pp. 83-90.

Pecina, S., Smith, K.S. & Berridge, K.C. (2006). Hedonic hot spots in the brain. *Neuroscientist*, Vol.12, No.6, (Dec 2006), pp. 500-511.

Pencea, V., Bingaman, K.D., Wiegand, S.J. & Luskin, M.B. (2001). Infusion of brain-derived neurotrophic factor into the lateral ventricle of the adult rat leads to new neurons in the parenchyma of the striatum, septum, thalamus, and hypothalamus. *J Neurosci*, Vol.21, No.17, (Sep 1 2001), pp. 6706-6717.

Perlis, R.H., Moorjani, P., Fagerness, J., Purcell, S., Trivedi, M.H., Fava, M., Rush, A.J. & Smoller, J.W. (2008). Pharmacogenetic analysis of genes implicated in rodent models of antidepressant response: association of TREK1 and treatment resistance in the STAR(*)D study. *Neuropsychopharmacology*, Vol.33, No.12, (Nov 2008), pp. 2810-2819.

Perlis, R.H., Purcell, S., Fava, M., Fagerness, J., Rush, A.J., Trivedi, M.H. & Smoller, J.W. (2007). Association between treatment-emergent suicidal ideation with citalopram and polymorphisms near cyclic adenosine monophosphate response element binding protein in the STAR*D study. *Arch Gen Psychiatry,* Vol.64, No.6, (Jun 2007), pp. 689-697.

Peters, E.J., Slager, S.L., Kraft, J.B., Jenkins, G.D., Reinalda, M.S., McGrath, P.J. & Hamilton, S.P. (2008). Pharmacokinetic genes do not influence response or tolerance to citalopram in the STAR*D sample. *PLoS One,* Vol.3, No.4, 2008), pp. e1872.

Pezawas, L., Meyer-Lindenberg, A., Drabant, E.M., Verchinski, B.A., Munoz, K.E., Kolachana, B.S., Egan, M.F., Mattay, V.S., Hariri, A.R. & Weinberger, D.R. (2005). 5-HTTLPR polymorphism impacts human cingulate-amygdala interactions: a genetic susceptibility mechanism for depression. *Nat Neurosci,* Vol.8, No.6, (Jun 2005), pp. 828-834.

Pezawas, L., Meyer-Lindenberg, A., Goldman, A.L., Verchinski, B.A., Chen, G., Kolachana, B.S., Egan, M.F., Mattay, V.S., Hariri, A.R. & Weinberger, D.R. (2008). Evidence of biologic epistasis between BDNF and SLC6A4 and implications for depression. *Mol Psychiatry,* Vol.13, No.7, (Jul 2008), pp. 709-716.

Pineyro, G. & Blier, P. (1999). Autoregulation of serotonin neurons: role in antidepressant drug action. *Pharmacol Rev,* Vol.51, No.3, (Sep 1999), pp. 533-591.

Pizzagalli, D., Pascual-Marqui, R.D., Nitschke, J.B., Oakes, T.R., Larson, C.L., Abercrombie, H.C., Schaefer, S.M., Koger, J.V., Benca, R.M. & Davidson, R.J. (2001). Anterior cingulate activity as a predictor of degree of treatment response in major depression: evidence from brain electrical tomography analysis. *Am J Psychiatry,* Vol.158, No.3, (Mar 2001), pp. 405-415.

Porcelli, S., Drago, A., Fabbri, C., Gibiino, S., Calati, R. & Serretti, A. (2010). Pharmacogenetics of antidepressant response. *J Psychiatry Neurosci,* Vol.36, No.2, (Mar 2010), pp. 87-113.

Purba, J.S., Hoogendijk, W.J., Hofman, M.A. & Swaab, D.F. (1996). Increased number of vasopressin- and oxytocin-expressing neurons in the paraventricular nucleus of the hypothalamus in depression. *Arch Gen Psychiatry,* Vol.53, No.2, (Feb 1996), pp. 137-143.

Radcliffe, R.A., Lee, M.J. & Williams, R.W. (2006). Prediction of cis-QTLs in a pair of inbred mouse strains with the use of expression and haplotype data from public databases. *Mamm Genome,* Vol.17, No.6, (Jun 2006), pp. 629-642.

Raedler, T.J. & Wiedemann, K. (2006). CSF-studies in neuropsychiatric disorders. *Neuro Endocrinol Lett,* Vol.27, No.3, (Jun 2006), pp. 297-305.

Raikkonen, K., Matthews, K.A. & Kuller, L.H. (2007). Depressive symptoms and stressful life events predict metabolic syndrome among middle-aged women: a comparison of World Health Organization, Adult Treatment Panel III, and International Diabetes Foundation definitions. *Diabetes Care,* Vol.30, No.4, (Apr 2007), pp. 872-877.

Raison, C.L. & Miller, A.H. (2003). When not enough is too much: the role of insufficient glucocorticoid signaling in the pathophysiology of stress-related disorders. *Am J Psychiatry,* Vol.160, No.9, (Sep 2003), pp. 1554-1565.

Rajasethupathy, P., Fiumara, F., Sheridan, R., Betel, D., Puthanveettil, S.V., Russo, J.J., Sander, C., Tuschl, T. & Kandel, E. (2009). Characterization of small RNAs in

Aplysia reveals a role for miR-124 in constraining synaptic plasticity through CREB. *Neuron,* Vol.63, No.6, (Sep 24 2009), pp. 803-817.

Rajkowska, G. (2000). Postmortem studies in mood disorders indicate altered numbers of neurons and glial cells. *Biol Psychiatry,* Vol.48, No.8, (Oct 15 2000), pp. 766-777.

Rajkowska, G., Miguel-Hidalgo, J.J., Wei, J., Dilley, G., Pittman, S.D., Meltzer, H.Y., Overholser, J.C., Roth, B.L. & Stockmeier, C.A. (1999). Morphometric evidence for neuronal and glial prefrontal cell pathology in major depression. *Biol Psychiatry,* Vol.45, No.9, (May 1 1999), pp. 1085-1098.

Raju, T.N. (1998). The Nobel chronicles. 1927: Julius Wagner-Jauregg (1857-1940). *Lancet,* Vol.352, No.9141, (Nov 21 1998), pp. 1714.

Redrobe, J.P., Dumont, Y., Fournier, A. & Quirion, R. (2002). The neuropeptide Y (NPY) Y1 receptor subtype mediates NPY-induced antidepressant-like activity in the mouse forced swimming test. *Neuropsychopharmacology,* Vol.26, No.5, (May 2002), pp. 615-624.

Reiche, E.M., Morimoto, H.K. & Nunes, S.M. (2005). Stress and depression-induced immune dysfunction: implications for the development and progression of cancer. *Int Rev Psychiatry,* Vol.17, No.6, (Dec 2005), pp. 515-527.

Reichlin, S. (1993). Neuroendocrine-immune interactions. *N Engl J Med,* Vol.329, No.17, (Oct 21 1993), pp. 1246-1253.

Renthal, W., Maze, I., Krishnan, V., Covington, H.E., 3rd, Xiao, G., Kumar, A., Russo, S.J., Graham, A., Tsankova, N., Kippin, T.E., Kerstetter, K.A., Neve, R.L., Haggarty, S.J., McKinsey, T.A., Bassel-Duby, R., Olson, E.N. & Nestler, E.J. (2007). Histone deacetylase 5 epigenetically controls behavioral adaptations to chronic emotional stimuli. *Neuron,* Vol.56, No.3, (Nov 8 2007), pp. 517-529.

Riemann, D. (2007). Insomnia and comorbid psychiatric disorders. *Sleep Med,* Vol.8 Suppl 4, (Dec 2007), pp. S15-20.

Riemann, D., Berger, M. & Voderholzer, U. (2001). Sleep and depression--results from psychobiological studies: an overview. *Biol Psychol,* Vol.57, No.1-3, (Jul-Aug 2001), pp. 67-103.

Risch, N., Herrell, R., Lehner, T., Liang, K.Y., Eaves, L., Hoh, J., Griem, A., Kovacs, M., Ott, J. & Merikangas, K.R. (2009). Interaction between the serotonin transporter gene (5-HTTLPR), stressful life events, and risk of depression: a meta-analysis. *JAMA,* Vol.301, No.23, (Jun 17 2009), pp. 2462-2471.

Rizza, R.A., Mandarino, L.J. & Gerich, J.E. (1982). Cortisol-induced insulin resistance in man: impaired suppression of glucose production and stimulation of glucose utilization due to a postreceptor detect of insulin action. *J Clin Endocrinol Metab,* Vol.54, No.1, (Jan 1982), pp. 131-138.

Rosenkranz, J.A., Venheim, E.R. & Padival, M. (2010). Chronic stress causes amygdala hyperexcitability in rodents. *Biol Psychiatry,* Vol.67, No.12, (Jun 15 2010), pp. 1128-1136.

Rotzinger, S., Lovejoy, D.A. & Tan, L.A. (2010). Behavioral effects of neuropeptides in rodent models of depression and anxiety. *Peptides,* Vol.31, No.4, (Apr 2010), pp. 736-756.

Roybal, K., Theobold, D., Graham, A., DiNieri, J.A., Russo, S.J., Krishnan, V., Chakravarty, S., Peevey, J., Oehrlein, N., Birnbaum, S., Vitaterna, M.H., Orsulak, P., Takahashi, J.S., Nestler, E.J., Carlezon, W.A., Jr. & McClung, C.A. (2007). Mania-like behavior

induced by disruption of CLOCK. *Proc Natl Acad Sci U S A,* Vol.104, No.15, (Apr 10 2007), pp. 6406-6411.
Rubin, R.T., Heist, E.K., McGeoy, S.S., Hanada, K. & Lesser, I.M. (1992). Neuroendocrine aspects of primary endogenous depression. XI. Serum melatonin measures in patients and matched control subjects. *Arch Gen Psychiatry,* Vol.49, No.7, (Jul 1992), pp. 558-567.
Rubin, R.T., Rhodes, M.E. & Czambel, R.K. (2002). Sexual diergism of baseline plasma leptin and leptin suppression by arginine vasopressin in major depressives and matched controls. *Psychiatry Res,* Vol.113, No.3, (Dec 30 2002), pp. 255-268.
Sabol, S.Z., Hu, S. & Hamer, D. (1998). A functional polymorphism in the monoamine oxidase A gene promoter. *Hum Genet,* Vol.103, No.3, (Sep 1998), pp. 273-279.
Saletu, B., Anderer, P. & Saletu-Zyhlarz, G.M. (2010). EEG topography and tomography (LORETA) in diagnosis and pharmacotherapy of depression. *Clin EEG Neurosci,* Vol.41, No.4, (Oct 2010), pp. 203-210.
Salome, N., Stemmelin, J., Cohen, C. & Griebel, G. (2006). Differential roles of amygdaloid nuclei in the anxiolytic- and antidepressant-like effects of the V1b receptor antagonist, SSR149415, in rats. *Psychopharmacology (Berl),* Vol.187, No.2, (Aug 2006), pp. 237-244.
Santarelli, L., Gobbi, G., Debs, P.C., Sibille, E.T., Blier, P., Hen, R. & Heath, M.J. (2001). Genetic and pharmacological disruption of neurokinin 1 receptor function decreases anxiety-related behaviors and increases serotonergic function. *Proc Natl Acad Sci U S A,* Vol.98, No.4, (Feb 13 2001), pp. 1912-1917.
Santarelli, L., Saxe, M., Gross, C., Surget, A., Battaglia, F., Dulawa, S., Weisstaub, N., Lee, J., Duman, R., Arancio, O., Belzung, C. & Hen, R. (2003). Requirement of hippocampal neurogenesis for the behavioral effects of antidepressants. *Science,* Vol.301, No.5634, (Aug 8 2003), pp. 805-809.
Scharinger, C., Rabl, U., Sitte, H.H. & Pezawas, L. (2010). Imaging genetics of mood disorders. *Neuroimage,* Vol.53, No.3, (Nov 15 2010), pp. 810-821.
Schildkraut, J.J. (1965). The catecholamine hypothesis of affective disorders: a review of supporting evidence. *Am J Psychiatry,* Vol.122, No.5, (Nov 1965), pp. 509-522.
Schinka, J.A., Busch, R.M. & Robichaux-Keene, N. (2004). A meta-analysis of the association between the serotonin transporter gene polymorphism (5-HTTLPR) and trait anxiety. *Mol Psychiatry,* Vol.9, No.2, (Feb 2004), pp. 197-202.
Schule, C., Zill, P., Baghai, T.C., Eser, D., Zwanzger, P., Wenig, N., Rupprecht, R. & Bondy, B. (2006). Brain-derived neurotrophic factor Val66Met polymorphism and dexamethasone/CRH test results in depressed patients. *Psychoneuroendocrinology,* Vol.31, No.8, (Sep 2006), pp. 1019-1025.
Schwarz, M.J., Spath, M., Muller-Bardorff, H., Pongratz, D.E., Bondy, B. & Ackenheil, M. (1999). Relationship of substance P, 5-hydroxyindole acetic acid and tryptophan in serum of fibromyalgia patients. *Neurosci Lett,* Vol.259, No.3, (Jan 15 1999), pp. 196-198.
Scott, K.M., McGee, M.A., Wells, J.E. & Oakley Browne, M.A. (2008). Obesity and mental disorders in the adult general population. *J Psychosom Res,* Vol.64, No.1, (Jan 2008), pp. 97-105.
Sen, S., Burmeister, M. & Ghosh, D. (2004). Meta-analysis of the association between a serotonin transporter promoter polymorphism (5-HTTLPR) and anxiety-related

personality traits. *Am J Med Genet B Neuropsychiatr Genet,* Vol.127B, No.1, (May 15 2004), pp. 85-89.

Sen, S., Duman, R. & Sanacora, G. (2008). Serum brain-derived neurotrophic factor, depression, and antidepressant medications: meta-analyses and implications. *Biol Psychiatry,* Vol.64, No.6, (Sep 15 2008), pp. 527-532.

Sequeira, A., Mamdani, F., Ernst, C., Vawter, M.P., Bunney, W.E., Lebel, V., Rehal, S., Klempan, T., Gratton, A., Benkelfat, C., Rouleau, G.A., Mechawar, N. & Turecki, G. (2009). Global brain gene expression analysis links glutamatergic and GABAergic alterations to suicide and major depression. *PLoS One,* Vol.4, No.8, 2009), pp. e6585.

Sequeira, A. & Turecki, G. (2006). Genome wide gene expression studies in mood disorders. *OMICS,* Vol.10, No.4, (Winter 2006), pp. 444-454.

Serretti, A., Artioli, P., Lorenzi, C., Pirovano, A., Tubazio, V. & Zanardi, R. (2004). The C(-1019)G polymorphism of the 5-HT1A gene promoter and antidepressant response in mood disorders: preliminary findings. *Int J Neuropsychopharmacol,* Vol.7, No.4, (Dec 2004), pp. 453-460.

Serretti, A., Benedetti, F., Zanardi, R. & Smeraldi, E. (2005). The influence of Serotonin Transporter Promoter Polymorphism (SERTPR) and other polymorphisms of the serotonin pathway on the efficacy of antidepressant treatments. *Prog Neuropsychopharmacol Biol Psychiatry,* Vol.29, No.6, (Jul 2005), pp. 1074-1084.

Serretti, A., Zanardi, R., Cusin, C., Rossini, D., Lorenzi, C. & Smeraldi, E. (2001a). Tryptophan hydroxylase gene associated with paroxetine antidepressant activity. *Eur Neuropsychopharmacol,* Vol.11, No.5, (Oct 2001a), pp. 375-380.

Serretti, A., Zanardi, R., Rossini, D., Cusin, C., Lilli, R. & Smeraldi, E. (2001b). Influence of tryptophan hydroxylase and serotonin transporter genes on fluvoxamine antidepressant activity. *Mol Psychiatry,* Vol.6, No.5, (Sep 2001b), pp. 586-592.

Sharpley, A.L. & Cowen, P.J. (1995). Effect of pharmacologic treatments on the sleep of depressed patients. *Biol Psychiatry,* Vol.37, No.2, (Jan 15 1995), pp. 85-98.

Sheline, Y.I., Barch, D.M., Donnelly, J.M., Ollinger, J.M., Snyder, A.Z. & Mintun, M.A. (2001). Increased amygdala response to masked emotional faces in depressed subjects resolves with antidepressant treatment: an fMRI study. *Biol Psychiatry,* Vol.50, No.9, (Nov 1 2001), pp. 651-658.

Sher, L. (2006). Combined dexamethasone suppression-corticotropin-releasing hormone stimulation test in studies of depression, alcoholism, and suicidal behavior. *ScientificWorldJournal,* Vol.6, 2006), pp. 1398-1404.

Shieh, K.R., Chu, Y.S. & Pan, J.T. (1997). Circadian change of dopaminergic neuron activity: effects of constant light and melatonin. *Neuroreport,* Vol.8, No.9-10, (Jul 7 1997), pp. 2283-2287.

Shirayama, Y., Chen, A.C., Nakagawa, S., Russell, D.S. & Duman, R.S. (2002). Brain-derived neurotrophic factor produces antidepressant effects in behavioral models of depression. *J Neurosci,* Vol.22, No.8, (Apr 15 2002), pp. 3251-3261.

Shyn, S.I. & Hamilton, S.P. (2010). The genetics of major depression: moving beyond the monoamine hypothesis. *Psychiatr Clin North Am,* Vol.33, No.1, (Mar 2010), pp. 125-140.

Sibille, E., Wang, Y., Joeyen-Waldorf, J., Gaiteri, C., Surget, A., Oh, S., Belzung, C., Tseng, G.C. & Lewis, D.A. (2009). A molecular signature of depression in the amygdala. *Am J Psychiatry,* Vol.166, No.9, (Sep 2009), pp. 1011-1024.

Siuciak, J.A., Lewis, D.R., Wiegand, S.J. & Lindsay, R.M. (1997). Antidepressant-like effect of brain-derived neurotrophic factor (BDNF). *Pharmacol Biochem Behav,* Vol.56, No.1, (Jan 1997), pp. 131-137.

Sluzewska, A., Rybakowski, J., Bosmans, E., Sobieska, M., Berghmans, R., Maes, M. & Wiktorowicz, K. (1996). Indicators of immune activation in major depression. *Psychiatry Res,* Vol.64, No.3, (Oct 16 1996), pp. 161-167.

Smith, K.E., Walker, M.W., Artymyshyn, R., Bard, J., Borowsky, B., Tamm, J.A., Yao, W.J., Vaysse, P.J., Branchek, T.A., Gerald, C. & Jones, K.A. (1998). Cloned human and rat galanin GALR3 receptors. Pharmacology and activation of G-protein inwardly rectifying K+ channels. *J Biol Chem,* Vol.273, No.36, (Sep 4 1998), pp. 23321-23326.

Smith, R.S. (1991). The macrophage theory of depression. *Med Hypotheses,* Vol.35, No.4, (Aug 1991), pp. 298-306.

Song, C., Dinan, T. & Leonard, B.E. (1994). Changes in immunoglobulin, complement and acute phase protein levels in the depressed patients and normal controls. *J Affect Disord,* Vol.30, No.4, (Apr 1994), pp. 283-288.

Song, C., Merali, Z. & Anisman, H. (1999). Variations of nucleus accumbens dopamine and serotonin following systemic interleukin-1, interleukin-2 or interleukin-6 treatment. *Neuroscience,* Vol.88, No.3, 1999), pp. 823-836.

Spijker, S., Van Zanten, J.S., De Jong, S., Penninx, B.W., van Dyck, R., Zitman, F.G., Smit, J.H., Ylstra, B., Smit, A.B. & Hoogendijk, W.J. (2010). Stimulated gene expression profiles as a blood marker of major depressive disorder. *Biol Psychiatry,* Vol.68, No.2, (Jul 15 2010), pp. 179-186.

Srinivasan, V., Smits, M., Spence, W., Lowe, A.D., Kayumov, L., Pandi-Perumal, S.R., Parry, B. & Cardinali, D.P. (2006). Melatonin in mood disorders. *World J Biol Psychiatry,* Vol.7, No.3, 2006), pp. 138-151.

Stahl, S. (1994). 5HT1A receptors and pharmacotherapy. Is serotonin receptor down-regulation linked to the mechanism of action of antidepressant drugs? *Psychopharmacol Bull,* Vol.30, No.1, 1994), pp. 39-43.

Strobel, A., Gutknecht, L., Rothe, C., Reif, A., Mossner, R., Zeng, Y., Brocke, B. & Lesch, K.P. (2003). Allelic variation in 5-HT1A receptor expression is associated with anxiety- and depression-related personality traits. *J Neural Transm,* Vol.110, No.12, (Dec 2003), pp. 1445-1453.

Sullivan, P.F., Neale, M.C. & Kendler, K.S. (2000). Genetic epidemiology of major depression: review and meta-analysis. *Am J Psychiatry,* Vol.157, No.10, (Oct 2000), pp. 1552-1562.

Surguladze, S., Brammer, M.J., Keedwell, P., Giampietro, V., Young, A.W., Travis, M.J., Williams, S.C. & Phillips, M.L. (2005). A differential pattern of neural response toward sad versus happy facial expressions in major depressive disorder. *Biol Psychiatry,* Vol.57, No.3, (Feb 1 2005), pp. 201-209.

Szegedi, A., Rujescu, D., Tadic, A., Muller, M.J., Kohnen, R., Stassen, H.H. & Dahmen, N. (2005). The catechol-O-methyltransferase Val108/158Met polymorphism affects short-term treatment response to mirtazapine, but not to paroxetine in major depression. *Pharmacogenomics J,* Vol.5, No.1, 2005), pp. 49-53.

Tadic, A., Wagner, S., Schlicht, K.F., Peetz, D., Borysenko, L., Dreimuller, N., Hiemke, C. & Lieb, K. (2011). The early non-increase of serum BDNF predicts failure of antidepressant treatment in patients with major depression: a pilot study. *Prog Neuropsychopharmacol Biol Psychiatry,* Vol.35, No.2, (Mar 30 2011), pp. 415-420.

Takahashi, M., Terwilliger, R., Lane, C., Mezes, P.S., Conti, M. & Duman, R.S. (1999). Chronic antidepressant administration increases the expression of cAMP-specific phosphodiesterase 4A and 4B isoforms. *J Neurosci,* Vol.19, No.2, (Jan 15 1999), pp. 610-618.

Terman, M. & Terman, J.S. (2005). Light therapy for seasonal and nonseasonal depression: efficacy, protocol, safety, and side effects. *CNS Spectr,* Vol.10, No.8, (Aug 2005), pp. 647-663; quiz 672.

Tfilin, M., Sudai, E., Merenlender, A., Gispan, I., Yadid, G. & Turgeman, G. (2009). Mesenchymal stem cells increase hippocampal neurogenesis and counteract depressive-like behavior. *Mol Psychiatry,* Vol.15, No.12, (Dec 2009), pp. 1164-1175.

Thase, M.E. (2007). Molecules that mediate mood. *N Engl J Med,* Vol.357, No.23, (Dec 6 2007), pp. 2400-2402.

Thase, M.E., Kupfer, D.J., Fasiczka, A.J., Buysse, D.J., Simons, A.D. & Frank, E. (1997). Identifying an abnormal electroencephalographic sleep profile to characterize major depressive disorder. *Biol Psychiatry,* Vol.41, No.9, (May 1 1997), pp. 964-973.

Thompson, C., Mezey, G., Corn, T., Franey, C., English, J., Arendt, J. & Checkley, S.A. (1985). The effect of desipramine upon melatonin and cortisol secretion in depressed and normal subjects. *Br J Psychiatry,* Vol.147, (Oct 1985), pp. 389-393.

Trivedi, M.H., Rush, A.J., Wisniewski, S.R., Nierenberg, A.A., Warden, D., Ritz, L., Norquist, G., Howland, R.H., Lebowitz, B., McGrath, P.J., Shores-Wilson, K., Biggs, M.M., Balasubramani, G.K. & Fava, M. (2006). Evaluation of outcomes with citalopram for depression using measurement-based care in STAR*D: implications for clinical practice. *Am J Psychiatry,* Vol.163, No.1, (Jan 2006), pp. 28-40.

Tsai, S.J., Cheng, C.Y., Yu, Y.W., Chen, T.J. & Hong, C.J. (2003). Association study of a brain-derived neurotrophic-factor genetic polymorphism and major depressive disorders, symptomatology, and antidepressant response. *Am J Med Genet B Neuropsychiatr Genet,* Vol.123B, No.1, (Nov 15 2003), pp. 19-22.

Tsankova, N.M., Berton, O., Renthal, W., Kumar, A., Neve, R.L. & Nestler, E.J. (2006). Sustained hippocampal chromatin regulation in a mouse model of depression and antidepressant action. *Nat Neurosci,* Vol.9, No.4, (Apr 2006), pp. 519-525.

Tsuno, N., Besset, A. & Ritchie, K. (2005). Sleep and depression. *J Clin Psychiatry,* Vol.66, No.10, (Oct 2005), pp. 1254-1269.

Turnbull, A.V. & Rivier, C.L. (1999). Regulation of the hypothalamic-pituitary-adrenal axis by cytokines: actions and mechanisms of action. *Physiol Rev,* Vol.79, No.1, (Jan 1999), pp. 1-71.

Uher, R. & McGuffin, P. (2010). The moderation by the serotonin transporter gene of environmental adversity in the etiology of depression: 2009 update. *Mol Psychiatry,* Vol.15, No.1, (Jan 2010), pp. 18-22.

Verhagen, J.V. (2007). The neurocognitive bases of human multimodal food perception: consciousness. *Brain Res Rev,* Vol.53, No.2, (Feb 2007), pp. 271-286.

Videbech, P. & Ravnkilde, B. (2004). Hippocampal volume and depression: a meta-analysis of MRI studies. *Am J Psychiatry,* Vol.161, No.11, (Nov 2004), pp. 1957-1966.

Wan, Q., Xiong, Z.G., Man, H.Y., Ackerley, C.A., Braunton, J., Lu, W.Y., Becker, L.E., MacDonald, J.F. & Wang, Y.T. (1997). Recruitment of functional GABA(A) receptors to postsynaptic domains by insulin. *Nature,* Vol.388, No.6643, (Aug 14 1997), pp. 686-690.

Wang, S., Hashemi, T., Fried, S., Clemmons, A.L. & Hawes, B.E. (1998). Differential intracellular signaling of the GalR1 and GalR2 galanin receptor subtypes. *Biochemistry,* Vol.37, No.19, (May 12 1998), pp. 6711-6717.

Weaver, I.C., Cervoni, N., Champagne, F.A., D'Alessio, A.C., Sharma, S., Seckl, J.R., Dymov, S., Szyf, M. & Meaney, M.J. (2004). Epigenetic programming by maternal behavior. *Nat Neurosci,* Vol.7, No.8, (Aug 2004), pp. 847-854.

Weaver, I.C., D'Alessio, A.C., Brown, S.E., Hellstrom, I.C., Dymov, S., Sharma, S., Szyf, M. & Meaney, M.J. (2007). The transcription factor nerve growth factor-inducible protein a mediates epigenetic programming: altering epigenetic marks by immediate-early genes. *J Neurosci,* Vol.27, No.7, (Feb 14 2007), pp. 1756-1768.

Weiner, N., Clement, H.W., Gemsa, D. & Wesemann, W. (1992). Circadian and seasonal rhythms of 5-HT receptor subtypes, membrane anisotropy and 5-HT release in hippocampus and cortex of the rat. *Neurochem Int,* Vol.21, No.1, (Jul 1992), pp. 7-14.

Wermter, A.K., Laucht, M., Schimmelmann, B.G., Banaschweski, T., Sonuga-Barke, E.J., Rietschel, M. & Becker, K. (2010). From nature versus nurture, via nature and nurture, to gene x environment interaction in mental disorders. *Eur Child Adolesc Psychiatry,* Vol.19, No.3, (Mar 2010), pp. 199-210.

Wesemann, W. & Weiner, N. (1990). Circadian rhythm of serotonin binding in rat brain. *Prog Neurobiol,* Vol.35, No.6, 1990), pp. 405-428.

Wetterberg, L. (1999). Melatonin and clinical application. *Reprod Nutr Dev,* Vol.39, No.3, (May-Jun 1999), pp. 367-382.

Wichers, M. & Maes, M. (2002). The psychoneuroimmuno-pathophysiology of cytokine-induced depression in humans. *Int J Neuropsychopharmacol,* Vol.5, No.4, (Dec 2002), pp. 375-388.

Wilkie, M.J., Smith, D., Reid, I.C., Day, R.K., Matthews, K., Wolf, C.R., Blackwood, D. & Smith, G. (2007). A splice site polymorphism in the G-protein beta subunit influences antidepressant efficacy in depression. *Pharmacogenet Genomics,* Vol.17, No.3, (Mar 2007), pp. 207-215.

Will, M.J., Franzblau, E.B. & Kelley, A.E. (2003). Nucleus accumbens mu-opioids regulate intake of a high-fat diet via activation of a distributed brain network. *J Neurosci,* Vol.23, No.7, (Apr 1 2003), pp. 2882-2888.

Winokur, A., Maislin, G., Phillips, J.L. & Amsterdam, J.D. (1988). Insulin resistance after oral glucose tolerance testing in patients with major depression. *Am J Psychiatry,* Vol.145, No.3, (Mar 1988), pp. 325-330.

Winter, J., Jung, S., Keller, S., Gregory, R.I. & Diederichs, S. (2009). Many roads to maturity: microRNA biogenesis pathways and their regulation. *Nat Cell Biol,* Vol.11, No.3, (Mar 2009), pp. 228-234.

Wirz-Justice, A., Benedetti, F., Berger, M., Lam, R.W., Martiny, K., Terman, M. & Wu, J.C. (2005). Chronotherapeutics (light and wake therapy) in affective disorders. *Psychol Med,* Vol.35, No.7, (Jul 2005), pp. 939-944.

Wirz-Justice, A. & Van den Hoofdakker, R.H. (1999). Sleep deprivation in depression: what do we know, where do we go? *Biol Psychiatry,* Vol.46, No.4, (Aug 15 1999), pp. 445-453.

Witte, K. & Lemmer, B. (1991). Rhythms in second messenger mechanisms. *Pharmacol Ther,* Vol.51, No.2, 1991), pp. 231-237.

Wrenn, C.C. & Crawley, J.N. (2001). Pharmacological evidence supporting a role for galanin in cognition and affect. *Prog Neuropsychopharmacol Biol Psychiatry,* Vol.25, No.1, (Jan 2001), pp. 283-299.

Xia, Z., DePierre, J.W. & Nassberger, L. (1996). Tricyclic antidepressants inhibit IL-6, IL-1 beta and TNF-alpha release in human blood monocytes and IL-2 and interferon-gamma in T cells. *Immunopharmacology,* Vol.34, No.1, (Aug 1996), pp. 27-37.

Xu, Y., Day, T.A. & Buller, K.M. (1999). The central amygdala modulates hypothalamic-pituitary-adrenal axis responses to systemic interleukin-1beta administration. *Neuroscience,* Vol.94, No.1, 1999), pp. 175-183.

Xue, B. & Kahn, B.B. (2006). AMPK integrates nutrient and hormonal signals to regulate food intake and energy balance through effects in the hypothalamus and peripheral tissues. *J Physiol,* Vol.574, No.Pt 1, (Jul 1 2006), pp. 73-83.

Yirmiya, R. (2000). Depression in medical illness: the role of the immune system. *West J Med,* Vol.173, No.5, (Nov 2000), pp. 333-336.

Yoshitake, T., Reenila, I., Ogren, S.O., Hokfelt, T. & Kehr, J. (2003). Galanin attenuates basal and antidepressant drug-induced increase of extracellular serotonin and noradrenaline levels in the rat hippocampus. *Neurosci Lett,* Vol.339, No.3, (Mar 27 2003), pp. 239-242.

Zhang, M. & Kelley, A.E. (2000). Enhanced intake of high-fat food following striatal mu-opioid stimulation: microinjection mapping and fos expression. *Neuroscience,* Vol.99, No.2, 2000), pp. 267-277.

Zhang, X., Beaulieu, J.M., Sotnikova, T.D., Gainetdinov, R.R. & Caron, M.G. (2004). Tryptophan hydroxylase-2 controls brain serotonin synthesis. *Science,* Vol.305, No.5681, (Jul 9 2004), pp. 217.

Zhang, X., Gainetdinov, R.R., Beaulieu, J.M., Sotnikova, T.D., Burch, L.H., Williams, R.B., Schwartz, D.A., Krishnan, K.R. & Caron, M.G. (2005). Loss-of-function mutation in tryptophan hydroxylase-2 identified in unipolar major depression. *Neuron,* Vol.45, No.1, (Jan 6 2005), pp. 11-16.

Zheng, H., Lenard, N.R., Shin, A.C. & Berthoud, H.R. (2009). Appetite control and energy balance regulation in the modern world: reward-driven brain overrides repletion signals. *Int J Obes (Lond),* Vol.33 Suppl 2, (Jun 2009), pp. S8-13.

Zhou, J.N., Riemersma, R.F., Unmehopa, U.A., Hoogendijk, W.J., van Heerikhuize, J.J., Hofman, M.A. & Swaab, D.F. (2001). Alterations in arginine vasopressin neurons in the suprachiasmatic nucleus in depression. *Arch Gen Psychiatry,* Vol.58, No.7, (Jul 2001), pp. 655-662.

Zhou, Z., Zhu, G., Hariri, A.R., Enoch, M.A., Scott, D., Sinha, R., Virkkunen, M., Mash, D.C., Lipsky, R.H., Hu, X.Z., Hodgkinson, C.A., Xu, K., Buzas, B., Yuan, Q., Shen, P.H., Ferrell, R.E., Manuck, S.B., Brown, S.M., Hauger, R.L., Stohler, C.S., Zubieta, J.K. & Goldman, D. (2008). Genetic variation in human NPY expression affects stress response and emotion. *Nature,* Vol.452, No.7190, (Apr 24 2008), pp. 997-1001.

Zigova, T., Pencea, V., Wiegand, S.J. & Luskin, M.B. (1998). Intraventricular administration of BDNF increases the number of newly generated neurons in the adult olfactory bulb. *Mol Cell Neurosci,* Vol.11, No.4, (Jul 1998), pp. 234-245.

10

Depression During Pregnancy: Review of Epidemiological and Clinical Aspects in Developed and Developing Countries

Priscila Krauss Pereira, Giovanni Marcos Lovisi, Lúcia Abelha Lima, Letícia Fortes Legay, Jacqueline Fernandes de Cintra Santos, Simone Agadir Santos, Daianna Lima Thiengo and Elie Valencia
Federal University of Rio de Janeiro
Brazil

1. Introduction

Contrary to general belief, gestation is not always characterized by joy and accomplishments. Many women experience sadness or anxiety in these periods of their lives. Gestation and postpartum (puerperium) are periods of woman´s life which involve many physical, hormonal, psychic and social insertion changes which can have a direct effect on her mental health (Camacho et al., 2006). The changes caused by the newborn arrival are not limited to psychological and biochemical variables but also involve socioeconomic factors, especially in societies in which women are active in the labor market, contributing to the family income, and pursuing diverse professional and social interests (Maldonado, 1997).

The scientific literature indicates that in the gestational-postpartum period is the phase with the highest prevalence of mental disorders of women´s life, particularly in the first and third quarters of gestation and during the first 30 days of postpartum (Botega & Dias, 2006). The intensity of these mental health alterations depend and are regulated by interaction of multiple factors, including organic, family, marital, social, cultural aspects and the pregnant woman's personality (Falcone et al., 2005). Approximately one fifth of pregnant women and women in puerperium present symptoms of depression (Limlomwongse & Liabsuetrakul, 2006). Most of these women are not diagnosed neither adequately treated (Andersson et al, 2003).

Depression is the most prevalent mental disorder during pregnancy and the puerperium period (Bennett et al., 2004) and is associated with risk factors such as a psychiatric history, financial hardships, low education level, teenage pregnancy, lack of social support, stressful events and a history of domestic violence. There is evidence that pre-natal depression is not only more common, but it constitutes the main risk factor for postpartum depression. Indeed, in many cases it is the continuation of the depression that started during pregnancy (Alami et al., 2006; Andersson et al., 2006; Da Costa et al., 2000; Heron et al., 2004; Josefsson et al., 2001; Lovisi et al., 2005; Patel et al., 2003; Rich-Edwards et al., 2006; Ryan et al., 2005).

Current studies suggest that gestational depression needs to be addressed in a more consistent manner. Although there is a consensus that the factors that affect the relationship between mother and fetus begin in the prenatal period, there has been little research addressing this issue. Most studies focus on postpartum depression. Gestational depression needs to be considered as an important public health issue since it constitutes a strong risk factor that may lead to postpartum depression. Within this context, there is need to implement preventive interventions prior to childbirth. Some studies suggest that gestational depression is related to low birth weight, premature births and other problems in the development of the child (Patel & Prince, 2006; Rahman et al., 2004).

The belief that the pregnant woman's feelings may affect the baby's health is very old but only recently it has aroused scientific interest (Allister et al., 2001; Andersson et al., 2004; Chung et al., 2001; Dayan et al., 2006; Diego et al., 2004; Hoffman & Hatch, 2000; Patel & Prince, 2006; Patel et al., 2004; Rahman et al., 2002; Rahman et al., 2004). It is known that the mother's nutritional, hormonal, metabolic, psychological and social environment during gestation is related to the newborn's health. A woman suffering from gestational depression can be less concerned with her health in general. This can lead her to not follow through with prenatal care, to abuse alcohol, tobacco and other drugs, suffer from insomnia and diminished appetite, which results in a decrease in the quantity and quality of her nutrition. Furthermore, the literature indicates that there is also a relationship between maternal psycho-social stress and low fetal growth. Women with depression have higher cortisol rates which may lead to prematurity and low birth weight (Hobel et al., 1999; Wadhwa et al., 1996).

In developing countries, premature birth and low birth weight are the main causes of infant morbimortality. Studies suggest that depressive states that are not treated during pregnancy tend to decrease the frequency of prenatal consultations, which has been closely associated with neonatal mortality (Carvalho et al., 2007). Studies carried out in developed countries indicate that maternal depression is linked to long term emotional, cognitive and behavioral problems in children (Huot et al., 2004; Motta et al., 2005; Newport et al., 2002). In addition, the prevalence rates of depression during pregnancy have been significantly higher in developing countries than developed ones (Patel & Kleinman, 2003).

Within this context, the main objective of this chapter is to present a systematic review of epidemiological studies that investigated the prevalence and risks factors associated with depression during pregnancy in developing and developed countries.

2. Systematic review of epidemiological studies on the prevalence and factors associated with gestational depression

We carried out a literature review of epidemiological research on the prevalence of gestational depression or depression symptoms and their associated risk factors, including longitudinal research that estimated this prevalence before and after birth, in developed and low income countries.

2.1 Methods

The following bibliographical databases were consulted: PubMed/MEDLINE, ISIWEB, Scopus, LILACS, SciELO, with the last two databases used primarily to retrieve Latin American publications. The criteria for inclusion were: published articles in the last 10 years (from 2000 to April 2011) in English, Spanish or Portuguese with an observational epidemiological study design (cross-sectional, case-control, and cohort).

In searching the databases LILACS and SciELO used the following descriptors, according to their definition in DeCS (Health Descriptors): "depression" or "depressive disorder" or "mood disorders" and "pregnancy" and "prevalence" and "risk factors". In searching the databases PubMed/MEDLINE, ISIWEB and Scopus, we used keywords defined according to their description in MeSH (Medical Subject Headings): "depression" or "depressive disorder" or "unipolar depression" or "mood disorders" and "pregnancy" and "prevalence" and "risk factors". Different keywords were used in each database according to the definition that each database proposed in the descriptors. With this process, it was possible to find a greater number of articles related to the topic of interest in each database. Also, we also reviewed the bibliographical references of the principal articles found and specialized books on the subject.

The articles were evaluated and chosen according to methodological criteria proposed by Downs & Black (Downs & Black, 1998), applicable for the delineation of articles for the evaluation of their quality. These criteria evaluate the quality of information, the internal validity (bias and confounding), external validity and the ability of the study to detect a significant effect. The present article used the original version made up of 27 items, only excluding the item associated with experimental studies. Hence, in the end, 17 items were used for the cohort and case control studies, adding up to a maximum 18 points. Of these, 13 items referred to cross-sectional studies and represented at the most 14 points. These criteria were used by authors in national review articles (Araujo et al., 2010; Rossi & Vasconcelos, 2010).

The analysis of the methodological quality of the articles took the following items into consideration: clearly described hypotheses or objectives; an endpoint that was clearly described in the introduction or methodology; characteristics of the participants; distribution of main confounding variables; main results clearly described; information on estimates of the random variability of data; characteristics of losses; information on probability values of outcomes; representativeness of individuals included in the study; clear information on results that were not based on hypotheses established *a priori*; information on adjustments of the analysis for different follow-up durations in cohort studies; same amount of time allowed between intervention and the endpoint for cases and controls in case-control studies; adequacy of statistical tests; accuracy of the measures used for the main outcomes; recruitment of participants in different groups from the same population and in the same period of time; adequate inclusion of confounding factors in the analysis; and consideration of participant drop out during follow-up.

The study only included articles that obtained at least 50% of the maximum score on the Downs & Black scale (Downs & Black, 1998) - that is 9 points for cohort and case-control studies and 7 points for cross-sectional studies. Selected articles were compared on the following methodological aspects: year of publication, study location (developed or developing countries), study design, sample size, instruments used for assessment of depression, prevalence of depression during pregnancy, related factors (epidemiological and clinical aspects) and methodological assessment score (Downs & Black Scale).

2.2 Results and discussion

A total of 543 studies were identified in the database searches. However, only 51 articles met the pre-established criteria and were selected for inclusion in this comparison (Figure 1). Excluded studies were literature review and qualitative research reports and studies that had been repeated in different databases or because they were not associated with the subject. Thirty-seven studies were excluded for obtaining a score below the 50% of the maximum score on the Downs and Black methodological evaluation scale.

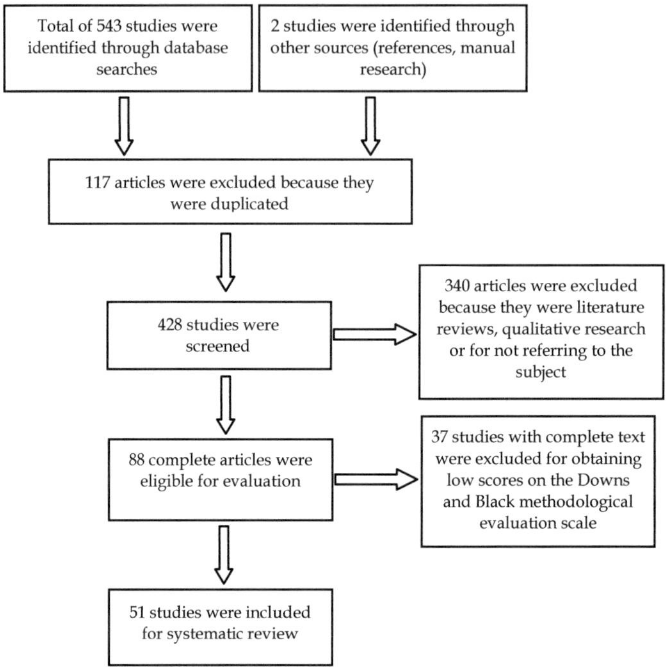

Fig. 1. Flowchart of inclusion and exclusion of original articles in the systematic review

The selected studies were divided into two categories: studies in developed countries (Chart 1) and studies in developing countries (Chart 2). This division was made with the purpose of observing possible variations in the prevalence of gestational depression and associated factors, since an unfavorable economic situation seems to be an important risk factor in the development of minor mental disorders such as depression, including depression during pregnancy (Patel & Kleinman, 2003). Together with the main methods and instruments used in collecting the comparison data in this study, this procedure allowed for the analysis of variations in depression frequency rates and associated factors reported in studies carried out in developed countries when compared to those carried out in developing countries.

2.2.1 Studies on the prevalence of gestational depression in developed countries

The prevalence of gestational depression reported in studies included in this review, originating in developed countries, showed a broad variation- oscillating from 5% to 30%. Few studies found prevalence rates above 20%. Prevalence rates were more frequently reported in the 10% to 15% range. Among the risk factors elucidated by these studies were psychiatric histories, use of substances, negative attitude towards pregnancy, lack of social support, presence of stressful events and marital conflicts (Chart 1). These factors were assessed through standardized questionnaires, including questions developed raised by the authors, and scales such as Stressful Life Event Scale (Holmes & Rahe, 1967), Intimate Bond Measure (Wilhelm & Parker, 1988), Parental Bonding Instrument (Parker et al., 1979), Index of Marital Satisfaction - IMS (Hudson, 1982), Social Desirability Scale (Crowne & Marlowe, 1960), Medical Outcome Studies Social Support Survey - SSS (Sherbourne & Stewart, 1991), Social Support Questionnaire - SSQ (Sarason et al., 1983) and TWEAK - Tolerance Worry

Eye-opener Annoyed Cut-down (Russell, 1994) - this latter scale being measures problematic alcohol use and risk of alcohol drinking during pregnancy.
Among the instruments used to evaluate gestational depression, more than half of these investigations used the Edinburgh Postnatal Depression Scale- EPDS (Cox et al., 1987), a self-administered questionnaire that evaluates the intensity of postpartum depression symptoms - which has also been validated to measure depression during pregnancy (Ortega et al., 2001; Murray & Cox, 1990). Standardized diagnostic interviews used included the Clinical Interview Schedule - CIS-R (Lewis et al., 1992), the Mini International Neuropsychiatric Interview - MINI (Sheehan et al., 1997), the Structure Clinical Interview - SCID (First et al., 1994) and the Composite International Diagnostic Interview - CIDI, based on DSM-III-R and DSM-IV diagnostic criteria (APA, 1987, 1994). Others administered instruments were The Primary Care Evaluation of Mental Disorders - PRIME-MD (Spitzer et al., 1994) and the Center for Epidemiologic Studies Depression (CES-D) Scale (Radloff, 1977). This latter was developed by the National Institute of Mental Health to assess depression symptoms using self-administered questionnaires. Another utilized instrument was the Beck Depression Inventory - BDI (Beck et al., 1998), which is also a self-administered questionnaire and measures the severity of depression symptoms.
Most of these studies had a longitudinal design. The majority of them were carried out in the USA and in European countries like England, Switzerland, Italy and Spain. There was a considerable variation in the size of the samples included in these investigations. However, many studies reported on samples that were relatively large, over 1000 women. Only one study used a sample below 100 women. Prenatal services and maternities were the most frequently selected research sites. A few studies were carried out at the participants' homes, usually using self-administered questionnaires sent by correspondence. The average score obtained on the Downs & Black scale by these studies was 14 points but four of them obtained the scale´s maximum score.

2.2.2 Studies on the prevalence of gestational depression in developing countries

Most gestational depression prevalence rates found in studies in developing countries were around 20%. Among the risk factors elucidated by these studies, most were associated with poverty such as low income, unemployment, financial hardships and poor educational backgrounds. Other reported factors associated with gestational depression were being single or divorced, having violence and psychiatry histories, stressful events and lack of social support (Chart 2). In order to evaluate these factors, most studies used structured questions and questionnaires developed by the authors. However, some scales were used such as the Krause-Markides Index (Krause & Markides, 1990) to evaluate social support received and the Paykel Life Events (Paykel, 1983) to assess stressful events during pregnancy and the puerperium period.
For the assessment of depression, half of these investigations used the Edinburgh Postnatal Depression Scale - EPDS (Cox et al., 1987). Some of these studies used standardized interviews to corroborate positive cases detected by this scale. This included the use the Mini International Neuropsychiatry Interview - MINI (Sheehan et al., 1997) that aims at reaching a diagnosis of Axis I mental disorder according to DSM-IV (APA, 1994) criteria. The Brazilian studies mainly used the Composite International Diagnostic Interview - CIDI (Wittchen et al., 1991), a standardized WHO instrument, and to a lesser extend the used

other scales such as the Beck Depression Inventory (Beck et al., 1998), the Hospital Anxiety and Depression Scale (Zigmond & Snaith, 1983) and the Primary Care Evaluation of Mental Disorders - PRIME-MD (Spitzer et al., 1994).

The majority of these investigations were carried out in Brazil and the rest in other low income countries such as Turkey, India, Nigeria and Mexico. Research with a cross-sectional design was more common among these studies in developing countries, particularly in the case of Brazilian studies. The sample size of these studies was mostly in the range of 100 to 500 women. There were only a few investigations with samples over 1000 women. Prenatal services and maternities were the predominant research sites and no study was carried out in residence of participants. The average score obtained through these studies on the Downs & Black scale was 12 points and few were close to the maximum score of the scale.

Authors	Country/ Publication year	Type of Study	Sample	Research Sites	Instruments	Prevalence	Risk Factors	Evaluation Score
Marcus et al	United States, 2011	Longitudinal	154	Hospital / Maternity	EPDS[1]; GHQ[2]; SCID (DSM IV)[3]; BDI[4]	8.0%	Development of the infant limbic-hypothalamic -pituitary axis (LHPA)	12
Wojcicki et al	United States, 2011	Longitudinal	201	Hospital / Maternity	EPDS; CES-D; MINI[5]	28.9%	Reduced weight gain in the first two years of life and greater risk for failure to thrive	12
Banti et al	Italy, 2010	Longitudinal	1066	Pre-natal service	EPDS; GHQ; SCID (DSM IV); BDI	12.4%	Not mentioned	14
Dhillon & MacArthur	England, 2010	Sectional	300	Pre-natal service	EPDS	30.7%	Unplanned pregnancy; history of anxiety and depression	12

[1] Edinburgh Postpartum Depression Scale
[2] General Health Questionnaire
[3] Structural Clinical Interview for DSM IV
[4] Beck Depression Inventory
[5] Mini International Neuropsychiatric Interview

Authors	Country/ Publication year	Type of Study	Sample	Research Sites	Instruments	Prevalence	Risk Factors	Evaluation Score
Gavin et al.	United States, 2010	Longitudinal	1997	Pre-natal service	PHQ[6]	5,1%	Black or Asian poor educational backgrounds; single or separated; stress; domestic violence; health problems	16
Micali et al.	England, 2010	Longitudinal	10887	Household	EPDS	6.3%	History of anxiety and depression	15
Price & Proctor	United States, 2009	Sectional	1086	Pre-natal service	PRIME-MD[7]; PHQ	13%	Low-income	13
Skouters et al	Australia, 2009	Longitudinal	207	Pre-natal service	BDI	28.3%	Anxiety disorder	16
Spoozak et al	United States, 2009	Sectional	783	Hospital / Maternity	CIDI[8]	9.0%	Poor educational background; low income, over 35 years	13
Leigh & Milgrom	Australia, 2008	Longitudinal	367	Hospital / Maternity	BDI	16,9%	Anxiety disorders; stressful events; low income and sexual abuse history	15
Martinéz et al	Spain, 2008	Sectional	200	Pre-natal service	EPDS	15,0%	Low income, poor educational background; over 35 years; large number of children	14
Rodriguez et al	United States, 2008	Sectional	210	Pre-natal service	BDI	41,0%	Domestic violence; stressful events	14

[6] Patient Health Questionnaire
[7] Primary Care Evaluation of Mental Disorders
[8] Composite International Diagnostic Interview

Authors	Country/ Publication year	Type of Study	Sample	Research Sites	Instruments	Prevalence	Risk Factors	Evaluation Score
Kitamura et al	Japan, 2006	Longitudinal	290	Hospital / Maternity	SDI (DSM-III-R)[9]	5.6%	Being young. negative attitude towards pregnancy	14
Rich-Edwards et al	USA, 2006	Longitudinal	1662	Pre-natal service	EPDS	9.0%	Psychiatric history; financial hardships; unwanted pregnancy	16
Chee et al	Singapore, 2005	Longitudinal	559	Hospital / Maternity	EPDS; SCID-IV (DSM-IV)	12.2%	Psychiatric history; unwanted pregnancy; low social support; family conflicts	18
Rubertsson et al	Sweden, 2005	Longitudinal	2430	Pre-natal service	EPDS	13.7%	Stressful events	15
Heron et al	England, 2004	Longitudinal	8323	Household	EPDS	11.4%	Pre-natal anxiety	16
Lee et al	Hong Kong, 2004	Longitudinal	157	Household and Maternity	BDI; SCID (DSM-IV)	6.4%	Not mentioned	15
Andersson et al	Sweden, 2003	Sectional	1795	Pre-natal service	PRIME-MD	6.9%	Not mentioned	12
Felice et al	Malta, 2003	Longitudinal	239	Hospital / Maternity	EPDS; CIS-R[10]	11.1%	Single; low social support; psychiatric history; unwanted pregnancy; marital conflicts	13
Marcus et al	USA, 2003	Sectional	3472	Pre-natal service	CES-D	20.4%	Psychiatric history; negative health perception ; substance abuse	12

[9] Structure Diagnostic Interview (DSM-III-R)
[10] Clinical Interview Schedule – revised edition (DSM-IV)

Authors	Country/ Publication year	Type of Study	Sample	Research Sites	Instruments	Prevalence	Risk Factors	Evaluation Score
Wu et al	USA, 2002	Longitudinal	1697	Hospital / Maternity	CES-D	15.6%	Age; race; marital status	16
Evans et al	England, 2001	Longitudinal	13.799	Household	EPDS	13.5%	Not mentioned	15
Josefsson et al	Sweden, 2001	Longitudinal	1558	Hospital / Maternity	EPDS	17.0%	Postpartum depression	15
Pajulo et al	Finland, 2001	Sectional	391	Pre-natal service	EPDS	7.7%	Substance abuse; difficulties with social relationships	14
Da Costa et al	Canada, 2000	Longitudinal	80	Pre-natal service	EPDS	25.0%	*Coping* strategies; anxiety; stress	15
Johanson et al	UK, 2000	Longitudinal	417	Hospital / Maternity	EPDS	9.8%	Marital conflicts; postpartum depression	16
Kurki et al	Finland, 2000	Longitudinal	623	Pre-natal service	BDI	30.0%	Not mentioned	15

Chart 1. Studies on the prevalence of gestational depression in developed countries

Authors	Country/ Publication year	Type of Study	Sample	Research Sites	Tools used	Prevalence	Associated Factors	Evaluation Score
Benute et al	Brazil, 2010	Sectional	326	Pre-natal service	PRIME-MD	9.0%	Unplanned pregnancy	11
Fisher et al	Vietnam, 2010	Sectional	364	Pre-natal service	SCID (DSM-IV)	10.0%	Rural household; violence and sexual abuse; stressful life events; poverty	12
Golbasi et al	Turkey, 2010	Sectional	258	Pre-natal service	EPDS	27.5%	Maternal age; multiparity; history of stillbirth; nuclear family; number of living children; social support	10

Authors	Country/ Publication year	Type of Study	Sample	Research Sites	Tools used	Prevalence	Associated Factors	Evaluation Score
Mohammad et al	Jordan, 2010	Sectional	353	Hospital / Maternity	EPDS	19%	Stress; anxiety; financial hardships; low social support; unplanned pregnancy; low self-esteem	13
Silva et al	Brazil, 2010	Sectional	1264	Pre-natal services	EPDS	21.1%	Advanced age; poor educational background; not living with companion; idealize abortion; previous psychological/ psychiatric treatment; tobacco and alcohol use during pregnancy; stressful events; multiparous; having planned the pregnancy	11
Karaçam & Ançel	Turkey, 2009	Sectional	1039	Hospital / Maternity	BDI	27.9%	Marital dissatisfaction; being a housewife; having an unwanted pregnancy; having a formal marriage.	12
Marcus et al	Peru, 2009	Sectional	222	Hospital / Maternity	EPDS	40.1%	Unplanned pregnancy; health problems during pregnancy	10
Mitsuhiro et al	Brazil, 2009	Sectional	1000	Hospital / Maternity	CIDI	12.9%	Psychiatric comorbidities	13

Authors	Country/ Publication year	Type of Study	Sample	Research Sites	Tools used	Prevalence	Associated Factors	Evaluation Score
Pereira et al	Brazil, 2009	Sectional	331	Pre-natal services Prenatal	CIDI	14.2%	Previous history of depression and psychiatric treatment; unplanned pregnancy; serious physical problem; formal work	12
Pottinger et al	Jamaica, 2009	Longitudinal	452	Pre-natal service	EPDS	25.0%	Previous history of depression; life style	15
Qiao et al	China, 2009	Sectional	527	Hospital / Maternity	HAD[11]	4.8%	Lower age; poor educational background	10
Adewuya et al	Nigeria, 2007	Sectional	180	Hospital / Maternity	EPDS	8.3%	Single, divorced or separated; low social support	13
Gulseren et al	Turkey, 2006	Longitudinal	125	Hospital / Maternity	EPDS	21.6%	Psychiatric history; stressful events	12
Alami et al	Morocco, 2006	Longitudinal	100	Pre-natal service	EPDS; MINI	19.2%	Obstetric history; unplanned pregnancy; marital problems; stressful events	14
Limlom-wongse & Liabsue-trakul	Thailand, 2006	Longitudinal	610	Hospital / Maternity	EPDS	20.5%	Single; negative attitude towards pregnancy	16
Patel et al	India, 2002	Longitudinal	270	Hospital / Maternity	EPDS	17.94%	Marital violence; psychiatric history; poor educational background; unwanted pregnancy	17

[11] Hospital Anxiety and Depression Scale

Authors	Country/ Publication year	Type of Study	Sample	Research Sites	Tools used	Prevalence	Associated Factors	Evaluation Score
Ortega et al	Mexico, 2001	Sectional	360	Pre-natal service	EPDS	21.7%	Not mentioned	10
Caputo & Bordin	Brazil, 2007	Sectional	207	Pre-natal service	Youth Self-Report	13%	Not mentioned	13
Ferri et al	Brazil, 2007	Sectional	930	Hospital / Maternity	CIDI	13%	physical violence	17
Faisal-Cury & Rossi Menezes	Brazil, 2007	Sectional	432	Pre-natal service	BDI	19.6%	Poor educational background; low family income, previous miscarriages	13
Mitsuhiro et al	Brazil, 2006	Sectional	1000	Hospital / Maternity	CIDI	12.9%	Dysfunctional family; unemployment; poor educational background	11
Lovisi et al	Brazil, 2005	Sectional	230	Hospital / Maternity	CIDI	19.1%	Financial hardships; poor educational background; domestic violence; psychiatric history	13
Freitas & Botega	Brazil, 2002	Sectional	120	Pre-natal service	CIS-R; HAD	20.8%	Suicidal ideation; single; low social support	12

Chart 2. Studies on the prevalence of gestational depression in developing countries

2.2.3 Epidemiological and clinical aspects of gestational depression in different socioeconomic contexts

In general, in this review the average prevalence of gestational depression found in developing countries was about 20% while in developed countries it ranged between 10% and 15%. Only a few studies in developed countries reported prevalence similar to that of developing countries. This fact suggests that this disorder ought to be of importance for world Public Health. The prevalence between 15% and 20% is significant and this higher rate seems to be associated with factors found in disadvantaged contexts such as poverty, violence, low education (Patel & Kleinmann, 2003). On one hand, it should be noted that the prevalence above this average was only found in some studies that used non-representative and non-randomized samples (Da Costa et al., 2000; Dhillon & MacArthur, 2010; Golbasi et al., 2010; Matos et al., 2009; Skouters et al., 2009; Wojcicki et al., 2011). On the other hand, gestational depression values a little below this prevalence average were found when standardized diagnostic interviews were used, particularly with the CID-10 (OMS, 1993) or DSM-IV (APA, 1994) diagnosis criteria, compared to studies that used inventories or symptomatology scales, such as the Beck Depression Inventory (Beck et al., 1998) and the Hospital Anxiety and Depression Scale (Zigmond & Snaith, 1983).

The gestational depression prevalence reported in the majority of these studies was approximately 20% (Alami et al., 2006; Bowen & Muhajarine, 2006; Faisal-Cury & Rossi Menezes, 2007; Freitas & Botega, 2002; Gulseren et al., 2006; Josefsson et al., 2001; Limlomwongse & Liabsuetrakul, 2006; Lovisi et al., 2005; Marcus et al., 2003; Mohammad et al., 2010; Ortega et al., 2001; Patel et al., 2002; Silva et al., 2010). This prevalence appears to be higher in the third gestational quarter and relatively higher in low income countries. It also tends to increase in high risk pregnancy cases (Lovisi et al., 2005). Studies have shown that depression symptoms are more common and severe during pregnancy than in the postnatal period (Andersson et al., 2006; Banti et al., 2010; Evans et al., 2001).

Depression tends to be higher among pregnant adolescents than in adult pregnant women. The same can be said of adolescent parents (Quinlivan & Condon, 2005). Depression is a frequent mental disorder in adolescence and pregnancy be an important risk factor in triggering its development in this stage of the life of woman. A study reported that anxiety and depression symptoms are more frequent in primiparous adolescents compared to non-pregnant adolescents (Caputo & Bordin, 2007). Another study carried out in Brazil reported high rates of prevalence of depression, anxiety and suicidal ideation in adolescent pregnant women: 20.8% for depression, 23.3% for anxiety and 16.7% for suicidal ideation (Freitas & Botega, 2002). It should be noted that adolescents between the ages of 10 and 19 account for approximately one quarter of the total number of childbirths that take place in developing countries such as Brazil, and constitutes the main cause of hospitalization in this population (Freitas & Botega, 2002).

In studies included in this review, investigations carried out in Eastern countries reported low rates of gestational depression. Investigations among Chinese women indicated a gestational depression rate of approximately 5% (Lee et al., 2004; Qiao et al., 2009). A Japanese study reported rates of 5.6% (Kitamura et al., 2006). These rates are lower than the average rates found in research studies carried out in Western societies. The explanation for this fact underlined in these studies consists in specific cultural aspects of these contexts whereby, among other factors, it was believed that pregnant women should refrain from having unhealthy behavior and feelings and this belief could favor the sub-notification of depressive symptoms (Lee et al., 2004).

It should be noted that there is an insufficiency of studies on the incidence of gestational depression since most studies address prevalence measures. In this review, only one incidence study was found (Kitamura et al., 2006). The importance of this kind of study lies in it enabling identification of new cases that really begin during the period being studied. In other words, that they are not pre-existing cases of depression and therefore can be rightly considered gestational depression cases. However, it is known that psychiatric incidence studies are hindered by the lack of a biological marker for mental disorders and by specific characteristics of the initiation, development and course of these disorders, which makes the exact moment of incidence almost impossible to determine.

In relation to the methodological quality of the articles, the studies carried out in developed countries did better on the Downs & Black scale than the studies carried out in developing countries, which may reflect, among other difficulties, the lack of governmental incentives for research in these countries. As for the instrument used assess depression, regardless of their country of origin, most authors used the Edinburgh Postnatal Depression Scale - EPDS (Cox et al., 1987) to detect the presence of depressive symptoms, both during the gestational and post-anatal periods. Some investigators used the Beck Depression Inventory - BDI (Beck et al., 1998), the Hospital Anxiety and Depression Scale - HAD (Zigmond & Snaith, 1983), among other instruments, to evaluate symptoms of depression. It should be noted that many of these instrument are self-administered and not appropriate for contexts with population with poor educational background, as it is the case in many developing countries. However, there are few standardized diagnostic interviews for assessing depressing during pregnancy in the reviewed study, such as for instance, the Composite International Diagnostic Interview - CIDI (Wittchen et al., 1991), the Mini International Neuropsychiatry Interview - MINI (Sheehan et al., 1997), the Clinical Interview Schedule-Revised - CIS-R (Lewis et al., 1992) and the clinical diagnostic interview based on the DSM-IV (APA, 1994), Structured Clinical Interview - SCID (First et al., 1994).

Among the risk factors that may lead to a gestational depressive condition, the studies on this reviewed identified a prior history of depression; financial hardships; low education levels; unemployment; lack of social support; instability in relationships; stressful life events; unwanted pregnancy; alcohol, tobacco or drug abuse; and a history of violence against women. It is highlighted that these factors are inter-related in varying degrees in the development of gestational depressive episodes. In general, the majority of risk factors associated with gestational depression were the same for developed and developing countries, with the exception of factors related to unfavorable economic contexts, low education, unemployment, financial hardships and violence which were predominant in studies carried out in low income countries.

In the last decades, epidemiological studies have significantly contributed to a greater understanding of the interrelation between social environment factors and the origin and course of mental disorders. A considerable amount of academic literature addresses the role that the so-called stressful life events play as risk factors in anxiety and depression (Lopes et al., 2003). Stressful events refer to life changes that require a social and psychological readjustment, such as the death of a loved one, marital conflicts, the loss of a job, having been a victim of a mugging. Several recent studies has reported an association between stressful events and the development of gestational depression (Alami et al., 2006; Fisher et al., 2010; Gulseren et al., 2006; Leigh & Milgrom, 2008; Lovisi et al., 2005; Pereira et al., 2009; Rodriguez et al., 2008; Rubertsson et al., 2005; Silva et al., 2010). On the other hand, stress seems also to be, in part, a result of the presence of gestational depression and anxiety (Da Costa et al., 2000).

Studies suggests that social support received before and during pregnancy, particularly support offered by the spouse, seems to be crucial to the pregnant woman's mental health since its absence has been associated with the manifestation of gestational depression symptoms (Adewuya et al., 2007; Chee et al., 2005; Felice et al., 2004; Freitas & Botega, 2002; Golbasi et al., 2010; Mohammad et al., 2010). It is also suggested that the perception of low level of spouse social support perception received is related to the prevalence of depression after childbirth (Cruz et al., 2005). Furthermore, marital problems also seem to be related to the prevalence of gestational depression (Alami et al., 2006; Felice et al., 2004; Johanson et al., 2000; Karaçam & Ançel, 2009). Single or divorced women report the higher level of symptoms of depression during this period (Adewuya et al., 2007; Faisal-Cury & Rossi-

Menezes, 2007; Felice et al., 2004; Freitas & Botega, 2002; Gavin et al., 2010; Limlomwongse & Liabsuetrakul, 2006; Lovisi et al., 2005; Silva et al., 2010).

A crucial factor in the development of gestational depression symptoms, which has a direct impact on the mother and the child's health, is violence against women, whether it is carried out by the spouse, a relative or a stranger. Although it is not restricted to poor areas, it is in these environments that we find the highest rates of violence. However, poverty and violence are both independent risk factors for gestational depression, which suggests that maternal mental health prevention strategies should include policies that aim at decreasing violence and offer financial aid to women in low income countries (Lovisi et al., 2005). Domestic violence against women during pregnancy, particularly when committed by the woman's partner, has several negative impacts on the baby's intra-uterine health and the mother's mental health, particularly in the development of gestational depression (Anderson et al., 2002; Ferri et al, 2007; Fisher et al., 2010; Gavin et al., 2010; Leigh & Milgrom, 2008; Lovisi et al., 2005; Patel et al., 2002; Rodriguez et al., 2008).

Financial hardships, unemployment, and low education levels stand out as risk factors for gestational depression (Faisal-Cury & Rossi-Menezes, 2007; Fisher et al., 2010; Gavin et al., 2010; Leigh & Milgrom, 2008; Martinéz et al., 2008; Mitsuhiro et al., 2006; Mohammad et al., 2010; Patel et al., 2002; Pereira et al., 2009; Pottinger et al., 2009; Qiao et al., 2009; Rich-Edwards et al., 2006; Silva et al., 2010; Spoozak et al., 2009). It has been suggested that a higher level of education rises the level of protection against gestational depression, (Lovisi et al., 2005; Patel et al., 2002). An unwanted or unplanned pregnancy can also be a strong cause for gestational depression symptoms (Alami et al., 2006; Benute et al., 2010; Dhillom & MacArthur, 2010; Karaçam & Ançel, 2009; Kitamura et al., 2006; Matos et al., 2009; Mohammad et al., 2010; Pereira et al., 2009). Moreover, women with depression usually have low level of quality of life (Nicholson et al., 2006).

Among the risk factors frequently associated with gestational and puerperal depression in the reviewed studies, it stands out a prior psychiatric history, particularly a prior history of depression (Chee et al., 2005; Dhillom & MacArthur, 2010; Felice et al., 2004; Marcus et al., 2003; Micali et al., 2010; Patel et al., 2002; Pereira et al., 2009; Rich-Edwards et al., 2006). Most women who developed gestational depression had had prior depressive episodes (Rich-Edwards et al, 2006). Additionally, alcohol, tobacco and drug abuse problems seem to be related to a considerable number of gestational anxiety and depression symptoms (Marcus et al., 2003; Pajulo et al., 2001; Silva et al., 2010).

In order to approach predictors of depression, reviewed studies used scales like the Stressful Life Events (Holmes & Rahe, 1967) and the Paykel Life Events Inventory (Paykel, 1983) to assess stressful events; the Social Support Questionnaire - SSQ (Sarason et al., 1983) to evaluate social support; the Index of Marital Satisfaction - IMS (Hudson, 1982) and the Abuse Assessment Screen - AAS (MacFarlane et al., 1992) to measure the satisfaction and violence suffered in a marital relationship and the Substance Abuse Subtle Screening Inventory - SASSI (Miller, 1994) to assess use of alcohol and drugs. Most studies only used questions and questionnaires elaborated by the study researchers to assess risk factors associated with depression.

Several longitudinal studies reported on the prevalence of gestational as well as postpartum depression (Alami et al., 2006; Andersson et al., 2006; Banti et al., 2010; Chee et al., 2005; Da Costa et al., 2000; Evans et al., 2001; Felice et al., 2004; Gulseren et al., 2006; Heron et al., 2004; Johanson et al, 2000; Josefsson et al., 2001; Kitamura et al., 2006; Limlomwongse & Liabsuetrakul, 2006; Patel et al., 2002; Rich-Edwards et al., 2006; Rubertsson et al., 2005). All these studies reported gestational depression rates greater than those found in postpartum depression, except one study which reported a higher rate for postpartum depression (Patel et al., 2002). According to the authors of this latter study, cultural aspects in India may have influenced the results since the birth of girls in that country is not appreciated. The birth of a girl brings about discontentment and represents a strong risk factor, raising the probability of maternal depression threefold.

The reviewed studies indicate that the prevalence of postpartum depression is usually lower than during pregnancy - below 15% (Banti et al., 2010; Chee et al., 2005; Evans et al., 2001; Felice et al., 2004; Heron et al., 2004; Johanson et al., 2000; Josefsson et al., 2001; Kitamura et al., 2006; Rich-Edwards et al., 2006; Rubertsson et al., 2005). The intensity of perinatal depression symptoms tend to decrease from the gestational period to the period after childbirth (Chee et al., 2005; Gulseren et al., 2006; Pottinger et al., 2009). Further, a study reported that out a rate of 8.7% postpartum depression prevalence only 3.9% were incidental - they had begun during this period. The other 4.8% represented cases that had started in the gestational period or before (Felice et al., 2004).

3. Diagnosis and treatment of gestational depression

The evaluation of gestational depression, particularly of mood disorders, may be confounded by the fact that some gestational period characteristics can be misinterpreted as depressive, as is the case of fatigue, changes in sleep habits, appetite and libido. Moreover, during pregnancy, a woman may present a high incidence of metabolic changes such as gestational diabetes, anemia and thyroid malfunction, all of which may suggest a secondary mental disorders (Botega & Dias, 2006; Camacho et al., 2006). Further, many women who suffer from depression do not reveal their symptoms for fear of possible stigmatization, since they perceive that society expects them to be content. They end up feeling guilty for having depressive symptoms at a time when they should be feeling happy (Epperson, 1999, as cited in Camacho, 2006).

The diagnostic criteria for gestational depression are the same as those for depressive disorders, regardless of the period of life in reference. There are no specific scales for the detection of gestational depression. However, there are symptoms which are particularly associated to gestational depression, such as depressed moods, diminished interest or pleasure, weight loss or gain, insomnia or hypersomnia, psychomotor agitation or retardation, fatigue or loss of energy, feeling of worthlessness or guilt, difficulty in concentrating and suicidal ideation. According to the DSM-IV (Diagnostic and Statistical Manual for Mental Disorders), classification of a Major Depressive Episode requires that at least five of the above symptoms be present during a period of at least two weeks. At least one of the symptoms must be depressed mood or diminished interest or pleasure (APA, 2002). The CID-10 Classification of Mental and Behavioral Disorders (International Classification of Diseases) uses the same criteria as the DSM-IV for diagnosis of a Major Depressive Episode. According to the CID-10 and the DSM-IV, the Major Depressive Episode, characterized by one or more Major Depressive Episodes, can also be classified as mild, moderate or severe (APA, 2002; WHO, 1993).

Treatment of gestational depression is a complex task. Cases need to be treated on an individual basis and taking in account the patients' autonomy and their social context, emphasizing early intervention (Coverdale et al., 1997; Marcus et al., 2001; Gold, 1999; Soares et al., 2001). The use of psychoactive medication during pregnancy and lactation must take needs to be carefully evaluated since treating may affect the fetus' health (Bonari et al., 2004; Cohen et al., 2004; Jablensky, 2005; O'Brien et al., 2007; Paton, 2008). The possible risks in using antidepressants include fetal toxicity, intra-uterine death, physical malformations, growth impairment, behavioral teratogenicity and neonatal toxicity (Camacho et al., 2006). However, these possible associations has not been adequately proven and several current studies have reported that the use of antidepressants during pregnancy is safe, especially the use of serotonin reuptake inhibitors.

Electroconvulsive therapy (ECT) is advised in more severe cases of gestational depression or in those in which all other forms of treatment have failed. It is the last resource used in treating gestational psychiatric disorders. Recent research has suggested that the risk of its use during gestation may be very small and that it can be a safe and effective alternative method in more severe cases (Camacho et al., 2006). Psychotherapy is recommended for women who develop a mild or moderate depressive condition, especially cognitive-behavioral and interpersonal therapy (Botega & Dias, 2006; Spinelli, 1997; Spinelli & Endicott, 2003; Weissman, 2007). This may be a good choice of treatment for women who do not agree to pharmacological treatment when they find out they are pregnant and in less severe cases of depression. However, it is not adequate to discontinue pharmacological treatment in more severe or recurrent cases. Pharmacological treatment and psychotherapy during pregnancy have also proven to be efficient in preventing postpartum depression (Zinga et al., 2005).

An intervention study reported that the participation of women in multi-professional educational groups contributed to decreasing the rate of gestational affective disorders (Falcone et al., 2005). The groups included a team of nurses, nutritionists, pedagogues, physiotherapists, social workers and community workers. They complemented formal prenatal care through monitoring the pregnancy, facilitating access to care and strengthening the mother-fetus relationship to safeguard maternal mental health. This study suggests that this sort of inter-disciplinary prenatal intervention is an effective approach for preventing, detecting and treating affective disorders in pregnant women and their children.

It is quite common for mental health problems, particularly depression, to complicate pregnancy. Depression is associated with certain risk factors and not treating this disorder may increase health risks factors to the mother and the fetus. Hence, preventive strategies that aim at detecting and preventing risk factors and early diagnosis of depression during prenatal care seem to be more effective than posterior therapeutic strategies. They ought to constitute a crucial aspect of preventive policies in the area of mother and child health (Austin, 2003; Gordon et al., 2006).

4. Conclusion

In this review, most gestational depression prevalence rates reported in developing countries were about 20%. The most common risk factors associated with depression in this stage of life were a psychiatric history- particularly a history of depression; factors related to poverty such as low income, financial difficulties, low education level, informal work and unemployment; lack of social, family or marital support, instability in relationships; stressful life events; unwanted pregnancy; alcohol, tobacco and other drug abuse; and a history of domestic violence. These factors are more frequent in disadvantaged socioeconomic contexts such as those found in developing countries where, many times, prenatal care is the only contact a woman in reproductive age will have with health services. Within this context, this prenatal period is a crucial to intervene in order to promote women's health and mental health in the long term (Neumann et al., 2003), as well as their children preventive health (Patel et al., 2004). The data reported in the reviewed studies support the need for integrating mental health and prenatal care for women in reproductive age. Postnatal depression prevention needs to be also started on the prenatal period (Patel et al, 2002). Lastly, the findings reported in these reviewed studies suggests that gestational depression is associated with poverty indicators, above all, to unemployment and low education levels, all for public policies which will address these social issues.

In sum, depression is a worldwide public health problem and tops the list of causes resulting on higher years lived with disability (YDLs) in the world (WHO, 2001). It affects approximately 154 million people all over the world and is twice as prevalent in women (5% to 9%) as it is in men (2% to 3%) (WHO, 2001). Further, since gestational depression can have negative consequences on the mother and baby's health during gestation, it needs to be addresses in development of public maternal and child health policies.

5. References

Adewuya, A.O.; Ola, B.A.; Aloba, O.O.; Dada, A.O. & Fasoto, O.O. (2007). Prevalence and correlates of depression in late pregnancy among Nigerian women. *Depress Anxiety*, 24(1): 15-21.

Alami, K.M.; Kadri, N. & Berrada, S. (2006). Prevalence and psychosocial correlates of depressed mood during pregnancy and after chilbirth in a Moroccan sample. *Arch. Womens Ment Health*, 9(6): 343-6.

Allister, L.; Lester, B.M.; Carr, S. & Liu, J. (2001). The effects of maternal depression on fetal heart rate response to vibroacoustic stimulation. *Dev Neuropsychol*, 20(3): 639-51.

American Psychiatric Association. (1994). *Manual Diagnóstico e Estatístico de Transtornos Mentais*. 4. ed. Porto Alegre: Artes médicas.

American Psychiatric Association. (2002). *Manual Diagnóstico e Estatístico de Transtornos Mentais*. 4. ed. rev. Porto Alegre: Artmed.

Anderson, B.A.; Marshak, H.H. & Hebbeler, D.L. (2002). Identifying intimate partner violence at entry to prenatal care: clustering routine clinical information. *J Midwifery Womens Health*, 47(5): 353-9.

Andersson, L.; Sundströn-Poromaa, I.; Aström, M. & Bixo, M. (2006). Depression and anxiety during pregnancy and six months postpartum: a follow-up study. *Acta Obstet Gynecol Scand*, 85(8): 937-44.

Araujo, D.M.R., Vilarim, M.M., Sabroza, A.R. & Nardi, A.E. (2010). Depressão no período gestacional e baixo peso ao nascer: uma revisão sistemática da literatura. *Cad Saúde Pública*. 26(2):219-227.

Banti, S., Mauri, M, Oppo, A, Borri, C, Rambelli, C, Ramacciotti, D, Montagnani, MS, Camilleri, V, Cortopassi, S, Rucci, P. & Cassan, GB. (2010). From the third month of pregnancy to 1 year postpartum. Prevalence, incidence, recurrence, and new onset of depression. Results from the Perinatal Depression–Research & Screening Unit study. *Compr Psychiatry*, 52(4): 343-51.

Beck, A.T.; Steer, R.A. & Garbin, M.G. (1998) Psychometric properties of the Beck Depression Inventory: twenty-five years of evaluation. *Clinical Psychology Review*, 8: 77–100.

Bennett, H.A.; Einarson, A.; Koren, G. & Einarson, T.R. (2004) Prevalence of Depression during Pregnancy: Sistematic Review. *Obstet Gynecol*, 103(4): 698-709.

Benute, G.R.G.; Nomura, R.M.Y.; Reis,J.S.; Junior,R.F.; Lucia, M.C.S. & Zugaib, M. (2010). Depression during pregnancy in women with a medical disorder: risk factors and perinatal outcomes. *CLINICS* 65(11): 1127-31.

Botega, N.J. & Dias, M.K. (2006). Gravidez e Puerpério. In: *Prática Psiquiátrica no Hospital Geral: Interconsulta e Emergência*. Botega, N.J et al. 2. ed. Porto Alegre: Artmed.

Camacho R.S.; Cantinelli F.S.; Ribeiro C.S.; Cantilino A.; Gonsales B.K.; Braguittoni E. et al. Transtornos Psiquiátricos na Gestação e no Puerpério: Classificação, Diagnóstico e Tratamento. *Rev Psiquiatr Clín*, 2006, 33(2): 92-102.

Caputo, V.G. & Bordin, I.A. Problemas de saúde mental entre jovens grávidas e não-grávidas. (2007). *Rev Saúde Pública*, 41(4): 573-81.

Carvalho, P.I.; Pereira, P.M.H.; Frias, P.G.; Vidal, S.A. & Figueiroa, J.N. (2007) Fatores de risco para a mortalidade neonatal em coorte hospitalar de nascidos vivos. *Epidemiol Ser Saúde*, 16(3): 185-194.

Chee, C.Y.I.; Lee, D.T.S.; Chong, Y.S.; Tan, L.K.; Ng, T.P. & Fones, C.S.L. (2005). Confinement and other psychosocial factors in perinatal depression: A transcultural study in Singapore. *Journal of Affective Disorders*, 89: 157–166.

Chung, T.K.; Lau, T.K.; Yip, A.S.; Chiu, H.F.; Lee, D.T. (2001). Antepartum depressive symptomatology is associated with adverse obstetric and neonatal outcomes. *Psychosom Med*, 63(5): 830-4.

Cohen, L.S.; Nonacs, R.; Viguera, A.C. & Reminick, A. (2004). Diagnosis and treatment of depression during pregnancy. *CNS Spectr*, 9(3): 209-16.

Cox, J.L.; Holden , J.M. & Sagovsky, R. (1987). Detection of postnatal depression. Development of the 10-item Edinburgh Postnatal Depression Scale . *British Journal of Psychiatry*, 1987, 150: 782-86.

Crowne, D.P. & Marlowe, D. (1960). A new scale of social desirability independent of psychopathology. *J Consul Psychol*, 24: 349-54.

Cruz, E.B.S.; Simões, G.L. & Faisal-Cury, A. (2005). Rastreamento da depressão pós-parto em mulheres atendidas pelo Programa de Saúde da Família. *Rev Bras Ginecol Obstet*, 27(4): 181-8.

Da Costa, D.; Larouche, J.; Dritsa, M. & Brender, W. (2000). Psychosocial correlates of prepartum and postpartum depressed mood. *Journal of Affective Disorders*, 59: 31-40.

Dhillon, N. & MacArthur, C. (2010). Antenatal depression and male gender preference in Asian women in the UK . *Midwifery*, 26(3): 286-293.

Downs S.H. & Black N. (1998). The feasibility of creating a checklist for the assessment of the methodological quality both of randomised and non-randomised studies of health care interventions. *J Epidemiol Community Health*. 52:377-84.

Evans, J.; Heron, J.; Francomb, H.; Oke, S. & Golding, J. (2001). Cohort study of depressed mood during pregnancy and after childbirth. *BMJ*, 323(7307): 257-60.

Faisal-Cury, A. & Rossi Menezes, P. (2007). Prevalence of anxiety and depression during pregnancy in a private setting sample. *Arch Womens Ment Health*, 10(1): 25-32.

Falcone, V.M., Mader, C.V.N., Nascimento, C.F.L.; Santos J.M.M.; Nóbrega F.J. Atuação multiprofissional e a saúde mental de gestantes. *Rev Saúde Pública*, 2005, 39(4): 612-18.

Felice, E.; Saliba, J.; Grech, V. & Cox, J. (2004). Prevalence rates and psychosocial characteristics associated with depression in pregnancy and postpartum in Maltese women. *Journal of Affective Disorders*, 82: 297–301.

Ferri, C.P.; Mitsuhiro, S.S.; Barros, M.C.M.; Chalem, E.; Guinsburg, R.; Patel, V. et al. (2007). The impact of maternal experience of violence and common mental disorders on neonatal outcomes: a survey of adolescent mothers in Sao Paulo, Brazil. *BMC Public Health*, 7(1): 209.

Freitas, G.V.S. & Botega, N.J. (2002). Gravidez na adolescência: prevalência de depressão, ansiedade e ideação suicida. *Rev Assoc Med Bras*, 48(3): 245-49.

Fisher, J.; Tran,T.; La,B.T.; Kriitmaa,K.; Rosenthal, D. & Tran, T. (2010). Common perinatal mental disorders in northern Viet Nam: community prevalence and health care use. *Bull World Health Organ*, 88: 737–745.

Gavin, A.R.; Melville, J.L.; Rue,T.; Guo, Y.; Dina, K.T. & Katon, W., J. (2011). Racial differences in the prevalence of antenatal depression. *General Hospital Psychiatry*, 33(2): 87-93.

Golbasi, Z., Kelleci, M., Kisacik, G. & Cetin, A. (2010). Prevalence and Correlates of Depression in Pregnancy Among Turkish Women. *Matern Child Health J*, 14: 485–491.

Gold, L.H. Treatment of depression during pregnancy. (1999). *J Womens Health Gend Based Med*, 8(5): 601-7.

Gordon, T.E.; Cardone, I.A.; Kim, J.J.; Gordon, S.M. & Silver, R.K. (2006). Universal perinatal depression screening in an Academic Medical Center. *Obstet Gynecol*, 107(2 Pt 1): 342-7.

Gulseren, L.; Erol, A.; Gulseren, S.; Kuey, L.; Kilic, B. & Ergor, G. (2006). From antepartum to postpartum: a prospective study on the prevalence of peripartum depression in a semiurbanTurkish community. *J Reprod Med*, 51(12): 955-60.

Heron, J.; O'connor, T.G.; Evans, J.; Golding, J. & Glover, V. (2004). The course of anxiety and depression trough pregnancy and the postpartum in a community sample. *Journal of Affective Disorders*, 80(1): 65-73.

Jablensky, A.V.; Morgan, V.; Zubrick, S.R.; Bower, C. & Yellachich, L. (2005). Pregnancy, delivery and neonatal complication in a population cohort of women with schizophrenia and major affective disorders. *Am J Psychiatry*, 162 (1): 79-91.

Johanson, R.; Chapman, G.; Murray, D.; Johnson, I. & Cox, J. (2000). The North Staffordshire Maternity Hospital prospective study of pregnancy-associated depression. *J Psychosom Obstet Gynaecol*, 21(2): 93-7.

Josefsson, A.; Berg, G.; Nordin, C. & Sydsjö, G. (2001). Prevalence of depressive symptoms in late pregnancy and postpartum. *Acta Obstet Gynecol Scand*, 80(3): 251-5.

Karaçam, Z. & Ançel, G. (2009). Depression, anxiety and influencing factors in pregnancy: a study in a Turkish population. *Midwifery*, 25: 344–356.

Kitamura, T.; Yoshida, K.; Okano, T.; Kinoshita, K.; Hayashi, M.; Toyoda, N. et al. (2006). Multicentre prospective study of perinatal depression in Japan: incidence and correlates of antenatal and postnatal depression. *Arch Womens Ment Health*, 9: 121-30.

Krause, N. & Markides, K. (1990). Measuring social support among older adults. *International Journal Aging and Human Development*, 30: 37-53.

Kurki, T.; Hiilesmaa, V.; Raitasalo, R.; Mattila, H. & Ylikorkala, O. (2000). Depression and anxiety in early pregnancy and risk for preeclampsia. *Obstet Gynecol*, 95(4): 487-90.

Lee, D.T.; Chan, S.S.; Sahota, D.S.; Yip, A.S.; Tsui, M. & Chung, T.K. (2004). A prevalence study of antenatal depression among chinese women. *J Affect Disord*, 82(1): 93-9.

Leigh, B. & Milgrom, J. (2008). Risk factors for antenatal depression, postnatal depression and parenting stress. *BMC Psychiatry*, 8(24): 1-11.

Lewis, G.; Pelosi, A.J.; Araya, R. & Dunn, G. (1992). Measuring psychiatric disorder in the community: a standardized assessment for use by lay interviewers. *Psychol Med*, 22: 465-86.

Limlomwongse, N.N. & Liabsuetrakul, T. (2006). Cohort study of depressive moods in Thai women during late pregnancy and 6–8 weeks of postpartum using the Edinburgh Postnatal Depression Scale (EPDS). *Arch Womens Ment Health*, 9: 131-38.

Lopes, C.; Faerstein, E. & Chor, D. (2003). Eventos de vida produtores de estresse e transtornos mentais comuns: resultados do Estudo Pró-Saúde. *Cad Saúde Pública*, 19(6): 1713-20.

Lovisi, G.M.; Lopes, J.R.; Coutinho, E. & Patel, V. (2005). Poverty, Violence and Depression during Pregnancy: a Survey of Mothers Attending a Public Hospital in Brazil. *Psychological Medicine*, 35: 1485-92.

Macfarlane, J.; Parker, B.; Soeken, K. & Bullock, L. (1992). Assessing for abuse during pregnancy. Severity and frequency of injuries and associated entry into prenatal care. *JAMA*, 267: 3176-78.

Maldonado, M.T. (1997). *Psicologia da Gravidez: Parto e Puerpério*. 17. ed. São Paulo: Saraiva.

Marcus, S.M.; Barry, K.L.; Flynn, H.A.; Tandon, R. & Greden, J.F. (2001). Treatment guidelines for depression in pregnancy. *Int J Gynaecol Obstet*, 72(1): 61-70.

Marcus, S.M.; Flynn, H.A.; Blow, F.C. & Barry, K.L. (2003). Depressive Symptoms among Pregnant Women Screened in Obstetrics Settings. *Journal of Women's Health*, 12(4): 373-80.

Marcus, S., Lopez, J.F., McDonough, S., MacKenzie, M.J., Flynn, H., Neal Jr., C.R., Gahagan, S., Volling, B., Kaciroti, N. & Vazquez, D.M. (2011). Depressive symptoms during pregnancy: Impact on neuroendocrine and neonatal outcomes. *Infant Behavior & Development*, 34: 26–34.

Martínez, J.R.L.; Ibarzabal, Z.U.; Doménech, S.P. & Soler, Y.H. (2008). Depresión durante el embarazo. *Revista Enfermaria Integral*, 8(1): 17-19.

Matos, M.L.L.; Piélago, J.S. & Figueroa, A.L. (2009). Depresión mayor en embarazadas atendidas en el Instituto Nacional Materno Perinatal de Lima, Perú. *Rev Panam Salud Publica/Pan Am J Public Health*, 26(4): 310-314.

Micali, N.; Simonoff, E. & Treasure, J. (2010). Pregnancy and post-partum depression and anxiety in a longitudinal general population cohort: The effect of eating disorders and past depression. *J Affect Disord*, 131(1-3): 150-157.

Miller, G.A. (1994). *The Substance Abuse Subtle Screening Inventory. Manual, and Supplement for SASSI-2*. Addiction Research and Consultation, Bloomington, IN.

Mitsuhiro, S.S.; Chalem, E.; Barros, M.M.; Guinsburg, R. & Laranjeira, R. (2006). Teenage pregnancy: use of drugs in the third trimester and prevalence of psychiatric disorders. *Rev Bras Psiquiatr*, 28(2): 122-5.

Mitsuhiro, S.S.; Chalem, E.; Barros, M.C.M.; Guinsburg, R. & Laranjeira, R. (2009). Brief report: Prevalence of psychiatric disorders in pregnant teenagers. *J Adolesc*, 32(3): 747-52.

Mohammad, K.I.; Gamble , J. & Creedy, D.K. Prevalence and factors associated with the development of antenatal and postnatal depression among Jordanian women. *Midwifery*, Article in Press [Epub ahead of print].

Motta, M.G.; Lucion, A.B. & Manfro, G.G. (2005). Effects of maternal depression on the neurobiological and psychological development of children. *Rev Psiquiatr Rio Gd Sul*, 27(2): 165-76.

Murray, D. & Cox, J.L. (1990). Screening for depression during pregnancy with the Edinburgh Depression Scale (EPDS). *J Reprod Inf Psychol*, 8: 99–107.

Neumann, N.A.; Tanaka, O.Y.; Victora, C.G. & Cesar, J.A. (2003). Qualidade e Eqüidade da atenção ao pré-natal e ao parto em Criciúma, Santa Catarina, Sul do Brasil. *Revista Brasileira de Epidemiologia*, 6(4): 307-18.

Newport, D.J.; Hostetter, A.; Arnold, A. & Stowe, Z.N. (2002). The treatment of postpartum depression: minimizing infant exposures. *J Clin Psychiatry*, 63(7): 31-34.

O'brien, L.; Schachtschneider, A.M.; Koren, G.; Walker, J.H. & Einarson, A. (2007). Longitudinal study of depression, anxiety, irritability and stress in pregnancy following evidence-based counseling on the use of antidepressants. *J Psychiatr Pract*, 13(1): 33-9.

Ortega, L.; Lartigue, T. & Figueroa, M.E. (2001). Prevalencia de depresión, a través de la Escala de Depresión Perinatal de Edinburgh (EPDS), en una muestra de mujeres mexicanas embarazadas. *Perinatol Reprod Hum*, 15(1): 11-20.

Pajulo, M.; Savonlahti, E.; Sourander, A.; Helenius, H. & Piha, J. (2001). Antenatal Depression, Substance Dependency and Social Support. *Journal of Affective Disorders*, 65: 9-17.

Parker, G.; Tupling, H. & Brown, L.B. (1979). A parental bonding instrument. *Br J Med Psychology*, 52: 1-10.

Patel, V.; Desouza, N. & Rodrigues, M. (2003). Postnatal Depression and infant growth and development in low income countries: a cohort study from Goa, Índia. *Archives of Disease in Childhood*, 88: 34-37.

Patel, V. & Kleinman, A. (2003). Poverty and common mental disorders in developing countries. *Bulletin of World Health Organization*, 81(8): 609-15.

Patel, V. & Prince, M. (2006). Maternal psychological morbidity and low birth in Índia. *Br J Psychiatry*, 188: 284-5.

Patel, V.; Rahman, A.; Jacob, K.S. & Hughes, M. (2004). Effect of maternal mental health on infant growth in low income countries: new evidence from South Asia. *BMJ*, 328(7443): 820-23.

Patel, V.; Rodrigues, M. & Desouza, N. (2002). Gender, Poverty and Postnatal Depression: a study of mothers in goa, Índia. *Am J Psychiatry*, 159(1): 43-47.

Paton, C. (2008). Prescribing in Pregnancy. *Br J Psychiatry*, 192(5): 321-22.

Paykel, E.S. (1983). Methodological aspects of life-events research. *J Psychom Res*, 27: 341–52.

Pereira, P.K.; Lovisi, G.M.;. Pilowsky, D.L.; Lima, L.A. & Legay, L.F. (2009). Depression during pregnancy: prevalence and risk factors among women attending a public health clinic in Rio de Janeiro, Brazil. *Cad. Saúde Pública*, 25(12): 2725-2736.

Pottinger, A.M.; Trotman-Edwards, H. & Younger, N. (2009). Detecting depression during pregnancy and associated lifestyle practices and concerns among women in a hospital-based obstetric clinic in Jamaica. *Gen Hosp Psychiatry*, 31(3): 254-61.

Qiao, Y-X., Wang, J., LI, J. & Ablat, A. (2009). The prevalence and related risk factors of anxiety and depression symptoms among Chinese pregnant women in Shanghai. *Australian and New Zealand Journal of Obstetrics and Gynaecology*, 49: 185–190.

Quinlivan, J.A. & Condon, J. (2005). Anxiety and depression in fathers in teenage pregnancy. *Aust N Z J Psychiatry*, 39(10): 915-20.

Radloff, L.S. (1977). The CES-D scale: a self-report depression scale for research in the general population. *Appl Psychol Meas*, 1: 385–401.

Rahman, A.; Harrington, R. & Bunn, J. (2002). Can maternal depression increase infant risk of illness and growth impairment in developing countries? *Child: Care, Health e Development*, 28(1): 51-56.

Rahman, A.; Iqbal, Z.; Bunn, J.; Lovel, H. & Harrington, R. (2004). Impact of maternal depression on infant nutritional status and illness: a cohort study. *Archives of General Psychiatry*, 61: 946-52.

Rich-Edwards, J.W.; Kleinman, K.; Abrams, A.; Harlow, B.L.; Mclaughlin, T.J.; Joffe, H. et al. (2006). Sociodemographic predictors of antenatal and postpartum depressive symptoms among women in a medical group practice. *J Epidemiol Community Health*, 60(3): 221-7.

Rodriguez, M. A.; Heilemann, M.V.; Fielder, E. A.; Nevarez, F. & Mangione, C.M. (2008). Intimate Partner Violence, Depression, and PTSD Among Pregnant Latina Women. *Annals of Family Medicine*, 6(1): 44-52.

Rossi C.E. & Vasconcelos, F.A.G. (2010). Peso ao nascer e obesidade em crianças e adolescentes: uma revisão sistemática. Rev Bras Epidemiol. 13(2):246-58.

Rubertsson, C.; Wickberg, B.; Gustavsson, P. & Radestad, I. (2005). Depressive symptoms in early pregnancy, two months and one year portpartum-prevalence and psychosocial risk factors in a national Swedish sample. *Arch Womens Ment Health*, 8: 97-104.

Russell, M. (1994). New assessment tools for risk drinking during pregnancy. *Alcohol World*, 18: 55.

Ryan, D.; Milis, L. & Misri, N. (2005). Depression during pregnancy. *Can Fam Physician*, 51: 1087-93.

Sarason, I.G.; Levine, H.M.; Basham, R.B. & Sarason, B.R. (1983). Assessment of social support: The Social Support Questionnaire. *J Pers Soc Psychol*, 44: 127-39.

Sheehan, D.V.; Lecrubier, Y.; Harnett Sheehan, K.; Janavs, J.; Weiller, E.; Keskiner, A. et al. (1997). The validity of the Mini International Neuropsychiatric Interview according to the SCID-P and its reliability. *Eur Psychiatry*, 12: 232-41.

Sherbourne, C.D. & Stewart, A.L. (1991). The MOS Social Support Survey. *Social Science and Medicine*, 32: 705-14.

Silva, R.A.; Jansen, K.; Souza, L.D.M.; Moraes, I.G.S.; Tomasi,E.; Silva, G.D.G.; Dias, M.S. & Pinheiro, R.T. Depression during pregnancy in the Brazilian public health care system. *Revista Brasileira de Psiquiatria*, 32(2): 139-44.

Skouteris, H.; Wertheim, E. H.; Rallis, S.; Milgrom, J. & Paxton, S. J. (2009). Depression and anxiety through pregnancy and the early postpartum: an examination of prospective relationships. *Journal of Affective Disorders*, 113(3): 303-308.

Soares, C.N.; Viguera, A.C. & Cohen, L.S. (2001). Mood disturbance and pregnancy: pros and cons of pharmacologic treatment. *Rev Bras Psiquiatr*, 23(1): 48-53.

Spinelli, M.G. (1997). Interpersonal psychoterapy for depressed antepartum women: a pilot study. *Am J Psychiatry*, 154(7): 1028-30.

Spinelli, M.G. & Endicott, J. (2003). Controlled clinical trial of interpessoal psychotherapy versus parenting education program for depressed pregnat women. *Am J Psychitry*, 160(3): 555-62.

Spitzer, R.L.; Williams, J.B.W.; Kroenke, K.; Linzer, M.; Degruy, F.V.; Hahn, S.R. et al. (1994). Utility of a New Procedure for Diagnosing Mental Disorders in Primary Care The PRIME-MD 1000 Study. *JAMA*, 272: 1749-56.

Spoozak, L.; Gotman, N.; Smith, M.V.; Belanger, K. & Yonkers, K.A. (2009). Evaluation of a social support measure that may indicate risk of depression during pregnancy. *Journal of Affective Disorders*, 114(1): 216–23.

Wadhwa, P.D.; Dunkel-Schetter, C.; Chicz-Demet, A.; Porto, M. & Sandman, C.A. (1996). Prenatal psychosocial factors and the neuroendocrine axis in human pregnancy. *Psychosomat Medicine*, 58: 432-46.

Weissman, M.M. (2007). Recent non-medication trials of interpersonal psychoterapy for depression. *Int J Neuropsychopharmacol*, 10(1): 117-22.

Wilhelm, K. & Parker, G. (1988). The development of a measure of intimate bonds. *Psychol Med*, 18: 225-34.

Wittchen, H.U.; Robbins, L.N.; Sartorius, N.; Burke, J.D. & Regier, D. (1991). Cross-cultural feasibility, reliabilty and sources of variance of the Composite International Diagnostic Interview (CIDI). *British Journal Psychiatry*, 159: 645-53.

Wojcicki, J.M., Holbrook, K., Lustig, R.H., Epel, E., Caughey, A.B., Muñoz, R.F., Shiboski, S.C. & Heyman, M.B. (2011). Chronic Maternal Depression Is Associated with Reduced Weight Gain in Latino Infants from Birth to 2 Years of Age. *PLoS ONE*, 6(2): e16737.

World Health Organization. (1993). *Classificação de Transtornos Mentais e de Comportamento da CID-10*. Porto Alegre: Editora Artes Médicas.

World Health Organization. (2001). *The World Health Report – Mental health: new understanding, new hope*. Genebra: World Health Organization.

Wu, J.; Viguera, A.; Riley, L.; Cohen, L. & Ecker, J. (2002). Mood disturbance in pregnancy and the mode of delivery. *Am J Obstet Gynecol*, 187(4): 864-7.

Zigmond, A. & Snaith, R. (1983). The Hospital Anxiety and Depression Scale. *Acta Psychiatr Scand*, 67: 361-70.

Zinga, D.; Shauna, D.P. & Born, L. (2005). Postpartum depression: we know the risks, can it be prevented? *Rev Bras Psiquiatr*, 27(Supl II): S56-64.

11

A New Class of Antidepressant Drugs in the Treatment of Psychiatric Disorders: The Triple Reuptake Inhibitors

B.P. Guiard
Laboratoire de Neuropharmacologie, Faculté de Pharmacie, Université Paris sud XI, Châtenay-Malabry, France

1. Introduction

It is well established that many antidepressant compounds with proven clinical efficacy act on the serotonergic and noradrenergic pathways. The monoaminergic hypothesis of major depression (MD) stipulates that a deficit in brain monoaminergic neurotransmission in various brain areas including the frontal cortex, hippocampus, amygdala or hypothalamus would account for some of signs and symptoms of the pathology (Katz et al., 2010a). For instance, abnormalities in the serotonin (5-HT) transmission are associated with impulsivity, aggressive, and anxious behaviors (Handley et al., 1995), whereas alteration in noradrenergic transmission, with motor activity, attention, and arousal (Morilak and Frazer, 2004). The role of dopamine (DA) on the other hand, attracted less attention in the mechanisms of action underlying MD. However, the observations that reserpine, which depletes catecholamines, results in lowering mood (Schidkrautn 1965) or that an inhibition of tyrosine hydroxylase induces a worsening of depressive symptoms (Miller et al., 1996), strongly suggest that decreasing DA function may be of particular relevance. The fact that several symptoms observed in MD, including impaired motivation, concentration, and pleasure result from an attenuation of dopaminergic neurotransmission, strengthens the hypothesis that DA also regulates mood (Dunlop and Nemeroff, 2007).

Most antidepressants approved, such as the selective serotonin reuptake inhibitors (SSRIs), the norepinephrine (NE) reuptake inhibitor (NRIs) or the dual serotonin/norepinephrine reuptake inhibitors (SNRIs), act by enhancing brain 5-HT and/or NE levels. Despite their therapeutic action, residual symptoms remain and may explain the fact that approximately 50% of depressive individuals do not respond adequately to these agents (Berton and Nestler, 2006). The question can be asked as to whether these remaining symptoms are caused by the antidepressants or if they result from dysfunction in other neurotransmitters such as a blunted DA neurotransmission. In this context, a new generation of antidepressant drugs, the triple reuptake inhibitors (TRIs), has been developed with the hope to offer a clinically relevant advantage over single- or dual-acting agents (Guiard et al., 2009). Indeed, since TRIs simultaneously enhance extracellular levels of 5-HT, NE and DA neurotransmissions in various brain regions, this class of antidepressants could exert their therapeutic activity by treating more symptoms of MD and/or by attenuating some side

effects observed in response to traditional antidepressants. As an example, it is believed that the dopaminergic component of TRIs may prevent sexual dysfunctions induced by an increase in brain 5-HT.
The present review describes the serotonergic, noradrenergic and dopaminergic pathways in the brain and the specific symptoms of depression under their control. Then it focuses on the preclinical *in vitro* and *in vivo* properties of TRIs. Indeed, the knowledge of their pharmacological properties may help better understand their mechanism of action and anticipate their putative efficacy over SSRIs, NRIs and SNRIs in humans. Finally, since over 75% of depressed patients suffer from painful symptoms and that monoaminergic pathways control many of the psychological functions that are disturbed in depression and pain perception (Hache et al., 2011), this review addresses the possibility that TRIs may exert part of their antidepressant activity by preventing/reversing algesia in depressed patients.

2. Monoaminergic pathways in the brain and their reciprocal interactions

2.1 The serotonergic system

Serotonin (5-HT) is present in most brain regions in the central nervous system. In the brain, serotonergic neurons originate within the brain stem. This system is comprised of a relatively small number of neurons that are clustered in nine phylogenetically conserved nuclei grouped into caudal (B1–B5) and rostral (B6–B9) nuclei including the dorsal and median raphe (DR and MR; respectively), with the former projecting to areas of the deep cerebellar nuclei, cortex, and spinal cord, whereas the latter extends an axonal network throughout the forebrain and cortices (Dahlström and Fuxe, 1964). Of particular relevance to mechanisms of MD are projections to structural correlates of emotionality including the amygdala, prefrontal and cingulated cortices, hypothalamus, and thalamus (Hornung 2003). Recently, 5-HT neurons have been classified based on genetic lineages. Specifically, 5-HT neuronal progenitors can be subdivided into subpopulations, which are discriminated by differing genetic transcription factors such as Pet-1 (Kiyasova et al., 2011; Hendricks, 2003). Indeed, this factor is required for the acquisition of serotonergic identity in a majority of neurons in the raphe nuclei including the dorsal and median raphe nuclei. However residual 5-HT neurons outline a unique subpopulation of raphe neurons with highly selective anatomical targets particularly the brain areas involved in stress responses with dense innervation to the basolateral amygdala, the paraventricular nucleus of the hypothalamus, and the intralaminar thalamic nuclei. It has thus been proposed the existence of Pet1-dependent and Pet1-resistant 5-HT neurons targeting different brain centers that might delineate the anatomical basis for a dual serotonergic control on stress responses (Kiyasova et al., 2011).

2.2 The noradrenergic system

The central noradrenergic neurotransmitter system originates from two distinct groups of cells in the brainstem (Dell'Osso et al., 2010). The main noradrenergic brain circuits are located in the locus coeruleus (corresponding to A4+A6 cell groups), which send noradrenergic projections throughout the neuroaxis innervating areas such as the frontal cortex, hippocampus and amygdala as well as the cerebellum (Dahlström and Fuxe, 1965). This ascending projection system is also referred to as the dorsal noradrenergic bundle. The locus coeruleus is basically involved in the responsiveness to external conditions and vigilance, providing pathways descending to the spinal cord and projecting throughout the limbic system and diencephalon (Racagni and Brunello). Efferents from the lateral tegmentum (corresponding to A1, A2, A5 and A7 cell groups) have less extensive projections (Dahlström and Fuxe, 1965). They provide predominant innervation of the hypothalamus and also innervate areas of the septum and the extended amygdala nuclei including the bed nucleus of the stria terminalis (Moore and Card, 1984). Interestingly, noradrenergic and serotonergic systems overlap at several levels and are far away to be independent, both distributing to broad cortical areas (Brühl et al., 2010). Reciprocal projections between the major groups of 5-HT and NE cell bodies have been reported, creating ample opportunity for cross-modulation between these systems. For example, it is well established that NE stimulates the neuronal activity of 5-HT neurons in the DR (Mongeau et al., 1997). In a marked contrast, 5-HT projections from the DR nucleus to the locus coeruleus, impose a tonic inhibitory tone on the firing of NE neurons (Dremencov et al., 2009).

2.3 The dopaminergic system

Most DA-producing neurons in the brain are located in brainstem nuclei: the retro-rubro field (A8), the substantia nigra pars compacta (A9), and the ventral tegmental area (VTA) (A10) (Dunlop and Nemeroff, 2007). Projection pathways of the axons arising from these cell bodies follow specific pathways via the medial forebrain bundle to innervate specific cortical and subcortical structures, unlike the more diffuse innervation patterns of serotonergic and noradrenergic cells. The nigrostriatal pathway projects from the substantia nigra pars compacta to the dorsal striatum (caudate and putamen) and has a prominent role in the motor planning and execution of movement, although it clearly also plays an important role in non-motor functions, such as cognition (McClure et al., 2003). The mesocortical pathway arises from the VTA and projects to the frontal and temporal cortices, particularly the anterior cingulate, enthorinal, and prefrontal cortices. This pathway is believed to be important for concentration and executive functions such as working memory. The mesolimbic pathway also arises from the VTA but projects to the ventral striatum (including the nucleus accumbens), bed nucleus of the stria terminalis, hippocampus, amygdala, and septum. It is particularly important for motivation, the experience of pleasure and reward. The tuberoinfundibular pathway arises from the arcuate nucleus of the hypothalamus (A12) and projects to the median eminence of the hypothalamus, where DA released into the portal vessels acts to inhibit the secretion of prolactin from the anterior pituitary (Ben-Jonathan and Hnasko, 2001). The incertohypothalamic pathway originates from cell bodies in the medial portion of the zona incerta (A13) and innervates amygdaloid and hypothalamic nuclei involved in sexual behavior. Unlike the other dopaminergic pathways, the "thalamic dopamine system" arises from multiple sites, including the periaqueductal gray matter and may contribute to the control of nociception (Hache et al., 2011). Importantly, serotonergic and noradrenergic neurons also display a high degree of anatomical and functional connectivity with the dopaminergic system. For instance, in addition to its tonic inhibition of NE transmission, 5-HT is believed to inhibit the firing of DA neurons in the VTA (Guiard et al., 2008a; 2008b). The influence of NE on DA neurons is more complex since both excitatory and inhibitory impacts have been reported (Guiard et al., 2008a; 2008b; Linner et al., 2001). On the other and, growing evidence suggest that DA may modulate the activity of 5-HT and NE neurons. It is suspected that DA directly increases the neuronal activity of 5-HT neurons in the DR (Haj-Dahmane, 2001; Martin-Ruiz et al., 2001), thereby enhancing local 5-HT outflow (Ferre et al., 1994; Ferre and Artigas, 1993; Martin-Ruiz et al., 2001). In contrast, multiple source of evidence demonstrates that DA inhibits the neuronal activity of NE neurons in the LC (Guiard et al., 2008a, 2008b; Deutch et al., 1986; Elam et al., 1986).

3. Depression: monoaminergic symptoms and disturbances

Based on the findings from studies of antidepressants, it may be possible to assign specific symptoms of depression to specific neurochemical mechanisms (Nutt, 2008a). Knowing which particular neurotransmitters are associated with particular symptoms of depression may help determine appropriate treatments that target specific mechanism that in turn target specific depression symptoms. 5-HT may be related to anxiety, compulsions and sleep disturbances; NE to alertness and energy as well as anxiety, attention, and interest in life; and DA to motivation, pleasure, and reward, as well as interest in life (Figure 1). Increasing any of these 3 neurotransmitters will elevate mood, but the other elements of depression may be particularly responsive to a certain neurotransmitter.

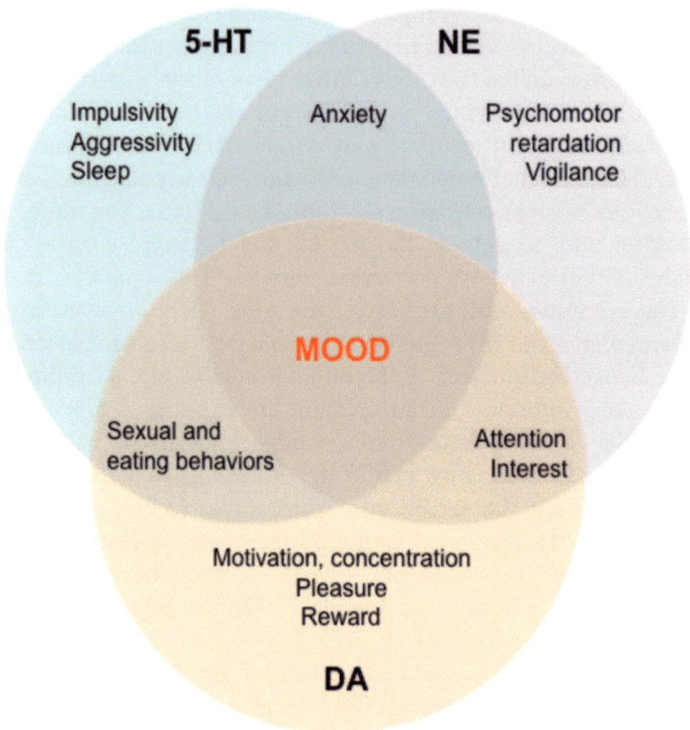

Fig. 1. Monoamine regulation of mood behavior (Adapted from Nutt, 2008).

3.1 Depressed mood and sadness

Neuroimaging studies have associated depressed mood and sadness with abnormal neuronal activity in the medial prefrontal cortex (Drevets, 1999). This brain region receives innervation from serotonergic (midbrain raphe), noradrenergic (locus coeruleus) and dopaminergic (ventral tegmental area) pathways. Low levels of these monoamines may decrease mood whereas antidepressants that enhance levels of monoamines have been shown to improve depressed mood and sadness (Morilak and Frazer, 2004). Other symptoms and/or comorbidities such as sleep or appetite disturbances as well as nociception may be affected in patients with MD and should draw attention of physicians when choosing antidepressants therapy. Clearly, an improved treatment of MD should start with a good diagnosis, based on the symptoms patients encounter as disturbances in different neurotransmitter systems.

3.2 Diminished interest and pleasure

Reduced dopaminergic activity has been linked to decreased motivation (Salamone et al., 2003), anhedonia (loss of pleasure) and loss of interest (Willner, 1983), whereas increased dopaminergic transmission has been linked to positive affect (Depue and Collins, 1999). The mesocortical dopaminergic pathway, in particular the nucleus accumbens is a key regulator of pleasure. The prefrontal cortex is believed to be important in motivation (Drevets, 2001). A dysfunction of the mesocorticolimbic dopaminergic system innervating limbic structures including the nucleus accumbens, amygdala, ventral hippocampus and cortical areas may underlie the symptoms of loss of motivation, loss of interest and the inability to experience pleasure observed in MD. Antidepressants that enhance DA release including bupropion, may thus improve these symptoms (Dunlop and Nemeroff, 2007).

3.3 Fatigue and loss of energy

Brains areas controlling motor function such as the striatum innervated by DA and 5-HT neurons may be involved in physical fatigue, (Stahl et al., 2008). Mental fatigue and lack of mental energy may be related to other symptoms of depression, such as apathy (absence in feeling, emotion, interest) and lack of motivation. Cortical brain regions, especially the dorsolateral prefrontal cortex, are more likely to be involved in mental fatigue (MacHale et al., 2000). Consequently, antidepressants that increase DA and 5-HT, or both, may be preferable for patients with predominant symptoms of fatigue and loss of energy (Stahl et al., 2008).

3.4 Anxiety

The neuronal pathway of fears involved the amygdala, which receives NE and 5-HT innervation from the LC and DR, respectively. High levels of amygdala activation are associated with an increased prevalence of anxiety (Davidson et al., 2002) raising the possibility that antidepressants targeting both NE and 5-HT, may be more appropriate for treating depressed patients with comorbid anxiety disorders (Morilak and Frazer, 2004).

3.5 Sleep disturbance

There is a very strong association between sleep disturbance and major depression. Depressed patients usually complain of insomnia, notably of difficulties in falling asleep, frequent awakenings during the night, early waking up, and non-refreshing sleep (Benca et al., 1992). As well as distressing symptoms of sleep experienced by patients, changes in sleep architecture have been reported. Compared with normal controls, sleep continuity of depressed subjects is often impaired, with increased wakefulness (more frequent and longer periods of wakefulness), and reduced sleep efficiency. Sleep onset latency is significantly increased and total sleep time reduced. Rapid eye movement (REM) latency is often shortened, and the duration of the first REM period is increased (Nutt et al., 2008b). The role of 5-HT in the regulation of sleep is well documented and studies indicate that the neuronal activity of 5-HT and its release is maximal during wakefulness (W), reduced during slow wave sleep (SWS), and minimal during rapid eye movement (REM) sleep (Adrien, 2002). Consequently, SSRIs, which increase 5-HT function increase REM latency, and reduce REM sleep (Wilson and Argyropoulos, 2005) may worsen sleep disturbance early in treatment (Hicks et al., 2002) and may leave residual sleep symptoms once mood is improved (Nelson et al., 2005). It is noteworthy that depressed patients may also display an excessive sleep and hypersomnia, particularly in atypical depression (Gold et al., 2002). This latter observation emphasizes the fact that a better diagnosis, based on the different subtypes of MD is a prerequisite to optimize and individualize antidepressant therapy.

3.6 Appetite and eating disorders

Eating disorders, the term now encompasses anorexia nervosa and bulimia nervosa (Jimerson et al., 1993), result from alteration, at least in part, in monoaminergic neurotransmission involved in the homeostatic control of appetite function. For example, positive correlations between mood disturbances and eating and weight concerns have been reported (Casper et al., 1998). Although, the background of eating disorders is complex, the involvement of impaired hypothalamic 5-HT function in these disorders is well documented (Wallin and Rissanen, 1994). In agreement with the observation that in this brain region, 5-HT contributes to post-ingestive satiety, several studies have shown that SSRIs, particularly fluoxetine, is effective in controlling bulimic episodes (Walsh, 1994). This is also the case for other serotoninergic drugs, among them fenfluramine, which was used in the treatment of obesity (Guy-Grand, 1992). There is growing notion that mesolimbic dopaminergic neurotransmission also contributes to the effect of DA on feeding behavior (Volkow and Wise, 2005). Sibutramine, in addition to its effect on 5-HT, inhibits the reuptake of other monoamines and has been shown to enhance postprandial satiety, reduce total calorie intake and to diminish the decline in energy expenditure usually associated with a diet-induced negative energy balance (Hansen et al., 1999). Consequently, combined blockade of NE and 5-HT reuptake by SNRIs results in reduced food intake and body weight that neither monoamine reuptake inhibitor could achieve on its own. Interestingly, bupropion the dual NE releaser and DAT inhibitor (Dong and Blier, 2001), cause weight loss by combined induction of hypophagia and thermogenesis (Billes and Cowley, 2007).

Recently there has been interest in investigating the use of SSRIs in the treatment of patients with anorexia nervosa. Although fluoxetine has been associated with weight loss, it was proposed that this medication, because of a favorable side effect profile, could have advantages for treating depressive symptoms in patients with anorexia (Gwirtsman et al., 1990).

3.7 Nociception

This is specifically illustrated in the fifth chapter of the present review.

4. Pharmacological properties of TRIs

As described in the precedent chapter some comorbid symptoms of depression such as anhedonia, loss of motivation and concentration are directly connected to a deficit in central dopaminergic transmission. Consequently, triple reuptake inhibitors (TRIs) that simultaneously inhibit the reuptake of the three monoamines 5-HT, NE, DA (Chen & Skolnick, 2007) may provide greater symptomatic relief than SSRIs, NRIs or SNRIs. The interest of TRIs may also rely on the excitatory effect of DA upon the serotonergic system (Haj-Dahmane, 2001; Martin-Ruiz et al., 2001), thus suggesting that an increase in dopaminergic neurotransmission would facilitate that of 5-HT. In accordance with this hypothesis, it was shown that combination of SSRIs with bupropion lead to a synergy on monoamine transmission (Ghanbari et al. 2010; Prica et al. 2008; Li et al. 2002), as well as producing a robust antidepressant effect especially in treatment-resistant depressed patients

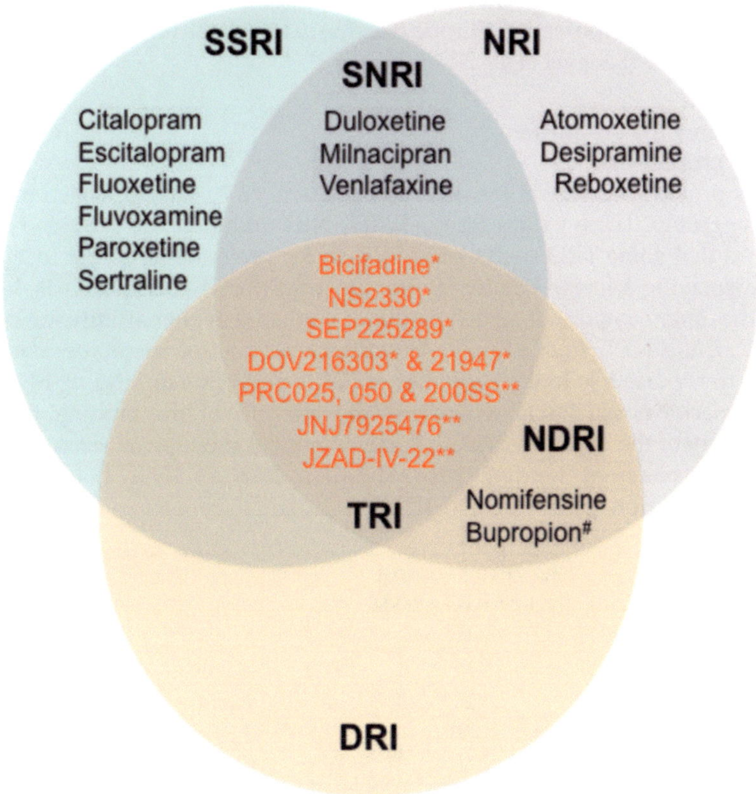

Fig. 2. Monoaminergic antidepressants blocking the serotonin, norepinephrine and/or dopamine transporter. These agents are in various clinical* or preclinical** phases of development in MD or comorbidities. Selective serotonin reuptake inhibitor (SSRI), norepinephrine reuptake inhibitor (NRI), dopamine reuptake inhibitor (DRI), serotonin/norepinephrine reuptake inhibitor (SNRI), norepinephrine/dopamine reuptake inhibitor (NDRI), triple reuptake inhibitor (TRI). #This agent is a dopamine reuptake inhibitor and a norepinephrine releaser (Dong and Blier, 2001).

(Leuchter et al. 2008; Zisook et al. 2006). A number of compounds with the ability to bind and block all three monoamine transporters have been developed. DOV Pharmaceutical, Inc. is the first company having provided *in vitro* and *in vivo* preclinical data with their triple reuptake inhibitors DOV216303 and DOV21947. New molecules have followed such as NS2330 (tesofensine, GlaxoSmith-Kline/NeuroSearch), SEP225289 (Sepracor Inc.), CNS-1 and CNS-2 (Albany Molecular Research Institute Inc), PRC-025, PRC-050, PRC-200SS (Mayo Foundation), JNJ7925476 (Johnson & Johnson Pharmaceutical Research & Development), WF-23 (Eli Lilly) and JZAD-IV-22 (PsychoGenics). Lundbeck laboratories develop their own compounds such as LuAA24530 but with the difference that they also antagonize monoaminergic receptors. Others compounds will undoubtedly emerge in a near future. Indeed, it is interesting to note that in 2010-2011, the pharmacological profiles of nine new compounds, studying the structure activity relationship (SAR), have been reported (Shao et al., 2011a; 2001b; 2011c; Caldarone et al., 2010; Carter et al., 2010; Lee et al., 2010; Lucas et al., 2010; Micheli et al., 2010a, 2010b; Schoedel et al., 2010). Despite the emergence of these compounds, older molecules with the abilities to inhibit all three monoamines transporters were already available such as the tryciclic agent nefopam approved in Europe (Heel et al., 1980), bicifadine in phase III (Basile et al., 2007) or indatraline (Lengyel et al., 2008) (Figure 2).

4.1 Preclinical in vitro properties

4.1.1 Binding properties

Many studies provide Kd values for their compounds, or Ki values, which are sometimes used interchangeably. These values for the SERT, NET and DAT are provided in Table 1. It can be noticed that some TRIs such as the PRC series preferentially bind to the SERT and NET while displaying a lower affinity for the DA transporter (DAT). This is, however, not the case for the other compounds which display a similar or higher affinity for the DAT than for the SERT or the NET. Interestingly, the affinity of most of these new compounds for monoamines transporters is lower than that of SSRIs and NRIs at binding SERT and NET, respectively (Hache et al., 2011). Therefore, the analysis of the binding properties and functional activity of the TRIs indicates that the novelty of these pharmacological agents lies in their relative balanced binding profile rather than in their potency at blocking monoamines transporters (Hache et al., 2011).

TRIs	In vitro binding (Ki or Kd in nM)			References
	SERT	NET	DAT	
Bicifadine[a]	2400	5000	5200	Basile et al., 2007
Indatraline[a]	0.6	2	4	Lengyel et al., 2008
DOV216303[a]	190	380	190	Chen and Skolnick, 2007
DOV21947[a]	110	260	210	Skolnick et al., 2003
JNJ7925476[a]	0.9	16	5	Aluisio et al., 2008
PRC025[b]	6	10	53	Shaw et al., 2007
PRC050[b]	12	1.2	43	Shaw et al., 2007
PRC200-SS[b]	2.1	1.5	61	Liang et al., 2008

Table 1. In vitro binding affinities of triple reuptake inhibitors (TRIs). [a]Ki values are expressed in nM (Ki for inhibition of radioligand binding). [b]Kd values are expressed in nM and represent the equilibrium dissociation constant. The smaller the Kd values, the higher affinity of a drug is for the corresponding monoaminergic transporter.

4.1.2 Functional activity: Synaptosomes

Inhibition of [^{3}H]-5-HT or [^{3}H]-NE reuptake in synaptosomes, is one of the most widespread method to assess the *in vitro* potency of reuptake inhibitors (Sanchez and Hytell, 1999) and to predict indirectly, their selectivity on biogenic amines transporters. In addition, it is noteworthy that the binding properties of triple reuptake inhibitors do not necessarily correspond to their *in vitro* functional activity assessed from rat brain synaptosomes (Tables 1 and 2). For example, although *in vitro* studies with PRC compounds (PRC025, PRC050 and PRC200SS: *1S,2S*-isomer of racemic PRC050), revealed a perfect correlation between binding affinity and functional activity towards monaminergic transporters (i.e. the rank of potency is NET>SERT>DAT), DOV216303 which preferentially binds to SERT and DAT, mainly inhibits the uptake of [^{3}H]5-HT and [^{3}H]NE (Chen and Skolnick, 2007; Skolnick et al., 2003). Such a discrepancy could be explained by the fact that the uptake of [^{3}H]NE from synaptosomal fractions involved the DAT. Indeed, unselective reuptake mechanisms have been previously reported with monoaminergic systems. In particular, it is well established that the clearance of DA from the extracellular space can occur through the NET in various brain regions including the hippocampus, the FC and the NAcc (Carboni et al., 2004; Bymaster et al., 2002; Moron et al., 2002). More recent evidence shows that DA may also be taken up by the SERT (Larsen et al., 2011).

4.2 Preclinical in vivo properties

In vivo strategies for characterizing the selectivity and potency of monoamines reuptake inhibitors examine the electrophysiological and neurochemical effects of these compounds, generally in rat or mouse brain. At presynaptic level, when the 5-HT or NE transporters are blocked on the serotonergic or noradrenergic cell bodies, respectively, there results an accumulation of 5-HT or NE in the vicinity of somatodendritic 5-HT1A or α2 autoreceptors in the dorsal raphe (DR) or locus coeruleus (LC). This lead to an attenuating firing of DR 5-HT or LC NE neurons in a dose-dependent manner due to the activation of these neuronal elements exerting a negative feedback influence (Tremblay and Blier 2006). This parameter can be used to characterize the pharmacological profile of reuptake inhibitors. At nerve terminals, an accumulation of 5-HT or NE also occurs in response to the inactivation of the 5-HT or the NE transporter by SSRIs or NRIs, and the enhancement of extracellular levels of monoamines can be probed by microdialysis in various brain regions (Guiard et al., 2009). This approach constitutes a second parameter to study the functional activity of reuptake inhibitors. Nevertheless, since microdialysis methodology may vary between laboratories, the electrophysiological approach seems to be more appropriate to establish relevant comparisons between compounds.

4.2.1 Functional activity: Electrophysiology

Electrophysiological recordings with TRIs (in comparison with single- or dual-acting agents) on monoamines neuronal activities have yet to be determined. Nevertheless, an initial study reported, that relative high intravenous doses of the TRIs SEP225289 and DOV216303 were required to inhibit the electrical activities of DR 5-HT, LC NE and VTA DA neurons. Although this may result from a lower affinity for the monoaminergic transporters than selective reupake inhibitors or from a poor brain penetration, 5 mg/kg; iv of DOV216303, produced an inhibition of 80% of LC NE neuronal activity but only of 30% and 40% of DR 5-HT and VTA DA neurons; respectively (Guiard et al., 2011). The observation that both TRIs exerted a predominant effect in the LC, while producing only a partial decrease in DR 5-HT firing activity was puzzling given the equal *in vitro* affinity and potency of the former drugs for all three transporters. The reciprocal interactions between monoaminergic neurons might have thus contributed to alter the functional *in vivo* activity of TRIs because the majority of SSRIs, NRIs and SNRIs produce a complete suppression of DR 5-HT neurons firing (Hache et al., 2011). The possibility has been raised that the lesser than expected effect of SEP225289 or DOV216303 on the firing activity of 5-HT neurons resulted, at least in part, from the accumulation of DA and NE in the DR, which are supposed, as abovementioned to be excitatory on the neuronal activity of 5-HT neurons (Katz et al., 2010b).

4.2.2 Functional activity: Intracerebral microdialysis

With respect to microdialysis data, as expected all TRIs increase extracellular monoamines levels with distinct intensities, depending on their pharmacological properties, on the brain regions studied and their relative equipment in monoamines transporters and, on the model used "naïve" *vs* depressed animal (Table 2). In a recent study performed in control rats, PRC200-SS was shown to increase the extracellular levels of the three monoamines in the medial prefrontal cortex cortex (mPFC) and the Nucleus accumbens (NAcc) (Liang et al., 2008). In the mPFC, in agreement with its *in vitro* pharmacological profile, PRC200-SS (5 and 10 mg/kg; ip) significantly increased extracellular levels of NE and 5-HT with a more pronounced effect for NE. Nevertheless, in this brain region PRC200-SS failed to modify the extracellular levels of DA. This result is somewhat surprising given the dense dopaminergic innervation and the high expression of DAT in the frontal cortex (Kuikka et al., 1995). The lack of increase in cortical DA extracellular levels may be explained by its heterologous reuptake from the NET (Moron et al., 2002; Giros et al., 1994). However the observations that catecholamine uptake blockers such as nomifensine, desipramine or GBR12909 increase DA levels (Devoto et al., 2004; Valentini et al., 2004; Gresh et al., 1995) could emphasize the importance of the reciprocal interactions between the DA and NE or 5-HT system at nerve terminal. Indeed if NE and/or 5-HT exert an inhibitory influence on cortical dopaminergic projections, as describe in the VTA (Guiard et al., 2008a), this might have produced counter-productive effects. However, in the core of the NAcc, where the density of DAT is relatively high, PRC200-SS (10 mg/kg; ip) increased DA and, to a lower extent, 5-HT outflow without affecting NE, probably because of the absence of noradrenergic innervation in this brain area (Carboni et al., 2006). Using microdialysis in the cortex of freely moving rats, confirmation of the blocking activity of JNJ7925476 on the SERT, NET and DAT has also been provided. A robust and dose-dependent increase in all three monoamines, lasting for several hours, was detected with a maximal effect for DA compared to 5-HT and NE at the highest dose tested (10 mg/kg; sc) (Aluisio et al., 2008). These results strongly contrast with *in vitro* data showing that JNJ7925476 displayed a better *in vitro* binding affinity and blocking activity for SERT than for DAT (Aluisio et al., 2008). Differences in transporter occupancy cannot explain these findings since this parameter followed the same trend observed with cortical extracellular monoamines levels. It has therefore been proposed that the high cortical levels of DA might have resulted from the blockade of the NET by this drug, which displays a high affinity for the DAT (Moron et al., 2002; Giros et al., 1994). Another possibility would be that JNJ7925476 acted by stimulating the release of DA but this property has not been demonstrated yet. Indirect effects might have also involved functional interaction between monoaminergic neurons leading to high extracellular levels of cortical DA. Together, these findings illustrate the fact that the *in vivo* activity of TRIs does

not necessarily reflect their *in vitro* functional activity, probably due, at least in part, to functional interactions between monoaminergic neurons. Another interesting example of unexpected results comes from neurochemical studies with bicifadine. Indeed, microdialysis studies in normal waking rats indicated that bicifadine preferentially increase DA and 5-HT than NE extracellular levels in the nucleus accumbens at the highest dose tested (60 mg/kg; i.p.) despite the higher potency of this TRI at binding and inhibiting the SERT and NET (Nicholson et al., 2009; Basile et al., 2007). Although the selectivity of this compound at the dose tested can be questioned, it is possible that the combined elevation in 5-HT and DA produce robust inhibitory effect on the noradrenergic system.
In olfactory bulbectomized rats, a model of depression (Song et al., 2005), it has been shown that the removal of olfactory bulbs results in a significant decreased in DA, but not 5-HT and NE, cortical extracellular levels when compared to sham operated. Interestingly, although after acute administration, DOV216303 increased DA, 5-HT and NE outflow in sham and bulbectomized rats, chronic administration resulted in a blunted rise in neurotransmitter (Prins et al., 2011; Prins et al., 2010). In the hippocampus, no changes in monoamines levels were observed in bulbectomized rats, DOV216303 increase DA, 5-HT and NE in both sham and bulbectomized rats either after acute or chronic treatment (Prins et al., 2011). This raises the possibility that monamines homeostasis in response to TRIs is regulated in a region-dependant manner. In the search for new drugs, adaptations in receptor and transporter density pre- and post-synaptically after chronic drug administration should be investigated as well.

TRI	In vitro uptake (Kd or IC50 in nM)			In vivo uptake			References
	SERT	NET	DAT	5-HT	NE	DA	
Bicifadine[a]	117	55	910	+++	++	+++	Nicholson et al., 2009 ; Basile et al., 2007
DOV216303[a]	30	45	80	+++	++	++	Caldarone et al., 2010 ; Prins et al., 2010
DOV21947[a]	12	23	96	ND	ND	ND	Skolnick et al., 2003
JNJ7925476[a]	1	1	2.5	+++	+++	+++	Aluisio et al., 2008
JZAD-IV-22[a]	15	84	120	++	+++	+++	Caldarone et al., 2010
PRC025[b]	6	19	100	ND	ND	ND	Shaw et al., 2007
PRC050[b]	6	0.4	120	ND	ND	ND	Shaw et al., 2007
PRC200-SS[b]	2	0.6	18	+	+++	++	Liang et al., 2008
SEP225289[a]	14	4	2	ND	ND	ND	Guiard et al., 2011

Table 2. In vitro and in vivo functional activity of triple reuptake inhibitors (TRIs) from synaptosomes and intracerebral microdialysis; respectively. [a]Values are expressed in IC50. [b]Values are Kd expressed in nM and represent the equilibrium dissociation constant. The smaller the Kd values, the higher inhibitory effect of a drug is for the corresponding monoaminergic transporter. In microdialysis experiments, signs "+" reflects the relative increase in 5-HT, NE and DA obtained with the highest acute dose used. ND: not determined.

4.3 Antidepressant-like activity

In humans, it is accepted that antidepressant and more particularly SSRIs, typically inhibit 80% of the SERT binding sites at minimally effective doses (Blier, 2008). It is, however, not known how much inhibition or occupancy for each transporter is required for antidepressant action. Correlation between *in vitro* binding profile towards monoamines transporters and *in vivo* behavioral studies may help shed light on some important and often debated issues.

4.3.1 In test predictive of antidepressant-like activity

The most frequently paradigms used to screen the antidepressant-like activity of pharmacological agents are the forced swimming and the tail suspension tests (FST and TST, respectively). Interestingly in the FST a further distinction can be made in swimming and climbing behaviors. Swimming is a parameter that reflects the activation of the brain serotonergic system in rodents (Cryan and Lucki, 2000; Reneric and Lucki, 1998; Detke et al., 1995). Such an association comes from the observation that pretreatment with the tryptophan hydroxylase inhibitor parachlorophenylalanine, prevents SSRIs-induced increase in swimming behavior (Page et al., 1999). On the other hand, climbing behavior has been shown to reflect the activation of noradrenergic system, particularly the subpopulation of neurons arising from the lateral tegmentum (Cryan et al., 2002). Surprisingly, none of the studies evaluating the antidepressant-like activity of TRIs has examined the climbing response, to compare for example, their *in vivo* potency at stimulating brain serotonergic and noradrenergic neurotransmissions. It is also important to mention that only one test in animals cannot cover all the complex depressive aspects. Ideally, novel compounds should be tested in several behavioral paradigms and animal models in order to address their putative antidepressant-like activity on a wide variety of symptoms of MD. In this prospect, Guilloux et al., (2011) have recently developed a score integrating measures from different tests to provide a robust characterization of the underlying "emotionality" of individual mouse, similarly as mood and related syndromes are defined in humans through various related symptoms over time.

Behavioral data currently available, have clearly demonstrated the antidepressant-like effect of triple reuptake inhibitors that act by increasing the time of mobility and/or by reducing the time of immobility in the FST or the TST (Aluisio et al., 2008; Liang et al., 2008; Shaw et al., 2007; Skolnick et al., 2003) (Table 3). Among the TRIs tested, PRC200-SS and JNJ7925476 produced the most robust antidepressant-like effects in these tests. For example, JNJ7925476 (0.3 mg/kg; sc) or PRC200-SS (10mg/kg; ip) produced a greater increase in the time of mobility in the mouse TST than that observed with PRC025, PRC050 (Aluisio et al., 2008; Bannwart et al., 2008; Liang et al., 2008; Shaw et al., 2007; Skolnick et al., 2003). In the rat FST, PRC200-SS is also the compound exhibiting the best performance since at the dose of 10 mg/kg; ip, it produced a more pronounced increase in the time of immobility than that observed with the corresponding doses of DOV21947, PRC025 and PRC050. Interestingly, both compounds (i.e. JNJ7925476 and PRC0200-SS) display a higher affinity for the SERT and the NET compared to the others compounds, suggesting that this double action is an important prerequisite to produce maximal effects. Since DA is known to enhance locomotor activity, the possibility cannot be excluded that triple reuptake inhibitors increased the time of immobility in these various studies, through a psychostimulant effect. In various studies, however, TRIs did not modify locomotor activity at doses that produce antidepressant-like effects (Aluisio et al., 2008; Liang et al., 2008; Shaw et al., 2007; Skolnick et al., 2003), thus suggesting that the antidepressant-like activity of TRIs does not appear to be from "false-positive" results.

4.3.2 In animal models of depression

An important drawback in the development of antidepressants is the fact that the new compounds are tested after acute administration in "naïve" non-depressed animals. Their chronic use in animal models is likely more relevant and would provide more informative results to determine whether or not a new pharmacological agents worth being tested in clinical trials. A recent study in bulbectomized rats has provided some interesting results. In this model, a 14-day regimen of DOV216303 (20 mg/kg/day; po), normalized bulbectomy-induced hyperactivity in the open field, similar to the effect of imipramine at the same dose (Breuer et al., 2008). Further studies in these animal models are required to precise the potential of TRIs and dissect their mechanism of action in pathological conditions.

TRIs	Doses, routes	Tests	Mobility (% of baseline increase)	Immobility (% of baseline decrease)	References
DOV 216,303	10 mg/kg; po 15 mg/kg; po 20 mg/kg; po	FST (mice)	ND ND ND	-20% (*) -20% (*) -40% (*)	Skolnick et al., 2003
DOV 21,947	5 mg/kg; po 10 mg/kg; po 15 mg/kg; po 20 mg/kg; po	TST (mice)	ND ND ND ND	-25% (***) -40% (***) -40% (***) -55% (***)	Skolnick et al., 2003
	5 mg/kg; po 10 mg/kg; po 15 mg/kg; po 20 mg/kg; po	FST (rats)	ND ND ND ND	-20% (*) -25% (***) -30% (***) -40% (***)	
JNJ-7925476	0.3 mg/kg; po	TST (mice)	115%	ND	Aluisio et al., 2008
PRC025	5 mg/kg; ip 10 mg/kg; ip	TST (mice)	+60% (*) +60% (*)	-40% (*) -40% (*)	Shaw et al., 2007
	5 mg/kg; ip 10 mg/kg; ip	FST (rats)	+145% (*) +100% (*)	-40% (*) -30% (*)	
PRC200-SS (active enantiomere of PRC050)	5 mg/kg; ip 10 mg/kg; ip	TST (mice)	+80% (*) +70% (*)	-40% (*) -80% (*)	Shaw et al., 2007
	5 mg/kg; ip 10 mg/kg; ip	FST (rats)	+110% (*) +165% (*)	-30% (*) -55% (*)	

TRIs	Doses, routes	Tests	Mobility (% of baseline increase)	Immobility (% of baseline decrease)	References
PRC200-SS (active enantiomere of PRC050)	0.5 mg/kg; ip 1 mg/kg; ip 10 mg/kg; ip 1 mg/kg; ip 5 mg/kg; ip 10 mg/kg; ip	TST (mice) FST (rats)	+40% (*) +95% (**) +95% (**) +130% (*) +246% (*) +226% (*)	-40% (*) -90% (**) -90% (**) -45% (*) -85% (*) -75% (*)	Liang et al., 2008
JZAD-IV-22	15 mg/kg; ip 30 mg/kg; ip 60 mg/kg; ip 15 mg/kg; ip 30 mg/kg; ip 60 mg/kg; ip	TST (mice) FST (mice)	ND ND ND ND ND ND	-15% (ns) -30% (*) -35% (*) -20% (ns) -40% (*) -70% (*)	Caldarone et al., 2010
6-(3,4-dichlorophenyl)-1-[(methyloxy) methyl]-3-azabicyclo[4.1.0] heptane	3 mg/kg; ip 10 mg/kg; ip 30 mg/kg; ip	FST (mice)	ND ND ND	-30% (**) -70% (**) -90% (**)	Micheli et al., 2010a
1-(Aryl)-6-[alkoxyalkyl]-3-azabicyclo[3.1.0] hexanes and 6-(aryl)-6-[alkoxyalkyl]-3-azabicyclo[3.1.0] hexanes	1 mg/kg; ip 3 mg/kg; ip 10 mg/kg; ip	FST (mice)	ND ND ND	-20% (ns) -40% (*) -90% (**)	Micheli et al., 2010b
3-aryl-3-azolylpropan-1-amines	3 mg/kg; po 10 mg/kg; po	TST (mice) FST (mice)	ND ND	-60% (*) -15% (*)	Lee et al., 2010

TRIs	Doses, routes	Tests	Mobility (% of baseline increase)	Immobility (% of baseline decrease)	References
4-(3,4-dichlorophenyl)-N-methyl-1,2,3,4-tetrahydronaphthalenyl amines (compound#10)	3 mg/kg; ip 10 mg/kg; ip 30 mg/kg; ip	TST (mice)	ND	-15% -20% (*) -50% (*)	Shao et al., 2011a
N-methyl-1-(1-phenylcyclohexyl) methanamine (compound #1)	3 mg/kg; ip 10 mg/kg; ip 30 mg/kg; ip	TST (mice)	ND	-5% -10% -25% (*)	Shao et al., 2011b
N-methyl-1-(1-phenylcyclohexyl) methanamine (compound #31)	3 mg/kg; ip 10 mg/kg; ip 30 mg/kg; ip	TST (mice)	ND	-10% -14% (*) -30% (*)	Shao et al., 2011c

Table 3. Antidepressant-like activity of triple reuptake inhibitors (TRIs) in rodents assessed in the forced swimming test (FST) or the tail suspension test (TST). Po: per os; ip: intraperitoneal; ND: not determined. *$p<0.05$, **$p<0.01$ and $p<0.001$: significantly different from vehicle-treated group.

4.4 Clinical properties of TRIs

On the basis of preclinical data, TRIs are in process of development (Millan, 2009) and most are now in Phase II clinical trials (Table 4). A small citalopram-controlled trial of DOV216303 in severely depressed patients yielded significant improvements in Hamilton Depression Rating Scale (HAM-D) scores in both groups at both one-week and two week time points (Skolnick et al., 2006). Since the optimal selectivity of TRIs at the three transporter sites remains undetermined, it is plausible that different potency ratios may result in different clinical effects. It can be envisaged to adapt the treatment to the nature of depressive symptoms. Drugs with high affinities for the 5-HT and NE transporters could be prescribed to patients displaying anxious symptoms, whereas compounds with a high affinity for the DAT could be more beneficial to patients having a loss of motivation and/or anhedonia. Despite these encouraging data, further investigations failed to demonstrate the beneficial therapeutic effect of NS2359 resulting in discontinued development. Of particular importance, a concern with drugs that block DA transporters is their potential reinforcing property and abuse liability. This comes from the fact that drugs that block DAT do not necessarily lead to dependence. Indeed, Volkow and collaborators showed that DA-transporter-blocking drugs must induce more than 50% DAT blockade to produce reinforcing effects (Volkow et al., 2005). Hence, DA reuptake inhibitors have been classified into two groups: type 1 blockers, which produce addiction and euphoria, and type 2 blockers, which do not (Rothman, 1990). It is thus possible that the capacity of DA reuptake blockers to produce dependence may involve other mechanisms that should carefully be considered with multi-targets agents such as TRIs. Nevertheless, although rigorous clinical feedback is yet to come, it can be hoped that TRIs will prove to have acceptable abuse and dependence potential and will offer improved efficacy in the management of depression. Accordingly a recent study involving comparing tesofensine vs. placebo, D-amphetamine and bupropion, in recreational stimulant users shows that although the effects of D-amphetamine were significantly greater than those of placebo on all primary and secondary subjective measures, tesofensine were not significantly different from those of placebo and lower than those of D-amphetamine and bupropion suggesting that the abuse potential for tesofensine is no greater than that of bupropion (Schoedel et al., 2010). Similar conclusions were reported with bicifadine, which display a low abuse potential (Nicholson et al., 2009). With respect to MD and eating disorders, weight loss has also been observed as an adverse event in studies with tesofensine (Hauser et al., 2007; Hansen et al., 2010), prompting further research for the indication of obesity. This effect is believed to result from appetite suppression (Axel et al., 2010; Sjodin et al., 2010). Recently published data from the first randomized, double-blind, Pl-controlled phase-II trial in primarily healthy, obese subjects showed that tesofensine was able to produce a greater weight loss after 24 weeks about twice that of currently approved drugs (Astrup et al., 2008a, 2008b). Appetite was significantly suppressed after an overnight fast after treatment with tesofensine in this study (Astrup et al., 2008a, 2008b).

5. Pain relief by TRIs, an example of symptom of depression

Acute and chronic pains may result from reduced levels of endogenous 5-HT, NE and DA activities, at both the spinal and supraspinal levels (Ren and Dubner, 2002). Indeed, pain is a bi-directional process of ascending and descending neuronal pathways involving monoaminergic systems whose activation may have an inhibitory influence on nociception. Despite the complexity of pharmacological interactions between monoaminergic neurons, that sometimes may attenuate monoaminergic neurotransmission, one would expect a better efficacy of dual-or triple-acting agents over selective 5-HT or NE reuptake inhibitors in analgesia (Hache et al., 2011). Indeed, since all three monoamines are involved in antinociception, the recruitment of more than one system may produce additional effects. Selected antidepressants suppress pain by diverse mechanisms and are now considered as an essential component of the therapeutic strategy for treatment of many types of persistent pain (Sawnyok et al., 2001). Their main mechanism of action involves reinforcement of the descending inhibitory pathways by increasing the amount of 5-HT and NE, but also DA in the synaptic cleft at both supraspinal and spinal levels (Hache et al., 2011). Several open-label randomized controlled clinical trials, meta-analyses, and systematic reviews have confirmed the clinical efficacy of selected antidepressants in persistent pain conditions (Dharmshaktu et al., 2011). Precedent for the use of TRIs in the treatment of clinical pain exists with nefopam, a tricyclic agent with non-narcotic analgesic (Heel et al., 1980). It was reported that DA played a critical role in nefopam analgesia as indicated by the observation that rats with selective loss of DA neurons, have a marked reduction in nefopam-induced analgesia. In a marked contrast, the lesion of the serotonergic or noradrenergic systems induced by 5,7-duhydroxytryptamine (5,7-DHT) or DSP4, respectively, failed to affect nefopam-induced analgesia in rats (Esposito et al., 1986; Girard et al., 2006; Girard et al., 2011). The potential interest of TRIs in the relief of pain has been corroborated by a recent publication characterizing the antinociceptive effects of the TRI bicifadine in acute, persistent and chronic models of pain (Basile et al., 2007). In this study, bicifadine potently suppressed pain responses in two models of acute inflammatory pain in both rats and mice. It also normalized the nociceptive threshold in the complete Freund's adjuvant model of persistent inflammatory pain and suppressed mechanical and thermal hyperalgesia and mechanical allodynia in the spinal nerve ligation model of chronic neuropathic pain. Mechanical hyperalgesia was also reduced by bicifadine in the STZ model of neuropathic pain (Basile et al., 2007). Clinical (phase II/III) studies have demonstrated that bicifadine is an effective analgesic in the treatment of postoperative pain (Krieter et al., 2008). The impact of bicifadine on 5-HT, NE and DA neurotransmissions was confirmed by *in vitro* binding assays and intracerebral *in vivo* microdialysis study in freely moving rats. In a second study, another TRI, NS7051, has shown comparable antinociceptive properties to tramadol confirming the interest of these antidepressants in the relief of pain (Munro et al., 2008). The molecule has undergone several Phase II and III trials for the treatment of pain, including acute postsurgical pain and chronic low back pain, and is being evaluated for painful diabetic neuropathy (clinical trial.gov). However, bicifadine has failed to meet endpoints in a number of trials such as diabetic neuropathy (clinical trial.gov) suggesting that TRIs may be used in specific pain. Other TRIs currently under development for depression should draw attention for future investigations in the field of pain and confirm whether or not they display any activity in diabetic neuropathy.

6. Conclusion

Numerous arguments support the contention that multi-target mechanisms may be more effective and better tolerated than their highly selective counterparts in the management of MD (Millan, 2009). Hence, drugs in preclinical and clinical studies (Table 4) include, but are not limited to TRIs, which simultaneously increase brain 5-HT, NE and DA neurotransmissions. Several lines of evidence specifically substantiate interest in dual-and triple-acting antidepressants. First there is no single cause of major depression. A vast array

TRIs	Comparator(s)	Phases	Conditions
Tesofensine	placebo	I	Obesity
Tesofensine	placebo	II	Obesity
DOV21947	placebo	II	Major Depressive Disorder
SEP225289	placebo venlafaxine	II	Major Depressive Disorder
Bicifadine	placebo standard analgesic treatment	III	Chronic low back pain
Nefopam	dexmedetomidine fentanyl	IV	Post operative analgesia

Table 4. Clinical studies with triple reuptake inhibitors (TRIs) in major depressive disorder or related morbidities. Details of these studies can be found on http://www.clinicaltrials.gov using the Boolean research for the following keywords: "Triple reuptake inhibitors".

of interacting genes, epigenetic influences, developmental events, and environmental factors collectively compromise mood. Second, agents that have complementary components of action may have a greater chance of controlling both the mood deficits of depression and other residual symptoms such as sleep disturbances, eating, sexual disorders or pain. This review particularly focuses on nocicpetion since over 75% of depressed patients suffer from painful symptoms (Hache et al., 2011), predicting a greater severity and a less favorable outcome of depression. In addition, imaging, anatomical and functional studies have demonstrated the existence of common brain structures, neuronal pathways and neurotransmitters in depression and pain raising the possibility that managing pain in depressed patients may help them recover more rapidly and efficiently. This is an example illustrating the fact that MD does not rely on only one impaired system and that an improved antidepressant therapy requires a diagnosis taking into considerations symptom profiles.

7. References

Adrien J (2002). Neurobiological bases for the relation between sleep and depression. *Sleep Med Rev* 6(5): 341-351.

Aluisio L, Lord B, Barbier AJ, Fraser IC, Wilson SJ, Boggs J, *et al.* (2008). In-vitro and in-vivo characterization of JNJ-7925476, a novel triple monoamine uptake inhibitor. *Eur J Pharmacol* 587(1-3): 141-146.

Astrup A, Madsbad S, Breum L, Jensen TJ, Kroustrup JP, Larsen TM (2008a). Effect of tesofensine on bodyweight loss, body composition, and quality of life in obese patients: a randomised, double-blind, placebo-controlled trial. *Lancet* 372(9653): 1906-1913.

Astrup A, Meier DH, Mikkelsen BO, Villumsen JS, Larsen TM (2008b). Weight loss produced by tesofensine in patients with Parkinson's or Alzheimer's disease. *Obesity (Silver Spring)* 16(6): 1363-1369.

Axel AM, Mikkelsen JD, Hansen HH (2010). Tesofensine, a novel triple monoamine reuptake inhibitor, induces appetite suppression by indirect stimulation of alpha1 adrenoceptor and dopamine D1 receptor pathways in the diet-induced obese rat. *Neuropsychopharmacology* 35(7): 1464-1476.

Bannwart LM, Carter DS, Cai HY, Choy JC, Greenhouse R, Jaime-Figueroa S, *et al.* (2008). Novel 3,3-disubstituted pyrrolidines as selective triple serotonin/norepinephrine/dopamine reuptake inhibitors. *Bioorg Med Chem Lett* 18(23): 6062-6066.

Basile AS, Janowsky A, Golembiowska K, Kowalska M, Tam E, Benveniste M, *et al.* (2007). Characterization of the antinociceptive actions of bicifadine in models of acute, persistent, and chronic pain. *J Pharmacol Exp Ther* 321(3): 1208-1225.

Ben-Jonathan N, Hnasko R (2001). Dopamine as a prolactin (PRL) inhibitor. *Endocr Rev* 22(6): 724-763.

Benca RM, Obermeyer WH, Thisted RA, Gillin JC (1992). Sleep and psychiatric disorders. A meta-analysis. *Arch Gen Psychiatry* 49(8): 651-668; discussion 669-670.

Berton O, Nestler EJ (2006). New approaches to antidepressant drug discovery: beyond monoamines. *Nat Rev Neurosci* 7(2): 137-151.

Billes SK, Cowley MA (2007). Inhibition of dopamine and norepinephrine reuptake produces additive effects on energy balance in lean and obese mice. *Neuropsychopharmacology* 32(4): 822-834.

Blier P (2008). Resiliency of monoaminergic systems: the 80% rule and its relevance to drug development. *J Psychopharmacol* 22(6): 587-589.

Breuer ME, Chan JS, Oosting RS, Groenink L, Korte SM, Campbell U, *et al.* (2008). The triple monoaminergic reuptake inhibitor DOV 216,303 has antidepressant effects in the rat olfactory bulbectomy model and lacks sexual side effects. *Eur Neuropsychopharmacol* 18(12): 908-916.

Bruhl AB, Kaffenberger T, Herwig U (2010). Serotonergic and noradrenergic modulation of emotion processing by single dose antidepressants. *Neuropsychopharmacology* 35(2): 521-533.

Bymaster FP, Zhang W, Carter PA, Shaw J, Chernet E, Phebus L, *et al.* (2002). Fluoxetine, but not other selective serotonin uptake inhibitors, increases norepinephrine and dopamine extracellular levels in prefrontal cortex. *Psychopharmacology (Berl)* 160(4): 353-361.

Caldarone BJ, Paterson NE, Zhou J, Brunner D, Kozikowski AP, Westphal KG, *et al.* (2010). The novel triple reuptake inhibitor, JZAD-IV-22, exhibits an antidepressant pharmacological profile without locomotor stimulant or sensitization properties. *J Pharmacol Exp Ther.*

Carboni E, Silvagni A, Vacca C, Di Chiara G (2006). Cumulative effect of norepinephrine and dopamine carrier blockade on extracellular dopamine increase in the nucleus accumbens shell, bed nucleus of stria terminalis and prefrontal cortex. *J Neurochem* 96(2): 473-481.

Carboni E, Silvagni A (2004). Dopamine reuptake by norepinephrine neurons: exception or rule? *Crit Rev Neurobiol* 16(1-2): 121-128.

Carter DS, Cai HY, Lee EK, Iyer PS, Lucas MC, Roetz R, *et al.* (2010). 2-Substituted N-aryl piperazines as novel triple reuptake inhibitors for the treatment of depression. *Bioorg Med Chem Lett* 20(13): 3941-3945.

Casper RC (1998). Depression and eating disorders. *Depress Anxiety* 8 Suppl 1: 96-104.

Chen Z, Skolnick P (2007). Triple uptake inhibitors: therapeutic potential in depression and beyond. *Expert Opin Investig Drugs* 16(9): 1365-1377.

Cryan JF, Page ME, Lucki I (2002). Noradrenergic lesions differentially alter the antidepressant-like effects of reboxetine in a modified forced swim test. *Eur J Pharmacol* 436(3): 197-205.

Cryan JF, Lucki I (2000). Antidepressant-like behavioral effects mediated by 5-Hydroxytryptamine(2C) receptors. *J Pharmacol Exp Ther* 295(3): 1120-1126.

Dahlstrom A, Fuxe K (1965). Evidence for the existence of an outflow of noradrenaline nerve fibres in the ventral roots of the rat spinal cord. *Experientia* 21(7): 409-410.

Dahlstrom A, Fuxe K (1964). Localization of monoamines in the lower brain stem. *Experientia* 20(7): 398-399.

Davidson RJ (2002). Anxiety and affective style: role of prefrontal cortex and amygdala. *Biol Psychiatry* 51(1): 68-80.

Dell'osso B, Palazzo MC, Oldani L, Altamura AC (2010). The Noradrenergic Action in Antidepressant Treatments: Pharmacological and Clinical Aspects. *CNS Neurosci Ther.*

Depue RA, Collins PF (1999). Neurobiology of the structure of personality: dopamine, facilitation of incentive motivation, and extraversion. *Behav Brain Sci* 22(3): 491-517; discussion 518-469.

Detke MJ, Rickels M, Lucki I (1995). Active behaviors in the rat forced swimming test differentially produced by serotonergic and noradrenergic antidepressants. *Psychopharmacology (Berl)* 121(1): 66-72.

Deutch AY, Goldstein M, Roth RH (1986). Activation of the locus coeruleus induced by selective stimulation of the ventral tegmental area. *Brain Res* 363(2): 307-314.

Devoto P, Flore G, Pira L, Longu G, Gessa GL (2004). Alpha2-adrenoceptor mediated co-release of dopamine and noradrenaline from noradrenergic neurons in the cerebral cortex. *J Neurochem* 88(4): 1003-1009.

Dharmshaktu P, Tayal V, Kalra BS (2011). Efficacy of Antidepressants as Analgesics: A Review. *J Clin Pharmacol.* (In press)

Dremencov E, El Mansari M, Blier P (2009). Effects of sustained serotonin reuptake inhibition on the firing of dopamine neurons in the rat ventral tegmental area. *J Psychiatry Neurosci* 34(3): 223-229.

Drevets WC (2001). Neuroimaging and neuropathological studies of depression: implications for the cognitive-emotional features of mood disorders. *Curr Opin Neurobiol* 11(2): 240-249.

Drevets WC (1999). Prefrontal cortical-amygdalar metabolism in major depression. *Ann N Y Acad Sci* 877: 614-637.

Dong J, Blier P (2001). Modification of norépinephrine and serotonin, but not dopamine, neuron firing by sustained bupropion treatment. *Psychopharmacol (Berl)* 155(1): 52-57.

Dunlop BW, Nemeroff CB (2007). The role of dopamine in the pathophysiology of depression. *Arch Gen Psychiatry* 64(3): 327-337.

Elam M, Clark D, Svensson TH (1986). Electrophysiological effects of the enantiomers of 3-PPP on neurons in the locus coeruleus of the rat. *Neuropharmacology* 25(9): 1003-1008.

Esposito E, Romandini S, Merlo-Pich E, Mennini T, Samanin R (1986). Evidence of the involvement of dopamine in the analgesic effect of nefopam. *Eur J Pharmacol* 128(3): 157-164.

Ferre S, Cortes R, Artigas F (1994). Dopaminergic regulation of the serotonergic raphe-striatal pathway: microdialysis studies in freely moving rats. *J Neurosci* 14(8): 4839-4846.

Ferre S, Artigas F (1993). Dopamine D2 receptor-mediated regulation of serotonin extracellular concentration in the dorsal raphe nucleus of freely moving rats. *J Neurochem* 61(2): 772-775.

Ghanbari R, El Mansari M, Blier P (2010). Electrophysiological effects of the co-administration of escitalopram and bupropion on rat serotonin and norepinephrine neurons. *J Psychopharmacol* 24(1): 39-50.

Girard P, Niedergang B, Pansart Y, Coppe MC, Verleye M (2011). Systematic evaluation of the nefopam-paracetamol combination in rodent models of antinociception. *Clin Exp Pharmacol Physiol.*

Girard P, Coppe MC, Verniers D, Pansart Y, Gillardin JM (2006). Role of catecholamines and serotonin receptor subtypes in nefopam-induced antinociception. *Pharmacol Res* 54(3): 195-202.

Giros B, Wang YM, Suter S, McLeskey SB, Pifl C, Caron MG (1994). Delineation of discrete domains for substrate, cocaine, and tricyclic antidepressant interactions using chimeric dopamine-norepinephrine transporters. *J Biol Chem* 269(23): 15985-15988.

Gold PW, Chrousos GP (2002). Organization of the stress system and its dysregulation in melancholic and atypical depression: high vs low CRH/NE states. *Mol Psychiatry* 7(3): 254-275.

Gresch PJ, Sved AF, Zigmond MJ, Finlay JM (1995). Local influence of endogenous norepinephrine on extracellular dopamine in rat medial prefrontal cortex. *J Neurochem* 65(1): 111-116.

Guiard BP, Chenu F, El Mansari M, Blier P (2011). Characterization of the electrophysiological properties of triple reuptake inhibitors on monoaminergic neurons. *Int J Neuropsychopharmacol* 14(2): 211-223.

Guiard BP, El Mansari M, Blier P (2009). Prospect of a dopamine contribution in the next generation of antidepressant drugs: the triple reuptake inhibitors. *Curr Drug Targets* 10(11): 1069-1084.

Guiard BP, El Mansari M, Merali Z, Blier P (2008a). Functional interactions between dopamine, serotonin and norepinephrine neurons: an in-vivo electrophysiological study in rats with monoaminergic lesions. *Int J Neuropsychopharmacol* 11(5): 625-639.

Guiard BP, El Mansari M, Merali Z, Blier P (2008b). Cross-talk between dopaminergic and noradrenergic systems in the rat ventral tegmental area, locus coeruleus, and dorsal hippocampus. *Mol Pharmacol.* 74(5): 1463-1475.

Guiard BP, Lanfumey L, Gardier AM (2006). Microdialysis approach to study serotonin outflow in mice following selective serotonin reuptake inhibitors and substance P (neurokinin 1) receptor antagonist administration: a review. *Curr Drug Targets* 7(2): 187-201.

Guilloux JP, Seney M, Edgar N, Sibille E (2011). Integrated behavioral z-scoring increases the sensitivity and reliability of behavioral phenotyping in mice: relevance to emotionality and sex. *J Neurosci Methods* 197(1): 21-31.

Guy-Grand B (1992). Clinical studies with d-fenfluramine. *Am J Clin Nutr* 55(1 Suppl): 173S-176S.

Gwirtsman HE, Guze BH, Yager J, Gainsley B (1990). Fluoxetine treatment of anorexia nervosa: an open clinical trial. *J Clin Psychiatry* 51(9): 378-382.

Hache G, Coudore F, Gardier AM, Guiard BP (2011). Monoaminergic antidepressant in the relief of pain : potential therapeutic utility of triple reuptake inhibitors (TRIs). *Pharmaceuticals* 4: 285-342.

Haj-Dahmane S (2001). D2-like dopamine receptor activation excites rat dorsal raphe 5-HT neurons in vitro. *Eur J Neurosci* 14(1): 125-134.

Handley SL (1995). 5-Hydroxytryptamine pathways in anxiety and its treatment. *Pharmacol Ther* 66(1): 103-148.

Hansen HH, Hansen G, Tang-Christensen M, Larsen PJ, Axel AM, Raben A, *et al.* (2010). The novel triple monoamine reuptake inhibitor tesofensine induces sustained weight loss and improves glycemic control in the diet-induced obese rat: comparison to sibutramine and rimonabant. *Eur J Pharmacol* 636(1-3): 88-95.

Hansen DL, Toubro S, Stock MJ, Macdonald IA, Astrup A (1999). The effect of sibutramine on energy expenditure and appetite during chronic treatment without dietary restriction. *Int J Obes Relat Metab Disord* 23(10): 1016-1024.

Hauser RA, Salin L, Juhel N, Konyago VL (2007). Randomized trial of the triple monoamine reuptake inhibitor NS 2330 (tesofensine) in early Parkinson's disease. *Mov Disord* 22(3): 359-365.

Heel RC, Brogden RN, Pakes GE, Speight TM, Avery GS (1980). Nefopam: a review of its pharmacological properties and therapeutic efficacy. *Drugs* 19(4): 249-267.

Hendricks TJ, Fyodorov DV, Wegman LJ, Lelutiu NB, Pehek EA, Yamamoto B, *et al.* (2003). Pet-1 ETS gene plays a critical role in 5-HT neuron development and is required for normal anxiety-like and aggressive behavior. *Neuron* 37(2): 233-247.

Hicks JA, Argyropoulos SV, Rich AS, Nash JR, Bell CJ, Edwards C, *et al.* (2002). Randomised controlled study of sleep after nefazodone or paroxetine treatment in out-patients with depression. *Br J Psychiatry* 180: 528-535.

Hornung JP (2003). The human raphe nuclei and the serotonergic system. *J Chem Neuroanat* 26(4): 331-343.

Jimerson DC, Herzog DB, Brotman AW (1993). Pharmacologic approaches in the treatment of eating disorders. *Harv Rev Psychiatry* 1(2): 82-93.

Katz MM, Bowden CL, Frazer A (2010a). Rethinking depression and the actions of antidepressants: uncovering the links between the neural and behavioral elements. *J Affect Disord* 120(1-3): 16-23.

Katz NS, Guiard BP, El Mansari M, Blier P (2010b). Effects of acute and sustained administration of the catecholamine reuptake inhibitor nomifensine on the firing activity of monoaminergic neurons. *J Psychopharmacol* 24(8): 1223-1235.

Kiyasova V, Fernandez SP, Laine J, Stankovski L, Muzerelle A, Doly S, *et al.* (2011). A genetically defined morphologically and functionally unique subset of 5-HT neurons in the mouse raphe nuclei. *J Neurosci* 31(8): 2756-2768.

Krieter PA, Gohdes M, Musick TJ, Duncanson FP, Bridson WE (2008). Pharmacokinetics, disposition, and metabolism of bicifadine in humans. *Drug Metab Dispos* 36(2): 252-259.

Larsen MB, Fontana AC, Magalhaes LG, Rodrigues V, Mortensen OV (2011). A catecholamine transporter from the human parasite Schistosoma mansoni with low affinity for psychostimulants. *Mol Biochem Parasitol* 177(1): 35-41.

Lee KH, Park CE, Min KH, Shin YJ, Chung CM, Kim HH, *et al.* (2010). Synthesis and pharmacological evaluation of 3-aryl-3-azolylpropan-1-amines as selective triple serotonin/norepinephrine/dopamine reuptake inhibitors. *Bioorg Med Chem Lett* 20(18): 5567-5571.

Lengyel K, Pieschl R, Strong T, Molski T, Mattson G, Lodge NJ, *et al.* (2008). Ex vivo assessment of binding site occupancy of monoamine reuptake inhibitors: methodology and biological significance. *Neuropharmacology* 55(1): 63-70.

Leuchter AF, Lesser IM, Trivedi MH, Rush AJ, Morris DW, Warden D, *et al.* (2008). An open pilot study of the combination of escitalopram and bupropion-SR for outpatients with major depressive disorder. *J Psychiatr Pract* 14(5): 271-280.

Li SX, Perry KW, Wong DT (2002). Influence of fluoxetine on the ability of bupropion to modulate extracellular dopamine and norepinephrine concentrations in three mesocorticolimbic areas of rats. *Neuropharmacology* 42(2): 181-190.

Liang Y, Shaw AM, Boules M, Briody S, Robinson J, Oliveros A, *et al.* (2008). Antidepressant-like pharmacological profile of a novel triple reuptake inhibitor, (1S,2S)-3-(methylamino)-2-(naphthalen-2-yl)-1-phenylpropan-1-ol (PRC200-SS). *J Pharmacol Exp Ther* 327(2): 573-583.

Linner L, Endersz H, Ohman D, Bengtsson F, Schalling M, Svensson TH (2001). Reboxetine modulates the firing pattern of dopamine cells in the ventral tegmental area and selectively increases dopamine availability in the prefrontal cortex. *J Pharmacol Exp Ther* 297(2): 540-546.

Lucas MC, Weikert RJ, Carter DS, Cai HY, Greenhouse R, Iyer PS, *et al.* (2010). Design, synthesis, and biological evaluation of new monoamine reuptake inhibitors with potential therapeutic utility in depression and pain. *Bioorg Med Chem Lett* 20(18): 5559-5566.

MacHale SM, Lawrie SM, Cavanagh JT, Glabus MF, Murray CL, Goodwin GM, *et al.* (2000). Cerebral perfusion in chronic fatigue syndrome and depression. *Br J Psychiatry* 176: 550-556.

Martin-Ruiz R, Ugedo L, Honrubia MA, Mengod G, Artigas F (2001). Control of serotonergic neurons in rat brain by dopaminergic receptors outside the dorsal raphe nucleus. *J Neurochem* 77(3): 762-775.

McClure SM, Berns GS, Montague PR (2003). Temporal prediction errors in a passive learning task activate human striatum. *Neuron* 38(2): 339-346.

Micheli F, Cavanni P, Andreotti D, Arban R, Benedetti R, Bertani B, *et al.* (2010a). 6-(3,4-dichlorophenyl)-1-[(methyloxy)methyl]-3-azabicyclo[4.1.0]heptane: a new potent and selective triple reuptake inhibitor. *J Med Chem* 53(13): 4989-5001.

Micheli F, Cavanni P, Arban R, Benedetti R, Bertani B, Bettati M, *et al.* (2010b). 1-(Aryl)-6-[alkoxyalkyl]-3-azabicyclo[3.1.0]hexanes and 6-(aryl)-6-[alkoxyalkyl]-3-azabicyclo[3.1.0]hexanes: a new series of potent and selective triple reuptake inhibitors. *J Med Chem* 53(6): 2534-2551.

Millan MJ (2009). Dual- and triple-acting agents for treating core and co-morbid symptoms of major depression: novel concepts, new drugs. *Neurotherapeutics* 6(1): 53-77.

Miller HL, Delgado PL, Salomon RM, Berman R, Krystal JH, Heninger GR, *et al.* (1996). Clinical and biochemical effects of catecholamine depletion on antidepressant-induced remission of depression. *Arch Gen Psychiatry* 53(2): 117-128.

Mongeau R, Blier P, de Montigny C (1997). The serotonergic and noradrenergic systems of the hippocampus: their interactions and the effects of antidepressant treatments. *Brain Res Brain Res Rev* 23(3): 145-195.

Moore RY and Card JP (1984). Noradrenaline-containing neuron systems. Editors, *Handbook of Chemical Neuroanatomy. Vol. 2: Classical Transmitters in the CNS Part 1*, Elsevier, Amsterdam : 123–156.

Morilak DA, Frazer A (2004). Antidepressants and brain monoaminergic systems: a dimensional approach to understanding their behavioural effects in depression and anxiety disorders. *Int J Neuropsychopharmacol* 7(2): 193-218.

Moron JA, Brockington A, Wise RA, Rocha BA, Hope BT (2002). Dopamine uptake through the norepinephrine transporter in brain regions with low levels of the dopamine transporter: evidence from knock-out mouse lines. *J Neurosci* 22(2): 389-395.

Munro G, Baek CA, Erichsen HK, Nielsen AN, Nielsen EO, Scheel-Kruger J, *et al.* (2008). The novel compound (+/-)-1-[10-((E)-3-Phenyl-allyl)-3,10-diaza-bicyclo[4.3.1]dec-3-yl]-

propan -1-one (NS7051) attenuates nociceptive transmission in animal models of experimental pain; a pharmacological comparison with the combined mu-opioid receptor agonist and monoamine reuptake inhibitor tramadol. *Neuropharmacology* 54(2): 331-343.

Nelson CA, Wolk R, Somers VK (2005). Sleep-disordered breathing: implications for the pathophysiology and management of cardiovascular disease. *Compr Ther* 31(1): 21-27.

Nicholson KL, Balster RL, Golembiowska K, Kowalska M, Tizzano JP, Skolnick P, *et al.* (2009). Preclinical evaluation of the abuse potential of the analgesic bicifadine. *J Pharmacol Exp Ther* 330(1): 236-248.

Nutt DJ (2008a). Relationship of neurotransmitters to the symptoms of major depressive disorder. *J Clin Psychiatry* 69 Suppl E1: 4-7.

Nutt D, Wilson S, Paterson L (2008b). Sleep disorders as core symptoms of depression. *Dialogues Clin Neurosci* 10(3): 329-336.

Page ME, Detke MJ, Dalvi A, Kirby LG, Lucki I (1999). Serotonergic mediation of the effects of fluoxetine, but not desipramine, in the rat forced swimming test. *Psychopharmacology (Berl)* 147(2): 162-167.

Popik P, Krawczyk M, Golembiowska K, Nowak G, Janowsky A, Skolnick P, *et al.* (2006). Pharmacological profile of the "triple" monoamine neurotransmitter uptake inhibitor, DOV 102,677. *Cell Mol Neurobiol* 26(4-6): 857-873.

Prica C, Hascoet M, Bourin M (2008). Is co-administration of bupropion with SSRIs and SNRIs in forced swimming test in mice, predictive of efficacy in resistant depression? *Behav Brain Res* 194(1): 92-99.

Prins J, Westphal KG, Korte-Bouws GA, Quinton MS, Schreiber R, Olivier B, *et al.* (2011). The potential and limitations of DOV 216,303 as a triple reuptake inhibitor for the treatment of major depression: a microdialysis study in olfactory bulbectomized rats. *Pharmacol Biochem Behav* 97(3): 444-452.

Prins J, Denys DA, Westphal KG, Korte-Bouws GA, Quinton MS, Schreiber R, *et al.* (2010). The putative antidepressant DOV 216,303, a triple reuptake inhibitor, increases monoamine release in the prefrontal cortex of olfactory bulbectomized rats. *Eur J Pharmacol* 633(1-3): 55-61.

Racagni G, Brunello N (1999). Physiology to functionality: the brain and neurotransmitter activity. *Int Clin Psychopharmacol* 14 Suppl 1: S3-7.

Ren K, Dubner R (2002). Descending modulation in persistent pain: an update. *Pain* 100(1-2): 1-6.

Reneric JP, Lucki I (1998). Antidepressant behavioral effects by dual inhibition of monoamine reuptake in the rat forced swimming test. *Psychopharmacology (Berl)* 136(2): 190-197.

Rothman RB (1990). High affinity dopamine reuptake inhibitors as potential cocaine antagonists: a strategy for drug development. *Life Sci* 46(20): PL17-21.

Salamone JD, Correa M, Mingote S, Weber SM (2003). Nucleus accumbens dopamine and the regulation of effort in food-seeking behavior: implications for studies of natural motivation, psychiatry, and drug abuse. *J Pharmacol Exp Ther* 305(1): 1-8.

Sanchez C, Hyttel J (1999). Comparison of the effects of antidepressants and their metabolites on reuptake of biogenic amines and on receptor binding. *Cell Mol Neurobiol* 19(4): 467-489.

Sawynok J, Reid A (2001). Antinociception by tricyclic antidepressants in the rat formalin test: differential effects on different behaviours following systemic and spinal administration. *Pain* 93(1): 51-59.

Schildkraut JJ (1965). The catecholamine hypothesis of affective disorders: a review of supporting evidence. *Am J Psychiatry* 122(5): 509-522.

Schoedel KA, Meier D, Chakraborty B, Manniche PM, Sellers EM (2010). Subjective and objective effects of the novel triple reuptake inhibitor tesofensine in recreational stimulant users. *Clin Pharmacol Ther* 88(1): 69-78.

Shao L, Hewitt MC, Wang F, Malcolm SC, Ma J, Campbell JE, *et al.* (2011a). Discovery of N-methyl-1-(1-phenylcyclohexyl)ethanamine, a novel triple serotonin, norepinephrine and dopamine reuptake inhibitor. *Bioorg Med Chem Lett* 21(5): 1434-1437.

Shao L, Hewitt MC, Wang F, Malcolm SC, Ma J, Campbell JE, *et al.* (2011b). Discovery of N-methyl-1-(1-phenylcyclohexyl)ethanamine, a novel triple serotonin, norepinephrine and dopamine reuptake inhibitor. *Bioorg Med Chem Lett* 21(5): 1438-1441.

Shao L, Wang F, Malcolm SC, Ma J, Hewitt MC, Campbell UC, *et al.* (2011c). Synthesis and pharmacological evaluation of 4-(3,4-dichlorophenyl)-N-methyl-1,2,3,4-tetrahydronaphthalenyl amines as triple reuptake inhibitors. *Bioorg Med Chem* 19(1): 663-676.

Shaw AM, Boules M, Zhang Y, Williams K, Robinson J, Carlier PR, *et al.* (2007). Antidepressant-like effects of novel triple reuptake inhibitors, PRC025 and PRC050. *Eur J Pharmacol* 555(1): 30-36.

Sjodin A, Gasteyger C, Nielsen AL, Raben A, Mikkelsen JD, Jensen JK, *et al.* (2010). The effect of the triple monoamine reuptake inhibitor tesofensine on energy metabolism and appetite in overweight and moderately obese men. *Int J Obes (Lond)* 34(11): 1634-1643.

Skolnick P, Krieter P, Tizzano J, Basile A, Popik P, Czobor P, *et al.* (2006). Preclinical and clinical pharmacology of DOV 216,303, a "triple" reuptake inhibitor. *CNS Drug Rev* 12(2): 123-134.

Skolnick P, Popik P, Janowsky A, Beer B, Lippa AS (2003). Antidepressant-like actions of DOV 21,947: a "triple" reuptake inhibitor. *Eur J Pharmacol* 461(2-3): 99-104.

Song C, Leonard BE (2005). The olfactory bulbectomised rat as a model of depression. *Neurosci Biobehav Rev* 29(4-5): 627-647.

Stahl S (2008). Stahl's Essential Psychopharmacology: Neuroscientific Basis and Practical Applications (Essential Psychopharmacology Series). Cambridge University Press.

Tremblay P, Blier P (2006). Catecholaminergic strategies for the treatment of major depression. *Curr Drug Targets* 7(2): 149-158.

Valentini V, Frau R, Di Chiara G (2004). Noradrenaline transporter blockers raise extracellular dopamine in medial prefrontal but not parietal and occipital cortex: differences with mianserin and clozapine. *J Neurochem* 88(4): 917-927.

Volkow ND (2005). What do we know about drug addiction? *Am J Psychiatry* 162(8): 1401-1402.

Volkow ND, Wise RA (2005). How can drug addiction help us understand obesity? *Nat Neurosci* 8(5): 555-560.

Wallin MS, Rissanen AM (1994). Food and mood: relationship between food, serotonin and affective disorders. *Acta Psychiatr Scand Suppl* 377: 36-40.

Walsh BT (1991). Fluoxetine treatment of bulimia nervosa. *J Psychosom Res* 35 Suppl 1: 33-40.

Willner P (1983). Dopamine and depression: a review of recent evidence. I. Empirical studies. *Brain Res* 287(3): 211-224.

Wilson S, Argyropoulos S (2005). Antidepressants and sleep: a qualitative review of the literature. *Drugs* 65(7): 927-947.

Zisook S, Rush AJ, Haight BR, Clines DC, Rockett CB (2006). Use of bupropion in combination with serotonin reuptake inhibitors. *Biol Psychiatry* 59(3): 203-210.

Part 3

Addiction Psychiatry

12

Drug Use Disorders and Recovery

Arthur J. Lurigio
Department of Psychology
Department of Criminal Justice
Loyola University Chicago
USA

1. Introduction

Drug abuse and dependence disorders are chronic but treatable brain diseases, involving compulsive drug-seeking and -using behaviors that persist despite immediate or potentially harmful consequences for users and their families and communities. Drug abuse and dependence are serious threats to public health and safety, costing hundreds of billions of dollars in yearly healthcare expenditures, crime, poor work productivity, and job loss (Hoffman & Fromeke, 2007). For example, illegal drug use in the United States cost nearly 200 billion dollars in 2002; approximately two-thirds of the costs (129 billion) were economic losses attributable to people's inability to work because of drug-precipitated illness, premature death, or incarceration. The treatment of the healthcare problems of drug addicts cost 16 billion dollars, while drug-related criminal justice and welfare costs totaled 36 billion dollars in 2002 (Office of National Drug Control Policy, 2004). Addiction also can result in intangible costs, such as homelessness, academic failure, and troubled relationships, and is one of the most pervasive and intransigent mental health disorders in the world, affecting the thoughts, feelings, and behaviors of millions of people annually (World Health Organization, 2004).

2. Drug effects and classification

Drugs are psychoactive substances that change moods and behaviors by altering brain chemistry and function (Hyman & Malenka, 2001). Drugs of abuse include medically prescribed (e.g., barbiturates and pain relievers), legal (e.g., alcohol and nicotine), and illegal (e.g., marijuana and heroin) substances. Some drugs, such as alcohol, have been used since ancient times, whereas others, such as methamphetamine and designer drugs (e.g., Ecstasy), are relatively new. People consume drugs to feel good (some drugs produce euphoria, confidence, and relaxation), to keep from feeling bad (some drugs combat anxiety, depression, and hopelessness), to accelerate performance (some drugs sharpen attention and enhance physical strength and athletic prowess), and to experience altered sensory perceptions (some drugs cause visual, auditory, or tactile hallucinations) (National Institute on Drug Abuse [NIDA], 2007).

Drugs of abuse can be classified into five groups according to effects. The first class consists of stimulants, which increase alertness and decrease fatigue; examples include amphetamines, Benzedrine, caffeine, Dexedrine, ephedrine, and nicotine. The second class consists of depressants, which reduce tension, alleviate nervousness, and induce sedation. Among these drugs are Nembutal, Seconal, Tunial, Veronal, Valium, and Xanax. The third class, hallucinogens, changes sensory perceptions; examples include cannabis, Lysergic Acid Diethylamide (LSD), Mescaline, Phencyclidine (PCP), and psilocybin. The fourth class consists of opiates, which induce sleep, euphoria, and relaxation as well as relieve pain and anxiety; opiates include codeine, heroin, opium, OxyContin, Percodan, and morphine. The fifth class consists of performance enhancers; they increase athletic strength and speed and stimulate the growth and recovery of skeletal muscles. Anadrol, Depo-Testosterone, Dianabol, and Winstrol are some examples of such performance enhancers (Abadinsky, 2007).

Drug abusers typically prefer one class of drugs over others. However, when they have difficulty obtaining their drug of choice, they often turn to other drugs in the same class that produce similar effects. Psychoactive drugs in the same class can be compared on the basis of their potency and efficacy. The potency of a drug is the amount that must be ingested to produce a desired effect whereas efficacy is a drug's ability to produce a desired effect regardless of dosage. Both the strength and the potency of a substance can determine an abuser's drug of choice as well as the drug's potential for abuse and dependence (see below) (NIDA, 2007).

3. The addictive process

Drug use can escalate to substance use disorders: abuse or dependence. The progression to uncontrolled use depends on several risk factors. For example, biological factors play a role in addiction; in other words, genetics can predispose a person to addictive behavior—a predisposition that is shared among close biological relatives. Scientists estimate that genes account for nearly half of a person's vulnerability to a substance use disorder (NIDA, 2007). Age of first use and psychiatric history are also important factors for explaining drug use problems. Younger users are more likely to become addicted because developing adolescent brains are more susceptible to a drug's ability to change brain chemistry and functions. Likewise, people with mental illness are also more likely to abuse or become dependent on drugs. In addition, a person's exposure to a parent's or a peer's use of drugs can increase his or her risk of addiction. The mode of drug ingestion can also raise the potential for abuse and dependence: a drug that is inhaled or injected is more addictive than one that is ingested orally. Inhalation and injection send the drug to the brain faster and produce more intense highs and lows. Drug-seeking behavior intensifies in response to the cycle of peaks and valleys that the user experiences (Hoffman & Fromeke, 2007).

Psychoactive drugs are thought to become addictive through their activation of the brain's mesocorticolimbic dopamine pathway, extending from the brain's ventral tegmental area to the nucleus accumbens to the frontal cortex. Drugs of abuse stimulate this pleasure circuit by increasing the amount of dopamine in the brain two- to ten-fold, creating an extremely pleasurable experience for users that compels them to repeat the incident. Drugs of abuse either mimic the effects of dopamine on neurotransmitters (i.e., they act as agonists) or block the re-absorption of dopamine so that it can continue to activate neurons (i.e., they act as antagonists). Eventually, the brain shuts down its own production of dopamine, causing the user to ingest the drug merely to stave off feelings of listlessness, depression, and other withdrawal symptoms. Drugs of abuse also affect the brain's frontal regions, impairing judgment and leading addicts to crave drugs even as the rewards of use steadily diminish. Hence, relapses—a return to drug use after a period of abstinence—are common among people with substance use disorders and can be triggered by stress, mood changes, and cues that remind the abuser of the substance (Karch, 2007; NIDA, 2007).

4. Substance use disorders

Substance abuse and dependence disorders are diagnosed according to criteria in the American Psychiatric Association's Diagnostic and Statistical Manual IV-TR (American Psychiatric Association, 2007). A substance abuse disorder is diagnosed when drug use in the previous 12 months has led to significant distress and impairment in functioning and meets at least one of several diagnostic criteria—namely, failure to fulfill obligations at work, school, or home; recurring use of substances in dangerous situations (e.g., driving while intoxicated); recurring substance use-related criminal justice involvement; and continued substance use that leads to interpersonal conflicts.

A drug-dependence disorder—more serious than a drug-abuse disorder—is diagnosed when drug use in the previous 12 months has reached the level of abuse and meets at least three of seven criteria that include tolerance (i.e., increasing amounts of the drug must be taken to achieve desired effects), physical withdrawal (i.e., symptoms that accompany the cessation of drug use, such as tremors, chills, drug craving, restlessness, bone and muscle pain, sweating, and vomiting), and persistent failure to reduce drug consumption.

5. Prevalence of drug use and substance use disorders

The National Survey on Drug Use and Health assesses the prevalence of substance use and substance use disorders in the United States. In 2005, an estimated 20 million Americans age 12 or older (or 8 percent of the total population in this age group) reported having used an illicit substance in the previous month; marijuana was the most commonly used drug (15 million), followed by cocaine (2 million), hallucinogens (1 million), methamphetamine (580,000), and heroin (166,000). Meanwhile, an estimated 22 million people age 12 or older were classified with a substance abuse or dependence problem (9 percent of the population). Among them, more than 3 million were classified with abuse of or dependence on both alcohol and illicit drugs; more than 3.5 million had abused or were dependent on illicit drugs but not alcohol; and more than 15 million had abused or were dependent on alcohol but not illicit drugs (Substance Abuse and Mental Health Services Administration, 2007).

In 2005, the order of lifetime illicit drug use among members of the general population paralleled past-month illicit drug use in 2005. Nearly half (46 percent) of people age 12 or older reported the lifetime use of any illicit substance. The most popular drug was marijuana (40 percent), followed by powder or crack cocaine (17 percent), hallucinogens (14 percent), methamphetamine (4 percent), and heroin (2 percent).

6. A public health approach to addiction

The most widely used definition of *health* is found in the World Health Organization's (WHO) 1948 charter: "Health is a state of complete physical, mental, and social well-being and not merely the absence of disease or infirmity." This definition was expanded by the WHO in its 1986 *Ottawa Charter for Health Promotion* in order to underscore the notion that health is "a resource for everyday life, not the objective of living. Health is a positive concept emphasizing social and personal resources as well as physical capacities" (WHO, 1986, p. 11). By this definition, drug addiction is a serious public health problem that adversely affects all of these domains. As I have discussed in this chapter, drug abuse and dependence are formidable threats to public health and safety, costing hundreds of billions of dollars in yearly healthcare expenditures, crime, poor work productivity, and job loss (Hoffman & Fromeke, 2007; United Nations Office on Drugs and Crime, 2006). Treating addiction as a crime rather than a health problem compounds its negative impact on individuals and communities in terms of public health and safety. Not only do most addicted ex-offenders emerge from behind bars with untreated substance use disorders, but they are likely to have been exposed to a variety of contagious diseases in prison, to have learned criminogenic behaviors that discourage contributive citizenship, and to have lost connections with family and friends whose support is critical for their healthy reintegration into society.

7. Importance of treatment

Prevention and education programs for nonusers and treatment programs for users are widely recognized as the most effective means of decreasing the demand for drugs. However, throughout the long history of the drug war, approximately two-thirds of government expenditures have been on supply reduction efforts. Numerous experts acknowledge that supply-side interventions have done little to curtail drug use or the violence that accompanies the sale and distribution of illegal drugs in the United States (MacCoun & Reuter, 2001). Moreover as I noted above, prohibition and strict penalties for drug possession and sales have spawned many unanticipated problems. Nonetheless, few government officials are willing to shift the emphasis of the war on drugs away from punitive measures and toward treatment and rehabilitation programs for people with substance use disorders. Most politicians are particularly reluctant to decry punitive drug policies out of fear of being labeled as "soft on crime" and losing the support of their constituents (Kleinman, 1992; Nadelmann, 1989).

Offenders with drug use problems are a diverse group, and the relationship between drugs and crime is complicated (Bureau of Justice Statistics, 1991). Offenders become addicted to drugs and commit crimes as a result of various events in their lives (Lurigio & Swartz, 1999). Whatever the road to addiction and criminality, drug control policies must fully incorporate what research has consistently shown: drug addiction is a chronic relapsing brain disease with biological, psychological, social, and behavioral concomitants. Therefore, programs for drug-abusing offenders should be comprehensive and include a wide range of treatment and adjunctive social services (Gerstein & Harwood, 1990).

One of the most successful examples of drug treatment as an alternative to incarceration has been Arizona's Proposition 200, the Drug Medicalization, Prevention and Control Act of 1996. This initiative prohibits incarceration for first- and second-time non-violent drug offenders, mandating probation and drug treatment instead of prison. A 1999 evaluation of the initiative by the Arizona Supreme Court found that it saved taxpayers 2.6 million dollars annually. Furthermore, nearly 75% of the drug offenders who had been sentenced to probation and drug treatment as a result of Proposition 200 remained drug-free during their participation in the program and paid their own money to offset the cost of treatment (Arizona Supreme Court, 1999).

A similar initiative in California has also significantly reduced incarceration rates and criminal justice expenditures. California's Proposition 36, the Substance Abuse and Crime Prevention Act (SACPA), allows first- and second-time non-violent drug offenders to enter substance abuse treatment programs as opposed to being incarcerated. Although the impact of SACPA varied by county based on the characteristics of drug treatment programs (in-patient vs. outpatient, duration of treatment), results showed that after 5 years, SACPA reduced the prison population of those convicted of drug possession by 27%. This resulted in an estimated savings of $350 million in prison costs alone (Ehlers & Ziedenberg, 2006). The costs associated with arrests and convictions were also significantly lower among drug offenders who completed treatment, compared to those who never entered treatment and those who entered but did not complete treatment (Longshore, Hawken, Urada, & Anglin, 2006). California saved more than $2.50 for every dollar spent on drug treatment; for those who completed treatment, the savings increased to $4 saved for every dollar spent (UCLA, 2007).

Studies of substance abuse treatment for drug offenders have repeatedly demonstrated the success of these programs in reducing drug use and its attendant problems, as well as in significantly decreasing the costs associated with crime and the criminal justice system. Drug treatment programs have proven effective as an alternative to incarceration and as a prison-based, post-release, or work-release intervention for addicted offenders. Hence, drug treatment is suitable for a wide range of offenders, and it is a cost-effective intervention at various points in the criminal justice process.

Considerable research shows the crime-reducing benefits and cost effectiveness of treatment relative to other antidrug measures (e.g., interdiction) and supports a greater investment in drug treatment (Anglin & Hser, 1990). Nonetheless, the treatment infrastructure in the criminal justice system has eroded over the past several years, a disheartening development that bodes ill for future efforts to control crime and reduce illegal drug use (Lipton, 1995). For example, despite record numbers of people incarcerated for drug crimes, the proportion of drug offenders who received drug treatment in prison declined throughout the 1990s and remained at a low level during the early 2000s (Belenko, Patapis, & French, 2005; Inciardi, 1996).

The economic benefits of drug treatment accrue mostly from reductions in incarceration, criminal victimization, medical treatment, and lost wages (Hoffman & Fromeke, 2007). A recent study in California found that the state saved $7,500 in aggregate reductions in crime and incarceration for every addicted person treated (Ettner, Huang, Evans, Ash, Hardy, Jourabchi, & Hser, 2007). A similar study found that every dollar spent on drug treatment resulted in an average savings of seven dollars, stemming from decreased crime and its corollaries (e.g., increased employment and major reductions in healthcare expenditures) (McCarthy, 2007). In an extensive review of hundreds of studies of drug treatment programs, Belenko, Patapis, and French (2005) found that drug treatment reduces drug use and crime, incarceration, and victimization as well as health care expenses and other medical costs. Belenko et al. (2005) concluded that "it is clear from research on the economic impacts of substance abuse addictions on health, crime, social stability, and community well-being that the costs to society of *not* (authors' italics) treating persons with substance abuse problems would be quite substantial" (p. 58).

8. Types of drug treatment: A brief overview

As I mentioned previously in this chapter, addiction is a recurring disease that often requires repeated episodes of treatment. The ultimate goal of treatment is sustained abstinence. During the process of recovery, treatment is designed to improve overall functioning while minimizing the social and medical consequences of substance abuse and dependence disorders. The recovery process begins with treatment and progresses as addicts gain insights into their uncontrolled use of alcohol and drugs and start to manage their thoughts, feelings, and behaviors (Center for Health and Justice, 2006).

The course of treatment for drug-dependent persons follows a general therapeutic process and lies on a continuum of care (NIDA, 2006b). Drug treatment encompasses a broad range of services, including detoxification, educational and vocational training, urine testing, counseling, HIV education and prevention, life and interpersonal skills training, psychiatric care, pharmacotherapy, psychotherapy, relapse prevention strategies, and self-help groups (see section on drug treatment principles below) (Anglin & Hser, 1990; Hoffman & Fromeke, 2007; Peters, 1993). Depending on the nature and severity of the addiction and an individual's progress toward recovery, treatment can occur at various levels and in diverse settings: inpatient, intensive outpatient, outpatient, or sobriety maintenance (Center for Health and Justice, 2006). NIDA (2006b) classifies treatment into two broad categories: pharmacological and behavioral.

The use of medication in recovery typically begins during detoxification. Persons who are physically dependent on alcohol and drugs are placed on medications to safely alleviate the painful symptoms and control the adverse physical consequences of withdrawal. Medication is used in the treatment and relapse prevention process to "help re-establish normal brain function and to prevent relapse and diminish [drug] cravings" (NIDA, 2006b, p. 3). For example, buprenorphine and methadone effectively treat opiate addiction by blocking withdrawal symptoms and reducing drug cravings. The passage of the Drug Addiction Treatment Act in 2000, permits physicians to prescribe these medications in medical settings; previously, such medications could be dispensed only in specialized drug treatment clinics. Promising new medications for drug addiction are pending FDA approval, including Baclofen (for cocaine addiction), Nalemfene (for opiate addiction), Topitamate (for alcohol, opiate, and cocaine addiction), and Disulfiram (for cocaine addiction [although for many years used for alcohol addiction]) (Hoffman & Fromeke, 2007).

Behavioral therapy consists of interventions designed to change addicts' attitudes and behaviors as well as help them acquire the skills and competencies they need to avoid relapses. Several behavioral approaches have proved successful in treating addicts—used by themselves or in combination with medications. The most common are cognitive behavioral therapy (helps addicts avoid relapse triggers), multidimensional family therapy (focuses on adolescents and their peers and family members), motivational enhancement therapy (capitalizes on addicts' readiness to change their behaviors and begin treatment), and motivational incentive therapy (employs positive reinforcement and contingency management techniques to promote abstinence) (NIDA, 2006b).

9. Drug treatment studies

Abundant research demonstrates that drug treatment reduces illegal drug use, crime, and recidivism in the general and correctional population (Anglin & Hser, 1990; Anglin et al., 1996; Gerstein & Harwood, 1990; Office of Technology Assessment, 1990). Since the 1960s, numerous studies at the local, state, and federal levels have shown that drug treatment works (Lurigio, 2000). The best research on drug treatment consists of large-scale, federally funded studies that involve large samples of participants and employ longitudinal designs and a comprehensive range of outcome measures. These studies have provided the most compelling evidence that addiction is a treatable disease and have identified the principles of drug treatment that characterize the most useful and effective programs (see below).

10. Large-scale studies of drug treatment

Three large-scale, multisite investigations, funded by NIDA, strongly support the conclusion that drug treatment works: the Drug Abuse Reporting Program (DARP), the Treatment Outcome Prospective Study (TOPS), and the Drug Abuse Treatment Outcome Study (DATOS). These evaluations of community-based treatment have contributed greatly to our knowledge about the benefits of drug treatment and significantly influenced drug treatment policies, programs, and research (Gerstein & Harwood, 1990; McLellan, Metzger; Alterman, Cornish, & Urschel, 1992; Simpson, Chatham, & Brown, 1995). As Lillie-Blanton (1998) stated, "these studies are generally considered by the research community to be the major evaluations of drug abuse treatment effectiveness, and much of what is known about 'typical' drug abuse treatment outcomes comes from these studies" (p. 3).

10.1 Drug abuse reporting program

DARP involved more than 44,000 persons admitted to drug treatment between 1969 and 1973. Participants were in 52 federally funded treatment programs that administered four types of treatment modalities: methadone maintenance, therapeutic communities, outpatient drug-free treatment, and detoxification. Conducted by researchers at Texas Christian University, data were collected through client interviews with treated clients and persons who applied for treatment but never returned for services (intake-only clients). Information was also collected from clients' progress reports and other program records. Follow-up intervals occurred from 3 to 12 years after treatment. "The DARP findings have been widely used to support continued public funding of drug-abuse treatments and to influence federal drug policy in the United States" (DARP, 2007, p.3)

DARP found that clients' daily use of opiates declined from 100 percent prior to treatment to 36 percent in the first year after treatment and to 24 percent 3 years after treatment. In the DARP study, addicts who were in treatment for more than 90 days were significantly less likely to use drugs in the year after treatment than those who were in treatment for fewer than 90 days (Simpson & Sells, 1982). Outpatient drug-free treatment, methadone maintenance, and therapeutic communities were equally effective at producing positive outcomes; clients in detoxification programs or those who dropped out of treatment within 3 months showed no positive outcomes. Moreover, among drug treatment clients in general, arrest rates declined 74 percent and employment rates increased 24 percent after treatment. Twelve years after treatment, daily heroin use remained 74 percent lower (Simpson, 1993; Simpson & Sells, 1982, 1990).

Approximately three-fourths of the opiate addicts studied in DARP reported at least one relapse to daily use after they had experienced a period of sobriety. The highest percentage of addicts (85%) who quit using drugs, did so while in treatment. The most common reasons reported for staying sober referred primarily to the adverse consequences of addiction. For example, 83 percent of the treatment participants indicated that they quit because they were "tired of the hustle," 56 percent, because they were "afraid of going to jail," and 54 percent, because they had to "meet family responsibilities" (Simpson & Sells, 1990).

10.2 Treatment outcome prospective study

TOPS involved 11,000 people admitted from 1979 through 1981 to 41 drug treatment programs in 10 cities. Three types of programs were examined—outpatient drug free, residential, and methadone maintenance—and clients were followed 1, 2, and 3 to 5 years after treatment. TOPS found that drug treatment reduced drug use for as many as 5 years after a single treatment episode; different treatment modalities appeared to be equally effective in helping drug users recover. Declines in drug use were most dramatic among heroin and cocaine users (Hubbard et al., 1989)

TOPS also produced solid evidence that drug treatment reduces drug users' criminal activities. Three to 5 years after treatment, the proportion of clients engaged in pretreatment predatory crimes decreased by one-third to one-half among the three treatment modalities. Moreover, TOPS demonstrated that drug treatment is cost-effective and cost-beneficial; data showed that the costs of treatment were recouped largely during treatment and that additional cost savings accrued with reductions in post-treatment drug use. Criminal justice savings were significant. Researchers reported a 30 percent decline in costs to victims of drug-related crimes and a 24 percent decline in costs to the criminal justice system (Harwood, Collins, Hubbard, Marsden, & Rachal, 1988). TOPS' principal investigators, Hubbard et al. (1989), concluded that "publicly funded drug abuse treatment is essential to our national effort to reduce the demand for drugs and its related social and economic costs" (p. 12)

10.3 Drug abuse treatment outcome study

DATOS, the third NIDA-funded comprehensive evaluation of drug abuse treatment (Leshner, 1997), followed a sample of 10,000 clients in 96 programs located in 11 large- and medium-sized cities in the United States for 36 months, from 1991 through 1993. DATOS participants were selected from four treatment programs: outpatient drug-free, outpatient methadone maintenance, short-term inpatient, and long-term residential. According to Leshner (1997), DATOS was "the first national study of treatment outcomes since the AIDS epidemic began, the first to examine outcomes for community-based cocaine abuse treatment, the first since the transition to NIDA block grants in 1981, and the first to include public and private short-term inpatient hospitals as a treatment modality" (p. 211) (also see Hubbard, Craddock, Flynn, Anderson, & Etheridge, 1997).

DATOS found that a larger percentage of drug-free outpatients than similar TOPS participants were involved in the criminal justice system and that clients with psychiatric disorders were more likely to be poly-drug users (Flynn, Craddock, Luckey, Hubbard, & Dunteman, 1996). Drug treatment significantly reduced drug use from pretreatment baseline levels to 12-month post-treatment levels for persons addicted to heroin, cocaine, and other types of drugs (Hubbard, et al., 1997; Simpson, Brown, & Joe 1997). DATOS also found that ancillary services for addicts had declined, but drug treatment programs were delivering core services (i.e., assessment, treatment, and aftercare) more effectively than they had in the DARP and TOPS studies (Etheridge, Hubbard, Anderson, Craddock, & Flynn, 1997).

In a five-year study of cocaine addicts, DATOS researchers reported that treatment reduced cocaine use from 100 percent at intake to 25 percent 5 years after discharge from treatment. Illegal activity declined from 40 percent in year 1 post-treatment to 25 percent in year 5 post-treatment. In general, the study found that clients with more serious drug and psychosocial problems at intake had poorer outcomes in treatment. However, more exposure to treatment was related to more positive long-term outcomes (Simpson, Brown, & Joe, 1997).

11. National treatment improvement evaluation study

Another federally funded, national evaluation of drug treatment was the National Treatment Improvement Evaluation Study (NTIES). Funded by the Center for Substance Abuse Treatment and conducted by the National Opinion Research Center and the Research Triangle Institute, NTIES used a highly rigorous methodology and extensive outcome measures. The purpose of the project was to investigate the impact of drug treatment on more than 4,000 clients in publicly supported drug treatment programs across the country.

NTIES found that drug treatment had numerous favorable effects on clients, including reductions in drug use. For example, one year after treatment, clients' use of heroin dropped from 73 to 38 percent while cocaine use dropped from 40 to 18 percent. The study also found post-treatment reductions in arrests rates, self-reported criminal activities, drug selling, and illegal earnings. Among treatment participants, homelessness, unemployment, and welfare dependency declined while overall physical and mental health problems became less severe. Moreover, participants engaged in safer sex practices after drug treatment than before; specifically, the percentage of participants who reported having sex for money declined 56 percent, and the number who had sex with an intravenous drug user declined 51 percent (Substance Abuse and Mental Health Services Administration [SAMHSA], 2007).

12. Services research outcome study

The Services Research Outcome Study (SROS), conducted by the Substance Abuse and Mental Health Services Administration (SAMHSA), was the first nationally representative study of drug treatment in the United States. SROS involved 1,800 participants in inpatient, outpatient, and residential care who were discharged in 1990 from a random sample of 100 facilities in rural, suburban, and urban areas nationwide. Five years after treatment, participants were interviewed; the results showed consistent reductions in drug use – namely, 45 percent in cocaine use, 28 percent in marijuana use, 17 percent in crack cocaine use, and 14 percent in alcohol and heroin use. The study also reported 23 to 38 percent reductions in criminal activity, such as burglary, the selling of drugs, and prostitution. Finally, after completing drug treatment, participants were less likely to be involved in physically abusive relationships or to attempt suicide and were more likely to live in secure housing (SAMHSA, 1998).

13. Principles of effective drug treatment

Several basic principles underlie and characterize successful drug treatment practices. These principles have largely been derived from studies of whether and how drug treatment works to change addicts' behaviors; many of these studies were discussed earlier in this chapter (Anglin et al., 1996, 1998; Prendergast, Anglin, & Wellisch, 1995; Taxman & Spinner,

1997). With funding and guidance from NIDA, researchers explored the implementation of drug treatment programs and their effects on a variety of populations. Their aggregate findings led to the identification of core program elements that assist addicts in achieving sobriety and improving their lives in many areas of functioning (NIDA, 2006a; 2006b). The following is a synthesis and distillation of NIDA's principles of effective drug-treatment programs.

13.1 Drug assessment and treatment matching

The first principle is that no single drug treatment regimen is useful for all addicts (NIDA, 2006a). To develop successful treatment approaches, tailored to each client's addiction and service needs, clinical evaluations must be conducted to assess the specific nature and extent of clients' substance use disorders. The fundamental clinical question is what type of treatment or intervention is most appropriate for what type of client, in which type of setting, and for what length of time (NIDA, 2006a.

A crucial first step in the formulation of an individualized treatment plan is the use of comprehensive and standardized assessment protocols that collect accurate information about a client's current and previous drug use; criminal history; medical conditions; drug and psychiatric treatment experiences; education and employment records; cognitive, psychological, and interpersonal adjustment; and social support networks (Anglin et al., 1996). Before treatment begins, a client's readiness and motivation for change must also be thoroughly evaluated (NIDA, 1999).

At intake, clients should be tested for communicable diseases (e.g., HIV/AIDS, tuberculosis, and Hepatitis B and C), which are significantly more prevalent among people who use drugs (NIDA, 2006a). If they test positive, clients should be counseled on treatment options and the importance of avoiding behaviors that can spread infections to others. If they test negative, clients should be counseled on ways to prevent infection through safer sex and drug-use practices (so-called harm reduction strategies) as they strive for recovery.

Following assessment, clients' problems and needs should be matched to treatment settings and strategies (NIDA, 2006a). Addicts who openly acknowledge their drug problems and commit fully to the recovery process can benefit greatly from drug treatment and adjunctive social and medical services (Simpson, 1998b). Repeated, unfavorable consequences from substance abuse can lead addicts to realize that professional interventions are necessary to achieve sobriety (Hoffman & Fromeke, 2007). Thus, addicts with extensive drug use and criminal histories are often amenable to treatment (Anglin et al., 1996).

Clients in the early stages of drug use can also be excellent candidates for drug treatment programs (Center for Substance Abuse Treatment, 1994). With the implementation of proper assessment and treatment-matching techniques, most persons with substance use disorders can be helped by treatment at any juncture in their addiction careers. The old adage that drug abusers must "hit rock bottom" before they can begin recovery is supported by neither research nor clinical experience (Hoffman & Fromeke, 2007).

13.2 Availability and length of participation

The second principle is that effective treatment takes time and must be highly accessible and readily available to take advantage of addicts' readiness for change (NIDA, 2006a). People with substance use disorders can lose their interest and willingness to enter treatment when they languish on waiting lists for services. Drug users must break through their denial and hesitancy and become motivated in the early stages of the recovery process, paving the way for long-term care (Anglin et al., 1996). Motivational interviewing techniques can be quite effective in encouraging engagement in the initial phases of treatment (NIDA, 2006a).

Treatment takes time. Addiction is an intractable disease and cannot be overcome with brief interventions. Hence, the goal of treatment should be the management of addiction, not its cure. Many studies show that the length of stay in treatment is positively related to outcomes (De Leon, 1991; Simpson, 1979, 1998a; Simpson, Joe, Lehman, & Sells, 1986). However, clients frequently leave drug treatment prematurely; therefore, different strategies must be used to engage and retain addicts in services long enough for them to gain therapeutic benefit from their participation. The threshold for achieving significant improvement in treatment is generally reached in three months, and several episodes of treatment, aftercare, and relapse are expected before abstinence is attained (Gendreau, 1996; Wexler, Falkin, Lipton, & Rosenblum, 1992).

Fletcher, Tims, and Brown (1997) observed that the "association between treatment duration and outcomes is strong enough to warrant research simply to improve retention." Furthermore, they stated that "time itself is a surrogate measure that might represent, for example, motivation, willingness to adhere to treatment, a process of behavioral change, or the ability of the practitioner to engage the patient" (p. 223). Therefore, favorable treatment outcomes depend not only on time spent in treatment but also on what happens during treatment to change clients' behaviors (Anglin et al., 1996). Recovery is a nonlinear process. Addicts learn to eschew old patterns of thinking (e.g., criminogenic attitudes and beliefs) and behaving and to replace them with new problem-solving skills for reducing cravings, avoiding relapse triggers (i.e., places, persons, and paraphernalia that remind the addict of drug use), and re-establishing healthy interpersonal relationships. Recovery involves steady progress toward a responsible, abstinent, and productive life (NIDA, 2006a).

13.3 Treatment structure and coercion

The third principle is that treatment should be both highly structured and adaptable, involving medical detoxification for persons with a substance dependence disorder and a contingency management component for all clients. Detoxification safely alleviates the acute physical symptoms of withdrawal and is a necessary (but not sufficient) precursor to successful drug treatment. Under a physician's care, detoxification is conducted in a hospital or residential setting and lasts from three to five days (Hoffman & Fromeke, 2007; NIDA, 2006a). After a client becomes stabilized through detoxification, progressive incentives can be incorporated into treatment. Different types of contingency contracts include positive and negative reinforcements to encourage addicts to remain drug free and engaged in the therapeutic process (Onken, Blain, & Boren, 1997). Voucher-based incentives can be combined with non-monetary rewards, such as verbal recognition, reward ceremonies, and certificates of completion (NIDA, 2006a).

Graduated sanctions should be leveled against participants who do not adhere to program regulations, and rewards should be given to those who do. To be most effective, positive and negative sanctions must be clearly specified, explicitly tied to behaviors, and swiftly administered (NIDA, 2006a). They should also be progressive and commensurate with the severity of clients' rule breaking or their degree of improvement. Clients should be monitored throughout treatment to overcome their struggles to identify and avoid the triggers for relapse. The continued use of drugs should be tracked through urinalysis or other objective drug tests (NIDA, 2006a).

Treatment success depends on the adaptability of services in meeting addicts' changing life circumstances (McLellan, Arndt, Metzger, Woody, & O'Brien, 1993). Interventions are most effective when they are responsive to addicts' evolving needs at different points in the recovery process (Anglin et al., 1996). Treatment and service plans should be continually renewed and modified throughout recovery. They must always be sensitive and responsive to differences in clients' age, gender, race, ethnicity, and sexual orientation. Practitioners should be skilled at combining several modalities, including medication, individual and group psychotherapy, family interventions, childcare assistance, and legal services.

Medications, such as methadone, LAAM, Naltrexone, and bupropion, can be essential aspects of care, especially when administered with psychotherapy and other supportive interventions (NIDA, 2006a). In addition, "self help can complement and extend the effects of professional treatment" (NIDA, 2006a, p. 20). Self-help interventions include 12-step programs (e.g., Alcoholics Anonymous, Narcotics Anonymous, and Cocaine Anonymous) (NIDA, 2006a).

Drug treatment programs must be flexible in their responses to relapses—expected, not exceptional, setbacks on the pathway to sobriety. Relapses can occur even after prolonged periods of abstinence, although addicts are most vulnerable to relapse in the first three to six months after treatment (Hoffman & Fromeke, 2007; NIDA, 2006a). Occasional drug use by participants, which minimally disrupts the recovery process, should be handled immediately through placement in detoxification, exposure to graduated sanctions, or return to a higher level of care. As a rule, one or two minor relapses should not result in participants being summarily dropped from drug treatment programs as the termination of treatment after relapse is ill-advised, unjustified, and unethical from a medical standpoint (Hoffman & Fromeke, 2007).

Addicts who are coerced into drug treatment by legal mandates are just as successful in recovery as those who enter treatment programs voluntarily, and legally coerced participants typically remain in treatment programs longer (Anglin et al., 1990). Whenever possible, legal mandates should be used to order offenders to participate in drug treatment programs and to hold them accountable for their progress in recovery (NIDA, 2006a). Coercion involves entering and complying with drug treatment or facing legal consequences. Participation is mandatory and noncompliance can result in sanctions, such as incarceration, the loss of child custody rights, or more stringent conditions of community supervision. Coerced treatment can be mandated at various stages of the criminal justice process and imposed with varying degrees of restrictiveness. Judges can offer a defendant the choice between treatment and incarceration. Probation officers can recommend and enforce treatment as a court-ordered condition of probation. Prison administrators can place inmates involuntarily into drug treatment programs (Lurigio, 2002).

A willingness to enter treatment is not a prerequisite for success (Hoffman & Fromeke, 2007). Legal coercion compels addicts make decisions that they might not be able to make on their own. Coercion is leverage that keeps addicted offenders in treatment long enough to benefit from the positive effects of a supportive therapeutic experience and become intrinsically motivated to remain and succeed in care. In short, coerced treatment provides services for addicts that would otherwise have been unavailable to them (Lurigio, 2002).

13.4 Evidence-based treatment

The fourth principle is that drug treatment must be evidence-based (science-validated) and implemented in accordance with proven models of recovery (Hoffman & Fromeke, 2007).

Evidence-based practices are never grounded in a drug treatment agency's traditions or the experiences or preferences of its staff; instead, they are supported by independent research that demonstrates their effectiveness in achieving outcomes that are broadly endorsed by experts and practitioners in the addiction field (Lurigio, 2006). As Brady states in Hoffman and Fromeke (2007, p. 135), "Evidence-based treatment is treatment that has been proven to work through rigorous scientific studies. Evidence-based treatment is particularly important in the addictions field because many myths and personal biases have infiltrated the treatment area and are often accepted without question."

The most compelling evidence of a program's effectiveness emerges from research that includes representative samples of participants, random assignment to treatment and control groups, and baseline and follow-up measures of client performance that are valid (accurate) and reliable (consistent). Moreover, the most useful results of studies—for the purpose of establishing evidence-based practices—are based on evaluations of programs that are manualized and implemented by trained, credentialed, and experienced staff persons. Practitioners must implement treatment protocols carefully and consistently, and participate regularly in professional development activities (Lurigio, 2006). Evidence-based drug treatment services include: relapse prevention therapy, supportive-expressive psychotherapy, individualized drug counseling, motivational enhancement therapy, multidimensional family therapy for adolescents, and the matrix model (NIDA 2006b).

13.5 Network of services

The fifth principle is that people with substance use problems should receive services that address their other difficulties (NIDA, 2006a). Drug abusers tend to suffer from a variety of psychological, medical, and social problems as well as deficits in education, employment, and housing (Swartz & Lurigio, 1999). Many of these problems persist throughout the recovery process (McLellan, et al., 1981). Drug treatment practitioners should collaborate with other service providers (e.g., psychiatrists and psychologists, vocational training experts, and housing advocates) in addressing the multifaceted problems of drug addicts, especially those with comorbid psychiatric disorders who need integrated substance use and psychiatric treatment services. Addicts must be treated comprehensively; their various problems should be addressed simultaneously, not sequentially (Waller & Weiner, 1989).

13.6 Continuity of care

The sixth principle is that residential (short- or long-term) treatment must be followed by a continuum of care, namely, intensive outpatient treatment, aftercare, and relapse prevention services. Seamless interventions are instrumental in achieving sobriety (NIDA, 2006a; Russell, 1994). As mentioned throughout this chapter, drug abuse and dependence disorders are chronic, and several cycles of treatment and aftercare services—often "with a cumulative impact"—are required to minimize relapses and sustain recovery (NIDA, 1999, p. 16). If drug abusers remain in intensive treatment for at least 90 days and receive continuous care after treatment, they are more likely to attain sobriety, get a job, and stop committing crimes (NIDA, 2006b).

Continuity of care is particularly crucial to the recovery of drug-involved offenders leaving correctional settings (NIDA, 1999; Peters, 1993). Offenders who complete structured drug treatment programs in jails or prisons should be assisted in their transition to community-based services by engaging in prerelease planning and programming activities. Without aftercare services (i.e., continuity of care), the gains that offenders make in prison or jail treatment programs are frequently diminished or lost altogether (Lipton, 1995; NIDA, 2006a).

Prison inmates who participated in a drug treatment program with follow-up services in work release centers demonstrated significantly lower drug use and recidivism rates than those who participated in institutional treatment only (Inciardi, 1998). Similarly, offenders participating in both prison- and community-based treatment programs were less likely to commit subsequent crimes than offenders who participated in drug treatment without follow-up care (Wexler, 1996; Wexler, De Leon, Thomas, Kressel, & Peters, 1999).

Numerous obstacles can impede the delivery of aftercare services, including the fragmented nature of the criminal justice system, the lack of coordination between criminal justice practitioners and treatment providers, and the absence of incentives and sanctions for offenders to remain drug free after unsupervised release from jails and prisons. The paucity of community treatment programs and treatment providers' inexperience with offenders are also impediments to recovery (Field, 1998). Relapse prevention services for offenders should be more thoroughly studied and understood (Vigdal, 1995) as suggested by the following under-investigated and unresolved issues:

- Reasons why offenders are especially vulnerable to relapse, including stressors related to release from correctional facilities and psychosocial factors related to crime and drug use;
- The evolving recovery process at its various stages;
- The destabilized and stabilized relapse-prone individual;
- Methods to overcome recovery plateaus;
- Basic components of relapse prevention therapy (e.g., self-knowledge and identification of warning signs, coping skills and management of warning signs, and involvement of family members and others in the relapse prevention plan; and
- The timing of relapse prevention efforts, particularly in advance of release from jail and prison.

13.7 Service coordination

The seventh principle is that drug treatment programs for offenders work best when criminal justice professionals (e.g., probation, parole, and detention officers) and service providers communicate with one another and coordinate their efforts (NIDA, 2006a). Cross-training can help both groups understand the competencies and limitations of the other and work more effectively as a case management team. As stated in NIDA (2006a), "The coordination of drug abuse treatment with correctional planning can encourage participation in drug abuse treatment and can help treatment providers incorporate correctional requirements as treatment goals." (p. 3)

Treatment Alternatives for Safe Communities (TASC) was the culmination of a federal effort to establish and promote coordination between criminal justice agencies and treatment providers at the local level. Seeded in 1972 with funding from the Law Enforcement and Assistance Administration, TASC's first pilot program was implemented in Wilmington, Delaware. By 2007, more than 220 TASC programs were operating in 30 states. TASC identifies, assesses, and refers offenders at the pretrial and post-adjudication levels to treatment and adjunctive services. TASC monitors clients' treatment progress through case management, urine testing, and other techniques, and reports violations of the conditions of release to the court.

Case managers establish linkages between treatment providers and correctional staff in order to develop coordinated strategies that hold offenders accountable and protect community safety (Anglin et al., 1996; Inciardi & McBride, 1991; Swartz, 1993; Weinman, 1990). The critical elements of TASC operations include "a process to coordinate justice, treatment, and other systems; procedures for providing information and cross-training to justice, treatment, and other systems; policies and procedures for regular staff training; clearly defined client eligibility criteria; and performance of client-centered case management" (National TASC, 2007).

13.8 Program evaluation

The eighth principle is that drug treatment programs should be routinely examined by outside evaluators to determine whether services are being implemented as planned (treatment fidelity) and to measure the overall impact of services (treatment effectiveness). Process evaluations should provide program staff members with real-time information that can be used to improve service delivery and preserve treatment integrity. Outcome evaluations should be based on internally valid research designs that incorporate random assignment and control groups; such designs yield data that permit confident conclusions about program effectiveness. Researchers should also consider client selection criteria and attrition (i.e., program dropouts) when interpreting results.

Evaluations of program impact must include a variety of outcome measures, such as number and type of drugs used; frequency of drug use; treatment retention; desistence from criminal activities; length of time to relapse and rearrest; vocational skills; employment; social, psychological, and family functioning; reliance on social service agencies; physical and emotional health; HIV risk behaviors; and mortality rates (Anglin & Hser, 1990; Swartz, 1993; Vigdal, 1995). Finally, researchers should test different treatment modalities to ascertain which approaches work best with which groups of clients; they should also employ longitudinal and nested research designs to understand more precisely the effectiveness of interventions as well as the trajectories of participants' addiction and criminal careers (Leukefeld & Tims, 1992).

14. Conclusions

The use of illicit substances is common in the United States. The casual use of drugs can escalate to misuse, abuse, and dependence, resulting in distress and impairment in functioning as well as hardship for users' families and the larger community. The criteria for rendering a clinical diagnosis of drug abuse and dependence are enumerated in the 4th Edition of the Diagnostic and Statistical Manual of the American Psychiatric Association (DSM-IV-TR). These criteria help diagnosticians in evaluating the nature and severity of substance use disorders. Although substance use disorders produce serious harm for those affiliated with such problems, they are considered treatable conditions. Many studies have demonstrated the effectiveness of drug treatment in leading to recovery. Substance use changes brain chemistry and functioning; therefore addiction is a chronic disease that requires a life-long commitment to achieve long-term sobriety.

Since the War on Drugs was declared 40 years ago, people arrested for drug crimes have been the fastest-growing subpopulations at every step in the criminal justice process from arrest to post-incarcerative release from prison. The criminal justice system often provides the first and only opportunity for criminally involved drugs users to obtain substance abuse treatment and other recovery services. NIDA has discussed several principles of effective care for drug-involved members of the general and correctional populations, including assessment, treatment matching, relapse prevention, the use of medications and adjunctive services, and the evaluation of services to identify evidence-based practices.

15. References

Abadinsky, H. (2007). *Drug use and abuse: A comprehensive introduction*. Pacific Grove, CA: Wadsworth Publishing.

American Psychiatric Association. (2007). *Diagnostic and statistical manual of mental disorders IV-TR*. Washington, DC; Author.

Anglin, M.D., Brecht, M.L. & Maddahian, E. (1990). Pretreatment characteristics and treatment performance of legally coerced versus voluntary methadone maintenance admissions *Criminology*, 27, 537-557.

Anglin, M.D., & Hser Y. (1990). Treatment of drug abuse. In M. Tonry & J.Q. Wilson (Eds.), *Drugs and crime* (pp.393-460). Chicago: University of Chicago Press.

Anglin, M.D., Longshore, D., Turner, S. McBride, D., Inciardi, J.A., & Prendergast, M.L. (1996). *Studies of the functioning and effectiveness of Treatment Alternatives to Street Crime (TASC) programs*. Los Angeles: University of California, Los Angeles Drug Abuse Research Center.

Anglin, M D., Prendergast, M .L., & Farabee. D (1998). *The effect of coerced drug treatment for drug-abusing offenders*. Paper presented at the Office of National Drug Control Policy's Conference of Scholars and Policy Makers, Washington, DC.

Arizona Supreme Court (1999). Proposition 200 working, saving money. Phoenix, AZ: Author

Belenko, S., Patapis, N., & French, M.T. (2005). *Economic Benefits of Drug Treatment: A critical review of evidence for policy makers*. Philadelphia, PA: Treatment Research Institute, University of Pennsylvania.

Bureau of Justice Statistics. (1991). *Drugs and crime data. Fact sheet: Drug data summary*. Washington, D.C.: Author.

Center for Health and Justice. (2006). *Understanding treatment and recovery*. Chicago, IL: Treatment Alternatives for Safe Communities.

Center for Substance Abuse Treatment. (1994). *Screening and assessment for alcohol and other drug abuse among adults in the criminal justice system* (DHHS Publication Number SMA 94-2076). Rockville, MD: Author.

De Leon, G. (1991) Retention in drug-free therapeutic communities In R W Pickens, C. G. Leukefeld, & C. R. Shuster (Eds.), *Improving drug abuse treatment* (pp 21-38) Rockville, MD: National Institute on Drug Abuse.

Drug Abuse Reporting Program. (2007). *DATOS background*. Washington, DC: Author. http://www.datos.org/background.html. Retrieved on December 16, 2007.

Ehlers, S. & Zeidenberg, J. (2006). *Proposition 36: Five years later*. Washington, DC: Justice Policy Institute.

Etheridge, R.M., Hubbard, R. L., Anderson, J., Craddock, S.G., & Flynn, P.M. (1997). Treatment structure and program services in the Drug Abuse Treatment Outcome Study. *Psychology of Addictive Behaviors, 11*, 244-260.

Ettner, S.L., Huang, D., Evans, E., Ash, D.R., Hardy, M., Jourabchi, M., & Hser, Y. (2006). *Health Services Research, 41,* 192-213.

Field, G. (1998). *Continuity of offender treatment: Institution to the community* Paper presented at the Office of National Drug Control Policy's Conference of Scholars and Policy Makers, Washington, DC.

Fletcher, B.W., Tims, F.M., & Brown, B.S. (1997). The Drug Abuse Treatment Outcome Study (DATOS): Treatment evaluation research in the United States *Psychology of Addictive Behaviors, 11,* 216-229.

Flynn, P.M., Craddock, S. G. Luckey, J. W., Hubbard, R.L., Dunteman, G.H. (1996). Comorbidity of antisocial personality and mood disorders among psychoactive substance-dependent treatment clients. *Journal of Personality Disorders, 10,* 56-67.

Gendreau, P. (1996). The principles of effective intervention with offenders. In A T. Harland (Ed.), *Choosing correctional options that work* (pp 121-146) Thousand Oaks, CA: Sage

General Accounting Office. (1995). Drug courts: Information on a new Washington, DC: GAO.

Gerstein, D., & Harwood, H.J. (Eds.). (1990) *Treating drug problems: A study of the evolution, effectiveness, and financing of public and private drug treatment systems.* Washington, DC: National Academy Press.

Hardwood, H.J., Collins, J.J., Hubbard, R.L., Marsden, M.E., & Rachal, J.V. (1988). The costs of crime and benefits of drug abuse treatment: A cost benefit analysis using TOPS data. In C.G. Leukefeld & F.M. Tims (Eds.), Compulsory treatment of drug abuse: Research and clinical practice (NIDA Research Monograph 86, NIH Publication Number 94-3713) (pp. 209-235). Washington, DC: Government Printing Office.

Hoffman, J., & Froemke, S. (2007). *Addiction: New knowledge, new treatments, new hope.* New York: Rodale.

Hubbard, R.L., Craddock, S.G., Flynn, P.M., Anderson, J., & Etheridge, R.M. (1997). Overview of 1-year follow-up outcomes in the Drug Abuse Treatment Outcome Study (DATOS). *Psychology of Addictive Behaviors, 11,* 261-278.

Hubbard, R.L., Marsden, M.E., Rachal, J.V., Hardwood, H.J., Cavanaugh, E.R., & Ginzburg, H.M. (1989). *Drug Abuse treatment: A national study of effectiveness.* Chapel Hill: University of North Carolina Press.

Hyman S.E. & Malenka R.C. (2001). Addiction and the brain: the neurobiology of compulsion and its persistence. *Nature Reviews: Neuroscience, 2,* 695–703.

Inciardi, J. A. (1996). *A corrections-based continuum of effective drug abuse treatment.* Washington, DC: National Institute of Justice.

Inciardi, J. A., & McBride, D. C. (1991). Treatment alternatives to street crime History, experiences, and issues. *Rockville, MD: National Institute on Drug Abuse.*

Karch, S. (Ed.). (2007). *Drug abuse handbook.* Boca Raton, FL: CRC Press.

Kleiman, M. A. R. (1992). *Against excess: drug policy for results.* New York: Basic Books.

Leshner, A. I. (1997) Drug abuse and addiction treatment research. The next generation. *Archives of General Psychiatry, 54,* 730-735.

Leukefeld, C.G., & Tims, F M. (1992). *Drug abuse treatment in prisons and jails.* Rockville, MD: National Institute on Drug Abuse.

Lillie-Blanton, M. (1998). *Studies show treatment is effective, but benefits may be overstated.* Washington, DC: General Accounting Office.

Lipton, D.S. (1995). *The effectiveness of treatment for drug abusers under criminal justice supervision.* Washington, DC: National Institute of Justice.
Longshore, D., Hawken, A., Urada, D., & Anglin, M.D. (2006). *Evaluation of the Substance Abuse and Crime Prevention Act: SACPA cost-analysis report. Los Angeles: UCLA.*
Lurigio, A. J. (2002). Coerced drug treatment for offenders: Does it work? *GLATTC Research Update, 4,* 1-2.
Lurigio, A.J. (2000). Drug treatment availability and effectives: Studies of the general and criminal justice populations. *Criminal Justice and Behavior, 27,* 495-528.
Lurigio, A.J. (2000). Drug treatment availability and effectives: Studies of the general and criminal justice populations. *Criminal Justice and Behavior, 27,* 495-528.
Lurigio, A. J., & Swartz, J. A. (1999). The nexus between drugs and crime: Theory, research, and practice. *Federal Probation, 63,* 67-72.
MacCoun, R. J., & Reuter, P. (2001). *Drug war heresies.* New York: Cambridge University Press.
McCarthy, D. (2007). *Substance abuse treatment benefits and costs: Knowledge assets policy brief.* Greenburo, NC: Substance Abuse Policy Research Program.
McLellan, A.R., Arndt, I.O., Metzger, D. S., Woody, G.E., & O'Brien, C.P. (1993). The effects of psychosocial services in substance abuse treatment. *Journal of the American Medical Association, 269,* 1953-1996.
McLellan, A.T., Luborsky, L., Woody, G.E., O'Brien, C.P., & Kron, R. (1981). Are the "addiction-related" problems of substances abuses really related? *The Journal of Nervous and Mental Disease, 173,* 94-102.
McLellan, A. T., Metzger, D., Alterman, A.I., Cornish, J., & Urschel, H. (1992). How effective is substance abuse treatment-Compared to what? In C. P. O'Brien & J. Jaffe (Eds.), *Advances in understanding the addictive states* (pp. 231-252). New York: Raven Press.
Nadelmann, E. (1989). Drug prohibition in the United States: Costs, consequences, and alternatives. *Science, 245,* 939-947.
National Institute on Drug Abuse (2007). *Drugs, brains, and behavior.* Washington, DC: National Institutes of Health: U.S. Department of Health and Human Services.
National Institute on Drug Abuse. (2006a). *Principles of drug abuse treatment for criminal justice populations: A research based guide.* Washington, DC: Author.
National Institute on Drug Abuse. (2006b). *Treatment approaches for drug addiction.* Washington, DC: Author.
National TASC. (2007). *National TASC: Treatment Accountability for Safer Communities.* www.nationaltasc.org.
Office of National Drug Control Policy. (2004). *National drug control strategy: Update.* Washington, DC: White House.
Office of Technology Assessment. (1990). *The effectiveness of drug abuse treatment: Implications for controlling AIDS/HIV infection.* Washington, DC: Government Printing Office.
Onken, L.S., Blain, J.0., & Boren, J. J. (Eds.) (1997). *Beyond the therapeutic alliance: Keeping the drug-dependent individual in treatment* (NIDA Research Monograph 165, NIH Publication Number 97-4142). Washington, DC: Government Printing Office.
Peters, R.H. (1993). Drug treatment in jails and detention settings. In J.A. Inciardi (Ed.), *Drug treatment and criminal justice* (pp. 44-80) Newbury Park, CA: Sage.
Prendergast, M., Anglin, M D , & Wellisch, J. (1995). Treatment for drug-abusing offenders under community supervision. *Federal Probation, 59,* 66-75.

Simpson, D.D. (1993). Drug treatment evaluation in the United States. *Psychology of Addictive Behaviors, 7,* 120-128.
Simpson, D. D (1998a). *Ingredients of effective treatment* Fort Worth, IX: Institute of Behavioral Research, Texas Christian University.
Simpson, D. D. (1998b). *Patient engagement and duration of treatment.* Paper presented at the Office of National Drug Control Policy's Conference of Scholars and Policy Makers, Washington, DC.
Simpson, D. D. (1979). The relation of time spent in drug abuse treatment to post-treatment outcome *American Journal of Psychiatry, 36,* 1449-1453.
Simpson D. D., Brown B. S., Joe, G. W. (1997) Treatment retention and follow-up outcomes in the Drug Abuse Treatment Outcome Study (DATOS). *Psychology of Addictive Behaviors* 11:294-307.
Simpson, D.D. Chatham, L.R., & Brown, B.S. (1995) The role of evaluation research in drug abuse policy. *Current Directions in Psychological Science, 4,* 123-126.
Simpson, D. D., Joe, G.W., Lehman W. E. K., & Sells, S B. (1986). Addiction careers: Etiology, treatment, and 12-year follow-up procedures. *Journal of Drug Issues, 16,* 107-121.
Simpson, D.D., & Sells, S.B. (Eds.). (1982). Effectiveness of treatment for drug abuse: An overview of the DARP research program. *Advances in Alcohol and Substance Abuse, 2,* 7-29.
Simpson, D. D., & Sells, S. B. (Eds.). (1990), *Opioid addiction and treatment: A twelve year follow-up.* Malabar, FL: Robert E. Krieger Publishing Co.
Substance Abuse and Mental Health Services Administration. (2007). *Results of the 2005 national survey on drug use and health: National findings.* Washington, DC: Department of Health and Human Services.
Swartz. J. A. (1993) TASC—the next 20 years: Extending, refining, and assessing the model. In J A. Inciardi (Ed.), *Drug treatment and criminal justice* (pp. 127-148). Newbury Park, CA: Sage.
Swartz, J A., & Lurigio, A. J (1999). Psychiatric illness and comorbidity among adult male detainees in drug treatment. *Psychiatric Services, 50,* 1628-1630.
Taxman, F., & Spinner, D. (1997). *Fail Addiction Services· (JAS) Demonstration Project in Montgomery County, MD. Jail and community-based substance abuse treatment program model.* College Park: University of Maryland. College Park.
United Nations Office on Drugs and Crime. (2006). *World drug report: Volume I analysis.* Vienna, Austria: United Nations.
University of California, Los Angeles Integrated Substance Abuse Programs (2007). *Evaluation of the substance abuse and crime prevention act: Final report.* Prepared for the California Department of Alcohol and Drug Programs (ADP), California Health and Human Services Agency.
Vigdal, G L. (1995). Planning for alcohol and other drug abuse treatment for adults in the criminal justice system. Rockville, MD: Department of Health and Human Services.
Waller, M., & Weiner, H. (1989). The dually diagnosed patient in an inpatient chemical dependency treatment program *Alcoholism Treatment Quarterly, 5,*197-218.
Weinman, B. (1990). Treatment Alternatives to Street Crime (TAW) In J. A. Inciardi (Ed.), *Handbook of drug control in the United States* (pp 139-150).Westport CT: Greenwood.

Wexler, H. K. (1996). *The Amity Prison TC evaluation: Inmate profiles and reincarceration outcomes.* Presentation for the California Department of Corrections, Sacramento, CA.

Wexler, H K, De Leon, G. Thomas, G., Kiessel, D., & Peters, 3. (1999) .The Amity Prison T'C evaluation: Reincarceration outcomes. *Criminal Justice and Behavior, 26,* 147-.167.

Wexler, H. K., Falkin, G P., Lipton, D. S & Rosenblum, A. B. (1992). Outcome evaluation of a prison therapeutic community for substance abuse treatment In C. G Leukefeld & F. M Tims *(Eds.), Drug abuse treatment in prisons and jails* (NIDA Research Monograph 118, DIMS Publication Number ADM 92-1884, pp. 54-72). Washington, DC: National Institute on Drug Abuse.

World Health Organization. (2004). *Neuroscience of psychoactive substance use and dependence.* Geneva, Switzerland:Author.

World Health Organization. (1986). *Ottawa charter for health promotion.* Presented at the first international conference on health promotion. Ottawa, Canada. (November 21, 1986).

http://www.intechweb.org/booksprocess/authorguidelines/chapter/36007

13

Contributions of Non-Human Primates to the Understanding of Cocaine Addiction

Rafael S. Maior, Marilia Barros and Carlos Tomaz
University of Brasilia
Brazil

1. Introduction

In this review, we aim to highlight the importance of neuropharmacological data, originated in non-human primate studies, towards our understanding of the mechanisms of cocaine addiction. Most studies in this field are undertaken with rodents as animal models, having provided over the years important knowledge on the behavioral, neurological and pharmacological mechanisms of drug addiction. There are, nonetheless, significant hormonal, neurochemical and neuroanatomical discrepancies between rodents and primates, particularly in reference to humans. Although the phylogenetic distance between humans-rodents, as opposed to humans-non-human primates may seem obvious, the impact this has on research findings is not always very evident. The gap in brain chemistry, neuronal organization and development, as well as behavioral diversity has serious implications in rodent models and limits somewhat their significance and generalization potential when trying to understand cocaine addiction - a phenomenon typical in humans. Due to ethical and important methodological restrictions on human testing, non-human primate (NHP) models are not only insightful, but also crucial to further the current scientific knowledge on this topic.

2. Addiction and cocaine

Cocaine is one of the most prevalent drugs of abuse. Data from the World Health Organization (WHO) estimated that, until 2008, approximately 19 million people worldwide had made use of cocaine (WHO, 2010). While the illicit retail market of cocaine is deemed to be worth around US$ 88 billions per year (WHO, 2009), its economic burden is difficult to measure. In terms of health treatment costs, there were 31,800 drug-related deaths in the United States alone in 2007 - a rate twice as high as that for murder in that year - with cocaine being related to about 40% of this toll. From 2002 to 2007, the WHO estimates that these premature deaths cost around 33 billion dollars. The American Drug Control program's budget for all drug-related control efforts in 2011 corresponds to US$15 billion, including treatment, prevention and illicit trade combat (National Drug Control Budget, 2011). Most of this will be spent on cocaine control, as the USA is the major destination of cocaine exports (WHO). On the other hand, the global cost of cocaine is less clear, considering that data from several countries are less reliable or regular.

Cocaine addiction is a psychological substance dependence where addicts have great difficulty in abstaining from drug-seeking, even at the cost of evident negative consequences (Vanderschuren & Everitt, 2004). It is a relapsing disorder with pervading effects on the human brain (O'Brien, 1997). Repeated use of cocaine leads to sensitization, i.e. enhanced response to the stimulus. In this case, repeated cocaine intake induces increased motor response and motivation (Robinson & Berridge, 2008). Sensitization is a long-lasting behavioral phenomenon with several implications to addiction (Paulson et al., 1991). The enduring sensitization induced by cocaine is linked to the relapsing properties of this disorder. Relapse or reinstatement is the return of drug-seeking or drug-taking behavior after a drug-free interval. In animal models, reinstatement has been shown to take place with priming injections of the drug (de Wit & Stewart, 1981), other compounds (Crombag et al., 2002), re-exposure to environmental cues associated with drug-taking (Meil & See, 1996) or even by stressful events (Anker & Carroll, 2010). In fact, cocaine relapse is one of the most difficult obstacles for the rehabilitation of addicts (O'Brien, 1997), possibly being related to cocaine sensitization of motivation or stimulus salience and not sensitization of locomotor activity (Robinson & Berridge, 2008).

Although progress in understanding the function of the brain and addiction has been made, there is still no pharmacological treatment that effectively blocks cocaine dependence, even after 30 years or so of research. Therefore, it is evident that cocaine addiction is a lingering and crippling health issue that warrants continued attention from the scientific community.

3. The case for non-human primates as models

As in the case of most biomedical fields, rodent models stand as the primary source of data in the study of addiction. Their small size and short reproductive cycle makes them easy to maintain, handle and reproduce, as well as relatively inexpensive in up keeping in laboratories around the world. Nevertheless, rats and mice did not reach this ubiquity in biomedical research on these merits alone. Rodent models have proved reliable in a wide range of topics, from drug screening to cognitive tests (eg. Fouquet et al., 2010; Heinrichs, 2010; Schmidt et al., 2011). Naturally, the versatility of these subjects has reflected on the enormous amount of scientific literature and experimental apparatus that have been generated over the course of the last five decades. The extensive amount of rodent research also spurs a faster refinement of the techniques, which in turn, makes rodents an even more practical and useful model. In terms of cocaine addiction, rats have been employed in several paradigms (self-administration, conditioned place-preference, open field; Mello & Negus, 1996; Ator & Griffiths, 2003) and also make up the majority of cocaine-related studies. Unfortunately, there is a significant genetic gap between humans and rodents: the actual figure being 66-82% homology (Nilsson et al., 2001). This difference has several implications in the understanding of cocaine abuse in humans.

NHP have been employed in addiction paradigms for approximately 40 years (Thompson and Schuster, 1964; Griffiths et al., 1980; Mello and Negus, 1996). Although the primate database on addiction is less abundant than that of rodents', there is considerable information available for comparison and interpretation. The genetic homology between NHP and human falls within 95%, depending on the species considered (Hacia et al., 1998). A greater phylogenetic proximity reflects on a more similar anatomy, physiology and behavior. In the sections below, we will examine the most important discrepancies between rodents and NHP and the contributions of primate research to the understanding of cocaine addiction. The importance of NHP however does not lie solely on their genetic distance to rodents. There is rather a powerful tool in primate research that allows for a greater and more refined analysis of the intricacies of cocaine effects: primate behavior.

In this sense, one of the most widespread and reliable tests for cocaine addiction is the self-administration paradigm (Griffiths et al., 1980; Ator & Griffiths, 2003). In this model, the animal subject is trained to press a lever or push a button to receive a rewarding stimulus (e.g. electrical stimulation to "rewarding centers" in the brain or a direct infusion of an addictive substance). There are several schemes under which this paradigm may work for both rodents and NHP. Nevertheless, there is a limit to how many response parameters one may expect to gather from rats and mice. The great advantage of primate research is the plethora of behaviors that may be drawn upon, ranging from simple self-directed behaviors, to very complex social behaviors. All apes and monkey species present high cognitive indices and good manipulatory skills (Pouydebat et al., 2009, 2011). They may form large social structures, including even non-kin members. As a result, there are quite complex social situations that entail a variety of social cues and behaviors. For instance, they display (and react appropriately to) facial expressions signaling emotional states or intentions beyond only aggressiveness, as in the case of most non-primates species (Schimidt & Cohn, 2001). They may even engage in very cognitively demanding behaviors such as deception (Reader et al., 2011). Thus, the use of a species-appropriated ethogram may add a wealth of new data even to simple reaction time experiments. Models may be improved to resemble very closely human social conditions or complex cognitive tasks that models human drug-seeking behavior. As pointed out by Nader and coworkers (2008), "...all animal models are, as a minimum, predictive of some clinical outcome... When social behaviors of NHP and cocaine self-administration (for example) are included, these models are homologous models of human drug abuse." Indeed, some paradigms have included social variables in the study of cocaine abuse (Czoty et al., 2005; Morgan et al. 2002).

Furthermore, physical reactions to compounds or the abstinence thereof mirrors very closely those of humans. For example, NHP demonstrate all key signs of opioid withdrawal seen in humans, including retching, hiccups, pallor and abdominal cramps (see Weerts et al., 2007). Rodents, on the other hand, lack those and several other symptoms. Likewise, more subtle and yet relevant drug effects, such as hallucinatory behavior, are only clearly discernible in NHP (Castner & Goldman-Rakic, 2003; Ellison et al., 1981).

In the case of addiction, NHP longevity is also another advantage. Most ape and monkey species tend to live quite long; a few may even live beyond the age of 40 (Judge & Carey, 2000). This has important implications for the study of long-term effects of drug abuse. It means, among other aspects, that long-term effects of cocaine consumption may be more easily modeled for a specific developmental stage, such as adolescence. It also allows studies of a drug's cumulative effects or cross-drug comparisons in the same subject (Ator & Griffiths, 2003). Together with their greater physiological similarities and behavioral diversity, longevity makes NHP models key for addiction research.

At this point, it is important to add a caveat to our argument. Although NHP might prove crucial to research in most biomedical fields, for several reasons it may not always be the ideal model for many laboratories worldwide. First, primates require appropriate facilities that cater to their size, locomotion, habits and social needs. This makes primate research considerably more expensive than working with rats or mice. Longer reproductive cycles and development stages also reduce the pace of any experimental output. Even small species offers difficulty in handling and training. Another restriction refers to the lack of background research on the behavior and/or physiology for several primate species. Behavioral ethograms, for instance, are not always readily available in the literature. Lastly, ethical considerations regarding the availability of specimens and the threat of extinction for some species may also limit the use of primates. Therefore, we are not advocating the use of primates as the primary source of scientific data. Biomedical research will still rely heavily on rodent studies, and rightly so. One of the aims of the present review is to advise that caution should be taken before generalizing rodent findings to human and to show how NHP research may help bridge the gap between them.

3.1 Dopamine

The primary focus of cocaine research, as well as most drug of abuse, is the brain's dopaminergic system. Dopamine (DA) is a neurotransmitter produced in the substantia nigra, ventral tegmental area (VTA) and hypothalamus. The projection of VTA dopaminergic neurons reaches two main targets in the brain: the prefrontal cortex (mesocortical pathway) and the ventral striatum (mesolimbic pathway). Both comprise what is called the reward system, with the mesolimbic pathway playing a major role (see Berridge, 2007 and Wise, 1996 for review). Not surprisingly, the rewarding and psychostimulant effects of cocaine are mediated by its ability to enhance dopaminergic activity within the meso-cortico-limbic circuit (Roberts et al., 1977). Briefly, cocaine binds to and blocks the pre-synaptic transporter responsible for DA re-uptake (Heikkila et al., 1975; Ritz et al., 1987,). This dopamine transporter is referred to as DAT. As DA reuptake is inhibited, the synaptic cleft is overflown with DA that will bind to post-synaptic receptors, inducing a prolonged or enhance signaling effect.

The DA receptors are classically divided into 5 subtypes, classified as: D_1, D_2, D_3, D_4 and D_5. These subtypes have been further divided and organized into two main groups, the 'D_1-like' receptors: D_1/D_{1a}, D_5/D_{1b}, D_{1c} and D_{1d}; and the 'D_2-like' receptors: $D_{2\text{long and short}}$, D_3, D_4 or $D_{2\text{al and s}}$, D_{2b} and D_{2c} (Sibley and Monsma, 1992). D_1-like and D_2-like are traditionally involved in the rewarding properties of stimuli such as cocaine (Hummel & Unterwald, 2002; Di Chiara et al., 2004). In this regard, several studies have reported critical differences between rodents and primates. NHP post-synaptic D_1-like receptors show higher levels and their laminar distribution is more complex than in rodents, but similar to humans (Smiley et al., 1994). Regarding the densities of D_2-like receptors, Lidow and coworkers (1989) showed a distinct pattern of distribution in the primate cortex: a rostro-caudal gradient, with the prefrontal cortex showing the highest concentration and the occipital cortex the lowest. Rats, on the other hand, were found to have a more diffuse distribution of these receptors. More specifically, the ratio between D_1-like and D_2-like receptors in the NHP striatum is almost 1:1 (Madras et al, 1988; Weed et al, 1998), whereas D_1-like receptors are three times more prevalent than D_2-like (Hyttel and Arnt, 1987; Weed et al, 1998). The density ratio in humans seems to follow the same pattern as that observed in NHP (Hall et al, 1994; Piggott et al, 1999). There is also greater similarity between humans and NHP in the distribution of D_1-like (Hersi et al., 1996) and D_2-like receptors in the hippocampal formation (Kohler et al., 1991). These are also reflected in low ligand efficacy of D_1-like receptor agonists in the primate brain (Izenwasser & Katz, 1993; Pifl et al., 1991; Vermeulen et al., 1994).

The distribution and the organization of DA receptors are not the only discrepancies concerning the DA system. An early review from Berger and coworkers (1991) noted important differences in the organization of primate and rodent DA cells. They indicated larger and differentially organized terminal fields in the DA mesocortical pathway in primates. DA cells arriving in the rat striatum are clearly organized into two tiers, ventral and dorsal, whereas no such distinction is found in monkeys (Joel & Weiner, 2000). Cytoarchitecture of midbrain DA cells in monkeys and humans is noticeably different with large and dense dendritic plexuses (Gonzalez-Hernandez et al., 2004). The primate cortex shows a higher density of DA innervation, as compared to rodents (Goldman-Rakic et al., 1992; Goldman-Rakic et al., 1989). Goldman-Rakic and coworkers (1992) emphasized that the cortical DA system in rhesus monkeys is near identical to that of humans. Both species show a bi-laminar innervation of the prefrontal cortex with projections reaching upper and deep cortical areas. These discrepancies bear important consequences for cocaine addiction studies. For instance, the development of compounds that may block cocaine addictive effects will probably depend on receptor specificity.

It is noteworthy that greater focus is generally given to rodent pathways that show high homology with humans. Nevertheless, a few promising options may remain unexplored if NHP are not employed. For instance, the rat thalamus is very poorly innervated by DA neurons (Groenewegen, 1988). Only recently has some attention been given to the multiple DA projections to the thalamus in the monkey and human brain (Sanchez-Gonzalez et al., 2005). Likewise, drug screening may be severely restricted by results in rodents. As pointed out by Weerts and coworkers (2007), "unacceptable performance in the rat can result in termination of further examination of a compound or an entire chemical series".

All the physiological and anatomical dissimilarities between primates and rodents seem to bear on the dynamics of DA circuits and its associated metabolism. Cocaine infusion in NHP was shown to reduce glucose metabolism in several brain regions, including the prefrontal cortex and the ventral striatum, in a manner similar to that reported in human studies (London et al., 1990; Pearlson et al., 1993; Lyons et al. 1996). The effect seems to reduce metabolism also in cortical areas projecting to the ventral striatum (Lyons et al. 1996; Porrino et al., 2002). This is in clear opposition to rodent findings, where metabolic activity is increased, not decreased, being also restricted to dopaminergic circuits (Hammer & Cooke, 1994; Porrino et al., 1988).

The pharmacokinetics of the DA system also shows important differences in behavioural profiles. In NHP, rate-increasing effects of cocaine seem not to be important for the reinstatement of behavior after extinction (Banks et al. 2007). Odum and Shahan (2004) had found earlier that also the psychostimulant amphetamine significantly increased extinguished responding. Lile and co-workers also reported that cocaine and DA agonists induce different behavioural effects in monkeys and challenged the accepted influence of neurotransmitters transporters in reinforcement, as previously established in rats (Lile et al. 2003; Roberts et al. 1999). This became clearer when Letchworth and coworkers (2001) found long-term cocaine-induced increases in DAT densities in monkey striatum, which is not seen in rodents but is quite similar to human studies.

Regarding drug abuse in general, the DA system has been the most extensively investigated pathway. Despite this, its causal role in the reward system is still under debate. In short, three competing hypotheses have been put forward: (1) DA mediates the hedonic aspects of reward (i.e. 'liking'; Wise, 1980); (2) DA mediates the prediction of rewards concordant with associative learning (Schultz, 2004); and (3) DA mediate the motivational aspect of drug-seeking behavior by attributing incentive salience to reward-related stimuli (i.e. 'wanting'; Berridge & Robinson, 1998). In a detailed review of mostly rodent literature, Berridge (2007) examined the findings from the last 30 years and concluded that there is more support for the incentive salience hypothesis. However, there is also support from a few electrophysiological studies in monkeys showing that DA neurons cease to fire after reward-related cues have been learned (Schultz, 2006).

Nonetheless, primate studies have yielded a few other contributions. The study of cocaine-induced response sensitization also showed striking differences between primate and rodents. Rats generally display a dose-dependent sensitization of DA reinforcing responses (Liu et al., 2005). Chronic exposure to cocaine or amphetamine, on the other hand, has failed to produce sensitization in NHP (Castner et al., 2000; Bradberry & Rubino, 2006; Castner & Williams, 2007), which is in agreement with human imaging studies (Volkow et al. 1997; Martinez et al. 2003). Similarly, cocaine-associated cues have been shown to induce DA release in the rat striatum (Ito et al., 2002; Weiss et al. 2000). Similar studies with monkeys were unable to produce significant increases in extracellular DA in either the striatum or cortex (Bradberry, 2000; Kimmel et al. 2005). Human findings, via imaging studies, seem to agree with NHP results, although DA release was not measured directly (see Bradberry, 2007 for review). It is beyond the scope of the present review to try to settle the issue of DA causal role in drug abuse. Instead, the data shown here underscores critical NHP findings that put rodent studies in perspective.

Overall, the data reviewed above indicates that rodent DA system differs significantly from humans'. This is important to keep in mind when analyzing results from rats and mice studies. Although rodent studies provide the initial step of investigation, data obtained from such models are not easily generalized to humans. In some cases they may even bias investigation towards rodent-related issues. As we shall see further, there are also important differences concerning serotonin (5-HT), neuropetides and hormones. However, these systems have been studied less extensively in the framework of cocaine abuse, but their importance is gradually becoming clearer.

3.2 Serotonin

Serotonin or (5-hydroxytryptamine [5-HT]) is an important neurotransmitter in the brain. It is mostly synthesized in the raphe nuclei in the midbrain and from there 5-HT neurons project to several regions in the brain (Kazakov et al., 1993). There are at least 14 types of 5-HT receptors grouped into seven families (see Roth, 2006), with 5-HT_1 and 5-HT_2 being the most relevant and widespread in the human brain (Glennon et al., 2000). The release of 5-HT is modulated by the inhibition of two types of 5-HT auto-receptors: cell body and fiber terminal (Price et al., 1996).

As in the case of DA receptors, discrepancies between rodent and primate 5-HT auto-receptor distribution have been reported. 5-HT_{1A} distribution in rats and humans seem to be highly congruent (Hartig et al., 1992). Autoradiographic assays, however, have shown an abundance of 5-HT_{1A} mRNA expression in the superficial layers of monkeys' prefrontal cortex (de Almeida & Mengod, 2008; Marazziti et al. 1994; Mengod et al. 1996). This suggests that raphe nuclei efference may modulate high-level cortico-cortical communication in primates. In rodents, 5-HT_{1A} mRNA seems to be restricted to the deeper layers of the prefrontal cortex (Pompeiano et al., 1992; Santana et al., 2004) and therefore would not exert the same influence on cortical activity.

Although data on 5-HT_{1A} distribution throughout the brain is still lacking for NHP, there is little reason to suppose it differs much from humans and rodents. The same does not hold true, for example, in the case of 5-HT_{2A} receptors. High densities of this receptor were found in the rat caudate, putamen and accumbens nuclei, as well as 5-HT_{2A} mRNA in the caudate, putamen and substantia nigra (Lopez-Gimenez et al., 2001). This may reflect the fact that 5-HT neurons in the rat striatum are not as evenly distributed as in NHP (Ikemoto et al., 1996; Van Bockstaele et al. 1993). A similar pattern emerges from immunohistochemical assays on 5-HT transporting proteins (SERT), where rats show a more heterogeneous distribution than primates (Owashi et al., 2004). In spite of some efforts, there is as serious lack of data regarding the distribution specific 5-HT receptors in NHP brains. At this point, the involvement of 5-HT in cocaine behavioral effects still seems quite complicated (eg. Dic Dhonnchadha & Cunningham, 2008) and unfolding the intricacies of serotonergic system in the primate brain may prove crucial.

Nevertheless, the basic interaction between cocaine and 5-HT seems to be the same as DA. Besides its effects on DAT, cocaine is also a potent inhibitor of 5-HT reuptake: it binds strongly to SERT, thereby preventing their reuptake by pre-synaptic cells (Heikkila et al., 1975; Ritz et al., 1987; Ritz et al., 1990). There are, once again, discrepancies in how cocaine affects rodent and primate serotonergic transmission. Work from Miller and coworkers (2001) showed that although both rodents and NHP share a high similarity in DAT sequence homology with humans (≅ 98.9%). In the case of SERT, NHP to human homology is slightly lower (98.3%), and even lower in for rodents (95%). Not surprisingly, SERT inhibition has an inverted effect on rats and primates, where it strengthens the discriminative stimulus of cocaine and has no impact on self-administration on the former (Tella, 1995), while it reduces the discriminative stimulus and self-administration in the latter (Howell & Byrd, 1995; Spealman, 1995).

Although the effects of cocaine on 5-HT inhibition were already well established by the early 1990s (Cunningham & Lakoski, 1990; Cunningham et al., 1992), it was only more recently that 5-HT neurotransmission was implicated in the cocaine-increased locomotor activity in rats (Hergers & Taylor, 1998). These findings were further explored by Carey and coworkers (2000, 2001 and 2005) showing that cocaine-induced locomotor activity in rats was mediated more specifically by 5-HT_{1A} receptors. Although self-administration of cocaine seems unaffected by 5-HT_{1A} manipulations in rats (Parsons, Weiss, & Koob, 1998), low doses of highly selective 5-HT_{1A} antagonist WAY100635 were shown to block cocaine-induced hyperlocomotion, whereas pre-treatment with 8-OHDPAT (5-HT_{1A} partial agonist) enhanced it. These findings were corroborated in NHP, where WAY100635 also blocked increases in locomotion induced by diethylpropion, an amphetamine-like drug (Mello Jr. et al., 2005). Pharmacological antagonism of this particular subtype of receptor showed conflicting results in rodent stress and anxiety tests (Fletcher et al., 1996; Griebel et al., 2000; Bell et al., 1999; Groenink et al., 1996). In monkeys, WAY100635 reduced anxiety behaviors in a confrontation model (Barros et al., 2003). These results are important if one considers the fact that stress and anxiety may trigger relapse in cocaine addicts (Steketee & Kalivas, 2011). Also 5-HT_{1A} agonism has been shown to enhance cocaine's reinforcing effects in NHP (Czoty et al., 2002).

The role of 5-HT on cocaine relapse seems to be related not only to its involvement in anxiety and stress processes. 5-HT may influence cocaine relapse due to its role in memory retrieval (Molodtsova, 2008). In rodents, the non-selective 5-$HT_{1B/1A}$ agonist RU24969 was shown to reduce the retrieval of cocaine induced cues (Acosta et al., 2005). This effect was reversed by 5-HT_{1B} antagonism which indicates prevalence of 5-HT_{1B} receptor in this case. Antagonism of 5-HT_{1B} receptors receptors seems to have no effect of their own on cocaine-related memories or behavior reinstatement. There are no reports on the effects of 5-HT_{1A}

agonists on retrieval of cocaine operant behavior *per se*, but one study found a reinstatement of cocaine-induced locomotor behavior (Carey et al., 2009). Retrieval of cocaine-associated memories in rats was also shown to be impaired by 5-HT_{2A} antagonism (Burmeister et al., 2004; Fillip, 2005) and 5-HT_{2C} agonism (Burbassi & Cervo, 2008; Fletcher et al., 2008; Neisewander & Acosta, 2007).

Although the understanding of 5-HT receptor's modulation of cocaine-related memory is still inceptive, Nic Dhonnchadha & Cunningham (2008) argued that future research should focus on 5-HT_{1B}, 5-HT_{2A} and 5-HT_{2C}. To our knowledge, the effects of 5-$HT_{1A/1B}$ and 5-$HT_{2A/2C}$ pharmacological manipulation on cocaine-associated memories have yet to be tested. Nevertheless, disparities of primate and rodent serotonergic system warrant a broader stance for future research. Although 5-HT_{1B} and 5-$HT_{2A/2C}$ modulation enhance self-administration in both species (Bubar & Cunningham, 2006; Czoty et al., 2005; Fletcher et al., 2002; Howell & Byrd, 1995; Parsons, Weiss, & Koob, 1998), 5-HT_{1A} agonism has shown to enhance the reinforcing properties of cocaine only in primates (Gold & Balster, 1992; Nader and Barrett, 1990). Therefore, differences in 5-HT reinforcing effects between rodents and NHP may very well transpose to cocaine-associated memories or even provide a entirely distinct pattern.

3.3 Peptides

Compared to DA and 5-HT, the role of neuropeptides in the effects of cocaine remains largely unknown. Nonetheless the past 20 years have witnessed important advances, especially in two fronts: tachykinin receptors and cocaine-and-amphetamine regulated transcript (CART). As shown below, the differences in primate and rodent brain regarding these two neuropeptides should exact caution from researchers.

Tachykinins comprise a group of neuropeptides that share a common C-terminal sequence (Phe-X-Gly-Leu-Met-NH2), with five known mammalian tachykinins: substance P - SP, neurokinin A (NKA), neurokinin B (NKB), neuropeptide K and neuropeptide g. They have been shown to bind to three specific tachykinin receptors: NK1, NK2 and NK3. NK1-Rs and NK3-Rs are widely distributed in the brain, while the NK2-Rs are found only in restricted areas. Although SP, NKA and NKB have a high binding affinity to the NK1-R, NK2-R and NK3-R, respectively, all tachykinins bind to all three receptor types (Severini et al., 2002).

In rats, cocaine administration induced the expression of tachykinin-related mRNA in the striatum (Adams et al., 2001; Arroyo et al., 2000; Johansson et al., 1994; Hurd et al., 1992; Mathieu-Kia & Besson, 1998). It also increased SP immunoreactivity in the striatum, substantia nigra and frontal cortex (Alburges et al., 2000). Nevertheless, results from NK1 manipulations on cocaine effects in rodents have been controversial so far. NK1 antagonism was shown to block cocaine-induced hyperlocomotion (Kraft et al., 2001), reverse sensitization (Davidson et al., 2004) and reduce cocaine-induced DA increases in the striatum (Loonam et al., 2003). NK1 agonism reinstated cocaine operant behaviors, yet SP – which binds preferentially to NK1 – failed to replace cocaine (Ukai et al., 1995). NK1 knockout mice showed no difference in cocaine self-administration and sensitization, as compared to controls (Ripley et al., 2002).

In the case NK3 receptors, there are a few reports implicating its activity in alcohol addiction in rats (Ciccocioppo et al., 1998; Massi et al., 2000). Also, NK3 activation in the VTA has been shown to reinstate cocaine-seeking behavior (Placenza et al., 2004) and its antagonism seems to block cocaine sensitization (Nwaneshiudu & Unterwald, 2010). In a joint effort from Huston and Tomaz's groups, a series of comparative studies regarding the involvement of

NK3 receptors in the effects of cocaine in rats and marmoset monkeys has been carried out. In rats, NK3 antagonist SR142801 reduced behavioral effects of cocaine, but increased DA action in the ventral nucleus accumbens and showed no significant effect on conditioned place preference (Jocham et al., 2006). It also had no individual effect on DA content in the striatum. In monkeys, the same antagonist blocked cocaine-induced effects in a range of behaviors, including locomotion and vigilance (De Souza Silva et al., 2006b). It also had no effect *per se*. In contrast, NK3 agonist senktide showed discrepancies between the two species. In rats, senktide increased both cocaine-induced hyperlocomotion and the DA response in the nucleus accumbens (Jocham et al., 2007). Senktide alone induced a brief increase in activity but no neurochemical changes. On the other hand, this same compound blocked cocaine-induced hyperlocomotion in monkeys, although it enhanced cocaine's effects on exploratory activity and some vigilance behaviors dose-dependently (Fig. 1; De Souza Silva et al., 2006a). Furthermore, unlike rats, senktide did not induce significant

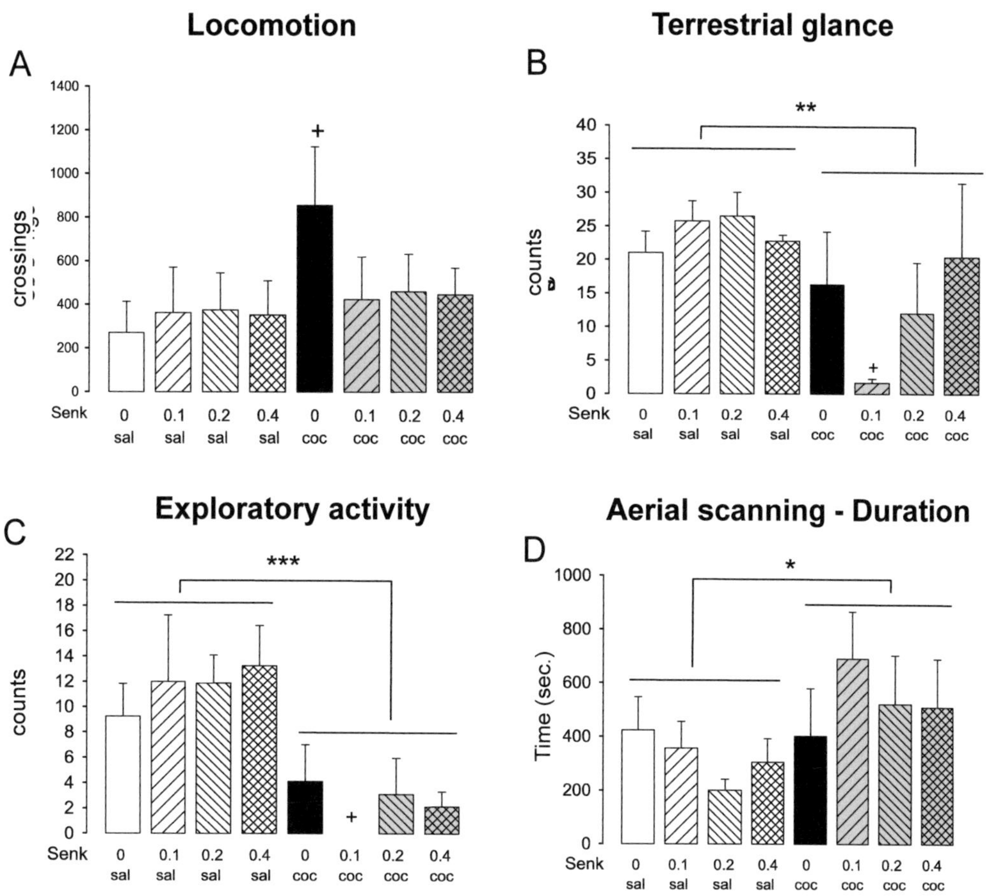

Fig. 1. The effects of cocaine (10 mg/kg, i.p.) on marmoset locomotor activity (A), terrestrial glance (B), exploratory activity (C) and aerial scanning duration (D; mean ± S.E.M.) and its modulation by the NK3-receptor agonist, senktide (0.1–0.4 mg/kg, s.c.), during a 20 min test trial ($n = 8$). +p < 0.05 vs. saline–saline, *p < 0.05, **p < 0.01, ***p < 0.001, two-way ANOVA (Modified from de Souza Silva et al., 2006a).

behavioral changes on its own (Fig 1A). These conflicting findings may be due to relevant differences in NK3 receptor distribution between rodents and NHP (Langlois et al., 2001). Despite that, NK3 receptor seems to be an interesting target for investigation and future therapeutic intervention of cocaine addiction.

CART is an mRNA identified in 1995, whose transcription seems to be modulated by psychostimulants (Douglas et al., 1995). It encodes two proteins in the rat (short and long CART), but only one in humans (short). In CART knockout mice, cocaine and amphetamine locomotor and reinforcing effects were reduced (Couceyro et al., 2005). The literature on CART research in primates, however, is scarce. There is one recent comparative report on the cocaine-induced expression of CART in the rat and monkey brain (Fagergren & Hurd, 2007). They report a higher expression of CART mRNA in the primate frontal and temporal cortices, positive labeling confined to the shell-like region of the striatum, different distribution in the hippocampal formation and more markedly differences in the thalamus. These aspects are different from those in rats, yet seem to be in agreement with human studies. Limbic distribution of CART mRNA was overall very similar to that of rodents'. However, the authors point that they were unable to investigate the nucleus accumbens where cocaine had been shown to induce increases in CART mRNA in humans (Albertson et al., 2004).

In summary, neuropeptidic involvement in cocaine-induced effects is beginning to provide important insights. The scarcity of primate studies on the subject is unsettling, considering that the discrepancies with rodents' anatomy and physiology are not trivial. There is, for instance, an absence of co-localization of several neuropeptides with DA in primates (Gaspar et al., 1990; Oeth & Lewis, 1992). Although the discovery of CART is fairly recent, compounds acting on NK1- and NK3-receptors have been under investigation for quite some time. Regardless, the understanding of tachykinins' influence on cocaine addiction seems to be progressing in a very slow pace.

3.4 Hypothalamic-pituitary-adrenal (HPA) axis

Another key aspect of psychostimulant effects concerns the neuroendocrine system. Stressful stimuli or situations trigger a series of neuroendocrine steps in the HPA axis; i.e., the release of corticotropin-releasing factor (CRF) from the hypothalamus, adrenocorticotropic hormone (ACTH) from the pituitary gland and finally glucocorticoids from the adrenal cortex. There is increasing evidence that this physiological response to stress is related to several aspects of drug addiction (Piazza & Le Moal, 1997; Sinha, 2001; Spealman et al., 2004). The work from Piazza and coworkers revealed that glucocorticoids were implicated in the DA response to cocaine and opioids (Marinelli et al., 1998; Marinelli et al., 1997; Piazza &Le Moal, 1997) and, therefore, the HPA axis was a possible target for addiction treatment. Glucocorticoid stress response seems to be essential for the acquisition, maintenance and reinstatement of stimulant self-administration (Goeders, 2002; Piazza et al., 1991; Piazza and Le Moal, 1998).

There are major and pervasive differences in the rodent and primate HPA system. First, the activation of the HPA in rodents relies predominantly on corticosterone, as opposed to cortisol in humans and NHP. There also seems to be discrepant age-related influences on hormones and cocaine. Rats display an increase in basal glucocorticoids as they age (Haugert et al., 1994; Meany et al., 1992), whereas no such difference was observed in NHP or humans (Goncharova & Lapin, 2002). More importantly, the distribution of corticotropin-releasing-factor (CRF) reactivity and that of corticoid receptors in the brain show great discrepancies in the amygdala (Bassett & Foote, 1992; Sanchez et al., 1999), hippocampus and pre-frontal cortex (PFC; Sanchez et al., 2000). The discrepancies in the amygdala and hippocampus are similar to the differences in the distribution of norepinephrine in those regions (Smith et al., 2006). These structures are important for learning and memory (McGaugh 2002; Tomaz et al., 1992) which, in turn, are also implicated in addictive behaviors (Garavan et al., 2000; Kilts et al., 2001; O'Brien et al., 1998). The amygdala also sends critical inputs to the striatum and PFC.

The discrepancies in receptor distribution in the PFC are of particular interest. The PFC is another area relevant for cocaine effects. It is a critical structure in decision-making and is involved in stress responses (Weinberg et al., 2010). It has undergone a massive expansion in primates, with NHP sharing a high similarity with humans in terms of structure, neurochemistry and connections (Carmichael and Price, 1994, 1996; Hardman et al., 2002; Ongur et al., 2003; Porrino & Lyons, 2000). The predominance of glucocorticoid receptors in the primate PFC, compared to the hippocampus, suggests that in humans and NHP this structure plays an important role in the HPA negative feedback through GR-mediated mechanisms (Sanchez et al., 2000). Furthermore, increasing evidence has implicated PFC asymmetry with stimulant use and hormonal changes. Activity in the right PFC was positively correlated with elevated levels of cortisol and cocaine craving (Kalin et al., 1998; Volkow et al., 1999). Chronic use of cocaine was also correlated with greater volume loss of the right PFC (Liu et al., 1998).

Despite these differences, cocaine-induced effects have shown a considerably similar response in rodents and primates. Plasma levels of ACTH, endorphin and corticosterone in rats increase in response to cocaine administration (Forman & Estilow, 1988; Levy et al., 1991; Moldow & Fischman, 1987; Saphier et al., 1993) as also seen in NHP (Lima et al., 2008; Sarnyai et al., 1996). This same pattern is seen in humans, where ACTH and adrenaline levels were increased with cocaine infusions, along with its subjective effects such as euphoria (Mendelson et al., 2002). On the other hand, glucocorticoids show reinforcing properties of their own in rodents, whereas no such effect has been observed in primates (Broadbear et al., 1999). Broadbear and coworkers (2004) also reported that increases in ACTH and cortisol in NHP in response to cocaine infusion were in line with rodents studies, but the same did not hold true for opioid drugs, which induced an inhibition of HPA activity in monkeys.

Although rodent and primate research presents direct mechanisms for the cocaine-induced activation of HPA axis, the impact that stress may have on the maintenance and relapse into drug seeking behavior is not so clear (Sinha, 2001). Initial studies with footshock paradigms in rodents have suggested that corticosterone may play a role in relapse (Deroche et al. 1997; Shaham et al. 1998; Mantsch and Goeders 1999). Rodent studies on reinstatement, however, yielded conflicting results (Erb et al., 1998; Goeders, 2003; Lu et al., 2001). Studies with squirrel monkeys by Spealman and coworkers suggest that the HPA axis is not involved in cocaine relapse (Lee et al., 2003). Rather, their following work indicated that the noradrenergic system is more likely to mediate stress response in cocaine reinstatement (Lee et al., 2004; but see Platt et al., 2007). Nevertheless, a recent study with rats suggests that cocaine reinstatement may be dependent on the interplay of both the HPA and noradrenergic systems (Graf et al., 2011).

4. Current and future strategies against cocaine addiction

As mentioned above, an effective pharmacological treatment for cocaine addiction is still lacking. A recent study has attempted to implement a novel cocaine vaccine trial, with limited results (Martell et al., 2009), yet other trials are currently under way (Kinsey et al., 2010). There are, nonetheless, several ongoing efforts to develop pharmacological strategies in primates to block or reduce the reinforcing properties of cocaine. From the findings discussed above, DA and 5-HT receptors and their respective transporters seem to currently be the most likely candidates for such an endeavor. In fact, the co-administration of DAT and SERT inhibitors has yielded encouraging results in primates (Howell, 2008), with such joint infusion leading to a better outcome, when compared to DAT alone. Strategies that influence CART transcription may also exert an important modulatory effect on stimulant-seeking behavior and thus should not be overlooked in primate studies. On the other hand, NK1 and NK3 receptors seem to be more involved in the hyperlocomotor property of cocaine, even if the present lack of studies limits such a prediction, while the interaction of the stress response, via HPA axis, with the noradrenergic system seems promising in terms of preventing a relapse.

The development of drugs with such mechanisms will require confirmation and further testing in NHP models. Well-established testing paradigms are just now being combined with neuroimaging techniques in monkeys, such as PET scans (Howell, 2008; Howell & Murnane, 2011) and fMRI (Jenkins et al., 2004; Brevard et al., 2006). Besides the several aspects already pointed out in this chapter, other advantages for using NHP (specifically related to imaging studies) are worth mentioning, including a similar cerebral metabolism and pharmacokinetics profile between humans and NHP, as opposed to rodents (Banks et al., 2007; Lyons et al., 1996; Porrino et al., 2002). Therefore, the translational value of NHP neuroimaging is unparallel to any other animal model.

In summary, there is compelling evidence for the importance of NHP in cocaine research. In all neural pathways analyzed, the discrepancies detected between rodents and humans warrant some caution when generalizing the results observed in the former. Nevertheless, there are several lines of research related to cocaine that have few or no corresponding studies being held with primates. Besides the difficulty in handling and research costs, this may also be due to restrictions in the use of these animals for research, especially for large primates. The findings discussed in this chapter indicate that NHP will remain crucial for biomedical research for several years to come, as substitutes have not yet been made available. Therefore, the development of a clinically effective anti-cocaine or anti-relapse drug/vaccine will very likely depend on our ability to cope with the lack of studies and ever-mounting pressure against the use of animals in research.

5. Acknowledgements

The writing of this chapter was supported by CAPES/DAAD/PROBAL (324/09). CNPq/Brazil provided RSM with a doctoral fellowship and MB with a researcher fellowship (311621/2009-0).

6. References

Acosta, J.I., Boynton, F.A., Kirschner, K.F. & Neisewander, J.L. (2005). Stimulation of 5- HT_{1B} receptors decreases cocaine- and sucrose-seeking behavior. *Pharmacology Biochemistry and Behaviour*, Vol.80, pp. 297–307.

Adams, D.H., Hanson, G.R. & Keefe KA. (2001). Differential effects of cocaine and methamphetamine on neurotensin/neuromedin N and preprotachykinin messenger RNA expression in unique regions of the striatum. *Neuroscience*, Vol.102, pp. 843–851.

Albertson, D.N., Pruetz, B., Schmidt, C.J., Kuhn, D.M., Kapatos, G. & Bannon, M.J. (2004). Gene expression profile of the nucleus accumbens of human cocaine abusers: evidence for dysregulation of myelin. *Journal of Neurochemistry*, Vol.88, pp. 1211–1219.

Alburges, M.E., Ramos, B.P., Bush, L. & Hanson, G.R. (2000). Responses of the extrapyramidal and limbic substance P systems to ibogaine and cocaine treatments. *European Journal Pharmacology*, Vol.390, pp. 119–126.

Anker, J.J. & Carroll, M.E. (2010). Reinstatement of cocaine seeking induced by drugs, cues, and stress in adolescent and adult rats. *Psychopharmacology*, Vol.208, pp. 211-222.

Arroyo, M., Baker, W.A. & Everitt BJ. (2000). Cocaine self-administration in rats differentially alters mRNA levels of the monoamine transporters and striatal neuropeptides. *Molecular Brain Research*, Vol.83, pp. 107–120.

Ator, N.A. & Griffiths, R.R. (2003). Principles of drug abuse liability assessment in laboratory animals. *Drug and Alcohol Dependence*, Vol.70, No.3, pp. S55–S72.

Banks, M.L., Czoty, P.W. & Nader, M.A. (2007). The influence of reinforcing effects of cocaine on cocaine-induced increases in extinguished responding in cynomolgus monkeys. *Psychopharmacology*, Vol.192, pp. 449-456.

Barros, M., Mello, E.L., Maior, R.S., Muller, C.P., De Souza-Silva, M.A., Carey, R.J., Huston, J.P. & Tomaz, C. (2003). Anxiolytic-like effects of the selective 5-HT_{1A} receptor antagonist WAY 100635 in non-human primates. *European Journal of Pharmacology*, Vol.482, pp. 197–203.

Bassett, J.L. & Foote, S.L. (1992). Distribution of corticotropin-releasing factor-like immunoreactivity in squirrel-monkey (saimiri-sciureus) amygdala. *Journal of Comparative Neurology*, Vol.323, pp. 91-102.

Bell, R., Lynch, K. & Mitchell, P. (1999). Lack of effect of the 5-HT1A receptor antagonist WAY-100635 on murine agonistic behaviour. *Pharmacology Biochemistry and Behavior*, Vol.64, pp. 549–554.

Berger, B., Gaspar, P & Verney, C. (1991). Dopaminergic innervation of the cerebral cortex: unexpected differences between rodents and primates. *Trends in Neuroscience*, Vol.14, pp. 21–27.

Berridge, K.C. (2007). The debate over dopamine's role in reward: the case for incentive salience. *Psychopharmacology*, Vol.191, 391-431.

Berridge, K.C. & Robinson, T.E. (1998). What is the role of dopamine in reward: hedonic impact, reward learning, or incentive salience? *Brain Research Reviews*, Vol.28, pp. 309–369.

Bradberry, C.W. (2000). Acute and chronic dopamine dynamics in a nonhuman primate model of recreational cocaine use. *Journal of Neuroscience*, Vol.20, pp. 7109–7115.

Bradberry, C.W. (2007). Cocaine sensitization and dopamine mediation of cue effects in rodents, monkeys, and humans: areas of agreement, disagreement, and implications for addiction. *Psychopharmacology*, Vol191, pp. 705-717.

Bradberry, C.W. & Rubino, S.R. (2006). Dopaminergic responses to self-administered cocaine in rhesus monkeys do not sensitize following high cumulative intake. *European Journal of Neuroscience*, Vol.23, pp. 2773–2778.

Brevard, M.E., Meyer, J.S., Harder, J.A. & Ferris, C.F. (2006). Imaging brain activity in conscious monkeys following oral MDMA ("ecstasy"). *Magnetic Resonance Imaging*, Vol.24, pp. 707–714.

Broadbear, J.H., Winger, G. & Woods, J.H. (1999). Glucocorticoid-reinforced responding in the rhesus monkey. Psychopharmacology, Vol.147, pp. 46-55.

Broadbear, J.H., Winger, G. & Woods, J.H. (2004). Self-administration of fentanyl, cocaine and ketamine: effects on the pituitary-adrenal axis in rhesus monkeys. *Psychopharmacology*, Vol.176, pp. 398-406.

Bubar, M.J. & Cunningham, K.A. (2006). Serotonin 5-HT_{2A} and 5-HT_{2C} receptors as potential targets for modulation of psychostimulant use and dependence. *Current Topics on Medical Chemistry*, Vol.6, pp. 1971–1985.

Burbassi, S. & Cervo L. (2008). Stimulation of serotonin(2C) receptors influences cocaine-seeking behavior in response to drug-associated stimuli in rats. *Psychopharmacology* (Berl), Vol.196, pp. 15–27.

Burmeister, J.J., Lungren, E.M., Kirschner, K.F. & Neisewander JL. (2004). Differential roles of 5-HT receptor subtypes in cue and cocaine reinstatement of cocaine-seeking behavior in rats. *Neuropsychopharmacology*, Vol.29, pp. 660–668.

Carey, R.J., Damianopoulos, E.N. & DePalma G. (2000). The 5-HT1A antagonist WAY 100635 can block the low dose locomotor stimulant effects of cocaine. *Brain Research*, Vol.862, pp. 242–246.

Carey, R.J., Damianopoulos, E.N. & Shanahan, A.B. (2009). Cocaine conditioning: Reversal by autoreceptor dose levels of 8-OHDPAT. *Pharmacology Biochemistry and Behavior*, Vol.91, pp. 447-452.

Carey, R.J., DePalma, G. & Damianopoulos, E. (2001). Cocaine and serotonin: a role for the 5-HT_{1A} receptor site in the mediation of cocaine stimulant effects. *Behavioural Brain Research*, Vol.126, pp. 127-133.

Carey, R.J., DePalma, G., Damianopoulos, E., Shanahan, A., Muller, C.P. & Huston, J.P. (2005). Evidence that the 5-HT_{1A} autoreceptor is an important pharmacological target for the modulation of cocaine behavioral stimulant effects. *Brain Research*, Vol.1034, pp. 162-171.

Carmichael, S.T. & Price, J.L. (1994). Architectonic subdivision of the orbital and medial prefrontal cortex in the macaque monkey. *Journal of Comparative Neurology*, Vol.346, pp. 366–402.

Castner, S.A. & Goldman-Rakic, P.S. (2003). Amphetamine sensitization of hallucinatory-like behaviors is dependent on prefrontal cortex in nonhuman primates. *Biological Psychiatry*, Vol.54, pp. 105-110.

Castner, S.A. & Williams, G.V. (2007). From vice to virtue: Insights from sensitization in the nonhuman primate. *Progress in Neuro-Psychopharmacology & Biological Psychiatry*, Vol.31, pp. 1572-1592.

Castner, S.A., al-Tikriti, M.S., Baldwin, R.M., Seibyl, J.P., Innis, R.B. & Goldman-Rakic, P.S. (2000). Behavioral changes and [123I]IBZM equilibrium SPECT measurement of amphetamine-induced dopamine release in rhesus monkeys exposed to subchronic amphetamine. *Neuropsychopharmacology*, Vol.22, pp. 4–13.

Ciccocioppo, R., Panocka, I., Polidori, C., Froldi, R., Angeletti, S. & Massi, M. (1998). Mechanism of action for reduction of ethanol intake in rats by the tachykinin NK-3 receptor agonist aminosenktide. *Pharmacology Biochemistry and Behaviour*, Vol.61, pp. 459–464.

Couceyro, P.R., Evans, C., McKinzie, A., Mitchell, D., Dube, M., Hagshenas. L., White, F.J., Douglass, J., Richards, W.G. & Bannon, A.W. (2005). Cocaine- and amphetamine-regulated transcript (CART) peptides modulate the locomotor and motivational properties of psychostimulants. *Journal of Pharmacology and Experimental Therapeutics*, Vol.315, pp. 1091–1100.

Crombag, H.S., Grimm, J.W. & Shaham, Y. (2002). Effect of dopamine receptor antagonists on renewal of cocaine seeking by reexposure to drug-associated contextual cues. *Neuropsychopharmacology*, Vol.27, pp. 1006–1015.

Cunningham, K.A. & Lakoski, J.M. (1990). The interaction of cocaine with serotonin dorsal raphe neurons. *Neuropsychopharmacology*, Vol.3, pp. 41–50.

Cunningham, K.A., Paris, J.M. & Goeders, N.E. (1992). Chronic cocaine enhances serotonin autoregulation and serotonin uptake binding. *Synapse*, Vol.11, pp. 112–123.

Czoty, P.W., Ginsburg, B.C. & Howell, L.L. (2002). Serotonergic attenuation of the reinforcing and neurochemical effects of cocaine in squirrel monkeys. *Journal of Pharmacology and Experimental Therapeutics*, Vol.300, pp. 831–837.

Czoty, P.W., McCabe, C. & Nader, M.A. (2005). Assessment of the relative reinforcing strength of cocaine in socially housed cynomolgus monkeys using a choice procedure. *Journal of Pharmacology and Experimental Therapeutics*, Vol.312, pp. 96–102.

Davidson, C., Lee, T.H. & Ellinwood, E.H. (2004). NK1 receptor antagonist WIN51708 reduces sensitization after chronic cocaine. *European Journal of Pharmacology*, Vol.499, pp. 355–356.

de Almeida, J. & Mengod, G. (2008). Serotonin 1A receptors in human and monkey prefrontal cortex are mainly expressed in pyramidal neurons and in a GABAergic interneuron subpopulation: implications for schizophrenia and its treatment. *Journal of Neurochemistry*, Vol.107, pp. 488-496.

de Souza Silva, M.A.D., Mello, E.L., Muller, C.P., Jocham, G., Maior, R.S., Huston, J.P., Tomaz, C. & Barros, M. (2006a). Interaction of the tachykinin NK3 receptor agonist senktide with behavioral effects of cocaine in marmosets (Callithrix penicillata). *Peptides*, Vol.27, pp. 2214-2223.

de Souza Silva, M.A.D., Mello, E.L., Muller, C.P., Jocham, G., Maior, R.S., Huston, J.P., Tomaz, C. & Barros, M. (2006b). The tachykinin NK3 receptor antagonist SR142801 blocks the behavioral effects of cocaine in marmoset monkeys. *European Journal of Pharmacology*, Vol.536, pp. 269-278.

de Wit, H. & Stewart, J. (1981). Reinstatement of cocaine-reinforced responding in the rat. *Psychopharmacology*, Vol.75, pp. 134–143.

Deroche, V., Caine, S., Heyser, C., Polis, I., Koob, G., & Gold, L. (1997). Differences in the liability to self-administer intravenous co- caine between C57BL/6 and BALB/cByJ mice. *Pharmacology Biochemistry and Behavior*, Vol.57, pp. 429–440.

Di Chiara, G., Bassareo, V., Fenu, S., De Luca, M., Spina, L., Cadoni, C., Acquas, E., Carboni, E., Valentini, V. & Lecca, D. (2004). Dopamine and drug addiction: the nucleus accumbens shell connection. *Neuropharmacology,* Vol.47, Suppl 1, pp. 227–41.

Douglass, J., McKinzie, A.A. & Couceyro, P. (1995). PCR differential display identifies a rat brain mRNA that is transcriptionally regulated by cocaine and amphetamine. *Journal of Neuroscience*, Vol.15, 2471–2481.

Ellison, G., Nielsen, E.B. & Lyon, M. (1981). Animal-model of psychosis-hallucinatory behaviors in monkeys during the late stage of continuous amphetamine intoxication. *Journal of Psychiatric Research,* Vol.16, pp. 13-22.

Erb, S., Shaham, Y. & Stewart, J. (1998). The role of corticotropin-releasing factor and corticosterone in stress- and cocaine-induced relapse to cocaine seeking in rats. *Journal of Neuroscience*, Vol.18, pp. 5529- 5536.

Fagergren, P. & Hurd, Y. (2007). CART mRNA expression in rat monkey and human brain: Relevance to cocaine abuse. *Physiology & Behavior*, Vol.92, pp. 218-225.

Filip, M. (2005). Role of serotonin (5-HT)2 receptors in cocaine self-administration and seeking behavior in rats. *Pharmacological Report*, Vol.57, pp. 35–46.

Filip, M., Bubar, M.J. & Cunningham, K.A. (2006). Contribution of serotonin (5-HT) 5-HT_2 receptor subtypes to the discriminative stimulus effects of cocaine in rats. *Psychopharmacology*, Vol.183, pp. 482-489.

Fletcher, A., Forster, E.A., Bill, D.J., Brown, G., Cliffe, I.A., Hartley, J.E., Jones, D.E., McLenachan, A., Stanhope, K.J., Critchley, D.J., Childs, K.J., Middlefell, V.C., Lanfumey, L., Corradetti, R., Laporte, A.M., Gozlan, H., Hamon, M. & Dourish, C.T. (1996). Electrophysiological, biochemical, neurohormonal and behavioural studies with WAY- 100635, a potent, selective and silent 5-HT_{1A} receptor antagonist. *Behavioural Brain Research*, Vol.73, pp. 337–353.

Fletcher, P.J., Grottick, A.J. & Higgins, G.A. (2002). Differential effects of the 5-HT(2A) receptor antagonist M100907 and the 5-HT(2C) receptor antagonist SB242084 on cocaine-induced locomotor activity, cocaine self-administration and cocaine-induced reinstatement of responding. *Neuropsychopharmacology,* Vol.27, pp. 576–586.

Fletcher, P.J., Rizos, Z., Sinyard, J., Tampakeras, M. & Higgins, G.A. (2008). The 5-HT(2C) receptor agonist Ro60-0175 reduces cocaine self-administration and reinstatement induced by the stressor yohimbine, and contextual cues. *Neuropsychopharmacology,* Vol.33, pp. 1402–1412.

Forman, L.J. & Estilow, S. (1988). Cocaine influences beta-endorphin levels and release. *Life Sciences*, Vol.43, pp. 309–315.

Fouquet, C., Tobin, C. & Rondi-Reig, L. (2010). A new approach for modeling episodic memory from rodents to humans: The temporal order memory. *Behavioural Brain Research*, Vol.215, pp. 172-179.

Garavan, H., Pankiewicz, J., Bloom, A., Cho, J.K., Sperry, L., Ross, T.J., Salmeron, B.J., Risinger, R., Kelley, D. & Stein, E.A. (2000). Cue-induced cocaine craving:

neuroanatomical specificity for drug users and drug stimuli. *American Journal of Psychiatry*, Vol.157, pp. 1789–1798.

Gaspar, P., Berger, B. & Febvret, A. (1990). Neurotensin innervation of the human cerebral-cortex - lack of colocalization with catecholamines. *Brain Research* 530, pp. 181-195.

Gaspar, P., Berger, B., Febvret, A., Vigny, A. & Henry, J.P. (1989). Catecholamine innervation of the human cerebral-cortex as revealed by comparative immunohistochemistry of tyrosine-hydroxylase and dopamine-beta-hydroxylase. *Journal of Comparative Neurology*, Vol.279, pp. 249-271.

Glennon, R.A., Dukat, M., & Westkaemper, R.B. (2000). Serotonin receptor subtypes and ligands. In F. E. Bloom & D. J. Kupfer (Eds.), *Psychopharmacology: The fourth generation of progress* (4th rev. ed.). Philadelphia: Lippincott Williams & Wilkins.

Goeders, N.E. (2002). The HPA axis and cocaine reinforcement. *Psychoneuroendocrinology*, Vol.27, pp. 13-33.

Goeders, N.E. (2003). The impact of stress on addiction. *European Neuropsychopharmacology*, Vol.13, pp. 435-441.

Gold, L.H. & Balster, R.L. (1992). Effects of buspirone and gepirone on IV cocaine self-administration in rhesus monkeys. *Psychopharmacology*, Vol.108, pp. 289-294.

Goldman-Rakic, P.S., Leranth, C., Williams, S.M., Mons, N. & Geffard, M. (1989). Dopamine synaptic complex with pyramidal neurons in primate cerebral cortex. *Proceedings of the National Academy of Sciences of the United States of America*, Vol.86, No.22, pp. 9015–9019.

Goldman-Rakic, P.S., Lidow, M.S., Smiley, J.F. & Williams, M.S. (1992). The anatomy of dopamine in monkey and human prefrontal cortex. *Journal of Neural Transmission-General Section*, pp. 163-177.

Goncharova, N.D. & Lapin, B.A. (2002). Effects of aging on hypothalamic-pituitary-adrenal system function in non-human primates. *Mechanisms of Ageing and Development*, Vol,123, pp. 1191-1201.

Gonzalez-Hernandez, T., Barroso-Chinea, P., De La Cruz Muros, I., Del Mar Perez-Delgado, M. & Rodriguez, M. (2004). Expression of dopamine and vesicular mono- amine transporters and differential vulnerability of mesostriatal dopaminergic neurons. *Journal of Comparative Neurology*, Vol.479, pp. 198–215.

Graf, E.N., Hoks, M.A., Baumgardner, J., Sierra, J., Vranjkovic, O., Bohr, C., Baker, D.A. & Mantsch, J.R. (2011). Adrenal Activity during Repeated Long-Access Cocaine Self-Administration is Required for Later CRF-Induced and CRF-Dependent Stressor-Induced Reinstatement in Rats. *Neuropsychopharmacology*, Vol.36, pp. 1444-1454.

Griebel, G., Rodgers, R.J., Perrault, G. & Sanger, D.J. (2000). The effects of compounds varying in selectivity as 5-HT(1A) receptor antagonists in three rat models of anxiety. *Neuropharmacology*, Vol.39, pp. 1848–1857.

Griffiths, R.R., Bigelow, G.E. & Henningfield, J.E. (1980). Similarities in animal and human drug-taking behavior. In N. K. Mello (Ed.), *Advances in substance abuse* (pp. 1–90). Greenwich, CT: JAI Press.

Groenewegen, H.J. (1988). Organization of the afferent connections of the mediodorsal thalamic nucleus in the rat, related to the mediodorsal-prefrontal topography. *Neuroscience*, Vol.24, pp. 379–431.

Groenink, L., Mos, J., van der Gugten, J., Schipper, J. & Olivier, B. (1996). The 5-HT1A receptor is not involved in emotional stress-induced rises in stress hormones. *Pharmacology Biochemistry and Behavior*, Vol.55, pp. 303-308.

Hacia, J.G., Makalowski, W., Edgemon, K., Erdos, M.R., Robbins, C.M., Fodor, S.P., Brody, L.C. & Collins, F.S. (1998). Evolutionary sequence comparisons using high-density oligonucleotide arrays. *Nature Genetics*, Vol.18, pp. 155–158.

Hall, H., Sedvall, G., Magnusson, O., Kopp, J., Halldin, C. & Farde, L. (1994). Distribution of D_1- and D_2-dopamine receptors, and dopamine and its metabolites in the human brain. *Neuropsychopharmacology*, Vol.11, pp. 245–256.

Hammer, R.P. & Cooke, E.S. (1994). Gradual tolerance of metabolic-activity is produced in mesolimbic regions by chornic cocaine treatment, while subsequent cocaine challenge activates extrapyramidal regions of rat-brain. *Journal of Neuroscience*, Vol.14, pp.4289-4298.

Hardman, C.D., Henderson, J.M., Finkelstein, D.I., Horne, M.K., Paxinos, G. & Halliday, G.M. (2002). Comparison of the basal ganglia in rats, marmosets, macaques, baboons, and humans: volume and neuronal number for the output, internal relay, and striatal modulating nuclei. *Journal of Comparative Neurology*, Vol.445, pp. 238–255.

Hartig, P.R., Adham, N., Zgombick, J., Weinshank, R. & Branchek, T. (1992).Molecular biology of the 5-HT_1 Receptor family. *Drug Development Research*, Vol.26, pp. 215-224.

Haugert, B.L., Thrivikraman, K.V. & Plotsky, P.M. (1994). Age-related alterations of hypothalamic-pituitary-adrenal axis function in male Fischer 344 rats. *Endocrinology*, Vol.134, pp. 1528–1536.

Heikkila, R.E., Orlansky, H. & Cohen, G. (1975). Studies on distinction between uptake inhibition and release of h-3 dopamine in rat-brain tissue-slices. *Biochemical Pharmacology*, Vol.24, pp. 847-852.

Heinrichs, S.C. (2010). Neurobehavioral consequences of stressor exposure in rodent models of epilepsy. *Progress in Neuro-Psychopharmacology & Biological Psychiatry*, Vol.34, pp. 808-815.

Herges, S. & Taylor, D.A. (1998). Involvement of serotonin in the modulation of cocaine-induced locomotor activity in the rat. *Pharmacology Biochemistry and Behaviour*, Vol.59, pp. 595 - 611.

Hersi, A.I., Jacques, D., Gaudreau, P. & Quirion, R. (1996). Comparative distribution of D1-like receptors in the hippocampal formation of rat, monkey and human brains. Retrieved July 7, 2007, from http://www.neuroscience.com/manuscripts-1996/1996-005-quirion/1996-005-quirion.html

Howell, L.L. (2008). Nonhuman primate neuroimaging and cocaine medication development. *Experimental and Clinical Psychopharmacology*, Vol.16, pp. 446-457.

Howell, L.L. & Byrd, L.D. (1995). Serotonergic modulation of the behavioral effects of cocaine in the squirrel monkey. *Journal of Pharmacology and Experimental Therapeutics*, Vol.275, pp. 1551–1559.

Howell, L.L. & Murnane, K.S. (2011). Nonhuman Primate Positron Emission Tomography Neuroimaging in Drug Abuse Research. *Journal of Pharmacology and Experimental Therapeutics*, Vol.337, pp. 324-334.

Hummel, M. & Unterwald, E. (2002). D_1 dopamine receptor: a putative neurochemical and behavioral link to cocaine action. *Journal of Cell Physiology*, Vol.191, No.1, pp. 17–27.

Hurd, Y.L., Brown, E.E., Finlay, J.M., Fibiger, H.C. & Gerfen, C.R. (1992). Cocaine self-administration differentially alters messenger-RNA expression of striatal peptides. *Molecular Brain Research*, Vol.13, pp. 165–170.

Hyttel, J. & Arnt, J. (1987). Characterization of binding of 3*H*-SCH 23390 to dopamine D-1 receptors. Correlation to other D-1 and D-2 mea- sures and effect of selective lesions. *Journal of Neural Transmission*, Vol.68, pp. 171–189.

Ikemoto, K., Kitahama, K., Maeda, T. & Satoh, K. (1996). The distribution of noradrenaline, serotonin and gamma-aminobutyric acid in the monkey nucleus accumbens. *Progress in Neuro-Psychopharmacology & Biological Psychiatry*, Vol.20, pp. 1403-1412.

Ito, R., Dalley, J.W., Robbins, T.W. & Everitt, B.J. (2002). Dopamine release in the dorsal striatum during cocaine-seeking behavior under the control of a drug-associated cue. *Journal of Neuroscience*, Vol.22, pp. 6247–6253.

Izenwasser, S. & Katz, J.L. (1993). Differential efficacies of dopamine D1 receptor agonists for stimulating adenylyl cyclase in squirrel monkey and rat. *European Journal of Pharmacology*, Vol.246, pp. 39–44.

Jenkins, B.G., Sanchez-Pernaute, R., Brownell, A.L., Chen, Y.C. & Isacson, O. (2004). Mapping dopamine function in primates using pharmacologic magnetic resonance imaging. *Journal of Neuroscience*, Vol24, pp. 9553–9560.

Jocham, G., Lauber, A.C., Muller, C.P., Huston, J.P. & de Souza Silva, M.A. (2007). Neurokinin(3) receptor activation potentiates the psychomotor and nucleus accumbens dopamine response to cocaine, but not its place conditioning effects. *European Journal of Neuroscience*, Vol.25, pp. 2457-2472.

Jocham, G., Lezoch, K., Mueller, C.P., Kart-Teke, E., Huston, J.P. & de Souza Silva, M.A. (2006). Neurokinin(3) receptor antagonism attenuates cocaine's behavioural activating effects yet potentiates its dopamine-enhancing action in the nucleus accumbens core. *European Journal of Neuroscience*, Vol.24, pp. 1721-1732.

Joel, D. & Weiner, I. (2000). The connections of the dopaminergic system with the striatum in rats and primates: an analysis with respect to the functional and compartmental organization of the striatum. *Neuroscience*, Vol.96, pp. 451–74.

Johansson, B., Lindstrom, K. & Fredholm, B.B. (1994). Differences in the regional and cellular-localization of c-Fos messenger-RNA induced by amphetamine, cocaine and caffeine in the rat. *Neuroscience*, Vol.59, pp. 837–849.

Judge, D.S. & Carey, J.R. (2000). Postreproductive Life Predicted by Primate Patterns. *Journal of Gerontology: Biological Sciences*, Vol.55A, No.4, pp. B201–B209.

Kalin, N.H., Larson, C., Shelton, S.E. & Davidson, R.J. (1998). Asymmetric frontal brain activity, cortisol, and behavior associated with fearful temperament in rhesus monkeys. *Behavioural Neuroscience*, Vol.112, pp. 286–292.

Kazakov, V.N., Kravtsov, P.Y., Krakhotkina, E.D. & Maisky, V.A. (1993). Sources of cortical, hypothalamic and spinal serotonergic procjections - Topical organization within the nucleus-raphe-dorsalis. *Neuroscience*, Vol.56, pp. 157-164.

Kilts, C.D., Schweitzer, J.B., Quinn, C.K., Gross, R.E., Faber, T.L., Muhammad, F., Ely, T.D., Hoffman, J.N. & Dexter, K.P.G. (2001). Neural activity related to drug craving in cocaine addiction. *Archives of General Psychiatry*, Vol.58, pp. 334–341.

Kimmel, H.L., Ginsburg, B.C. & Howell, L.L. (2005). Changes in extracellular dopamine during cocaine self-administration in squirrel monkeys. *Synapse*, Vol.56, pp. 129–134.

Kinsey, B.M., Kosten, T.R. & Orson, F.M. (2010). Anti-cocaine vaccine development. *Expert Review of Vaccines*, Vol.9, pp. 1109-1114.

Kohler, C., Ericson, H., Hogberg, T., Halldin, C. & Chan-Palay, V. (1991). Dopamine D2 receptors in the rat, monkey and the post-mortem human hippocampus. An autoradiographic study using the novel D2-selective ligand 125I-NCQ 298. *Neuroscience Letters*, Vol.125, pp. 12–14.

Kraft, M., Ahluwahlia, S. & Angulo, J.A. (2001) Neurokinin-1 receptor antagonists block acute cocaine-induced horizontal locomotion. *Annual Reviews of the New York Academy of Sciences*, Vol.937, pp. 132–139.

Langlois, X., Wintmolders, C., te Riele, P., Leysen, J.E. & Jurzak, M. (2001). Detailed distribution of neurokinin 3 receptors in the rat, guinea pig and gerbil brain: a comparative autoradiographic study. *Neuropharmacology*, Vol.40, pp. 242–253.

Lee, B., Tiefenbacher, S., Platt, D.M. & Spealman, R.D. (2003). Role of the hypothalamic-pituitary-adrenal axis in reinstatement of cocaine-seeking behavior in squirrel monkeys. *Psychopharmacology*, Vol.168, pp. 177-183.

Lee, B., Tiefenbacher, S., Platt, D.M. & Spealman, R.D. (2004). Pharmacological blockade of alpha(2)-adrenoceptors induces reinstatement of cocaine-seeking behavior in squirrel monkeys. *Neuropsychopharmacology*, Vol.29, pp. 686-693.

Letchworth, S.R., Nader, M.A., Smith, H.R., Friedman, D.P. & Porrino, L.J. (2001). Progression of changes in dopamine transporter binding site density as a result of cocaine self-administration in rhesus monkeys. *Journal of Neuroscience*, Vol.21, pp. 2799–2807.

Levy, A.D., Li, Q., Kerr, J.E., Rittenhouse, P.A., Milonas, G., Cabrera, T.M., Battaglia, G., Alvarez Sanz, M.C. & Van De Kar, L.D. (1991). Cocaine-induced elevation of plasma adrenocorticotropic hormone and corticosterone is mediated by serotonergic neurons. *Journal of Pharmacology and Experimental Therapeutics*, Vol.259, pp. 495–500.

Lidow, M.S., Goldman-rakic, P.S., Rakic, P. & Innis, R.B. (1989). Dopamine-D_2 receptors in the cerebral-cortex - Distribution and pharmacological characterization with H-3 raclopride. *Proceedings of the National Academy of Sciences of the United States of America*, Vol.86, pp. 6412-6416.

Lile, J.A., Wang, Z.X., Woolverton, W.L., France, J.E., Gregg, T.C., Davies, H.M.L. & Nader, M.A. (2003). The reinforcing efficacy of psychostimulants in rhesus monkeys: The role of pharmacokinetics and pharmacodynamics. *Journal of Pharmacology and Experimental Therapeutics*, Vol.307, pp. 356-366.

Lima, D., Spindola, D.B., Dias, L.O., Tomaz, C. & Barros, M. (2008). Effects of acute systemic cocaine administration on the cortisol, ACTH and prolactin levels of black tufted-ear marmosets. *Psychoneuroendocrinology*, Vol.33, pp. 321-327.

Liu, X., Matochik, J.A., Cadet, J.L. & London, E.D. (1998). Smaller volume of prefrontal lobe in poly substance abusers: a magnetic resonance imaging study. *Neuropsychopharmacology*, Vol.18, pp. 243–252.

Liu, Y., Roberts, D.C. & Morgan, D. (2005). Sensitization of the reinforcing effects of self-administered cocaine in rats: effects of dose and intravenous injection speed. *European Journal of Neuroscience*, Vol.22, pp. 195–200.

London, E.D., Cascella, N.G., Wong, D.F., Phillips, R.L., Dannals, R.F., Links, J.M., Herning, R., Grayson, R., Jaffe, J.H. & Wagner, H.N. (1990). Cocaine-induced reduction of glucose utilization in human brain. *Archives in General Psychiatry*, Vol.47, pp. 567–574.

Loonam, T.M., Noailles, P.A.H., Yu. J., Zhu, J.P.Q. & Angulo, J.A. (2003). Substance P and cholecystokinin regulate neurochemical responses to cocaine and methamphetamine in the striatum. *Life Sciences*, Vol.73, pp. 727–739.

Lopez-Gimenez, J. F., Vilaro, M. T., Palacios, J. M. & Mengod, G. (2001). Mapping of 5-HT_{2A} receptors and their mRNA in monkey brain: [3H]MDL100,907 autoradiography and in situ hybridization studies. *Journal of Comparative Neurology*, Vol.429, pp. 571–589.

Lu, L., Liu, D. & Ceng, X. (2001). Corticotropin-releasing factor receptor type 1 mediates stress-induced relapse to cocaine-conditioned place preference in rats. *European Journal of Pharmacology*, Vol.415, pp. 203–208.

Lyons, D., Friedman, D.P., Nader, M.A. & Porrino, L.J. (1996). Cocaine alters cerebral metabolism within the ventral striatum and limbic cortex of monkeys. *Journal of Neuroscience*, Vol.16:, pp. 1230–1238.

Madras, B.K., Fahey, M.A., Canfield, D.R. & Spealman, R.D. (1988). D_1 and D_2 dopamine receptors in caudate-putamen of nonhuman primates *Macaca fascicularis*. *Journal of Neurochemistry*, Vol.51, pp. 934–943.

Mantsch, J.R. & Goeders, N.E. (1999). Ketoconazole blocks the stressor-induced reinstatement of cocaine-seeking behavior in rats: relationship to the discriminative stimulus effects of cocaine. *Psychopharmacology*, Vol.142, pp. 399–407.

Marazziti, D., Marracci, S., Palego, L., Rotondo, A., Mazzanti, C., Nardi, I., Ladinsky, H., Giraldo E., Borsini, F. & Cassano, G.B. (1994). Localization and gene expression of serotonin 1A ($5HT_{1A}$) receptors in human brain postmortem. *Brain Research*, Vol.658, pp. 55–59.

Marinelli, M., Aouizerate, B., Barrot, M., Le Moal, M. & Piazza, P.V. (1998). Dopamine-dependent responses to morphine depend on glucocorticoid receptors. *Proceedings of the National Academy of Sciences of the United States of America*, Vol.95, pp. 7742-7747.

Marinelli, M., RougePont, F., DeJesusOliveira, C., LeMoal, M. & Piazza, P.V. (1997). Acute blockade of corticosterone secretion decreases the psychomotor stimulant effects of cocaine. *Neuropsychopharmacology*, Vol.16, pp. 156-161.

Martell, B.A., Orson, F.M., Poling, J., Mitchell, E., Rossen, R.D., Gardner, T. & Kosten, T.R. (2009). Cocaine Vaccine for the Treatment of Cocaine Dependence in Methadone-Maintained Patients A Randomized, Double-blind, Placebo-Controlled Efficacy Trial. *Archives of General Psychiatry*, Vol.66, pp. 1116-1123.

Martinez, D., Foltin, R., Kegeles, L., Hwang, D., Huang, Y., Hackett, E., Frankle, G & Laruelle, M. (2003). PET imaging of dopamine transmission in the striatal substructures of humans and predictors of relapse. *Society for Neuroscience Abstracts*, Vol.29, pp. 354.8

Massi, M., Panocka, I. & de Caro, G. (2000). The psychopharmacology of tachykinin NK-3 receptors in laboratory animals. *Peptides*, Vol.21, pp. 1597–1609.

Mathieu-Kia, A.M. & Besson, M.J. (1998). Repeated administration of cocaine, nicotine and ethanol: effects on preprodynorphin, preprotachykinin A and preproenkephalin mRNA expression in the dorsal and the ventral striatum of the rat. *Molecular Brain Research*, Vol.54, pp. 141–151.

McGaugh, J.L. (2002). Memory consolidation and the amygdala: a systems perspective. *Trends Neuroscience*, Vol.25, pp. 456-461.

Meany, M.J., Aitken, D.H., Sharma, S. & Viau, V. (1992). Basal ACTH, corticosterone, and corticosterone-binding globulin levels over the diurnal cycle, and age-related changes in hippocampal type I and type II corticosteroid receptor binding capacity in young and aged, handled and nonhan- dled rats. *Neuroendocrinology*, Vol.55, pp. 204–213.

Meil, W.M. & See, R.E. (1996). Conditioned cued recovery of responding following prolonged withdrawal from self-administered cocaine in rats: an animal model of relapse. *Behavioural Pharmacology*, Vol.7, pp. 754–763.

Mello Jr., E.L., Maior, R.S., Carey, R.C., Huston, J.P., Tomaz, C. & Muller, C.P. (2005). Serotonin$_{1A}$-receptor antagonism blocks psychostimulant properties of diethylpropion in marmosets (*Callithrix penicillata*). *European Journal of Pharmacology*, Vol.511, pp. 43-52.

Mello, N.K., & Negus, S.S. (1996). Preclinical evaluation of pharmacotherapies for treatment of cocaine and opioid abuse using drug self-administration procedures. *Neuropsychopharmacology*, Vol.14, pp. 375–424.

Mendelson, J.H., Mello, N.K., Sholar, M.B., Siegel, A.J., Mutschler, N. & Halpern, J. (2002). Temporal concordance of cocaine effects on mood states and neuroendocrine hormones. *Psychoneuroendocrinology*, Vol.27, pp. 71-82.

Mengod, G., Vilaro, M.T., Raurich, A., Lopez-Gimenez, J.F., Cortes, R. & Palacios J.M. (1996). 5-HT receptors in mammalian brain: receptor autoradiography and in situ hybridization studies of new ligands and newly identified receptors. *Histochemical Journal*, Vol.28, pp. 747–758.

Miller, G.M., Yatin, S.M., De La Garza, R., Goulet, M. & Madras, B.K. (2001). Cloning of dopamine, norepinephrine and serotonin transporters from monkey brain: relevance to cocaine sensitivity. *Molecular Brain Research*, Vol.87, pp. 124-143.

Moldow, R.L. & Fischman, A.J. (1987). Cocaine induced secretion of ACTH, beta-endorphin, and corticosterone. *Peptides*, Vol.8, pp. 819–822.

Molodtsova, G.F. (2008). Serotonergic mechanisms of memory trace retrieval. *Behavioural Brain Research*, Vol.195, pp. 7-16.

Morgan, D., Grant, K.A., Gage, H.D., Mach, R.H., Kaplan, J.R., Prioleau, O., Nader, S.H., Buchheimer, N., Ehrenkaufer, R.L., & Nader, M.A. (2002). Social dominance in monkeys: dopamine D2 receptors and cocaine self-administration. *Nature Neuroscience*, Vol.5, pp. 169–174.

Nader, M.A. & Barrett, J.E. (1990). Effects of chlordiazepoxide, buspirone, and serotonin receptor agonists and antagonists on responses of squirrel monkeys maintained under second-order schedules of intramuscular cocaine injection or food presentation. *Drug Development Research*, Vol.20, pp. 5-17.

Nader, M.A., Czoty, P.W., Gould, R.W. & Riddick, N.V. (2008). Positron emission tomography imaging studies of dopamine receptors in primate models of addiction. *Philosophical Transactions of the Royal Academy of Science B Biological Sciences*, Vol.363, pp. 3223-3232.

National Drug Control Budget (2011). *FY 2011 Funding Highlights*, June 2011, Available from: http://www.whitehousedrugpolicy.gov/publications/policy/11budget/fy11Highlight.pdf

Neisewander, J.L. & Acosta, J.I. (2007). Stimulation of 5-HT_{2C} receptors attenuates cue and cocaine-primed reinstatement of cocaine-seeking behavior in rats. *Behavioural Pharmacology*, Vol.18, pp. 791–800.

Nic Dhonnchadha, B.A. & Cunningham, K.A. (2008). Serotonergic mechanisms in addiction-related memories. *Behavioural Brain Research*, Vol.195, pp. 39-53.

Nic Dhonnchadha, B.A., Fox, Sutz, S.J., R.G., Rice, K.C. & Cunningham, K.A. (2009). Blockade of the serotonin 5-HT_{2A} receptor suppresses cue-evoked reinstatement of cocaine-seeking behavior in a rat self-administration model. *Behavioural Neuroscience*, Vol.123, pp. 382-396.

Nic Dhonnchadha, B.A., Ripoll, N., Clenet, F., Hascoet, M. & Bourin, M. (2005). Implication of 5-HT_2 receptor subtypes in the mechanism of action of antidepressants in the four plates test. *Psychopharmacology*, Vol.179, pp. 418-429.

Nilsson, S., Helou, K., Walentinsson, A., Szpirer, C., Nerman, O. & Stahl, F. (2001). Rat–Mouse and Rat–Human Comparative Maps Based on Gene Homology and High-Resolution Zoo-FISH. *Genomics*, Vol.287, pp. 287-298.

Nwaneshiudu, C.A. & Unterwald, E.M. (2010). NK-3 receptor antagonism prevents behavioral sensitization to cocaine: a role of glycogen synthase kinase-3 in the nucleus accumbens. *Journal of Neurochemistry*, Vol.115, pp. 635-642.

O'Brien, C.P. (1997). A range of research-based pharmacotherapies for addiction. *Science*, Vol.278, pp. 66–70.

O'Brien, C.P., Childress, A.R., Ehrman, R. & Robbins SJ. (1998). Conditioning factors in drug abuse: can they explain compulsion? *Journal of Psychopharmacology*, Vol.12, pp. 15–22.

Odum, A.L. & Shahan, T.A. (2004). D-amphetamine reinstates behavior previously maintained by food: importance of context. *Behavioural Pharmacology*, Vol.15, pp. 513–516.

Oeth, K.M. & Lewis, D.A. (1992). Cholecystokinin-containing and dopamine-containing mesencephalic neurons provide distinct projections to monkey prefrontal cortex. *Neuroscience Letters*, Vol.145, pp. 87-92.

Ogren, S.O., Eriksson, T.M., Elvander-Tottie, E., D'Addario, C., Ekstrom, J.C., Svenningsson, P., Meister, B., Kehr, J. & Stiedl, O. (2008). The role of 5-HT_{1A} receptors in learning and memory. *Behavioural Brain Research*, Vol.195, pp. 54-77.

Owashi, T., Iritani, D., Niizato, K., Ikeda, K. & Kamijima, K. (2004). The distribution of serotonin transporter immunoreactivity in hippocampal formation in monkeys and rats. *Brain Research*, Vol.1010, pp. 166-168.

Parsons, L. H., Weiss, F., & Koob, G. F. (1998). Serotonin1B receptor stimulation enhances cocaine reinforcement. *Journal of Neuroscience*, Vol.18, pp. 10078–10089.

Paulson, P.E., Camp, D.M & Robinson, T.E. (1991). Time course of transient behavioral depression and persistent behavioral sensitization in relation to regional brain monoamine concentrations during amphetamine withdrawal in rats. *Psychopharmacology*, Vol.103, pp. 480–492.

Pearlson, G.D., Jeffery, P.J., Harris, G.J., Ross, C.A., Fischman, M.W. & Camargo, E.E. (1993). Correlation of acute cocaine-induced changes in local cerebral blood-flow with subjective effects. *American Journal of Psychiatry*, Vol.150, pp. 495-497.

Piazza, P.V. & Le Moal, M. (1998). The role of stress in drug self-administration. *Trends in Pharmacological Sciences*, Vol.19, pp. 67-74.

Pifl, C., Reither, H. & Hornykiewicz, O. (1991). Lower efficacy of the dopamine D1 agonist, SKF 38393, to stimulate adenylyl cyclase activity in primate than in rodent striatum. *European Journal of Pharmacology*, Vol.202, pp. 273–276.

Piggott, M.A., Marshall, E.F., Thomas, N., Lloyd, S., Court, J.A., Jaros, E., Costa, D., Perry, R.H. & Perry, E.K. (1999). Dopaminergic activities in the human striatum: rostrocaudal gradients of uptake sites and of D_1 and D_2 but not of D_3 receptor binding or dopamine. *Neuroscience*, Vol.90, pp. 433–445.

Placenza, F.M., Fletcher, P.J., Rotzinger, S. & Vaccarino FJ. (2004). Infusion of the substance P analogue, DiMe-C7, into the ventral tegmental area induces reinstatement of cocaine-seeking behaviour in rats. *Psychopharmacology*, Vol.177, pp. 111–120.

Placenza, F.M., Vaccarino, F.J., Fletcher, P.J. & Erb, S. (2005). Activation of central neurokinin-1 receptors induces reinstatement of cocaine-seeking behavior. *Neuroscience Letters*, Vol.390, pp. 42–47.

Platt, D.M., Rowlett, J.K. & Spealman, R.D. (2007). Noradrenergic mechanisms in cocaine-induced reinstatement of drug seeking in squirrel monkeys. *Journal of Pharmacology and Experimental Therapeutics*, Vol.322, pp. 894-902.

Pompeiano, M., Palacios, J.M. & Mengod, G. (1992). Distribution and cellular localization of mRNA coding for 5-HT1A receptor in the rat brain: correlation with receptor binding. *Journal of Neuroscience*, Vol.12, pp. 440–453.

Porrino, L.J. & Lyons, D. (2000). Orbital and medial prefrontal cortex and psychostimulant abuse: studies in animal models. *Cerebral Cortex*, Vol.10, pp. 326–333.

Porrino, L.J., Domer, F.R., Crane, A.M. & Sokoloff, L. (1988). Selective alterations in cerebral metabolism within the mesocorticolimbic dopaminergic system produced by acute cocaine administration in rats. *Neuropsychopharmacology*, Vol.1, pp. 109-118.

Porrino, L.J., Lyons, D., Miller, M.D., Smith, H.R., Friedman, D.P., Daunais, J.B. & Nader, M.A. (2002). Metabolic mapping of the effects of cocaine during the initial phases of self-administration in the nonhuman primate. *Journal of Neuroscience,* Vol.22, pp. 7687-7694.

Pouydebat, E., Gorce, P., Coppens, Y. & Bels, V. (2009). Biomechanical study of grasping according to the volume of the object: Human versus non-human primates. *Journal of Biomechanics*, Vol.42, pp. 266-272.

Pouydebat, E., Reghem, E., Borel, A. & Gorce, P. (2011). Diversity of grip in adults and young humans and chimpanzees (*Pan troglodytes*). *Behavioural Brain Research,* Vol.218, pp. 21-28.

Price, G.W., Roberts, C., Watson, J., Burton, M., Mulholland, K., Middlemiss, D.N. & Jones, B.J. (1996). Species differences in 5-HT autoreceptors. *Behavioural Brain Research* Vol.73, pp. 79-82.

Reader, S.M., Hager, Y. & Laland, K.N. (2011). The evolution of primate general and cultural intelligence. *Philosophical Transactions of the Royal Academy of Science B Biological Sciences*, Vol.366, pp. 1017-1027.

Ripley, T.L., Gadd, C.A., De Felipe, C., Hunt, S.P. & Stephens, D.N. (2002). Lack of self-administration and behavioural sensitisation to morphine, but not cocaine, in mice lacking NK1 receptors. *Neuropharmacology*, Vol.43, pp. 1258-1268.

Ritz, M.C., Cone, E.J. & Kuhar, M.J. (1990). Cocaine inhibition of ligand binding at dopamine, norepinephrine and serotonin transporters: a structure-activity study. *Life Sciences,* Vol.46, pp. 635-645.

Ritz, M.C., Lamb, R.J., Goldberg, S.R. & Kuhar, M.J. (1987). Cocaine receptors on dopamine transporters are related to self-administration of cocaine. *Science,* Vol.237, pp. 1219-1223.

Roberts, D.C.S., Corcoran, M.E. & Fibiger, H.C. (1977). Role of ascending catecholaminergic systems in intravenous self-administration of cocaine. *Pharmacology Biochemistry and Behavior*, Vol.6, pp. 615-620.

Roberts, D.C.S., Phelan, R., Hodges, L.M., Hodges, M.M., Bennett, B., Childers, S. & Davies, H. (1999). Self-administration of cocaine analogs by rats. *Psychopharmacology,* Vol.144, pp.389-397.

Robinson, T.E. & Berridge, K.C. (2008). The incentive sensitization theory of addiction: some current issues. *Philosophical Transactions of the Royal Society of London B: Biological Sciences*, Vol.363, pp. 3137-3146.

Roth, B.L. (2006). *The Serotonin Receptors* (1st edition), Humana Press, 1-58829-568-0, New Jersey (USA).

Sanchez-Gonzalez, M.A., Garcia-Cabezas, M.A., Rico, B. & Cavada, C. (2005). The primate thalamus is a key target for brain dopamine. *Journal of Neuroscience,* Vol.25, pp. 6076-6083.

Sanchez, M.M., Young, L.J., Plotsky, P.M. & Insel, T.R. (1999). Autoradiographic and in situ hybridization localization of corticotropin-releasing factor 1 and 2 receptors in nonhuman primate brain. *Journal of Comparative Neurology*, Vol.408, pp. 365-377.

Sanchez, M.M., Young, L.J., Plotsky, P.M. & Insel, T.R. (2000). Distribution of corticosteroid receptors in the rhesus brain: Relative absence of glucocorticoid receptors in the hippocampal formation. *Journal of Neuroscience*, Vol.20, pp. 4657-4668.

Santana, N., Bortolozzi, A., Serrats, J., Mengod, G. & Artigas, F. (2004). Expression of Serotonin(1A) and Serotonin(2A) receptors in pyramidal and GABAergic neurons of the rat prefrontal cortex. *Cerebral Cortex*, Vol.14, pp. 1100–1109.

Saphier, D., Welch, J.E., Farrar, G.E. & Goeders, N.E. (1993). Effects of intracerebroventricular and intra-hypothalamic cocaine administration on adrenocortical secretion. *Neuroendocrinology*, Vol.57, pp. 54–62.

Sarnyai, Z., Mello, N.K., Mendelson, J.H., Eros-Sarnyai, M. & Mercer, G. (1996). Effects of cocaine on pulsatile activity of the hypothalamic–pituitary–adrenal axis in male rhesus monkeys: neuroendocrine and behavioral correlates. *Journal of Pharmacology and Experimental Therapeutics*, Vol.277, pp. 225–234.

Schama, K.F., Howell, L.L. & Byrd, L.D. (1997). Serotonergic modulation of the discriminative-stimulus effects of cocaine in squirrel monkeys. *Psychopharmacology*, Vol.132, pp. 27-34.

Schmidt, K.L. & Cohn, J.F. (2001). Human facial expressions as adaptations: Evolutionary questions in facial expression research. *Yearbook of Physical Anthropology*. Vol.44, pp. 3-24.

Schmidt, M.V., Wang, X.D. & Meijer, O.C. (2011). Early life stress paradigms in rodents: potential animal models of depression? *Psychopharmacology*, Vol.214, pp. 131-140.

Schultz, W. (2004). Neural coding of basic reward terms of animal learning theory, game theory, microeconomics and behavioural ecology. *Current Opinion in Neurobiology*, Vol.14, pp.139–147.

Schultz, W. (2006). Behavioral theories and the neurophysiology of reward. *Annual Reviews in Psychology*, Vol.57, pp. 87–115.

Severini, C., Improta, G., Falconieri-Erspamer, G., Salvadori, S. & Erspamer, V. (2002). The tachykinin peptide family. *Pharmacological Reviews*, Vol.54, pp. 285–322.

Shaham, Y., Erb, S., Leung, S., Buczek, Y. & Stewart, J. (1998). CP-154,526, a selective, non-peptide antagonist of the corticotrophin-releasing factor receptor attenuates stress-induced relapse to drug seeking in cocaine and heroin-trained rats. *Psychopharmacology*, Vol.137, pp. 184–190.

Sibley, D.R. & Monsma, F.J. Jr. (1992). Molecular biology of dopamine receptors. *Trends Pharmacological Science*, Vol.13, pp. 61–69.

Sinha, R. (2001). How does stress increase risk of drug abuse and relapse? *Psychopharmacology*, Vol.158, pp. 343-359.

Smiley, J.F., Levey, A.I., Ciliax, B.J. & Goldman-Rakic, P.S. (1994). D_1 dopamine receptor immunoreactivity in human and monkey cerebral cortex: predominant and extrasynaptic localization in dendritic spines. *Proceedings of the National Academy of Sciences United States of America*, Vol.91, pp. 5720–5724.

Smith, H.R., Beveridge, T.J.R. & Porrino, L.J. (2006). Distribution of norepinephrine transporters in the non-human primate brain. *Neuroscience*, Vol.138, pp. 703–714.

Smith, Y., Kieval, J., Couceyro, P.R. & Kuhar, M.J. (1999). CART peptide-immunoreactive neurones in the nucleus accumbens in monkeys: Ultrastructural analysis, colocalization studies, and synaptic interactions with dopaminergic afferents. *Journal of Comparative Neurology*, Vol.407, pp. 491-511.

Spealman, R.D. (1995). Noradrenergic involvement in the discriminative stimulus effects of cocaine in squirrel-monkeys. *Journal of Pharmacology and Experimental Therapeutics*, Vol.275, pp. 53-62.

Spealman, R.D., Lee, B., Tiefenbacher, S., Platt, D.M., Rowlett, J.K. & Khroyan, T.V. (2004). Triggers of relapse: Nonhuman primate models of reinstated cocaine seeking. *Motivational Factors in the Etiology of Drug Abuse*, Vol.50, pp. 57-84.

Steketee, J.D. & Kalivas, P.W. (2011). Drug Wanting: Behavioral Sensitization and Relapse to Drug-Seeking Behavior. *Pharmacological Reviews*, Vol.63, pp. 348-365.

Tella, S.R. (1995). Effects of monoamine reuptake inhibitors on cocaine self-administration in rats. *Pharmacology Biochemistry and Behavior*, Vol.51, pp. 687-692.

Thompson, T. & Schuster, C.R. (1964). Morphine self-administration, food-reinforced and avoidance behaviors in rhesus monkeys. *Psychopharmacologia*, Vol.5, pp. 87-94.

Tomaz, C., Dickinsonanson, H. & McGaugh, J.L. (1992). Basolateral Amygdala lesions block diazepam-induced anterograde amnesia in an inhibitory avoidance task. *Proceedings of the National Academy of Sciences of the United States of America*, Vol.89, pp. 3615-3619.

Ukai, M., Mori, E. & Kameyama T. (1995). Effects of centrally administered neuropeptides on discriminative stimulus properties of cocaine in the rat. *Pharmacology Biochemistry and Behaviour*, Vol.51, pp. 705–708.

Van Bockstaele, E.J.V. & Pickel, V.M. (1993). Ultrastmcture of serotonin-immunoreactive terminals in the core and shell of rat nucleus accumbens: cellular substrates for interactions with catecholamine afferents. *Journal of Comparative Neurology*, Vol.344, pp. 603-617.

Vanderschuren, L. & Everitt, B.J. (2004). Drug seeking becomes compulsive after prolonged cocaine self-administration. *Science*, Vol.305, pp. 1017-1019.

Vermeulen, R.J., Jongenelen, C.A., Langeveld, C.H., Wolters, E.C., Stoof, J.C. & Drukarch, B. (1994). Dopamine D_1 receptor agonists display a different intrinsic activity in rat, monkey and human astrocytes. *European Journal of Pharmacology*, Vol.269, pp. 121–125.

Volkow, N.D., Wang G-J., Fowler, J.S., Logan, J., Gatley, S.J., Hitzemann, R., Chen, A.D., Dewey, S.L. & Pappas, N. (1997). Decreased striatal dopaminergic responsiveness in detoxified cocaine-dependent subjects. *Nature*, Vol.386, pp. 830–833.

Volkow, N.D., Wang, G.J., Fowler, J.S., Hitzemann, R., Angrist, B., Gatley, S.J., Logan, J., Ding, Y.S. & Pappas, N. (1999). Association of methylphenidate-induced craving with changes in right striato-orbitofrontal metabolism in cocaine abusers: implications in addiction. *American Journal of Psychiatry*, Vol.156, pp. 19–26.

Weed, M.R., Woolverton, W.L. & Paul, I.A. (1998). Dopamine D-1 and D-2 receptor selectivities of phenyl-benzazepines in rhesus monkey striata. *European Journal of Pharmacology*, Vol.361, pp. 129-142.

Weerts, E.M., Fantegrossi, W.E. & Goodwin, A.K. (2007). The value of nonhuman primates in drug abuse research. *Experimental and Clinical Psychopharmacology*, Vol.15, pp. 309-327.

Weinberg, MS; Johnson, DC; Bhatt, AP. & Spencer R.L. (2010). Medial prefrontal cortex activity can disrupt the expression of stress response habituation. *Neuroscience,* Vol.168, pp. 744-756.

Weiss, F., Maldonado-Vlaar, C.S., Parsons, L.H., Kerr, T.M., Smith, D.L. & Ben-Shahar, O. (2000). Control of cocaine-seeking behavior by drug-associated stimuli in rats: effects on recovery of extinguished operant-responding and extracellular dopamine levels in amygdala and nucleus accumbens. *Proceedings of the National Academy of Sciences of the United States of America,* Vol.97, pp. 4321–4326.

Wise, R.A. (1980). The dopamine synapse and the notion of 'pleasure centers' in the brain. *Trends in Neuroscience,* Vol.3, pp. 91–95.

Wise, R.A. (1996). Addictive drugs and brain stimulation reward. *Annual Review of Neuroscience,* Vol.19, pp. 319-340.

World Health Organization (2010). *World drug report 2010,* June 2010, Available from: http://www.unodc.org/unodc/en/data-and-analysis/WDR-2010.html

14

The Epidemiology and Treatment of Prescription Drug Disorders in the United States

Scott P. Novak,[1] Sara L. Calvin,[1] Cristie Glasheen[1] and Mark J. Edlund[2]
[1]RTI International, Department of Behavioral Epidemiology;
[2]University of Arkansas School of Medicine, Department of Psychiatry
USA

1. Introduction

The drug problem in the United States is a complex mosaic involving different types of drugs, consumption practices, and biological and psychological responses to their effects. Over the past two decades, the fields of psychiatry and neurology have witnessed dramatic scientific breakthroughs in understanding the actions of drugs that can be used to regulate the nervous system (Nestler, Hyman, & Malenka, 2009). This has led to a dramatic increase in use of these medications for treating a wide range of physical and mental disorders (Dasgupta et al., 2006). An unintended consequence of this increased level of availability is that a large proportion of these drugs are being consumed in excess of the dosage recommended by the manufacturer or prescriber, used to self-treat illnesses instead of seeking professional medical care, and/or combined with other drugs increase the desired effects. As a result, the numbers of unintentional poisonings and emergency room visits have nearly doubled. For instance, the latest figures from the Drug Abuse Warning Network (DAWN) indicate that in 2008, that nearly half of the 2 million emergency room visits to U.S. hospitals involved prescription medications. Approximately two-thirds of those visits that involved prescription medications were for prescription pharmaceuticals only and no co-occurring illicit drug or alcohol abuse (SAMHSA, 2006). In addition to the tremendous economic costs associated with overdoses involving prescription medications, the adverse social and mental/physical health effects, though difficult to directly quantify, are considerable.

The goal of this chapter is to present an overview of the current state of knowledge about the nonmedical use of prescription medications. Because of the sheer volume of the literature, this chapter cannot cover the entire breadth of this complex phenomenon. Therefore, the discussion is limited to those exhibiting features of dependence on prescription medications, as this is the most harmful pattern of use. Within the context of dependence, the goal is to present a concise review of the epidemiological data on the prevalence of dependence on prescription medications within various population sub-groups (e.g. youth, those with co-occurring illicit substance use disorders, and previous history of psychiatric illness). In addition, a brief summary is provided on the pharmacological properties that are likely to confer selective use of the particular drug class for nonmedical use. Information on the prevalence of seeking treatment for a substance use disorder involving prescription drugs, unmet need for treatment, and types of evidence-based treatment available for each drug class is also presented. Surveillance data also indicate that nonmedical use occurs in a wide range of medication classes (e.g., anabolic steroids, over-the-counter cough medicines, antihistamines) (Compton & Volkow, 2006; Kuehn, 2007; Lankenau, Sanders, Bloom, & Hathazi, 2008). However, this chapter focuses on the three classes of medications where the epidemiological and physiological literatures indicate that the likelihood of transitioning beyond experimentation to dependence is greatest—pain relievers, stimulants, and sedatives/tranquilizers (Blanco et al., 2007). Unless otherwise noted, the source of the surveillance data is the 2005-2009 National Survey on Drug Use and Health (NSDUH). It is a cross-sectional survey of non-institutionalized youth (age 12-17) and adults (age 18+) in the United States that is conducted on an annual basis and arguably contains the richest source of data covering topics related to the nonmedical use of prescription medications (Colliver, Kroutil, Dai, & Gfroerer, 2006).

2. Taxonomy of nonmedical prescription drug use

The term *nonmedical use of prescription drugs* has been criticized in the literature because studies typically define it use as a single item. However, NMPD is a multidimensional construct that encompasses a wide range of motivations to use prescription medications (Boyd & McCabe, 2008). Unlike heroin or other illicit drugs, prescription medications can be used to treat legitimate medical conditions. With the exception of cocaine, most illicit drugs are defined by the Drug Enforcement Agency in the United States as having no medical therapeutic value and therefore are considered illegal to possess or dispense (Table 1).

An important side note deserves mentioning. Marijuana and cocaine have some level of medically accepted therapeutic value and are available in certain States only under extremely unique circumstances. For instance, marijuana is currently treated by the US federal government as having no medically accepted therapeutic value and is therefore considered illegal (See Table 2). A small number of States (e.g., California, Colorado) consider marijuana an acceptable treatment, such as for patients with glaucoma. In those states, it is available from a licensed prescriber and may be obtained from a specialized pharmacy licensed to dispense limited quantities to patients. Cocaine is used as a topical anesthetic for conditions of the eye and nose, including nasal cauterization. However, prescriptions for cocaine and marijuana are highly regulated.

Substances: Categories and Names	Examples of *Commercial* and Street Names	DEA Schedule* / How Administered**	Intoxication Effects / Potential Health Consequences
Depressants			
barbiturates	*Amytal, Nembutal, Seconal, Phenobarbital;* barbs, reds, red birds, phennies, tooies, yellows, yellow jackets	II, III, V/injected, swallowed	Reduced pain and anxiety; feeling of well-being; lowered inhibitions; slowed pulse and breathing; lowered blood pressure; poor

Substances: Categories and Names	Examples of *Commercial* and Street Names	DEA Schedule* / How Administered**	Intoxication Effects / Potential Health Consequences
benzodiazepines (other than flunitrazepam)	*Ativan, Halcion, Librium, Valium, Xanax*; candy, downers, sleeping pills, tranks	IV/swallowed	concentration/confusion, fatigue; impaired coordination, memory, judgment; respiratory depression and arrest, addiction *For barbiturates* – sedation, drowsiness/depression, unusual excitement, fever, irritability, poor judgment, slurred speech, dizziness *For benzodiazepines* – sedation, drowsiness/dizziness *For flunitrazepam* – visual and gastrointestinal disturbances, urinary retention, memory loss for the time under the drug's effects
flunitrazepam***+	*Rohypnol*; forget-me pill, Mexican Valium, R2, Roche, roofies, roofinol, rope, rophies	IV/swallowed, snorted	
Opioids and Morphine Derivatives			
codeine	*Empirin with Codeine, Fiorinal with Codeine, Robitussin A-C, Tylenol with Codeine*; Captain Cody, Cody, schoolboy; (with glutethimide doors & hours, loads, pancakes and syrup	II, III, IV/injected, swallowed	Pain relief, euphoria, drowsiness/respiratory depression and arrest, nausea, confusion, constipation, sedation, unconsciousness, coma, tolerance, addiction *For codeine* – less analgesia, sedation, and respiratory depression than morphine
fentanyl	*Actiq, Duragesic, Sublimaze*; Apache, China girl, China white, dance fever, friend, goodfella, jackpot, murder 8, TNT, Tango and Cash	II/injected, smoked, snorted	
morphine	*Roxanol, Duramorph*; M, Miss Emma, monkey, white stuff	II/injected, swallowed, smoked	
opium	laudanum, paregoric; big O, black stuff, block, gum, hop	II, III, V/swallowed, smoked	

Substances: Categories and Names	Examples of *Commercial* and Street Names	DEA Schedule* / How Administered**	Intoxication Effects / Potential Health Consequences
other opioid pain relievers (oxycodone, meperidine, hydromorphone, hydrocodone, propoxypene)	*Tylox, OxyContin, Percodan, Percocet*; oxy 90s, oxycotton, oxycet, hillbilly heroin, percs *Demerol, meperidine hydrochloride*; demmies, pain killer *Dilaudid*; juice, dillies *Vicodin, Lortab, Lorcet, Darvon, Darvocet*	II, III, IV/swallowed, injected, suppositories, chewed, crushed, snorted	
Stimulants			
amphetamines	*Biphetamine, Dexedrine*; bennies, black beauties, crosses, hearts, LA turnaround, speed, truck drivers, uppers	II/injected, swallowed, smoked, snorted	Increased heart rate, blood pressure, metabolism; feelings of exhilaration, energy, increased mental alertness/rapid or irregular heart beat; reduced appetite, weight loss, heart failure *For amphetamines* – rapid breathing; hallucinations/tremor, loss of coordination; irritability, anxiousness, restlessness, delirium, panic, paranoia, impulsive behavior, aggressiveness, tolerance, addiction *For cocaine* – aggression, violence, psychotic behavior/memory loss, cardiac and neurological damage; impaired memory and learning, tolerance, addiction *For methylphenidate* – increase or decrease in blood pressure, psychotic episodes/ digestive problems, loss of appetite, weight loss
cocaine	*Cocaine hydrochloride*; blow, bump, c, candy, Charlie, coke, crack, flake, rock, snow, toot	II/injected, smoked, snorted	
methamphetamine	*Desoxyn*; chalk, crank, crystal, fire, glass, go fast, ice, meth, speed	II/injected, swallowed, smoked, snorted	
methylphenidate	*Ritalin*; JIF, MPH, R-ball, Skippy, the smart drug, vitamin R	II/injected, swallowed, snorted	

**Schedule I and II drugs have high potential for abuse. They require greater storage security and have a quota on manufacturing, among other restrictions. Schedule I drugs are available for research only and have no approved medical use; Schedule II drugs are available only by prescription (unrefillable) and require a form for ordering. Schedule III and IV drugs are available by prescription, may have five refills in 6 months, and may be ordered orally. Most Schedule V drugs are available over the counter.*

***Taking drugs by injections can increase the risk of infection through needle contamination with staphylococci, HIV, hepatitis, and other organisms.*

****Associated with sexual assaults.*

+Not available by prescription in the U.S.

Table 1. Selected Prescription Drugs with Potential for Abuse

Substance Category	Definition	Example Drugs
Schedule I	• Most restrictive level • Includes drugs or other substances with a high potential for abuse • No currently accepted medical use in the United States • Low level of safety • Not approved for use, distribution, manufacture, or importation	Heroin Marijuana Phencyclidine (PCP) Lysergic acid dithylamide (LSD)
Schedule II	• Drugs have high abuse potential • Have currently accepted medical use in treatment, with severe restrictions	Cocaine Methamphetamine Amphetamines Dextroamphetamine Adderall® Morphine Oxycodone OxyContin® Methylphenidate Ritalin®
Schedule III	• Drugs have abuse potential less than that of Schedule I or II drugs • Have currently accepted medical uses in treatment	Hydrocodone Vicodin® Butalbital Fiorinal®
Schedule IV	• Drugs have lower abuse potential than those of Schedule III drugs • Have currently accepted medical uses in treatment	Alprazolam Xanax® Diazepam Valium® Propoxyphene Darvon®
Schedule V	• Drugs have low abuse potential • Have recognized medical uses • Some pharmaceuticals contain drugs with higher abuse potential but in much lower concentrations relative to other ingredients	Cough medicines with codeine Robitussin AC®

Table 2. Drug Enforcement Agency's Controlled Substances Act Definitions of Substances Subject to Food and Drug Administration Regulation

Notwithstanding marijuana and cocaine, many illicit drugs were originally developed for medicinal purposes, but were deemed to have little or no efficacy, or having such a high abuse liability that they were prohibited as a legal medical treatment (e.g., heroin, LSD).

Therefore, prescription medications are unique in that their use is motivated by factors other than euphoria. For instance, prescription pain relievers are often used to treat legitimate medical injuries, but many patients self-treat without a doctor's prescription when a dosage of the drug is readily available to them (e.g., using a spouses prescription).

Attempts to develop survey items to capture the concept of nonmedical use has been challenging because there is no universally accepted definition as to what constitutes nonmedical use prescription drug use (NMPD). The National Survey on Drug Use and Health (NSDUH) frames the question as whether the respondent "used a particular drug that was not prescribed for you or was used only for the experience or feeling it caused." It is sometimes argued that the NSDUH definition of NMPD is overly inclusive, as it could include drugs that are used for self-treatment of a medical condition, but were not specifically prescribed by a physician (Huang et al., 2006). In contrast, another annual cross-sectional surveillance study focused on youth, the Monitoring the Future (MTF) study defines nonmedical prescription drug use as 'use of prescription medications without a doctor telling you to take them' (Johnston, O'Malley, Bachman, & Schulenberg, 2009). Then, the survey follows with queries about motivations about the most important reason for use, such as: experimentation, pain relief, euphoria. Understanding motivations for use are important because nonmedical users who use only for therapeutic value and those using for other reasons, such as for euphoria, are likely to have different profiles of risk and protective factors for use, abuse liabilities, and prevention and treatment needs (Zachny and Lichtor, 1998; Boyd and McCabe).

In the United States, there is a tremendous gulf among legislative stakeholders in terms of a formal taxonomy for nonmedical prescription drug use and problematic levels of use. The Food and Drug Administration has urged manufactured to focus on "Physical Dependence" and "Tolerance" (Dasgupta, Henningfield, Ertischek, & Schnoll, 2011) in the assessment of abuse liability for prescription medications. The National Institutes of Health (NIH) is concerned both the physical and psychological aspects of addiction that are linked to extant diagnostic criteria, such as the American Psychiatric Association's Diagnostic and Statistical Manual (DSM) or the International Classification of Diseases (ICD) categories of abuse and dependence (Compton & Volkow, 2006). The United States Drug Enforcement Agency (DEA) takes a more scientific approach, focusing on the legal requirements (e.g., number and timing of refills, quantity dispensed under a single prescription, written versus ePrescribing) that is tied to a drug's particular abuse liability (Katz et al., 2007). The words "abuse" and "misuse" have often been used interchangeably, but may be used to define separate acts of nonmedical use. The term Abuse may refer to use that involves seeking a euphoric "high" and misuse typically refers to "intentional use that involves a legitimate prescription that is used in amounts not directed by the prescriber or to treat another medical condition." An additional piece of this complicated taxonomy is whether the drug was prescribed for the user or whether they obtained it illicitly (e.g., stole/obtained from friends/family, forged written prescription, feigned symptoms to a prescriber with liberal prescribing habits [pill mills] (Boyd & McCabe, 2008).

In 2003, the College on Problems on Drug Dependence, the largest professional society in the United States dedicated solely to the advancement of knowledge about drug abuse, published a position statement about prescription pain relievers (Zacny et al., 2003). The statement urged for a formal clarification of the term nonmedical use that is broad enough to include motivations for use for inclusion on national surveillance surveys, such as the NSDUH. However, the purpose of this chapter focuses on the epidemiology and treatment of levels of use that are problematic and in need of specialty substance abuse treatment. Therefore, clarification of the term nonmedical use is less important than resolution of the diagnostic criteria that can be used to assess problem use, such as the DSM or ICD classifications of abuse or dependence. There is some debate about the degree to which opioids differ in their abuse liability and phenotypic expression of abuse and/or dependence symptoms (Wu, Woody, Yang, & Blazer, 2011; Wu, Woody, Yang, Mannelli, & Blazer, 2011). However, DSM and ICD criteria are generally accepted measures that can be easily translated onto epidemiological surveys to estimate the population in need of substance abuse treatment services for prescription drug-related problems. There are many clinical tools that are used to diagnose problem use for different therapeutic classes, as well as biological challenge tests of physical dependence (Kosten, Bianchi, & Kosten, 1989). At one end of the continuum, there is concern that the "one-size fits all" approach to defining the concepts of abuse and dependence may not operate similarly across all substances even within a therapeutic class (e.g., extended release having lower abuse liability than immediate release oxycodone) (Dasgupta, et al., 2011). At the other end of the continuum, there is an argument that abuse and dependence are a continuum, which is derived from an underlying biopsychosocial propensity (Krueger et al., 2002). Regardless of the placement on the spectrum, the term *Addiction* refers to a chronic and relapsing pattern of use and is defined by essentially three characteristics: compulsive use, loss of control in limiting intake, and altering behavioral activities in support of drug consumption. Medical professionals typically employ more specific terminology aligned within clinical (e.g., DSM or ICD criteria) criteria when referencing disordered patterns of substance use, such as abuse and/or dependence.

For the remainder of this chapter, we present data on problem levels of prescription drug use using the DSM-IV/ICD classification scheme of abuse and/or dependence. This scheme is the most widely employed diagnostic tool for problem use on national surveillance data systems, and are used to frame the nation's perspective and conversation related to research, prevention, treatment, and public policy toward the nonmedical use of prescription drugs. Within this diagnostic taxonomy, hierarchical criteria are used to ensure that substance use disorders are classified by whether symptoms are directly tied to substance use or a separate psychiatric disorder or illness. For example, mood and anxiety disorders (APA, 2006) have exclusionary criteria because a common symptom of withdrawal (e.g., "dope sick") may involve symptomotology that overlaps with mood and anxiety disorders, such as "feeling downhearted and blue" or "nervousness". This task is complicated by the high rate of comorbidity between mental (i.e., mood, anxiety, and personality) and substance use disorders (McLellan, Lewis, O'Brien, & Kleber, 2000; NIDA, 1999; O'Brien et al., 2004).

Evaluating a substance use disorder has been established using criteria that can be implemented by a clinician, or a trained interviewer using a semi-structured instrument, such as the Structured Clinical Interview for DSM Axis II disorders (First, 2002). There are also many diagnostic tools that are fully structured and can be implemented in the context of a research interview. These include the Composite International Diagnostic Interview [CIDI] (Green et al., 2011; Haro et al., 2006; Kessler et al., 2004)and the Associated Disabilities Interview Schedule [AUDADIS] (Grant et al., 2003; Grant, Harford, Dawson, Chou, & Pickering, 1995). Ascertaining the count of the population in need of services is a challenge because of the resources needed to execute a full diagnostic exam on a sufficiently large enough sample that permits generalization to the population as a whole. However, such a task is critical for policymakers to help identify and prioritize placement of finite resources that are funded through public monies. As mentioned earlier, there are a small number of surveys that collect data annually on nonmedical use of prescription drugs, but only one implements a fully-structured diagnostic interview for substance use disorders annually for youth (age 12-17) and adults (ages 18 or older—the National Survey on Drug Use and Health (SAMHSA, 2008). Other annual surveys administer brief screening scales that can be used to assess probable case based on a small number of items. A drawback is that they lack the sensitivity and specificity to accurately assess the number in need of treatment (Aldworth et al., 2010; Novak, Colpe, Barker, & Gfroerer, 2010). Therefore, in-depth diagnostic scales provide the best approach to capturing the complex phenomena of substance abuse disorders, despite the length and expense in their implementation.

The Diagnostic and Statistical Manual of Mental Disorders (DSM-IV) distinguishes problematic substance use along two categorical rubrics (shown in Table 3):

- ABUSE: Captures a maladaptive pattern of use that causes significant impairment in social, mental, and physical life-world domains. An example is missing work or failing to attend to household obligations because of use. Continued use despite consistent interpersonal or social problems associated with use is another hallmark system.
- DEPENDENCE: Is defined by a maladaptive pattern of use with adverse clinical consequences. Dependence involves two physical aspects: (1) *Tolerance*—refers to the decrease in the physical or psychological effects of a constant dosage of a drug over time; and (2) *Withdrawal*—refers to a physiological state of adverse mental and physical symptoms (e.g., nausea, insomnia, muscle aches/pains, These symptoms will vary depending upon how long the medication was taken and the type of medication.

In the next section, we summarize the epidemiology of nonmedical prescription drug use, with an emphasis on disordered patterns of use as defined by DSM-IV criteria (APA, 2002). Surveillance data are drawn from the National Survey on Drug Use and Health (SAMHSA, 2009). The NSDUH is an annual, nationally representative survey of youth (age 12-17) and adults (age 18 or older) in the United States. The procedures and characteristics of the sample have been published extensively elsewhere (SAMHSA, 2008). Briefly, the sample includes approximately 65,000 respondents each year. The target population is the civilian, noninstitutionalized population of the United States (including civilians living on military bases) and residents of noninstitutional group quarters (e.g., college dormitories, group homes, civilians dwelling on military installations) and persons with no permanent residence (homeless people in shelters and residents of single rooms in hotels). The NSDUH collects information on a large range of illicit substances, including consumption patterns, treatment utilization, and diagnoses aligned with the Diagnostic and Statistical Manual of Mental Disorders (DSM-IV) criteria for abuse and/or dependence (APA, 2000) for alcohol and selected drugs. For this paper, Substance use treatment was coded if the respondent reported any therapy or treatment, including detoxification and treatment for any medical problems associated with their drug use. Unmet treatment need was defined as the presence of a past-year DSM-IV diagnosis for abuse and/or dependence on prescription medications, but the respondent did not report receiving substance abuse treatment. Due to the complex sampling design of the NSDUH, all descriptive and inferential analyses were conducted with SUDAAN release 10.0 (RTI, 2009).

Disorders	Definition
Substance Use Disorders	
Substance Dependence	A maladaptive pattern of substance use with adverse clinical consequences. The DSM-IV has widened the concept of dependence to include the association of substance use with uncontrolled use or with use in spite of adverse consequences.
Substance Abuse	A maladaptive pattern of substance use that causes clinically significant impairment, not meeting dependence criteria. This may include impairments in social, family, or occupational functioning, in the presence of a psychological or physical problem, or in satiations in which use of the substance is physically hazardous, such as driving while intoxicated.
Substance Induced Disorders	
Substance Intoxication	Reversible, substance-specific physiological and behavioral changes due to recent exposure to a psychoactive substance. Produced by all substances.
Substance Withdrawal	A substance-specific syndrome that develops following cessation of or reduction in dosage of a regularly used substance. Occurs with chronic use of all substances, except perhaps cannabis and hallucinogens.
Substance Induced Delirium (confusion, psychosis)	Occurs with overdose of many substances
Substance Induced Psychotic Disorder (psychosis)	May occur with phenylcyclidine (PCP) and hallucinogens, stimulants, cannabis, and alcohol.
Substance Induced Mood Disorder (depression, mania) **Anxiety**	Common with many substances, especially alcohol and stimulants. Disorder must be distinguished from primary psychiatric disorder that preceded drug use.
Substance Induced Sleep Disorder	A sleep disturbance attributable to acute or chronic substance use. Common with alcohol, sedatives, and stimulants.
Substance Induced Sexual Dysfunction	Alcohol, benzodiazepines, and opioids commonly reduce sexual responsiveness and performance.
Substance Induced Persisting Disorders	Substance-specific syndromes that persist long after drug use ceases (e.g., hallucinogen "flashbacks," memory impairments, or dementia).

* dsm-iv criteria (american psychiatric association, 1994)

Table 3. Classification of Substance Use and Substance Induced Disorders*

3. Patterns of prescription drug use and disordered use in the United States

Although trend data indicate that the prevalence of nonmedical use of prescription drugs has nearly doubled over the past two decades (Blanco, et al., 2007), the rate of nonmedical use remained fairly consistent over the past 5 years (Figure 1). Among youth (aged 12-17), the NSDUH showed that approximately 8 percent (8,000 per 100,000) used any class of prescription medication in the prior year. Among those that used, about 16% met the criteria for abuse or dependence (Figure 2). The rate of use far exceeds that of adults (aged 18 or older) where approximately 6% used any prescription medication non-medically and the

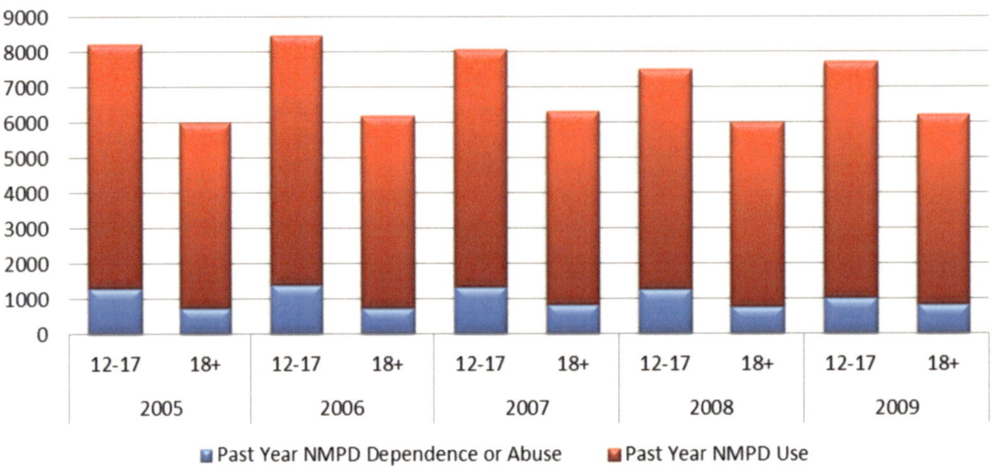

Fig. 1. Past Year Nonmedical Prescription Drug Use and Meeting Criteria for Dependence or Abuse of Nonmedical Prescription Drugs, by Age and Year: 2005-2009 NSDUH (per 100,000)

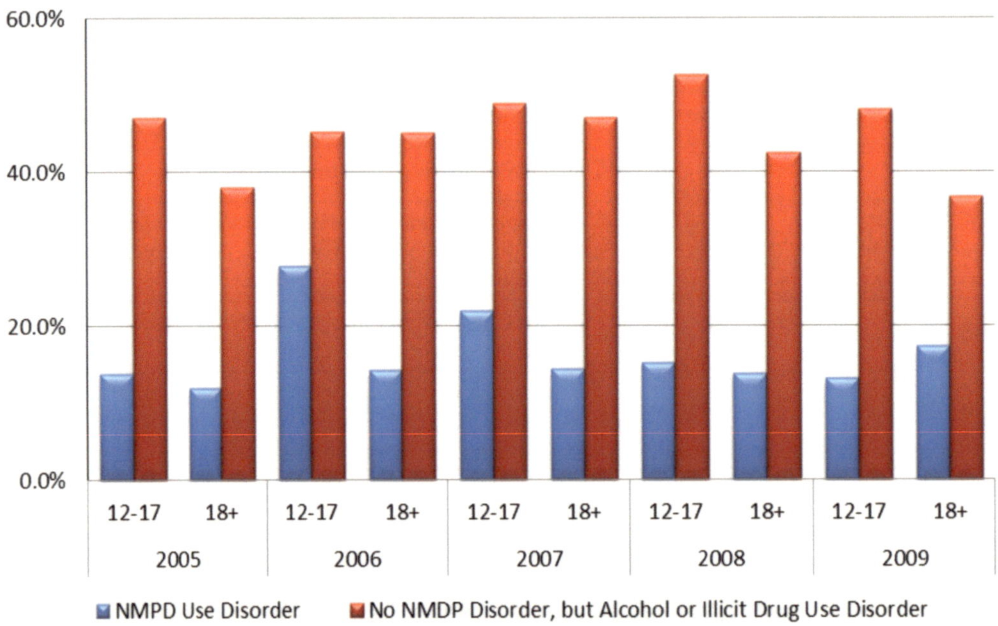

Fig. 2. Past Year Substance Use Disorder among Persons Receiving Drug Treatment in the Past Year, by Age and Year: 2005-2009 NSDUHs (In Percent)

rates of disordered use was about 16%, similar to adolescents. These data suggest that problematic levels of abuse are developing far earlier in lifecourse, especially compared to other drugs, such as heroin and cocaine where the median age of disordered use is in the mid 20s (SAMSHA, 2006). Additional data (Figure 2) indicate that adolescent females are progressing to abuse/dependence more rapidly than males. Among those that received any form of treatment for a substance use disorder in the United States (about 2.3 million in 2009), Figure 3 reveals that approximately 15% to 18% met the criteria for a prescription drug disorder. A concern about drug treatment is that care usually focuses on eliminating the most harmful substance in the client's drug-taking repertoire, so prescription drug disorders often go unrecognized and untreated compared to illicit drugs such as cocaine and heroin. When broken down by the amount of co-occurring disorders among those in treatment, Figure 4, shows that of those in drug treatment that have a prescription drug disorder, about 70% have a co-occurring drug and/or alcohol use disorder as well.

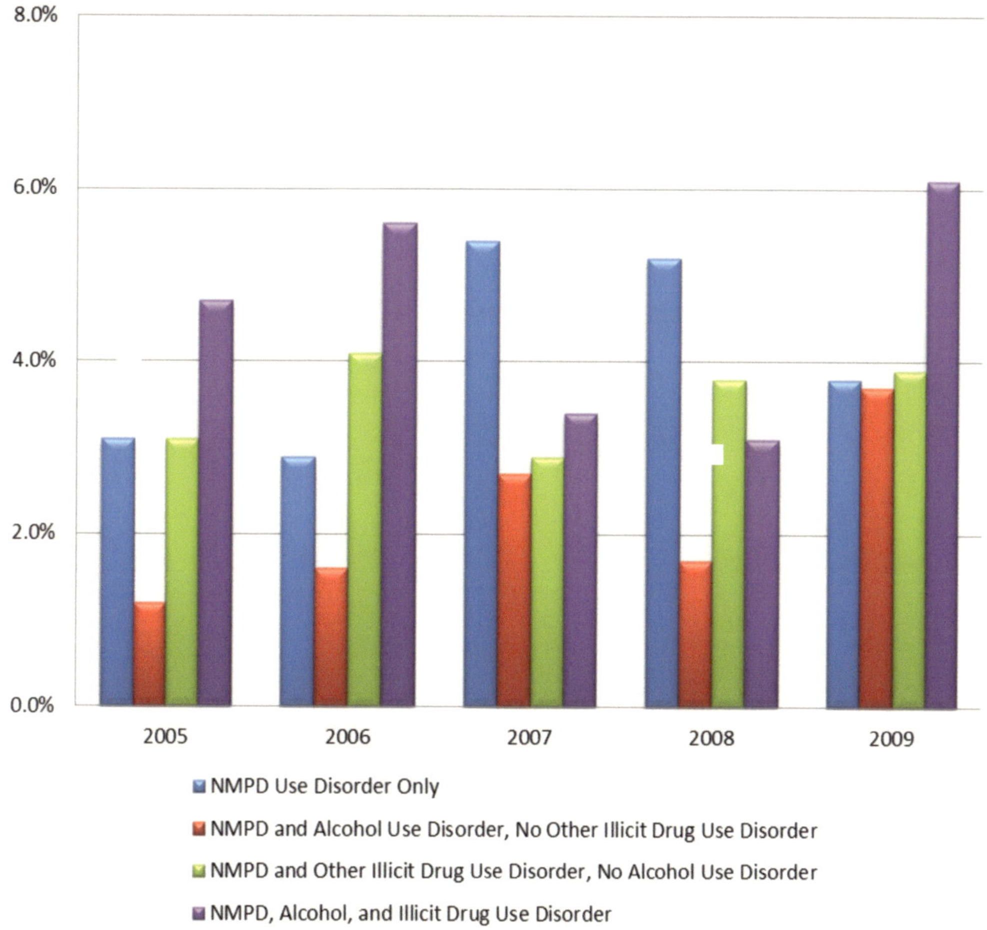

Fig. 3. Past Year Substance Use Disorders Among Persons Aged 18 or Older Receiving Past Year Drug Treatment, by Year: 2005-2009 NSDUHs

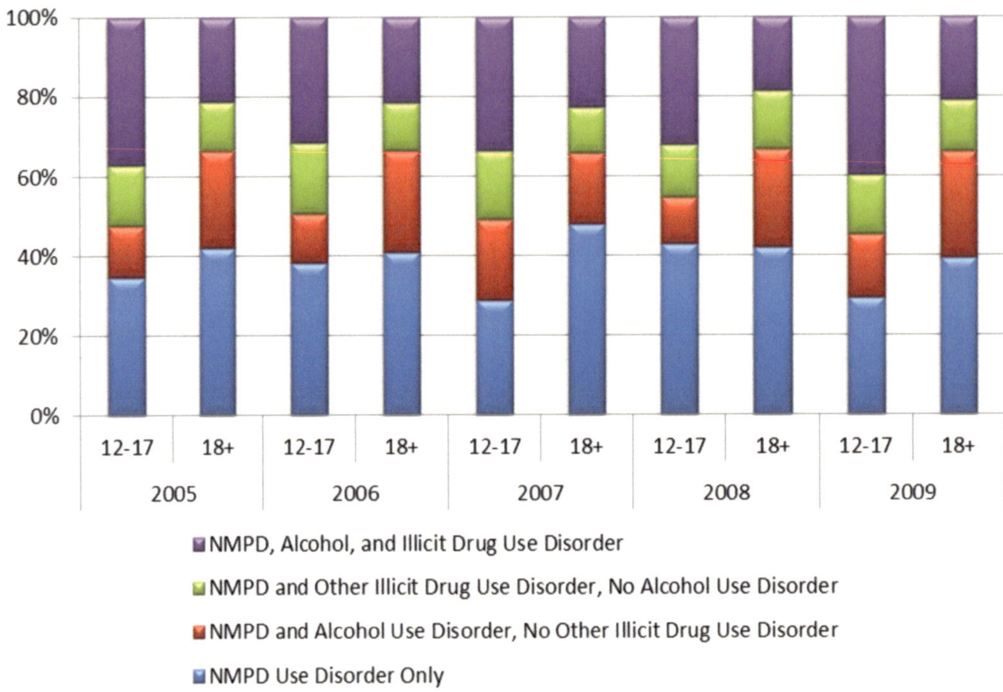

Fig. 4. Poly Drug Use Disorder among Persons with NMPD Use Disorder, by Age and Year: 2005-2009 NSDUHs

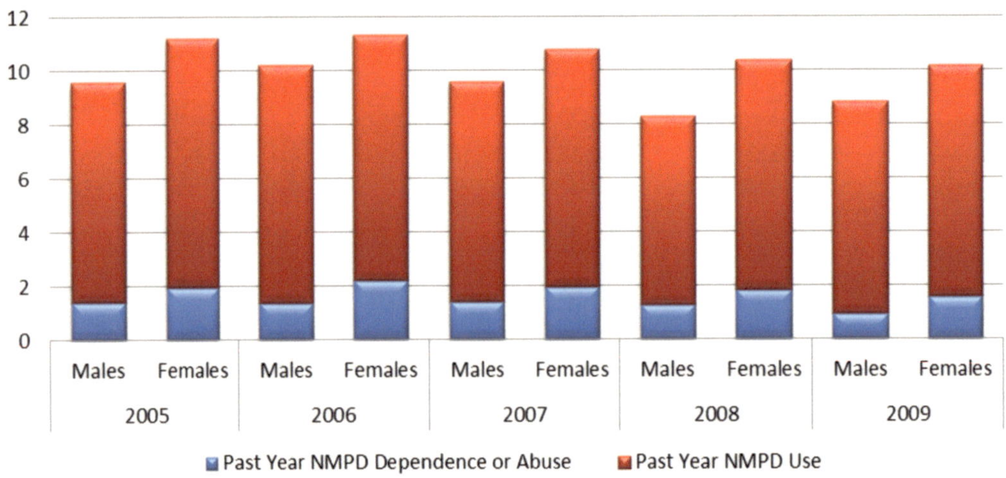

Fig. 5. Percent of Past Year Nonmedical Prescription Drug Use and Meeting Criteria for Dependence or Abuse of Nonmedical Prescription Drugs among 12-17 years olds, by Sex and year: 2005-2009 NSDUHs

4. Prescription pain relievers

Therapeutic Indications: Pain relievers as a therapeutic medication class are also referred to as analgesics. They are distinguished by the ways in which they act in the peripheral or central nervous system. Analgesics that are non-steroidal anti-inflammatory drugs (NSAIDS) are used to treat mild pain and act by reducing inflammation at the site of an injury or disease in the body. NSAIDS typically do not require a prescription in the United States and are available "over-the-counter" (OTC) at local pharmacies, drug stores, and even gas stations. Other types of (OTC) analgesics are not NSAIDS (e.g., acetaminophen), but act on the same physiological pathways to reduce the neuro-chemical sensation of pain.

Narcotic analgesics are used to treat moderate to severe pain, in many instances require a prescription from a prescriber that is licensed by the Drug Enforcement Agency (DEA). Perhaps the most widely used class of pain reliever in the United States is opioids, which can be subdivided into three types. First, naturally occurring (e.g., morphine or codeine) opioids are derived from the opium poppy plant. These drugs are typically altered into pro-drugs during the pharmaceutical manufacturing process, meaning that they are chemically converted to opioids as they are metabolized into the body. This manufacturing strategy is preferable to leaving the chemical structure unaltered (i.e., free base) because it increases the bioavailability of the drugs during metabolization and therefore maximizes their efficacy. Naturally occurring opioids are also used as chemical building blocks for semi-synthetic opiates (e.g., hydrocodone, oxycodone). Both naturally occurring and semi-synthetic opioids attach to specific opioid receptors in the brain (e.g., Mu, Kappa, Delta, and Epsilon). Heroin is a semi-synthetic opioid that is similar in chemical structure to morphine and was primarily developed as a legitimate treatment for pain in the 1800s. However, it was discovered to have high affinity to abuse because it quickly activates the brain's opioid neuro-receptors, thus producing a quick euphoric flush that is highly desirable by recreational abusers. Fully synthetic opioids (e.g., methadone, tramadol, dextropropoxyphene) are fully manufactured drugs and are not chemically related to opiates in structure, other than they selectively bind to the same neural receptors in the brain. There is controversy regarding the degree to which fully synthetic opioids have the same abuse liability as naturally occurring or semi-synthetic opioids (Aldworth, et al., 2010; Dasgupta, et al., 2011; Wu, Woody, Yang, Mannelli, et al., 2011). Overall, these drugs are known as exogenous opioids in that they are external stimuli, whereas endogenous opioids are produced internally (e.g., endorphins) in response to high levels of physical or emotional activity, and are secreted from the pituitary glands and attach to the opioid-like receptors in the brain.

Epidemiology of Nonmedical and Disordered Use: The United States has one of the highest levels per capital consumption of prescription opioids (United Nations, 2004). While the use of narcotic opioids is recognized as an important weapon in the physician's arsenal to combat mild to severe pain, studies have correlated high levels of exposure to nonmedical use and problematic levels to dependence (Dasgupta et al, 2006). Prescription pain relievers are the have the highest prevalence of nonmedical use, especially among youth aged 12-17 (Figure 6). Between 2005 to 2009, approximately 6.5% of youth (pop est. 6,000 per 100,000) used a prescription pain reliever non-medically in the prior year. About 1/6 of those who abused also used at levels consistent with DSM-IV abuse and/or dependence. Among adults aged 18 or older, the rates of nonmedical use were lower, approximately 4.5% (pop est. 4,500 per 100,000). The rates of disordered use were similar to youth, with about 16 percent reporting symptoms of abuse and/or dependence.

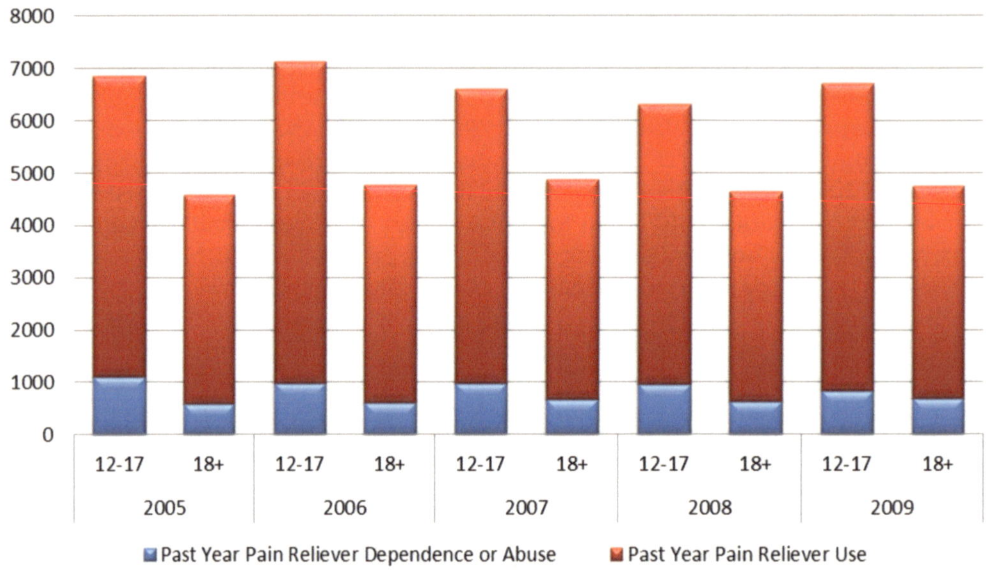

Fig. 6. Past Year Pain Reliever Use and Meeting Criteria for Dependence or Abuse of Pain Relievers, by Age and Year: 2005-2009 NSDUHs (Per 100,000)

Treatment: Treatment for opioid pain medications tend toward the pharmacological spectrum, although some behavioral therapies do exist. The most common pharmacological treatment therapies for opioid pain medications include methadone, Buprenorphine, and Naltrexone or buprenorhpine/suboxone. Of the three, methadone is the oldest and most frequently used pharmacology (Amato et al., 2005), although limited evidence has shown that Buprenorphine may be slightly advantageous to methadone in terms of lessening withdrawal symptoms faster and overall completion of treatment (Gowing, Ali, & White, 2004). In contrast, a systematic review of Naltrexone indicates that the treatment may not be very effective on treatment retention or abuse relapse rates (Minozzi et al., 2006). Although pharmacotherapies are popular with clinicians, trials on behavioral therapies have shown to be effective in the treatment of opioid pain medication abuse. These therapies have been found to increase treatment adherence as well as increase social support variables known to increase positive outcomes (Amato et al., 2008). Specific behavioral therapies like motivational interventions among prescription drug abusers have been shown to reduce use by 25% in over half of users (Zahradnik et al., 2009).

5. Sedatives/tranquilizers

This class of therapeutic medications is primary used to treat used to treat anxiety and sleep disorders. They are also a major source of drug overdoses and adverse drug reactions (DAWN, 2008). The effects of most sedative medications are mediated through the GABA-chloride receptor complex, and there have been specific neural-receptors that have a high affinity to benzodiazepines. These effects are potentiated with co-ingestion with other depressants, such as alcohol. At extremely high levels of use, sedatives/hypnotics produce a loss of coordination, euphoria, dyskinesia, and even hallucinations. There are primarily two classes of medications. Barbiturates are among the oldest sedative/hypnotics and are sub-classified into their mechanism of duration (ultrashort acting, short acting, and long acting pharmacokinetics). The second major class is benzodiazepines. Unlike barbiturates, benzodiazepines are not useful for producing deep sedation and therefore are considered less powerful and of lower addictive potential. Because sedative/hypnotic drugs reduce neural excitability in the brain, neural adaption may occur after a period of weeks or months of prolonged use. Therefore, tapering rather than immediate withdrawal is recommended for patients who may develop physical tolerance after long-term exposure.

Epidemiology of Nonmedical and Disordered Use: The rate of nonmedical use and disordered use is far lower for sedative/hypnotics than prescription pain relievers. As shown in Figure 7, approximately 2% of youth and adults reported nonmedical use in the prior year. Use also appeared stable between 2005 to 2009. Among those reporting use in the past year, approximately 16% of youth and adults met the criteria for abuse and/or dependence.

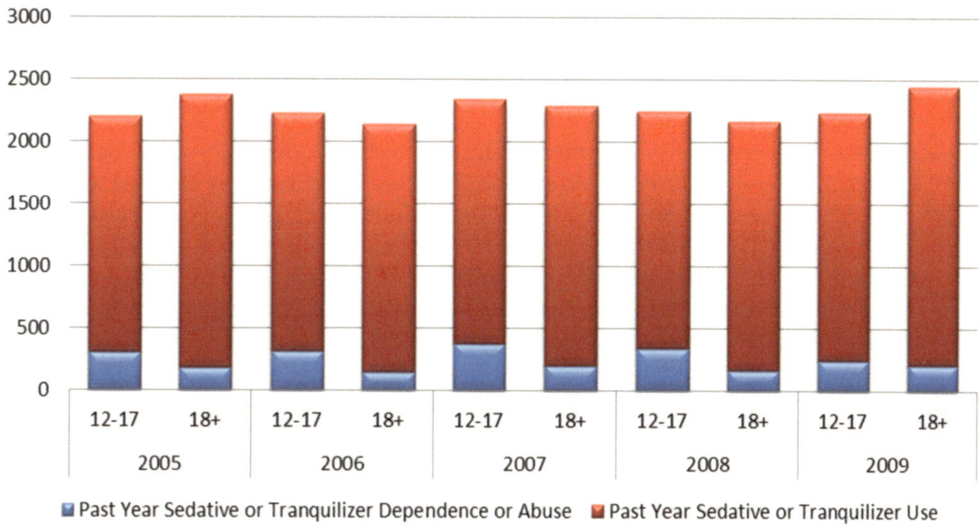

Fig. 7. Past Year Sedative and Tranquilizer Use and Meeting Criteria for Dependence or Abuse of Sedatives and Tranquilizers, by Age and Year: 2005-2009 NSDUHs (Per 100,000 |)

Treatment: Other than tapering, many types of treatment seem to be effective in treating benzodiazepine abuse. Minimal intervention, such as receiving physician advice or a form letter from a physician as well as treatment programs led by physicians or counselors are two effective treatments (Voshaar, Couvee, van Balkom, Mulder, & Zitman, 2006). Tailored behavioral interventions have also been found to be particularly effective in benzodiazepine abusers (Ten Wolde et al., 2008; Tyrer et al., 1996). Behavioral therapy programs augmented with pharmacotherapies, such as imipramine also help to reduce use among abusers. Other pharmacotherapies such as Carbamazepine have also significantly improved drug abstinence among benzodiazepine abusers (Voshaar, Couvee, et al., 2006; Voshaar et al., 2006; Voshaar et al., 2003). Behavioral interventions, such as cognitive behavioral therapy has also shown promise in reducing dependence (Denis, Fatseas, Lavie, & Auriacombe, 2006).

6. Psychostimulants

These drugs are typically used to treat attentional disorders (e.g., attention deficit disorder) and sleep disorders (e.g., narcolepsy). They are also compounds used in cold-medications because they are used to expand the nasal and esophageal airways and assist breathing (e.g., Ephedra). Ironically, low dosages of amphetamines actually produce a calming effect in those with attentional disorders. Drugs in this class are structurally related to a wide range of drugs that increase activation of the central nervous system. These include legitimate drugs such as caffeine and nicotine as illicit drugs such as crack cocaine. Prescription stimulants are typically referred to as amphetamines, and available in two chemical forms: I-amphetamine (e.g., Benzedrine) and d-amphetamine (aka dextroamphetamine). Amphetamines have a high resemblance to the dopamine (DA) transmitter in their chemical structure, therefore have a high affinity to DA receptors in binding. Methamphetamine is perhaps the most potent form of amphetamine in its effects on the central nervous system. Illicit forms of methamphetamine (e.g., crystallize methamphetamine or crystal meth) are manufactured using processes to increase the speed of uptake in the brain because amphetamine is first metabolized in the liver and has a slow uptake and a long half life (about 7-30 hours depending upon the formulation).

Epidemiology of Nonmedical and Disordered Use

The recent rise of diagnoses for attentional disorders in the United States (Birnbaum, 2004) has placed an increased volume of amphetamine stimulants used to treat ADHD/ADD within the public domain. An estimated 4% of youth aged 17 or younger have been projected to meet the diagnostic criteria for AHDH/ADD. Of importance is that much of the data indicate that youth and adults who use ADHD/ADD stimulants non-medically do so for its purported therapeutic value rather than euphoria or to "get high." (McCabe, et al., 2007; Novak et al., 2009). Epidemiological surveillance data from NSDUH (Figure 8) show

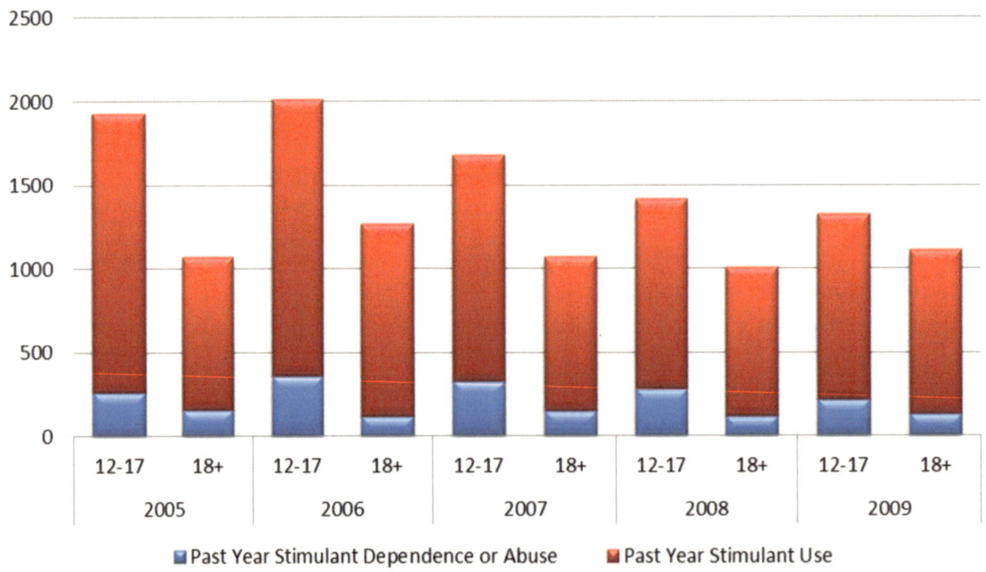

Fig. 8. Past Year Stimulant Use and Meeting Criteria for Dependence or Abuse of Stimulants, by Age and Year: 2005-2009 NSDUHs (Per 100,000)

that less than 2% of youth and 1% of adults reported nonmedical use, and of these, about 7% report levels consistent with abuse and/or dependence. Therefore, there may be a significant amount of nonmedical use of prescription psychostimulants, the level of problem use is far lower than prescription pain relievers and sedatives/hypnotics.

Treatment

Treatments for prescription stimulants and tranquilizers/sedatives are primarily limited to behavioral therapies (Rawson et al., 1995), though novel drug targets are being developed for cocaine and amphetamine use. Interventions such as cognitive behavioral therapy (CBT) and contingency management which have proven moderately effective for cocaine and methamphetamine use disorders in achieving drug abstinence can be applied to persons abusing or dependent upon prescription stimulants. Tapering can be used initially to begin treatment which will ease the symptoms of withdrawal, following by CBT and contingency management. An extensive review of the literature indicated that the behavioral therapies being applied to illicit stimulant abuse are currently the best options for treatment of prescription stimulant abuse (Vocci & Montoya, 2009). Currently, there is no Food and Drug Administration approved medication for the treatment of prescription stimulants.

7. Summary and future directions

Nonmedical prescription drug use had received a significant amount of policy and media attention in the past several years, with some using the term "epidemic" to describe the levels of use in the United States (Maxwell, 2011). In response, the Office of National Drug Control Policy (ONDCP), which is the policy arm of the President focused on substance abuse, issued a position statement in early 2011 (ONDCP, 2011). This policy release outlines the federal strategy for reducing nonmedical prescription drug abuse, and dictates various activities and a division of labor among federal agencies. The plan begins with patient and provider education programs across all federal health agencies. The content of which should focus on educating providers and patients on the safe and appropriate use of prescription medications, as well as the side effect profiles and the likelihood of abuse and diversion for nonmedical purposes. A more detailed understanding of the sequence of substance use initiation would help identify optimal points for prevention and treatment. For example, it is unknown how many persons develop a prescription drug disorder after long-term exposure to prescription medications used in the treatment of a legitimate medical condition. This pathway may be different in terms of etiology and treatment needs from a "garbage head" or poly-drug user who uses multiple illicit substances. For this latter type of user, prescription drugs are either substituted when illicit drugs are unavailable, used to self-treat withdrawal symptoms, or used concurrently to increase the feelings of euphoria. Research has shown differences in motivations to use based on therapeutic and euphoric reasons (McCabe, Cranford, Boyd, & Teter, 2007; McCabe, Teter, & Boyd, 2006; Novak, Kroutil, Williams, & Van Brunt, 2007; Novak, Reardon, & Buka, 2002), but additional knowledge is needed to articulate the pathways leading from initiation to regular use and dependence.

Tracking and enforcement are also primary goals outlined in the ONDCP Prescription Drug Control Strategy. While a large majority of the medications used for nonmedical purposes are obtained through friends and family, the highest volume consumers of prescription medications, who also meet the criteria for disordered use, obtain their medications through illicit channels such as doctor shopping, the internet, or theft (SAMHSA, 2009). There are a number of initiatives to reduce the availability of prescription medications for diversion, such as "Medication Take Back Days" sponsored by local law enforcement in various states. In addition, drugs with even modest abuse liability, such as Tramadol—a non-opioid prescription pain reliever, are being rescheduled by several States so that prescribing and refilling practices by doctors and patients is more restrictive.

In response to the public health threat that prescription drug abuse poses, federal and state initiatives in the United States have earmarked more than $500 million toward reducing the supply of NMPD through prescription monitoring programs, regulations for prescribing and dosing, and physician education programs (Fischer, Bibby, & Bouchard, 2010; Fishman, 2011; Manchikanti, 2007). These programs are implemented in more than 40 states, with some form of legislation pending in the rest. Several screening instruments have also been developed to help clinicians identify potential abuse liability for their patient. Unfortunately, these programs and assessments have been developed and implemented in the absence of a strong scientific understanding of characteristics of prescription drug abuse. Medical professionals need guidance about types of NMPD to identify those with the greatest potential for abuse of a particular medication. It is also unknown whether individuals are aware of these monitoring systems and programs and if they have significantly affected drug procuring behaviors.

This chapter began with an important statement about the complexities of the national drug problem involving prescription medications in the United States. This chapter presented descriptive epidemiological data on prescription drug disorders and their treatment. Unlike other drugs of abuse, the body of knowledge around prescription drug abuse is in its relative infancy. Many unresolved questions remain regarding the degree to which the risk factors for alcohol and tobacco and marijuana in adolescence are similar to prescription drug abuse. Resolution of this question would help frame primary prevention efforts toward either universal or specialized prevention programming in schools and in the community. Moreover, there are also many unknown questions about how the bio-pharmacological properties of prescription medications contribute toward abuse liability. Prescription drug manufacturers are developing abuse deterrent formulations (ADFs) of commonly abuse drugs. For example, several drugs in the FDA pipeline (Phase I to III) employ sequestered naltrexone, an opioid antagonist, to limit the nonmedical use of opioid-based pain medications. When the pill is crushed or tampered, the naltrexone becomes activated and counteracts the effects of the opioid concentrated in the medication. However, these methods are only effective against abuse by tampering (e.g., crushing, snorting, injecting), so additional methods are needed to curb routes of abuse that include oral ingestion as well. The health care delivery system for behavioral health is also under going tremendous transformation, which has wide-ranging implications for the prevention and treatment of prescription drug abuse. While the final proposed structure is likely to stay under significant and prolonged debate, experts agree that behavioral health, which is largely responsible for the delivery of substance abuse treatment services, will have greater integration into the primary and specialized health care systems. Taken together, it appears that a multi-pronged approach that involves effects at multiple systematic levels will be needed to reduce the epidemic of prescription drug abuse over the next several years.

8. Acknowledgements

The analyses for this paper were supported by a grant from the National Institute on Drug Abuse (R01DA030427, S. Novak, PI). The National Survey on Drug Use and Health was conducted by RTI International under a contract from the Substance Abuse and Mental Health Services Administration. The conclusions from this study are solely the authors. The authors would like to thank Richard Nowak, RPh. (CVS Pharmacy Group, USA) and David Brown, Ph.D. (Pfizer, Inc., USA) for their comments on early versions of this manuscript. The authors gratefully acknowledge the dedication of the NSDUH participants for their generosity and time.

9. References

Aldworth, J., Colpe, L. J., Gfroerer, J. C., Novak, S. P., Chromy, J. R., Barker, P. R., et al. (2010). The National Survey on Drug Use and Health Mental Health Surveillance Study: calibration analysis. *Int J Methods Psychiatr Res, 19 Suppl 1*, 61-87.

Amato, L., Davoli, M., Perucci, C. A., Ferri, M., Faggiano, F., & Mattick, R. P. (2005). An overview of systematic reviews of the effectiveness of opiate maintenance therapies: available evidence to inform clinical practice and research. *J Subst Abuse Treat, 28*(4), 321-329.

Amato, L., Minozzi, S., Davoli, M., Vecchi, S., Ferri, M. M., & Mayet, S. (2008). Psychosocial combined with agonist maintenance treatments versus agonist maintenance treatments alone for treatment of opioid dependence. *Cochrane Database Syst Rev*(4), CD004147.

APA. (2000). *Diagnostic and Statistical Manual of Mental Disorders* (4th ed.). Washington, DC: American Psychiatric Publishing, Inc.

Blanco, C., Alderson, D., Ogburn, E., Grant, B. F., Nunes, E. V., Hatzenbuehler, M. L., et al. (2007). Changes in the prevalence of non-medical prescription drug use and drug use disorders in the United States: 1991-1992 and 2001-2002. *Drug Alcohol Depend, 90*(2-3), 252-260.

Boyd, C. J., & McCabe, S. E. (2008). Coming to terms with the nonmedical use of prescription medications. *Subst Abuse Treat Prev Policy, 3*, 22.

Colliver, J. D., Kroutil, L. A., Dai, L., & Gfroerer, J. C. (2006). Misuse of prescription drugs: Data from the 2002, 2003, and 2004 National Surveys on Drug Use and Health (DHHS Publication No. SMA 06-4192, Analytic Series A-28). Rockville, MD: Substance Abuse and Mental Health Services Administration.

Compton, W. M., & Volkow, N. D. (2006). Abuse of prescription drugs and the risk of addiction. *Drug Alcohol Depend, 83 Suppl 1*, S4-7.

Dasgupta, N., Henningfield, J. E., Ertischek, M. D., & Schnoll, S. H. (2011). When drugs in the same controlled substance schedule differ in real-world abuse, should they be differentiated in labeling? *Drug Alcohol Depend.*

Dasgupta, N., Kramer, E. D., Zalman, M. A., Carino, S., Jr., Smith, M. Y., Haddox, J. D., et al. (2006). Association between non-medical and prescriptive usage of opioids. *Drug Alcohol Depend, 82*(2), 135-142.

Denis, C., Fatseas, M., Lavie, E., & Auriacombe, M. (2006). Pharmacological interventions for benzodiazepine mono-dependence management in outpatient settings. *Cochrane Database Syst Rev, 3*, CD005194.

Fischer, B., Bibby, M., & Bouchard, M. (2010). The global diversion of pharmaceutical drugsnon-medical use and diversion of psychotropic prescription drugs in North America: a review of sourcing routes and control measures. *Addiction, 105*(12), 2062-2070.

Fishman, S. M. (2011). Prescription drug monitoring programs serve a vital clinical need. *Pain Med, 12*(6), 845.

Gowing, L., Ali, R., & White, J. (2004). Buprenorphine for the management of opioid withdrawal. *Cochrane Database Syst Rev*(4), CD002025.

Grant, B. F., Dawson, D. A., Stinson, F. S., Chou, P. S., Kay, W., & Pickering, R. (2003). The Alcohol Use Disorder and Associated Disabilities Interview Schedule-IV (AUDADIS-IV): reliability of alcohol consumption, tobacco use, family history of depression and psychiatric diagnostic modules in a general population sample. *Drug Alcohol Depend, 71*(1), 7-16.

Grant, B. F., Harford, T. C., Dawson, D. A., Chou, P. S., & Pickering, R. P. (1995). The Alcohol Use Disorder and Associated Disabilities Interview schedule (AUDADIS): reliability of alcohol and drug modules in a general population sample. *Drug Alcohol Depend, 39*(1), 37-44.

Green, J. G., Avenevoli, S., Finkelman, M., Gruber, M. J., Kessler, R. C., Merikangas, K. R., et al. (2011). Validation of the diagnoses of panic disorder and phobic disorders in the US National Comorbidity Survey Replication Adolescent (NCS-A) supplement. *Int J Methods Psychiatr Res, 20*(2), 105-115.

Haro, J. M., Arbabzadeh-Bouchez, S., Brugha, T. S., de Girolamo, G., Guyer, M. E., Jin, R., et al. (2006). Concordance of the Composite International Diagnostic Interview Version 3.0 (CIDI 3.0) with standardized clinical assessments in the WHO World Mental Health surveys. *Int J Methods Psychiatr Res, 15*(4), 167-180.

Huang, B., Dawson, D. A., Stinson, F. S., Hasin, D. S., Ruan, W. J., Saha, T. D., et al. (2006). Prevalence, correlates, and comorbidity of nonmedical prescription drug use and drug use disorders in the United States: Results of the National Epidemiologic Survey on Alcohol and Related Conditions. *J Clin Psychiatry, 67*(7), 1062-1073.

Hubbard, R. L., Pantula, J., & Lessler, J. T. (1992). Effects of decomposition of complex concepts. In C. F. Turner & J. T. Lessler (Eds.), *Survey Measurement of Drug Use: Methodological Studies* (Vol. DHHS Publication no. (ADM) 92-1929). Washington, DC: Government Printing Office

Johnston, L. D., O'Malley, P. M., Bachman, J. G., & Schulenberg, J. E. (2009). *Monitoring the Future national results on adolescent drug use: Overview of key findings, 2008 (NIH Publication No. 09-7401). Bethesda, MD: National Institute on Drug Abuse, 73 pp.* : National Institute of Health (Number:)

Katz, N. P., Adams, E. H., Benneyan, J. C., Birnbaum, H. G., Budman, S. H., Buzzeo, R. W., et al. (2007). Foundations of opioid risk management. *Clin J Pain, 23*(2), 103-118.

Kessler, R. C., Abelson, J., Demler, O., Escobar, J. I., Gibbon, M., Guyer, M. E., et al. (2004). Clinical calibration of DSM-IV diagnoses in the World Mental Health (WMH) version of the World Health Organization (WHO) Composite International Diagnostic Interview (WMHCIDI). *Int J Methods Psychiatr Res, 13*(2), 122-139.

Kosten, T. A., Bianchi, M. S., & Kosten, T. R. (1989). Use predicts treatment outcome, not opiate dependence or withdrawal. *NIDA Res Monogr, 95*, 459-460.

Krueger, R. F., Hicks, B. M., Patrick, C. J., Carlson, S. R., Iacono, W. G., & McGue, M. (2002). Etiologic connections among substance dependence, antisocial behavior, and personality: modeling the externalizing spectrum. *J Abnorm Psychol, 111*(3), 411-424.

Kuehn, B. M. (2007). Many teens abusing medications. *JAMA, 297*(6), 578-580.

Lankenau, S. E., Sanders, B., Bloom, J. J., & Hathazi, D. (2008). Towards an Explanation of Subjective Ketamine Experiences among Young Injection Drug Users. *Addict Res Theory, 16*(3), 273-287.

Manchikanti, L. (2007). National drug control policy and prescription drug abuse: facts and fallacies. *Pain Physician, 10*(3), 399-424.

Maxwell, J. C. (2011). The prescription drug epidemic in the United States: a perfect storm. *Drug Alcohol Rev, 30*(3), 264-270.

McCabe, S. E., Cranford, J. A., Boyd, C. J., & Teter, C. J. (2007). Motives, diversion and routes of administration associated with nonmedical use of prescription opioids. *Addict Behav, 32*(3), 562-575.

McCabe, S. E., Teter, C. J., & Boyd, C. J. (2006). Medical use, illicit use, and diversion of abusable prescription drugs. *J Am Coll Health, 54*(5), 269-278.

McLellan, A. T., Lewis, D. C., O'Brien, C. P., & Kleber, H. D. (2000). Drug dependence, a chronic medical illness: implications for treatment, insurance, and outcomes evaluation. *Jama, 284*(13), 1689-1695.

Minozzi, S., Amato, L., Vecchi, S., Davoli, M., Kirchmayer, U., & Verster, A. (2006). Oral naltrexone maintenance treatment for opioid dependence. *Cochrane Database Syst Rev*(1), CD001333.

Nestler, E. J., Hyman, S. E., & Malenka, R. C. (2009). *Molecular Neuropharmacology: A foundation for clinical neuroscience* (Vol. II). New York: McGraw-Hill Companies

NIDA. (1999). *Principles of drug addiction treatment: a research based guide* (Vol. 2009). Rockville, MD: NIH.

Novak, S. P., Colpe, L. J., Barker, P. R., & Gfroerer, J. C. (2010). Development of a brief mental health impairment scale using a nationally representative sample in the USA. *Int J Methods Psychiatr Res, 19 Suppl 1*, 49-60.

Novak, S. P., Kroutil, L. A., Williams, R. L., & Van Brunt, D. L. (2007). The nonmedical use of prescription ADHD medications: results from a national Internet panel. *Subst Abuse Treat Prev Policy, 2*, 32.

Novak, S. P., Reardon, S. F., & Buka, S. L. (2002). How beliefs about substance use differ by socio-demographic characteristics, individual experiences, and neighborhood environments among urban adolescents. *J Drug Educ, 32*(4), 319-342.

O'Brien, C. P., Charney, D. S., Lewis, L., Cornish, J. W., Post, R. M., Woody, G. E., et al. (2004). Priority actions to improve the care of persons with co-occurring substance abuse and other mental disorders: a call to action. *Biol Psychiatry, 56*(10), 703-713.

ONDCP. (2011, June 21, 2011). Epidemic: Responding to America's Prescription Drug Abuse Crisis 5/11. Retrieved 5/11, 2011, from http://www.whitehousedrugpolicy.gov/publications/pdf/rx_abuse_plan.pdf

Rawson, R. A., Shoptaw, S. J., Obert, J. L., McCann, M. J., Hasson, A. L., Marinelli-Casey, P. J., et al. (1995). An intensive outpatient approach for cocaine abuse treatment. The Matrix model. *J Subst Abuse Treat, 12*(2), 117-127.

RTI. (2009). *SUDAAN User's Manual, Release 10.0.* Research Triangle Park, NC RTI International

SAMHSA. (2006). Drug Abuse Warning Network, 2005: National Estimates of Drug-Related Emergency Department Visits. *DAWN Series D-29, DHHS Publication No. (SMA)* 07-4256, Rockville, MD, 2007.

SAMHSA. (2008). *Results from the 2007 National Survey on Drug Use and Health: National Findings.*.

Ten Wolde, G. B., Dijkstra, A., van Empelen, P., van den Hout, W., Neven, A. K., & Zitman, F. (2008). Long-term effectiveness of computer-generated tailored patient education on benzodiazepines: a randomized controlled trial. *Addiction, 103*(4), 662-670.

Tyrer, P., Ferguson, B., Hallstrom, C., Michie, M., Tyrer, S., Cooper, S., et al. (1996). A controlled trial of dothiepin and placebo in treating benzodiazepine withdrawal symptoms. *Br J Psychiatry, 168*(4), 457-461.

Vocci, F. J., & Montoya, I. D. (2009). Psychological treatments for stimulant misuse, comparing and contrasting those for amphetamine dependence and those for cocaine dependence. *Curr Opin Psychiatry, 22*(3), 263-268.

Voshaar, R. C., Couvee, J. E., van Balkom, A. J., Mulder, P. G., & Zitman, F. G. (2006). Strategies for discontinuing long-term benzodiazepine use: meta-analysis. *Br J Psychiatry, 189*, 213-220.

Voshaar, R. C., Gorgels, W. J., Mol, A. J., van Balkom, A. J., Mulder, J., van de Lisdonk, E. H., et al. (2006). Predictors of long-term benzodiazepine abstinence in participants of a randomized controlled benzodiazepine withdrawal program. *Can J Psychiatry, 51*(7), 445-452.

Voshaar, R. C., Gorgels, W. J., Mol, A. J., van Balkom, A. J., van de Lisdonk, E. H., Breteler, M. H., et al. (2003). Tapering off long-term benzodiazepine use with or without group cognitive-behavioural therapy: three-condition, randomised controlled trial. *Br J Psychiatry, 182*, 498-504.

Wu, L. T., Woody, G. E., Yang, C., & Blazer, D. G. (2011). How do prescription opioid users differ from users of heroin or other drugs in psychopathology: Results from the National Epidemiologic Survey on Alcohol and Related Conditions. *J Addict Med, 5*(1), 28-35.

Wu, L. T., Woody, G. E., Yang, C., Mannelli, P., & Blazer, D. G. (2011). Differences in onset and abuse/dependence episodes between prescription opioids and heroin: results from the National Epidemiologic Survey on Alcohol and Related Conditions. *Subst Abuse Rehabil, 2011*(2), 77-88.

Zacny, J., Bigelow, G., Compton, P., Foley, K., Iguchi, M., & Sannerud, C. (2003). College on Problems of Drug Dependence taskforce on prescription opioid non-medical use and abuse: position statement. *Drug Alcohol Depend, 69*(3), 215-232.

Zahradnik, A., Otto, C., Crackau, B., Lohrmann, I., Bischof, G., John, U., et al. (2009). Randomized controlled trial of a brief intervention for problematic prescription drug use in non-treatment-seeking patients. *Addiction, 104*(1), 109-117.

15

Substance Use and Abuse Among Older Adults: A State of the Art

Marja Aartsen
VU-University Amsterdam
The Netherlands

1. Introduction

Substance abuse, defined here as the abuse of alcohol, cannabis, cocaine and heroin, in older adults is often neglected, both in science and in practice. Substance abuse is a serious public health issue as it not only affects physical and mental health of the abusers, it also leads to increased costs for society (Adams et al., 1993). Older adults with addiction problems deserve special attention. Compared to younger people, smaller amounts of substance may lead to intoxication and organ damage because of greater use of contraindicated medications, less efficient liver metabolism and decreases in lean body mass and total body water (Dufour & Fuller, 1995).

Substance use and abuse among people aged 50 and over is rapidly increasing in Europe and the United States (Beynon, 2009). For Europe, the number of older people with substance use problems is estimated to more than double between 2001 and 2020 (Gossop, 2008). This is partly due to the size of the baby-boom cohort (born between 1946 and 1964) and the higher rate of substance use among this group (Gfroerer et al., 2003). Estimates from the United States suggest that the number of adults aged 50 and over will double from 2.8 million (annual average) in 2002–06 to 5.7 million in 2020 (Han et al., 2009).

To reduce the negative trend in substance abuse, effective prevention is required. Cuijpers and Willemse (2005) distinguish four types of prevention in this context; universal prevention, selective prevention, indicated prevention and care based prevention. For each level of prevention, specific knowledge is needed. For universal prevention, targeted at the entire population regardless of the risk of addiction, knowledge about the prevalence, causes and adverse consequences of risk-full use are important. In selective prevention, aimed at groups at risk of becoming addicted, knowledge of risk factors is essential to identify the groups. For indicated prevention, aimed at people with limited symptoms, it is important to recognize signs of addiction and have knowledge of appropriate treatments. Finally, care based prevention, referring to people with an addiction according to DSM criteria, it is important to have insight into factors that influence the course of the disease. Insufficient knowledge of one or more levels of prevention can lead to under-recognition of addiction problems by social workers (Adams et al., 1992), lack of agreement between doctors on the causes and treatment of addiction (Brown, 1982), and people are still insufficiently aware of the importance and effects of proper treatment (McInnes & Powell, 1994).

In this chapter, an overview is given of what is known about the prevalence and the bio-psycho-social characteristics of older people who abuse substances. In addition, we will describe the known risk factors for the development and course of substance abuse.

2. Methods

2.1 Review

In addressing the aim of this chapter, three databases (PubMed, PsychINFO, and Socindex) were investigated for potentially relevant studies using the following keywords: "Alcohol", "drug abuse", "heroin", "cocaine", "cannabis", "substance abuse" each combined with AND (elderly OR older adults). Based on the title and abstract of each retrieved article the potential relevance for the current study was investigated. We selected only articles that were written in English, have appeared in peer-reviewed journals, were based on original quantitative empirical research, aiming at the older population (aged 50 years or older). Relevant information for answering the research questions was extracted from each selected article. For information on the prevalence and the bio-psycho-social characteristics of older people who abuse substances, studies containing information on one or more of the following characteristics were selected: prevalence, trends in use with age, bio-psycho-social characteristics of users, and risk-full use or addiction. For information on risk factors for the development and course of substance abuse, only longitudinal studies or case-control studies were selected.

2.2 Definitions

Substance abuse is defined in accord with the Diagnostic and Statistical Manual of Mental Disorders (DSM) if three or more of the following criteria were met: 1) tolerance, as defined by either a need for markedly increased amounts of the substance to achieve intoxication or the desired effect or markedly diminished effect with continued use of the same amount of the substance; 2) withdrawal, as manifested by the characteristic withdrawal syndrome for the substance or the same (or closely related) substance is taken to relieve or avoid withdrawal symptoms; 3) the substance is often taken in larger amounts or over a longer period than intended; 4) there is a persistent desire or unsuccessful efforts to cut down or control substance use; 5) a great deal of time is spent in activities necessary to obtain the substance, use the substance, or recover from its effects; 6) important social, occupational, or recreational activities are given up or reduced because of substance use; and 7) the substance use is continued despite knowledge of having a persistent physical or psychological problem that is likely to have been caused or exacerbated by the substance.

A limitation of the DSM classification is that it does not take account of the specific circumstances and life stage in which older people reside. The consequences of substance abuse are more visible in people who are still employed than in people who live alone, which is more prevalent among older people. Also milder forms of abuse or risky use can significantly affect the physical, cognitive and mental health of older adults. Therefore, also risk-full substance use will be addressed in this study.

3. Results

The literature search resulted in 432 studies potentially relevant to this investigation. Based on the title and abstract 81 studies were subsequently selected for further study and data extraction. Of the 81 selected studies, 75 studies were on alcohol consumption, 7 studies on alcohol use in combination with medicines and one study on cocaine and heroin use. Only a small fraction of all studies (n = 10) focused on addiction according to DSM-IV criteria. The results will be summarized around 6 themes: recognition of alcohol abuse, prevalence, changes in substance use with aging, bio-psycho-social characteristics of older substance users, risk factors, and consequences of abuse. In addition, also study results for risk-full of alcohol that does not fit the DSM criteria for an addiction will be summarized. The results will be described separately for alcohol, cannabis, heroin and cocaine.

3.1 Recognition of alcohol abuse

Assessing correct diagnosis regarding alcohol abuse is complicated (Aartsen et al., 2009). This is partly due to the reluctance of abusers and health care practitioners to discuss the drinking behavior. However, even without explicitly asking, there are signs that may indicate an underlying alcohol problem. For example, in some cases the breath of people can smell like alcohol, there may be complaints from the social environment of people about alcohol consumption, there may be convictions for driving with to much previous alcohol intake, and people may become annoyed once the subject is brought up to alcohol. Also, certain physical problems may indicate alcohol problems, such as hypertension, gastrointestinal problems, unexplained falls and psychological symptoms as anxiety and depression. There are screening instruments especially developed for older people that can help professionals to make a more deliberated diagnose. A simple, but not always adequate way is to ask how much alcohol is consumed on average per day. Besides the danger of under-reporting (people tend to underestimate their own drinking behavior), the average number of drinks per day is not always informative. Whether you drink two glasses a day, or once a week, 14 units, the average remains the same, but the social and physical consequences can vary widely. Moreover, one factor that affects the harmful effects of alcohol intake is the fat-moisture balance, and whether there are any concurrent medications or other chronic diseases that does not tolerate alcohol intake. A good alternative is the Alcohol Related Problem Survey (ARPS: Fink et al., 2002). The ARPS is a comprehensive questionnaire which not only questions drinking behavior, but also assesses health, life style, drug use and risky behaviors such as driving after alcohol use. Other screenings instruments are the Alcohol Use Disorders Identification Test (AUDIT), the Short Michigan Alcohol Screening Test-Geriatric (SMAST-G) and the Cut down, Annoyed, Guilty, Eye-opener test (CAGE).

3.2 Prevalence of substance use and abuse

Prevalence of risk-full alcohol consumption in the community ranged from 3 to 22% in men and 1 to 4% in women (Table 1). Men are two to five times more often risk-full alcohol consumers. The number of cannabis, heroin and cocaine users in the U.S. population is low (Blazer & Wu, 2009), of which the use of cannabis was the most prevalent. The annual prevalence of cannabis for people aged 50-64 year was 3,9%, and for people aged 65 0.7%. The annual prevalence of cocaine use by 50-64 year olds and 65 + was, respectively 0.68% and 0.04%. Heroin was used by 0.08% of 50-64 year old people. Heroin use is not observed among people aged 65 and over.

Prevalence rates of substance abuse, however, should be taken with caution. Taking into account that substance abuse among older adults is often under-diagnosed (Stewart & Oslin, 2001), and given the fact that only a small fraction of those with disorders related to substance abuse seek treatment, the actual number of older people with an alcohol use disorder in the general population must be much higher.

Alcohol First author and year of publication		**Country**
Breslow 2003	Prevalence of heavy drinking ranged from 9 to 10% in men and from 2% to 3% in women	US
Merrick 2008	16% of the men and 4% of the women are risk-full users	US
Du 2009	15% risk-full drinking, and 8% benzodiazepine and alcohol use	DE
Ganry 2001	3% of the 75+ women drank more than 30 grams per day	FR
Halme 2009	20% of the men and 1% of the women are heavy drinkers (more than 8 standard glasses per week)	FI
La Greca 1988	6% heavy users	US
Lang 2007	22% of the men and 4% of the women are heavy drinkers	GB
Rodgers 2005	7% of the men and 6% of the women drink hazardous amounts of alcohol	AU
Mirand 1996	13% of the men and 2% women were heavy drinkers	US
Cannabis, Cocaine, Heroin		
Blazer 2009	Prevalence of cannabis use: 3,9% for people aged 50-64 Prevalence of cannabis use: 0,7% 65 year old people Prevalence of cocaine use: 0,7% for people aged 50-64 Prevalence of cocaine use: 0,04% for 65 year old Prevalence of heroin use: 0,08% for people aged 50-64 Prevalence of heroin use: 0,0% 65 year old people	US

Table 1. Prevalence of alcohol, cannabis, cocaine and heroin use in society

In patient populations, prevalence rates of alcohol use were higher (Table 2). Estimates of the incidence of risk-full drinking range from 2% in women to 17% in men. Alcohol addiction in France varies in different patient populations from 3% in women and 18% in men (Lejoyeaux et al., 2003). Also Speckens et al., (1991) found high prevalence of alcohol in a university hospital in the Netherlands.

3.3 Developments in alcohol use with aging

Trends in alcohol use with aging were estimated in a number of longitudinal studies. Research in the United States (Adams et al., 1990) shows that older people generally reduce the number of drinks as they become older (each year a decrease of 2% drinkers). There is an indication for a gender effect. Men who drink heavily, but continue to drink, reduce drinking as opposed to heavily drinking women whose alcohol consumption remained stable (Breslow et al., 2003).

First author and year of publication		Country
Adams 1992	Prevalence of lifetime alcohol abuse: 24% Prevalence of current alcohol abuse: 14%.	US
Blow 2000	Prevalence of risk-full drinkers: 7%	US
Kahn 2001	Prevalence of risk-full alcohol use: 5%. Prevalence of lifetime alcohol abuse: men 37%, women 12%. Prevalence for last year alcohol abuse: 0.5%	NZ
Ganry 2000	Prevalence of risk-full alcohol use: men 17%, women 3%	FR
Kirchner 2007	Prevalence of risk-full drinkers: 5%	US
Lawley 1996	Prevalence of risk-full use: 12% Prevalence of abuse: 3%	GB
Lejoyeux 2003	Prevalence of alcohol abuse: 18% men and 3% women	FR
Onen 2005	Prevalence in Emergency Departments of alcohol abuse: 5,3%	BE
Speckens 1991	Prevalence of alcohol abuse: men 13%, women 7% women	NL

Table 2. Prevalence of alcohol abuse in patient population

3.4 Bio-psycho-social characteristics of older substance users

3.4.1 Alcohol

Older adults who are addicted to alcohol constitute a heterogeneous group consisting of people who have been addicted to alcohol before the age of 25 (early onset), people whose addiction started between the 25th and 45th year of life (late onset), and people who could remain at moderate levels of drinking till the age of 45, and became addicted at higher ages (very late onset). It is currently believed that the etiology and the course of alcohol disorders or risk-full drinking is complex and includes both genetic and environmental factors and the interaction of the two (Edenberg & Foroud, 2006). Genetic factors leading to differential risk for alcoholism were demonstrated using twin and family studies. In addition, functional polymorphisms of alcohol dehydrogenase (ADH2) and aldehyde dehydrogenase (ALDH2) genes have been shown to have a significant impact on alcohol metabolism in the liver, and thus, may contribute to vulnerability to alcohol abuse and dependence (Yokoyama & Omori, 2003). Antisocial personality is found to be a frequent cause of early onset (Watson et al., 1997), whereas very late onset seems to be more often induced by stressful life events (Hurt, 1988). Furthermore, early onset is more often seen among people who are homeless, who have family members with alcohol problems, and who have low socio-economic status, and people with very late onset often show better social functioning, have normal family lives and professional careers, rarely have a criminal history; furthermore, the course of very late onset is more favorable compared to early onset or late onset (Liberto & Oslin, 1995; Rigler, 2000).

Studies consistently show that there is a U-shaped relationship between alcohol use and mental and physical health. Abstainers, high-risk users and addicts have a poorer physical and mental health than moderate users (Blow et al., 2000; Brideveaux et al., 2004, Mukamal et al., 2001; Rodgers et al., 2005). Alcohol use appears to be related to prevailing beliefs about alcohol (Akers et al., 1989, Preston & Goodfellow, 2006; Graham & Braun, 1999).

Catholics, white people and non religious people drink significantly more than other ethnic groups or religions (Breslow et al., 2003; Forster et al., 1993, Merrick et al., 2008; Ruchlin, 1997). Higher education is associated with more, but also risk-full alcohol use (Breslow et al., 2003, Forster et al., 1993; Goodwin et al., 1987; Merrick et al., 2008; Ruchlin, 1997). Alcohol consumers smoke more than non-users (Mirand & Welte, 1996; Ganry et al., 2001), and alcoholics often live alone (Brennan, 2005; Onen et al., 2002).

First author	Main findings
Adlaf 1995	Men report more alcohol related problems then women
Aira 2005	Most alcohol drinkers used medications on a regular basis (86.9%) or as needed (87.8%).
Akers 1989	Drinking is related to the norms and behavior of one's primary groups, one's own attitudes toward (definitions of) alcohol, and the balance of reinforcement for drinking
Blow 2000	Low-risk drinkers were significantly better off than abstainers on the following domains: general health, physical functioning, bodily pain, vitality, mental health, emotional role, and social functioning. At-risk drinkers had significantly poorer mental health functioning than low-risk drinkers.
Brennan 2005	Nursing home residents with alcohol use disorders were more likely to have lived alone before admission and to have obtained mental health and social services. Residents with alcohol use disorders had somewhat better performance of basic activities than did residents in the demographically-matched sample group. Men with alcohol use disorders had shorter lengths of stay than did men without alcohol use disorders; women with alcohol use disorders had longer lengths of stay than did women without such disorders.
Breslow 2003	White people had the highest prevalence of moderate and heavier drinking compared with other racial/ethnic groups. Higher education was related to higher drinking levels. Moderate drinking was related to living with a partner.
Brideveaux 2004	Drinkers have a better health status than nondrinkers. Problem drinkers had lower health status than drinkers without drinking problems
Christie 2008	Controlling for age, gender, and vascular health, global Cerebral Blood Flow was greater in the lightest alcohol consumption group (<1 per week) and lower in the heaviest (>15 per week).
Forster 1993	Drinking is related to male gender, higher education, Catholic or no organized religious affiliation.
Ganry 2001	Smoking, good health status, higher socioeconomic status or single marital status are related to higher levels of alcohol use.
Gao 2009	Moderate current and lifetime alcohol consumption were found to be associated with reduced chronic atrophic arthritis compared to alcohol.
Geroldi 1994	Male gender, poorer cognitive function, and income dissatisfaction were significantly associated with alcohol problems.

First author	Main findings
Goodwin 1987	Alcohol intake was positively associated with male gender, income, cognitive functioning and amount of education and negatively associated with age.
Graham & Schmidt 1999	Depression was correlated with heavier drinking.
Graham & Braun 1999	Having a drinking spouse (versus an abstinent spouse) was associated with higher levels of drinking.
Kirchner 2007	Heavy drinking showed significant positive association with depressive/anxiety symptoms and less social support. Heavy drinking combined with binging was similarly positively associated with depressive/anxiety symptoms and perceived poor health.
Lang 2007	For both men and women, better cognition and subjective well-being, and fewer depressive symptoms, were associated with moderate levels of alcohol consumption than with never having drunk any.
Mattace-Raso 2005	Moderate alcohol consumption is associated with lower arterial stiffness in women but not in men independently of cardiovascular risk factors and atherosclerosis
Merrick 2008	Unhealthy drinking Is associated with higher education and income; better health status; male sex; younger age; smoking; being white; and being divorced, separated, or single. were associated with higher likelihood of unhealthy drinking. Among drinkers, in addition to socio-demographic variables, self reported depressive symptoms were positively associated with unhealthy drinking. Among unhealthy drinkers, race and ethnicity variables were associated with likelihood of heavy episodic drinking.
Midanik 1992	Sense of Coherence was a significant negative predictor of alcohol problems while controlling for alcohol consumption level, frequency of drunkenness and demographic characteristics.
Mirand 1996	Positive associations between heavy drinking and being male, having suburban residency, and currently using cigarettes. Negative relationships between heavy drinking and socioeconomic status, rural residency, and degree of health orientation.
Mukamal 2001	Moderate alcohol consumption is associated with a lower prevalence of white matter abnormalities and infarcts, thought to be of vascular origin, but with a dose-dependent higher prevalence of brain atrophy on MRI among older adults.
Mukamal 2004	Alcohol intake is associated with lower levels of inflammatory markers in older adults free of cardiovascular disease
Musick 2000	Alcohol use had no effect on depressive symptoms. One exception to this latter finding was that among rural Baptists who rarely attended religious services, using alcohol was associated with more depressive symptoms.

First author	Main findings
Onen 2002	Being homeless, living alone, being divorced and never married and being a man was associated with alcohol use disorders. Drinkers more commonly presented with gastrointestinal disorders.
Oslin 2005	Among people with alcohol use disorders, 22,3% has current depressive disorder, 44,9 physical disabilities, 13,6 anxiety disorder, 70,8% have college or higher education, 57% married. Compared to younger patients, they have less mental health problems, less severe alcohol use, and less outpatient treatment experience.
Preston 2006	Frequency of drinking and abuse is positively associated with personal approval of daily alcohol use and number of peers who use alcohol.
Rapuri 2000	Moderate alcohol intake was associated with higher bone mineral density in postmenopausal elderly women.
Rice 1995	Alcohol consumption was negatively associated with General Practitioners visits, controlling for gender and health
Riserus 2007	In men: self-estimated alcohol intake was not related to insulin sensitivity, early insulin response, or BMI, but was positively related to Waist Circumference.
Rodgers 2005	Abstainers have poorer cognitive function than light drinkers.
Ruchlin 1997	Everyday drinkers are more likely to being male, white, higher educated, living in the city centre and less likely to be in less than in excellent health, having diabetes, and believing that drinking has negative health consequences.
Schuckit 1978	Compared to younger alcoholics, older alcoholics had relatively more stable lives in early years and had developed alcohol-related problems in later years
Sheahan 1995	Alcohol use is not related to falls
Steunenberg 2008	Depression and alcohol use are not related in this very old, mostly female population. Alcohol use was related to extraversion and openness to experience. Chronic diseases was related to non-alcohol use and parental problem drinking was found to be a risk factor for late life problem drinking.
Sulander 2004	Higher alcohol use was more common among retired office workers than other former employees.
Westerterp 2004	Alcohol intake does not lead to increased body weight, probably due to the higher physical activity level

Table 3. Bio-Psycho-Social chraracteristics of older people who (ab)use alcohol

The relationship between cognitive functioning, cognitive pathology and drinking is more complicated. Risk-full use seems to be associated with worse cognitive function (Geroldi et al., 1994) and moderate use with better cognitive function (Goodwin et al., 1987; Lang et al., 2007; Rodgers et al., 2005). There are indications that the relationship is actually spurious, as the relation disappears when controlling for other potential influences (Cooper et al., 2009; Goodwin et al., 1987).

Several studies found a relationship with physical characteristics. Women who drink moderate levels of alcohol have a higher density of mineral in bone (Ilich et al., 2002; Rapuri et al., 2000). A positive correlation between alcohol use, reduced inflammation, lower prevalence of strokes

and white matter pathology, and the quality of blood vessels is found by Christie et al. (2008), Gao et al.(2009), Mattace-Raso et al. (2005) and Mukamal et al. (2001, 2004).
Risk-full drinkers appear to be more often depressed (Blow et al., 2000, Graham & Schmidt, 1999; Oslin et al., 2005), while moderate drinkers have fewer levels of depressive symptoms (Blow et al., 2000, Graham & Schmidt, 1999; Kirchner et al., 2007; Lang et al., 2007, Merrick et al, 2008). A relationship between alcohol and depression was however not found in very old nursing home residents (Steunenberg et al., 2008) and older Baptists (Musick, 2000).

3.4.2 Cannabis, cocaine and heroin

One study reported information on older cannabis, cocaine and heroin users. These users are more often male, single, and have depressive symptoms, but no differences in educational background are observed (Blazer & Wu, 2009).

3.5 Risk factors for substance abuse

Only one longitudinal study examined risk factors for risk-full drinking (Moos et al., 2010). The study revealed that a lower quality of marriage, lower participation in social activities, approval of drinking by friends and larger financial resources lead to an increased risk of risky alcohol use.

3.6 Consequences of substance use

In general, moderate consumption of alcohol has beneficial effects on physical and mental health, while risk-full use entails negative effects. Moderate alcohol use leads to higher bone density (Felson et al., 1995), longer life (Brideveaux et al., 2004; Colditz et al., 1985; Simons et al., 2000;), and reduced risk of Type 2 Diabetes (Djousse et al., 2007). Moderate alcohol consumption may also have some negative consequences as it may increase blood pressure, glycemia and body weight (Buja et al., 2010). Risk-full alcohol use leads to an increased risk of mental health problems (Friedman et al., 1999) and mortality (Gronbaek et al., 1998) and possibly an increased risk of acute pneumonia (Van der Horst Graat et al., 2007).

4. Conclusions

This study provides an overview of scientific knowledge in the field of substance abuse (alcohol, cannabis, heroin, and cocaine) in people aged 55 and older. Three databases were searched for relevant literature. There is useful information on alcohol use and risk-full use, but large gaps in knowledge about substance abuse exists. Research on alcohol addiction is limited and use of cannabis, cocaine and heroin in older adults is virtually absent. Moreover, many of the studies had a cross-sectional design, which limits conclusions about causes and effects. An additional problem is that most of the studies were conducted in the United States, while that information not necessarily applies to other countries because of cultural differences is (Vaz De Almeida et al., 2005).
Nevertheless, an outline of people who use risk-full amounts of alcohol became visible. First, there is a U-shaped relationship between amount of alcohol use and health. Moderate users are healthier than high-risk users and abstainers. The fact that abstainers were worse of than moderate users is possibly explained on the basis of the great heterogeneity in the non-using group. Not drinking is associated with certain medications and thus indicates the presence of disease, previous alcohol dependence, but also a healthy lifestyle.

High-risk alcohol users were more often male (2-5 times more), live in social environments where alcohol is not condemned, are higher educated, smoke more often, are more often single or depressed and may have poorer cognitive function. With age, the average consumption of alcohol decreases, except for risk-full drinking women. The consequences of risk-full alcohol use are decreased mental health and increased mortality. Very little is known about causes of alcohol addiction.

For information about use of cannabis, heroin and cocaine in older adults, we can only rely on one study conducted in the US. Of the three, cannabis is most often used, particularly 50-64 year olds (year prevalence 3.89% and 0.69% at 65). Less than 1 percent of older people use cocaine, while heroin use is not seen in people over 65 (Blazer & Wu, 2009).

In sum, it appears that knowledge of substance abuse in older adults is still mainly limited to the description of bio-psycho-social characteristics of older adults with alcohol abuse. Knowledge of prevalence, causes, consequences and characteristics of the elderly who according to DSM criteria are addicted to any of the tested agents is still virtually absent. The design of effective prevention of substance abuse in older adults, as well as effective therapies is therefore strongly hampered. With respect to universal and selective prevention at the population level, more research is required into causes and consequences of substance abuse. For effective care-oriented prevention research into the effects of treatments in patients populations such as in addiction clinics is needed in order to improve the effect of treatment programs.

5. Acknowledgements

The literature review was supported by The Netherlands Organization for Scientific Research NWO/ZonMW (project number 31160205).

6. References

Aartsen, M., Van Etten, D. & Spitsbaard, A. (2009). Older people and substance abuse [Ouderen en verslavingsproblematiek]. In: *Addiction, handbook for care, support and prevention,* Rutten, R., Loth, C. & Hulshof, A., pp.255-267, Elseviers gezondheidszorg, ISBN 978 90 352 3071 2, Maarssen, The Netherlands.

Adams, W. L., Garry, P. J., Rhyne, R., Hunt, W. C., & Goodwin, J. S. (1990). Alcohol intake in the healthy elderly. Changes with age in a cross-sectional and longitudinal study. *J.Am.Geriatr.Soc.,* 38, 211-216.

Adams, W. L., Magruder-Habib, K., Trued, S., & Broome, H. L. (1992). Alcohol abuse in elderly emergency department patients. *J.Am.Geriatr.Soc.,* 40, 1236-1240.

Adams, W. L., Yuan, Z., Barboriak, J. J., & Rimm, A. A. (1993). Alcohol-related hospitalizations of elderly people. Prevalence and geographic variation in the United States. *JAMA,* 270, 1222-1225.

Adlaf, E. M. & Smart, R. G. (1995). Alcohol use, drug use, and well-being in older adults in Toronto. *Int.J.Addict.,* 30, 1985-2016.

Aira, M., Hartikainen, S., & Sulkava, R. (2005). Community prevalence of alcohol use and concomitant use of medication. A source of possible risk in the elderly aged 75 and older? *Int.J.Geriatr.Psychiatry,* 20, 680-685.

Akers, R. L., La Greca, A. J., Cochran, J., & Sellers, C. (1989). Social learning theory and alcohol behavior among the elderly. *The Sociological Quarterly,* 30, 625-638.

Blazer, D. G. & Wu, L. T. (2009). The epidemiology of substance use and disorders among middle aged and elderly community adults: national survey on drug use and health. *Am.J.Geriatr.Psychiatry*, 17, 237-245.

Blow, F. C., Walton, M. A., Barry, K. L., Coyne, J. C., Mudd, S. A., & Copeland, L. A. (2000). The relationship between alcohol problems and health functioning of older adults in primary care settings. *J.Am.Geriatr.Soc.*, 48, 769-774.

Brennan, P. L. (2005). Functioning and health service use among elderly nursing home residents with alcohol use disorders: findings from the National Nursing Home Survey. *Am.J.Geriatr.Psychiatry*, 13, 475-483.

Breslow, R. A., Faden, V. B., & Smothers, B. (2003). Alcohol consumption by elderly Americans. *J.Stud.Alcohol*, 64, 884-892.

Bridevaux, I. P., Bradley, K. A., Bryson, C. L., McDonell, M. B., & Fihn, S. D. (2004). Alcohol screening results in elderly male veterans: association with health status and mortality. *J.Am.Geriatr.Soc.*, 52, 1510-1517.

Brown, B. B. (1982). Professionals' perceptions of drug and alcohol abuse among the elderly. *Gerontologist*, 22, 519-525.

Buja, A., Scafato, E., Sergi, G., Maggi, S., Suhad, M. A., Rausa, G. et al. (2010). Alcohol consumption and metabolic syndrome in the elderly: results from the Italian longitudinal study on aging. *Eur.J.Clin.Nutr.*, 64, 297-307.

Christie, I. C., Price, J., Edwards, L., Muldoon, M., Meltzer, C. C., & Jennings, J. R. (2008). Alcohol consumption and cerebral blood flow among older adults. *Alcohol*, 42, 269-275.

Colditz, G. A., Branch, L. G., Lipnick, R. J., Willett, W. C., Rosner, B., Posner, B. et al. (1985). Moderate alcohol and decreased cardiovascular mortality in an elderly cohort. *Am.Heart J.*, 109, 886-889.

Cooper, C., Bebbington, P., Meltzer, H., Jenkins, R., Brugha, T., Lindesay, J. E. et al. (2009). Alcohol in moderation, premorbid intelligence and cognition in older adults: results from the Psychiatric Morbidity Survey. *J.Neurol.Neurosurg.Psychiatry*, 80, 1236-1239.

Cuijpers, P., & Willemse, G. (2005) Preventie van depressie bij ouderen: Een overzicht van interventies. Trimbos Instituut, Utrecht 2005.

Djousse, L., Biggs, M. L., Mukamal, K. J., & Siscovick, D. S. (2007). Alcohol consumption and type 2 diabetes among older adults: the Cardiovascular Health Study. *Obesity.(Silver.Spring)*, 15, 1758-1765.

Du, Y., Scheidt-Nave, C., & Knopf, H. (2008). Use of psychotropic drugs and alcohol among non-institutionalised elderly adults in Germany. *Pharmacopsychiatry*, 41, 242-251.

Dufour, M & Fuller, R.K. (1995) Alcohol in the elderly. Annual Review of Medicine, 46, 123-132

Edenberg, H.J. & Foroud, T. (2006). The genetics of alcohol disorder: Identifying specific genes through family studies. *Addiction Biology*, 11, 386-396.

Felson, D. T., Zhang, Y., Hannan, M. T., Kannel, W. B., & Kiel, D. P. (1995). Alcohol intake and bone mineral density in elderly men and women. The Framingham Study. *Am.J.Epidemiol.*, 142, 485-492.

Fink, A., Morton, S.C., Beck, J.C., e.a. (2002). The alcohol-related problems survey: Identifying hazardous and harmful drinking in older primary care patients. *Journal of American Geriatrics Society*, 50, 1717-1722.

Forster, L. E., Pollow, R., & Stoller, E. P. (1993). Alcohol use and potential risk for alcohol-related adverse drug reactions among community-based elderly. *Journal of Community Health,* 18, 225-239.

Friedmann, P. D., Jin, L., Karrison, T., Nerney, M., Hayley, D. C., Mulliken, R. et al. (1999). The effect of alcohol abuse on the health status of older adults seen in the emergency department. *Am.J.Drug Alcohol Abuse,* 25, 529-542.

Ganry, O., Joly, J. P., Queval, M. P., & Dubreuil, A. (2000). Prevalence of alcohol problems among elderly patients in a university hospital. *Addiction,* 95, 107-113.

Ganry, O., Baudoin, C., Fardellone, P., & Dubreuil, A. (2001). Alcohol consumption by non-institutionalised elderly women: the EPIDOS Study. *Public Health,* 115, 186-191.

Gao, L., Weck, M. N., Stegmaier, C., Rothenbacher, D., & Brenner, H. (2009). Alcohol consumption and chronic atrophic gastritis: population-based study among 9,444 older adults from Germany. *Int.J.Cancer,* 125, 2918-2922.

Geroldi, C., Rozzini, R., Frisoni, G. B., & Trabucchi, M. (1994). Assessment of alcohol consumption and alcoholism in the elderly. *Alcohol,* 11, 513-516.

Gfroerer, J., Penne, M., Pemberton, M., & Folson, R. (2003). Substance abuse treatment need among older adults in 2020. The impact of the aging baby-boom cohort. *Drug and Alcohol Dependence,* 69, 127-135.

Goodwin, J. S., Sanchez, C. J., Thomas, P., Hunt, C., Garry, P. J., & Goodwin, J. M. (1987). Alcohol intake in a healthy elderly population. *Am.J.Public Health,* 77, 173-177.

Gossop, M (2008) *Substance Use among Older Adults: A Neglected Problem.* Lisbon: European Monitoring Centre for Drugs and Drug Addiction; 2008. Available from http://www.emcdda.europa.eu/attachements.cfm/att_50566_EN_TDAD08001EN C_web.pdf

Graham, K. & Schmidt, G. (1999). Alcohol use and psychosocial well-being among older adults. *J.Stud.Alcohol,* 60, 345-351.

Graham, K. & Braun, K. (1999). Concordance of use of alcohol and other substances among older adult couples. *Addictive Behaviors,* 24, 839-856.

Gronbaek, M., Deis, A., Becker, U., Hein, H. O., Schnohr, P., Jensen, G. et al. (1998). Alcohol and mortality: is there a U-shaped relation in elderly people? *Age Ageing,* 27, 739-744.

Halme, J. T., Seppa, K., Alho, H., Poikolainen, K., Pirkola, S., & Aalto, M. (2010). Alcohol consumption and all-cause mortality among elderly in Finland. *Drug Alcohol Depend.,* 106, 212-218.

Han, B, Gfroerer, J.C., Colliver, J.D. & Penne, M.A. (2009) Substance use disorder among older adults in the United States in 2020. *Addiction,* 104, 88-96

Hurt, R.D., Finlayson, R.E. Morse, R.M., & Davis, L.J. (1988), *Alcoholism in elderly persons: Medical aspects and prognosis of 216 inpatients,* in: Mayo Clinic Procedures, 63, 8, 761-768.

Ilich, J. Z., Brownbill, R. A., Tamborini, L., & Crncevic-Orlic, Z. (2002). To drink or not to drink: how are alcohol, caffeine and past smoking related to bone mineral density in elderly women? *J.Am.Coll.Nutr.,* 21, 536-544.

Khan, N., Wilkinson, T. J., Sellman, J. D., & Graham, P. (2001). Patterns of alcohol use and misuse among elderly rest home residents in Christchurch. *N.Z.Med.J.,* 114, 58-61.

Kirchner, J. E., Zubritsky, C., Cody, M., Coakley, E., Chen, H., Ware, J. H. et al. (2007). Alcohol consumption among older adults in primary care. *J.Gen.Intern.Med.,* 22, 92-97.

La Greca, A., Akers, R. L., & Dwyer, J. W. (1988). Life events and alcohol behavior among older adults. *Gerontologist*, 28, 552-558.

Lang, I., Wallace, R. B., Huppert, F. A., & Melzer, D. (2007). Moderate alcohol consumption in older adults is associated with better cognition and well-being than abstinence. *Age Ageing*, 36, 256-261.

Lawley, D. I., Reham, H., & Kendrick, D. (1996). The misuse of alcohol in elderly psychiatric patients. *Psychiatric Bulletin*, 20, 310.

Liberto, J.G. & Oslin, D.W. (1995). Early versus late onset alcohol disorder in the elderly. International Journal of Addiction, 30, 1799-1818.

Lejoyeux, M., Delaroque, F., McLoughlin, M., & Ades, J. (2003). Alcohol dependence among elderly French inpatients. *Am.J.Geriatr.Psychiatry*, 11, 360-364.

Mattace-Raso, F. U., van der Cammen, T. J., van den Elzen, A. P., Schalekamp, M. A., Asmar, R., Reneman, R. S. et al. (2005). Moderate alcohol consumption is associated with reduced arterial stiffness in older adults: the Rotterdam study. *J.Gerontol.A Biol.Sci.Med.Sci.*, 60, 1479-1483.

McInnes, E. & Powell, J. (1994). Drug and alcohol referrals: are elderly substance abuse diagnoses and referrals being missed? *BMJ*, 308, 444-446.

Merrick, E., Horgan, C. M., Hodgkin, D., Garnick, D. W., Houghton, S. F., Panas, L. et al. (2008). Unhealthy Drinking Patterns in Older Adults: Prevalence and Associated Characteristics. *Journal of American Geriatrics Society*, 56, 214-223.

Midanik, L. T., Soghikian, K., Ransom, L. J., & Polen, M. R. (1992). Alcohol problems and sense of coherence among older adults. *Soc.Sci.Med.*, 34, 43-48.

Mirand, A. L. & Welte, J. W. (1996). Alcohol consumption among the elderly in a general population, Erie County, New York. *Am.J.Public Health*, 86, 978-984.

Moos, R. H., Brennan, P. L., Schutte, K. K., & Moos, B. S. (2010). Social and financial resources and high-risk alcohol consumption among older adults. *Alcohol Clin.Exp.Res.*, 34, 646-654.

Mukamal, K. J., Longstreth, W. T., Jr., Mittleman, M. A., Crum, R. M., & Siscovick, D. S. (2001). Alcohol consumption and subclinical findings on magnetic resonance imaging of the brain in older adults: the cardiovascular health study. *Stroke*, 32, 1939-1946.

Mukamal, K. J., Cushman, M., Mittleman, M. A., Tracy, R. P., & Siscovick, D. S. (2004). Alcohol consumption and inflammatory markers in older adults: the Cardiovascular Health Study. *Atherosclerosis*, 173, 79-87.

Mukamal, K. J., Chung, H., Jenny, N. S., Kuller, L. H., Longstreth, W. T., Jr., Mittleman, M. A. et al. (2005). Alcohol use and risk of ischemic stroke among older adults: the cardiovascular health study. *Stroke*, 36, 1830-1834.

Musick, M. A. (2000). Religious Activity, Alcohol Use, and Depression in a Sample of Elderly Baptists. *Research on Aging*, 22, 91.

Onen, S.H., Onen, F., Mangeon, J. P., Abidi, H., Courpron, P., & Schmidt, J. (2005). Alcohol abuse and dependence in elderly emergency department patients. *Archives of Gerontology and Geriatrics*, 41, 191-200.

Oslin, D. W., Slaymaker, V. J., Blow, F. C., Owen, P. L., & Colleran, C. (2005). Treatment outcomes for alcohol dependence among middle-aged and older adults. *Addict.Behav.*, 30, 1431-1436.

Preston, P. & Goodfellow, M. (2006). Cohort comparisons: social learning explanations for alcohol use among adolescents and older adults. *Addict.Behav.*, 31, 2268-2283.

Rapuri, P. B., Gallagher, J. C., Balhorn, K. E., & Ryschon, K. L. (2000). Alcohol intake and bone metabolism in elderly women. *Am.J.Clin.Nutr.*, 72, 1206-1213.

Rice, C. & Duncan, D. F. (1995). Alcohol use and reported physician visits in older adults. *Preventive Medicine*, 24, 229-234.

Rigler, S.K. (2000), Alcoholism in the elderly. *American Family Physician* 61, 1710-1725.

Riserus, U. & Ingelson, E. (2007). Alcohol intake, insulin resistance, and abdominal obesity in elderly men. *Obesity*, 15, 1766-1773.

Rodgers, B., Windsor, T. D., Anstey, K. J., Dear, K. B., Jorm, F., & Christensen, H. (2005). Non-linear relationships between cognitive function and alcohol consumption in young, middle-aged and older adults: the PATH Through Life Project. *Addiction*, 100, 1280-1290.

Ruchlin, H. S. (1997). Prevalence and correlates of alcohol use among older adults. *Prev.Med.*, 26, 651-657.

Schuckit, M. A., Morrissey, E. R., & O'Leary, M. R. (1978). Alcohol problems in elderly men and women. *Addictive Diseases*, 3, 405-416.

Sheahan, S. L., Coons, S. J., Robbins, C. A., & Martin, S. S. (1995). Psychoactive medication, alcohol use, and falls among older adults. *Journal of Behavioral Medicine*, 18, 127-140.

Simons, L. A., McCallum, J., Friedlander, Y., Ortiz, M., & Simons, J. (2000). Moderate alcohol intake is associated with survival in the elderly: the Dubbo Study. *Med.J.Aust.*, 173, 121-124.

Speckens, A. E., Heeren, T. J., & Rooijmans, H. G. (1991). Alcohol abuse among elderly patients in a general hospital as identified by the Munich Alcoholism Test. *Acta Psychiatr.Scand.*, 83, 460-462.

Steunenberg, B., Yagmur, S., & Cuijpers, P. (2008). Depression and alcohol use among the Dutch residential home elderly: Is there a shared vulnerability? *Addiction Research & Theory*, 16, 514-525.

Stewart, D., & Oslin, D.W. (2001). Recognition and treatment of late-life addictions in medical settings. *Journal of Clinical Geropsychology*, 7, 145-158.

Sulander, T., Helakorpi, S., Rahkonen, O., Nissinen, A., & Uutela, A. (2004). Smoking and alcohol consumption among the elderly: trends and associations, 1985-2001. *Prev.Med.*, 39, 413-418.

Van der Horst Graat JM, Terpstra, J. S., Kok, F. J., & Schouten, E. G. (2007). Alcohol, smoking, and physical activity related to respiratory infections in elderly people. *J.Nutr.Health Aging*, 11, 80-85.

Vaz De Almeida, M. D., Davidson, K., De Morais, C., Marshall, H., Bofill, S., Grunert, K. G. et al. (2005). Alcohol consumption in elderly people across European countries: Results from the food in later life project. *Ageing International*, 30, 377-395.

Watson, C.G., Hancock,M.B.A., Gearhart, L.P.M., Malovrh, P., Mendez, C.B.S. & Raden, M.B.A (1997). A comparison of the symptoms associated with early and late onset alcohol dependence. *The Journal of Nervous and Mental Disease*, 185, 507-509.

Westerterp, K.R., Meijer, E.P., Goris, A.H.C., & Kester, A.D.M. (2004). Alcohol energy intake and habital physical activity in older adults. *British Journal of Nutrition*, 91, 149-152.

16

Tobacco Addiction

Stephan Muehlig
Chemnitz University of Technology
Germany

1. Introduction

"Tobacco is the single most preventable cause of death in the world today. This year, tobacco will kill more than five million people – more than tuberculosis, HIV/AIDS and malaria combined. By 2030, the death toll will exceed eight million a year. Unless urgent action is taken tobacco could kill one billion people during this century. Tobacco is the only legal consumer product that can harm everyone exposed to it – and it kills up to half of those who use it as intended." (WHO Report on the global tobacco epidemic, 2008, p. 8)

Although nearly all smokers are aware of the outstanding healthy risks of cigarette smoking and the majority of them is willing to quit, only a small proportion of regular smokers is able to stop smoking successfully. Within 12 months after a stop smoking trial, only 2-6% of quitters remain abstinent. This high relapse rate can only be explained by mechanisms of addiction. The term *"tobabacco addiction"* refers to the definition of substance use disorders, which includes harmful substance use as well as physiological and psychological dependence. This chapter aims to summarize the current state of knowledge regarding to the phenomenon of tobacco addiction and tobacco use related disorder.

2. Classification, epidemiology, etiology, and treatment of tobacco addiction

2.1 Diagnostic classification

Tobacco addiction states a mental disorder with severe somatic and mental symptoms and consequences. The term '*addiction*' was, due to its terminological vagueness, discarded as an official name for a diagnostic category by the WHO in 1964, however it is still used today in everyday speech and as part of the technical language. Within the current clinical classification systems DSM-IV and ICD-10 the phenomene of addiction caused by psychotropic substances is classified in two different diagnostic categories: DSM-IV differenciates '*substance dependence*' (303.xx) and '*substance abuse*' (305.xx) whereas ICD-10 refers to 'dependence' and '*harmful use*' (F1x.1). According to DSM, drug dependence is defined by seven diagnostic core criteria of which three must be met along with clinically important suffering in order to confirm the diagnosis. In contrast, abuse is determined by repeated, maladjusted substance use and psychosocial impairments (e.g., interpersonal problems, legal problems, high risk behaviour) over a period of at least 12 months (cf. Tab. 1).

There is a clinical and neurobiological distinction between somatic and mental addiction. *Somatic addiction* is primarily defined by development of tolerance and physiological withdrawal symptoms. That means, the organism "gets used" to the regular dose of the

DSM-IV-TR		**DSM-V**
Nicotine Abuse	**Nicotine Dependence**	**Tobacco Use Disorder**
at least one of the following *criteria* within the same 12 months period: (1) Severe problems regarding family, home, profession or school due to substance use (2) Substance use in dangerous situations (3)Legal problems due to substance use (4) Social and/or interpersonal problems due to substance use The symptoms have never fulfilled the criteria for substance addiction of the respective substance class.	*at least three* of the following *criteria* within the same 12 months period: (1) Development of tolerance (2) Withdrawal symptoms (3) Substance use longer or in larger quantities than intended (4) Permanent wish or failure to control substance use (5) Time-consuming procurement, use and recovery from substance (6) Important social, professional or recreational activities are given up or limited due to substance use (7) Continued substance use despite physical or psychic problems	*maladaptive pattern of substance use leading to clinically significant impairment or distress, as manifested by 2 (or more) of the following, occurring within a 12-month period:* 1. recurrent substance use resulting in a failure to fulfill major role obligations at work, school, or home 2. recurrent substance use in situations in which it is physically hazardous 3. continued substance use despite having persistent or recurrent social or interpersonal problems caused or exacerbated by the effects of the substance 4. tolerance, as defined by either of the following: a need for markedly increased amounts of the substance to achieve intoxication or desired effect b) markedly diminished effect with continued use of the same amount of the substance 5. withdrawal, as manifested by either of the following: a) the characteristic withdrawal syndrome for the substance; b) the same (or a closely related) substance is taken to relieve or avoid withdrawal symptoms 6. the substance is often taken in larger amounts or over a longer period than was intended 7. there is a persistent desire or unsuccessful efforts to cut down or control substance use 8. a great deal of time is spent in activities necessary to obtain the substance, use the substance, or recover from its effects 9. important social, occupational, or recreational activities are given up or reduced because of substance use 10. the substance use is continued despite knowledge of having a persistent or recurrent physical or psychological problem that is likely to have been caused or exacerbated by the substance 11. Craving or a strong desire or urge to use a specific substance.

Table 1. Tobacco-related Disorders according to DSM-IV-TR vs. DSM-V.

substance and thus needs ever increasing amounts to reach the desired state of intoxication (dose increase), however, also can tolerate higher doses than at the beginning of drug use (tolerance). In contrast, the *mental addiction* is characterized by behavioral patterns such as compulsive use, loss of control, addiction memory, craving and coping deficits. The term "addiction" refers more to the mental aspect of the dependency, i.e. to the continuing compulsive consumption of the drug despite negative effects and/or despite the wish to stop drug use. Whereas the somatic dependency syndrome is generally gone some weeks after the withdrawal, the addiction memory may remain active for years and decades and continue to trigger periodical craving or even relapses from time to time. Thus, a dependent smoker may have stopped to be dependent on tobacco after successful withdrawal therapy but he/she may remain addicted, possibly for his/her whole life.

Within the process for revising the Diagnostic and Statistical Manual of Mental Disorders *(DSM-V)* the work group which is responsible for addressing substance use disorders currently developed new recommendations to redefine these diagnostic categories. Among the work group's proposals are the following recommendations:

i. To move the categories of 'abuse' and 'dependence' in one common diagnosis category named 'Substance-Related Disorders';
ii. To include both substance use disorders and non-substance addictions (Gambling disorder, Internet addiction) in this new diagnostic category
iii. To tentatively re-title the category into the term 'Addiction and Related Disorders'.

In consequence, the diagnosis 'Nicotine Dependence' (305.1) should be replaced by *'Tobacco Use Disorder'* which includes 11 diagnostic criteria (s. table 1).

2.2 Epidemiology

2.2.1 Prevalence of cigarette smoking and nicotine dependence

The epidemiology of addictive smoking can be demonstrated by international *point prevalence* as well as *life-time prevalence* data of representative population-based health surveys. The rates of current smokers in adult population (> 14 years) are extremely varying by country and gender (figure 2).

Approximately one half of the smoking men and one-third of the women are classified as heavy smokers (>20 cig./day). However, not every chronic cigarette smoker will necessarily become addicted to nicotine or tobacco. A number of international epidemiological studies found that only a minority of persistent smokers become dependent according the diagnostic criteria for substance use disorders described above. In a currently conducted, well controlled population survey on nearly 8,000 representative participants in Germany, 6.3% participants among the total sample and 29.9% of all current smokers (smoking rate: 29,6%) met the DSM-IV criteria for a *nicotine dependence disorder* (Papst et al., 2010). Nevertheless, nicotine dependence has an outstanding significance from an epidemiological perspective since, with a lifetime prevalence of 17% and 21% (cf. Tab. 2), it is one of the most common mental disorders, compared to affective disorders (lifetime prevalence: 12-19%) or anxiety disorders (LT prevalence: 15%). By trend, nicotine dependence occurred more often in female smokers and in younger age groups compared with older cohorts. In Lifetime, 50% of all smokers succeed to quit, mostly after 5-10 ineffective attempts.

Approximately every second smoker who has tried to quit smoking reports somatic withdrawal symptoms that manifest themselves in psycho-vegetative conditions or cognitive-emotional adverse effects (cf. table 3). The *nicotine withdrawal syndrome* starts 2-4 hours after the last cigarette, reaches its intensity peak after 24-48 hours and gradually passes after 1-4 weeks. However, the primarily mental symptoms (craving, feeling of hunger, dysphoria) may persist for months.

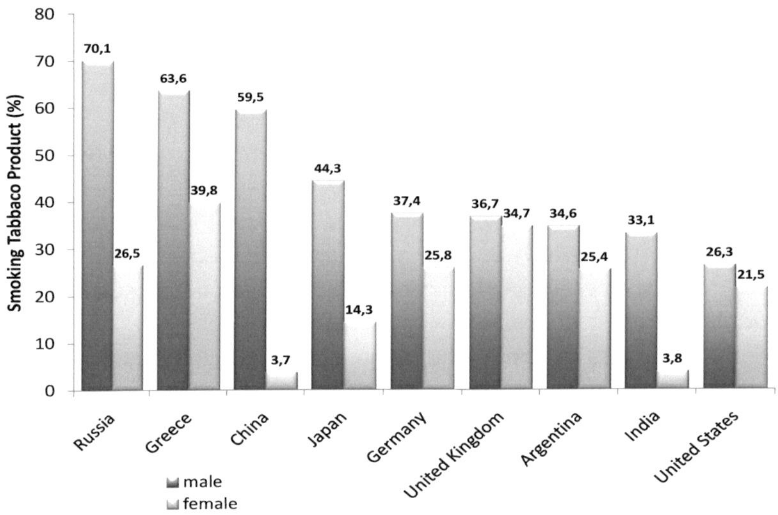

Fig. 1. WHO Report on the Global Tabacco Epidemic (2008)

	Total		Gender	
			Men	Women
Consumption prevalence (30 d)[1]	7,983		3,542	4,441
Non-Smokers	44.8%	(3,858)	38.8%	51.0%
Ex-smokers	26.0%	(1,771)	28.5%	23.6%
Smokers	29.2%	(2,354)	32.8%	25.5%
Consumption frequency (30 d)[2]	2,238		1,096	1,142
Not daily	29.6%	(714)	28.4%	31.0%
Daily up to 10	21.7%	(530)	17.4%	27.1%
Daily 11-19	23.5%	(517)	25.7%	20.9%
Daily more than 20	25.2%	(477)	28.5%	21.1%
DSM-IV (12M)[3]	7,984		3,521	4,427
Total sample	6.3%	(531)	6.8%	5.8%
Consumers[4]	19.9%	(531)	19.2%	20.9%

[1] Non-Smokers: have smoked a total of maximum 100 cigarettes; ex-smoker: have smoked more than 100 cigarettes, but not in the previous 30 days; smokers: smoked cigarettes in the previous 30 days.
[2] Referring to cigarette smokers during the previous 30 days.
[3] Nicotine dependence according to DSM-IV: unweighted number of cases regarding to total sample
[4] Referring to 12 months prevalence of smoking.

Table 2. Prevalence of smoking, of smoke frequency and nicotine dependence according to DSM-IV (Papst e al., 2010, p. 332)

- craving
- increased appetite, sensation of hunger, weight gain
- concentration problems
- nervousness, irritability, restlessness, insomnia
- feeling of frustration, unhappiness, depressive moods, depression, states of anxiety, anxieties
- circulation problems, sweating, digestive disorders

Table 3. Withdrawal symptoms during the smoke stop

The strength of the nicotine dependency can best be measured through specific withdrawal symptoms. The *Fagerstrom Test for Nicotine Dependence (FTND*; Heatherton et al., 1991; cf. table 4), which consists of six items, is recommended worldwide as a dimensional research tool for the measurement of nicotine dependency. This test has been validated in international studies and represents one of the best predictors for abstinence success.

Questions	Answers	Points
1 . How soon after you wake up do you smoke your first cigarette?	Within 5 minutes	3
	6 – 30 minutes	2
	31 – 60 minutes	1
	After 60 minutes	0
2. Do you find it difficult to refrain from smoking in places where it is forbidden, e.g., in church, at the library, in the cinema, etc.?	Yes	1
	No	0
3. Which cigarette would you hate most to give up?	The first one in the morning.	1
	Any other.	0
4. How many cigarettes/day do you smoke?	10 or less	0
	11 – 20	1
	21 – 30	2
	31 or more	3
5. Do you smoke more frequently during the first hours after awakening than during the rest of the day?	Yes	1
	No	0
6. Do you smoke if you are so ill that you are in bed most of the day?	Yes	1
	No	0
Score: Possible range is 0 – 10: Scores of 4 and greater indicating nicotine dependence Scores of 4 and greater indicating severe nicotine dependence		

Table 4. Fagerstrom Test for Nicotine Dependence (FTND; Heatherton et al., 1991)

2.2.2 Addiction and risk potential of the drug tobacco

The *'addiction potential'* of a drug describes the risk for developing a mental or physical dependence when using a drug and the subsequent failure to quit the use and to master a withdrawal. This addiction risk results from a) the pharmacological effects of the substance on the organism, b) the quality and intensity of the evoked subjective states of intoxication or well-being and c) the learned stimulus-response association between the drug use on the one hand and the 'kick' or flush response (positive reinforcement) and/or the avoidance of withdrawal symptoms on the other (negative reinforcement). The addiction potential of a psychotropic substance is not exclusively determined by its pharmacological characteristics and its potency for physical dependence but essentially, among other things, by the type of the substance intake (addiction potential decreasing with types of applications: injecting, sniffing, smoking and swallowing). This explains that smoked nicotine has a high addiction potential compared to nicotine patches at the same dose.

Alongside heroin, nicotine is seen as the substance with the highest *'pure addiction potential'*. This finding has been determined in animal studies wherein different substances are applied in standardised form (e.g. as an oral application). The measure for the addiction potential is typical addiction behaviour shown by the laboratory animals after a number of applications (e.g. number of lever actions or toleration of pain stimuli in order to get to the drug). However, the approaches for the determination of the addiction potential that are based on complex expert judgements on the addiction risk of persons under real using conditions seem to be more adequate. In a study conducted by the Swiss Institute for the Prevention of Alcohol and Drug Problems (SIPA), renowned addiction experts evaluated the addiction potential of seven different substances in direct comparison according to five evaluation criteria (cf., tab. 5). In the resulting ranking list heroin reached the highest addiction potential, followed by cocaine, alcohol and nicotine, whereby for nicotine especially a very high value for (mental) 'addiction' was declared (Fahrenkrug & Gmel, 1996).

Substance	Overall Evaluation	With-drawal Symptoms	Reinforce-ment	Increase of Tolerance	Addiction	Intoxication
Heroin	1	1	1	1	1	2
Cocaine	2	3	2	3	3	1
Alcohol	3	2	4	2	4	3
Nicotine	**4**	**4**	**3**	**4**	**2**	**6**
Caffeine	7	7	7	6	7	7
Ecstasy	5	5	5	5	5	4
Marihuana	6	6	6	7	6	5

1= highest addiction potential; 7= lowest addiction potential

Table 5. Addiction Potential of Different Psychotropic Substances (quoted in Fahrenkrug & Gmel, 1996).

The 'addiction potential' relates to the addiction risk, but does not state anything about the *overall biopsychosocial risk potential* of a drug. Nutt et al. (2007) determined three main factors of potential damage by a psychotropic substance: 1) physical damage, 2) addiction potential and 3) social effects. A three-dimensional risk categories matrix was derived from this, by means of which the different substances were evaluated by two independent expert groups regarding their overall risk potential. In this multi-dimensional evaluation of the biopsychosocial overall risks, tobacco smoking is positioned in the upper middle field (place 9).

2.2.3 Comorbidity: Tobacco smoking and mental disorders

Tobacco addiction is closely associated with the occurrence of *mental disorders* and their course of disease. Cigarette smoking is disproportionately prevalent amongst persons with mental disorders (population) and/or psychiatric patients (clinical populations; Breslau, 1995; Degenhardt & Hall, 2001; John et al., 2004; Meyer et al, 2004; Haug et al., Heinberg & Guarda, 2001; Kordon & Kahl, 2004). On the whole, prevalence of smoking in mentally comorbid persons is approximately twice as high (50%) when compared to the general population (25-30%) (Grant et al., 2004; Lasser et al., 2000). It even amounts to 71-90% in patients with addictions to other substances (Ker et al., 1996; Patten et al., 1996; Martin et al., 1997; Williams & Ziedonis, 2004); for other *severe types of disorders* such as schizophrenia and bipolar disorders prevalence is on average 80% (Hughes, 1993; Leon & Diaz, 2005). In the US, the market share of the overall cigarette consumption by persons with psychiatric diagnoses is currently between 44 and 46% (Lasser et al., 2000; Grant et al., 2004).

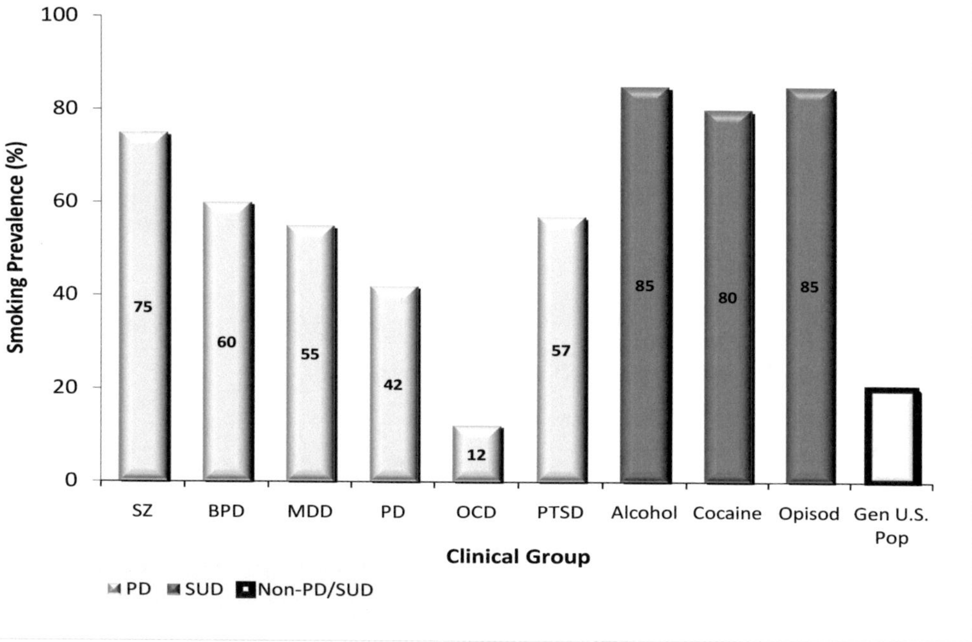

Fig. 2. Co-Morbidity of Smoking in Patients with Psychiatric and Substance Use Disorders (Kalman et al., 2005, p. 107)

Smokers with *mental comorbidity* mostly are heavy smokers, that means they are prone to smoke more cigarettes per day (days pack) and to smoke each cigagette more intensively (e.g. draws per cigarette, draw frequency, inhalation depth) (Lasser et al., 2000; Tidey et al., 2005). As a result, they do not only show increased physic long-term morbidity and mortality rates due to organic diseases associated with tobacco (Williams & Ziedonis, 2004), but they also have, amongst other things, a worse prognosis in relation to their mental disorder, a higher psychiatric lifetime-co-/multimorbidity, a more unfavourable course of disease (e.g. episodes in MDE that are more often, longer and more intensive), less successful therapy outcomes, a higher burden of disease, severe impairment of psychosocial functioning (Brown et al. 2000) as well as a lower *quality of life* (Schmitz et al., 2003). Smokers suffering from a mental disorder also show a lower self-efficacy and more negative attitudes towards a smoke stop (Carossella et al., 1999; Esterberg & Compton, 2005) as well as below average success rates for tobacco withdrawal that are often <15% (Glassman et al., 1993; Hall, Munoz, Reus, & Sees, 1993; Rohde et al., 2004; Ziedonis & George, 1997; Ziedonis et al., 1994). Moreover, smoking tobacco is a significant predictor for a *lifetime-suicidal tendency*, even when monitoring possible confounders (Breslau et al., 2005; Oquendo et al., 2004; Bronisch et al., 2009; Miller et al., 2000; figure 4).

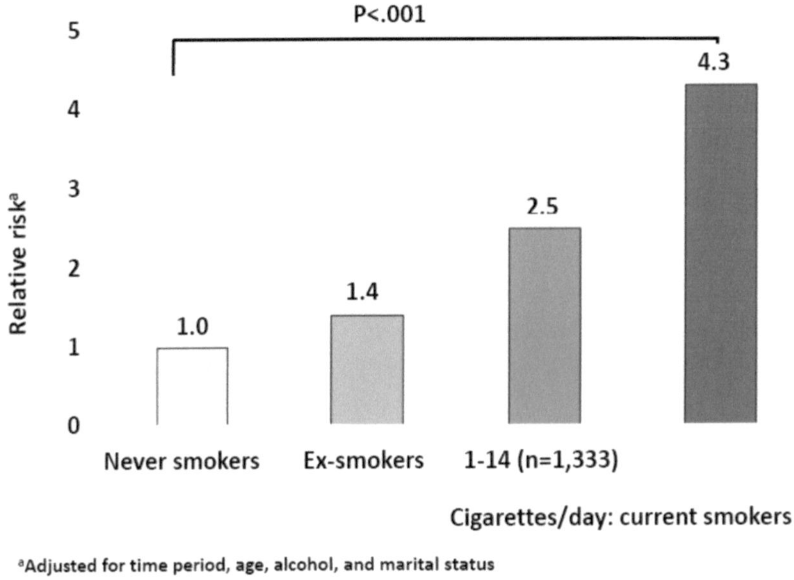

Fig. 3. Smoking and suicide risk (Miller et al., 2000)

The *etiological causality* of this coincidence between smoking tobacco and mental disorders is largely unresolved. Three competing theoretical models are being discussed: 1) According to the '*primary disorder model*' smoking is a reaction to the mental disorder (Guidelines of the American Psychiatric Association, 1996; Kendler et al., 1993; Pomerleau et al., 1997). In the sense of the '*self treatment hypothesis*', persons suffering from mental strain use nicotine for stress reduction (easing effect of nicotine) and for alleviating their subjective mental symptoms (effect of nicotine to soothe, enhance moods and improve the well-being of smokers) (Kendler et al., 1993; Hughes, 2004; Breslau, 2001). It is true that nicotine has specific anti-depressive effects (Tizabi et al., 1999; Balfour et al., 2000), since the serotonergic system is activated by nicotine similar to antidepressants (Vazquez-Palacios et al., 2005), and it is often used by psychiatric patients to specifically enhance their mood. According to this model, initial manifestation of the mental disorder would have to precede chronological tobacco smoking. 2) In contrast, the '*primary smoking model*' states that smoking can contribute to the development of a mental disorder. According to that, exposition to nicotine is a risk factor making individuals vulnerable to mental disorders due to the chronic impact on diverse transmitter systems that are involved in the development of mental disorders. This hypothesis is supported by the observation that the initial manifestation of mental symptoms often follows a longer break of regular smoking. Furthermore, for example, prenatal exposition to smoking is associated with the later occurrence of ADHD and depression in infancy and adolescence. 3) The '*bidirectional model*' assumes a long lasting interaction effect between smoking and mental disorders. Therefore, smoking triggers the development of mental symptoms in genetically disposed persons first and is later used for easing symptoms. In this way, regular nicotine consumption contributes to the chronification of the disorders in the long term (Mueser et al., 1998). It could be possible that smokers with mental disorders shy away from smoke stop because nicotine withdrawal symptoms contribute to an exacerbation of psychiatric symptoms and an increase of the relapse risk (Glassman, 2001; Balfour et al., 2000). Finally, it has been proven that e.g. schizophrenic patients often use nicotine to specifically counter regulate the effect of neuroleptics (Barnes et al., 2006; Glassman, 1994; Haring, Barnas, Saria, Humpel, & Fleischhaker, 1989; Hughes, 1993). 4) Finally, the '*common-factor model*' assumes a common etiology of nicotine dependence and other mental disorders (Breslau et al., 1998; Dierker, 2002; Covey, 1998). Since nicotine dependence itself is a mental disorder with manifold commonalities in terms of neurobiological, cognitive personal or social risk factors and mechanisms with a) other substance disorders (e.g. dopaminergic system) and also b) with other mental disorders (e.g. serotonergic system in MD), a common genetic disposition for e.g. depressions and susceptibility for the effects of nicotine positive seems likely (Kendler et al., 1993; Breslau et al., 1998).

2.3 Etiology: Neurobiological and psychological addiction mechanisms

2.3.1 Vulnerability and risk factors

Today, the average age of onset for smoking cigarettes ranges between eleven to thirteen years (Silagy et al., 1994; Nelson et al., 1998). The development of a tobacco addiction is dependent on a number of factors or causes. In addition to a *genetic disposition* (e.g. number of receptors, availability of specific enzymes, and function of transmitter systems), multiple acquired vulnerabilities and risk factors have been identified that comprise individual characteristics as well as specific environmental conditions (Brown et al., 1992; US Department of Health and Human Services, 1990). In the stage of initial or experimental use, despite of *availability of tobacco products* and *advertising influences, social factors like family models and the peer group* that are decisive for the start of one's smoking (Silagy et al., 1994). There are significant differences in *social classes* with the highest smoking rates in the lower social class, in unemployed people and social groups with lower educational achievement. Furthermore, an existing *psychiatric comorbidity* and unfavourable influences of the *family milieu* (parental psychopathology) primarily count towards the individual risk factors for the development of a tobacco addiction (WHO, 2001). Moreover, tobacco addiction and health risks towards smoking-related disorders correlate with the *early onset of smoking*. The physical addiction phenomena seem to develop especially rapidly in children and adolescents. In the stage of regular and dependent use, smokers try to manage their *psycho-social stress* or *daily hassles* by using nicotine ('self treatment'). In the long term run, the most important condition to maintain dependency is *negative reinforcement*, because every cigarette acts more and more to reduce withdrawal symptoms in the first line.

2.3.2 Neurobiological mechanisms

Like all psychotropic substances, nicotine stimulates the *mesolimbic dopamine system ('desire and reward system')* whose neurones are located in the area tegmentalis ventralis and project to the nucleus accumbens as well as the corpus striatum, among others. In contrast to other

drugs, nicotine exposition initiates a particular long term potentiation of specific neurons in this area of the brain, which causes a persistent increase of the dopamine level even after short term nicotine exposition.
In order to compensate for the artificial biochemical flooding and to maintain the normal functions, the brain reacts on two levels: 1) with a neuroanatomical change of the number and responsiveness of specific receptors (*neuroplastic down or up regulation*) and 2) with an inhibiting feedback on the level of transmitters, restricting the effect of nicotine by releasing *counter-regulative molecules* (Kunze et al., 1998). Both reactions lead to a weakening of the effect of nicotine. If the smoker subsequently tries to compensate the diminishing effect by means of more intensive smoking, the brain respectively produce more inhibiting molecules in that ever-increasing doses of nicotine are necessary to achieve 'intoxication' (*tolerance*). If the organism is then suddenly deprived of the substance (*withdrawal*), the balance of the system is forcefully disturbed. On the one hand, too few bodily-owned transmitters are available since the body has limited its own production and, on the other hand, a surplus of compensatorily released inhibitory molecules, which further inhibit the normal remaining functions of the transmitter balance, exist for a number of weeks. A strong *state of deprivation* results thereof and causes torturing mental and physical acute withdrawal conditions (withdrawal syndrome). The body is now not able to exist without tobacco any more and, therefore, an *addiction* has formed.

2.3.3 Psychological and neuropsychological mechanisms

Addicted ex-smokers are still at *risk to relapse* in face of any smoking-associated cues which trigger an irresistible desire (craving) for nicotine, even many years and decades after the withdrawal, probably for their whole lifetime. This long time active '*addiction memory*' cannot be explained by mechanism of physical dependence, which normalise within a few weeks after quitting. In the first line, complex *learned conditioning processes* are responsible for the continuing sensitisation to nicotine and the ongoing high relapse rates.
Simultaneously to dopamine release in the '*desire and reward system*' nicotine stimulates specific *areas in the brain which are involved in association learning processes*. That is why smoking tobacco has a particularly strong link to *situational* (smoking break, coffee drinking, after work beer), *behavioural* (reaching for the box of cigarettes), *sensory* (smell, taste) or *affective* (mood) *cues* that are associated with smoking. Insofar, persistent addiction can be primarily traced back to *respondent* and *operant conditioning*. In the case of smoking *positive reinforcement* is generated by the fateful association between the inhalation (stimulus) and the subsequent state of well-being (response) that permanently becomes engraved in memory ('*addiction memory*') within a short time. Despite the missing intensive intoxication, the high addiction potential of tobacco smoking results from the brain of a regular smoker being flooded with nicotine 200 to 400 times per day (per year: 73,000 to 146,000 times) – and the stimulus-response connection is thereby continuously enforced.
The high *risk of a relapse* and the actual *relapse process* after a smoke stop can be explained by means of *neuropsychological* and *cognitivepsychological models*. However, one of the main - questions, why the addiction behaviour and craving is not extinguished after a certain time was not resolved satisfactorily. The latest research in cognitive learning shows that the *extinction* of a respondent conditioning is, in a neurobiological sense, no unlearning in terms of a decoupling of synaptic links but a *new learning and/or re-learning* where new stimulus-reaction-links are generated while the old ones are principally still available (Conklin &

Tiffany, 2002). That is why old addiction conditionings can, if certain triggers emerge, be reactivated even after a long time (e.g. by reinstatement or spontaneous recovery).
Furthermore, the hypersensitivity to the addiction cues (*cue reactivity*), which is profoundly resistant against extinction and overwriting, can be explained with *neuroplastic changes* in the dopamine system. In the case of chronic substance intake a neurobiological hyper reactivity to the drug and their trigger cues develops in the mesolimbic dopamine system (*subcortical dysfunction*) and, at the same time, the areas that are responsible for executive control (*frontal cortical dysfunction*) are weakened. Finally, the relapse can be described by the different levels of information processing of addiction-related cues on the one hand, and by the intentional control of action on the other (Tiffany und Conklin, 2000). The addicts' reaction to drug-associated cues is an example of *'automatic processing'*, i.e. it is made unconsciously quick, linked to certain trigger situations, with a low use of cognitive capacity and can only be influenced to a small degree. In contrast, abstinence demands an intentional regulation of action with conscious information processing and executive control functions (*'controlled processing'*), which is consciously, intention controlled and flexible, but relatively slow, cognitively demanding and limited by the processing capacity. In case of chronic substance abuse an increasing disequilibrium between the growing influence of automatic stimulus processing (*'implicit cognitions'*), as well as a weakening of executive control and regulation of emotions that makes the person trying to quit increasingly vulnerable to addiction triggers and, finally, relapse.

2.4 Treatment

Almost all smokes are aware of the smoke-related health risks and a majority of them repeatedly tries to stop smoking. The *willingness to quit* depends on the individual stage of motivation. According to the widely known *transtheoretical model* (Prochaska & DiClimente, *1993)* smokers move through a discrete series of five motivational stages before they quit successfully: (i) *precontemplation* (no thoughts of quitting), (ii) *contemplation* (thinking about quitting), (iii) *preparation* (planning to quit in the next 30 days), (iv) *action* (quitting successfully for up to six months), and (v) *maintenance* (no smoking for more than six months). The transtheoretical theory has not been empirically supported, and some authors cast doubt its practical value (Etter & Sutton, 2002; Sutton, 2001).
However, most smokers will succeed to quit at one point in their life: There are more ex-smokers than current smokers to be found in the age cohort over 50 years old. However, tobacco withdrawal often requires a multitude of stop smoking trials to be successful when no professional help is sought. The success rate of unassisted smoke stop trials is at a mere 3-6% during the 12-months period. However, less than 5 % of all smokers willing to stop make use of professional help, despite the availability of effective smoking cessation therapies (WHO, 2001; Nelson & Wittchen, 1998).
Professional smoking cessation treatments include a wide range of interventions, from medical advice through to brief motivational interventions to complex withdrawal programs. In practice, less effective methods such as hypnosis and acupuncture are used alongside motivational interviewing, cognitive-behavioural therapy interventions (CBT) and medicinal approaches in withdrawal and substitution treatment. Professional smoking cessation treatment is first and foremost based on behavioural group interventions (cf. Box 1) and approaches of motivational interviewing, and often offered in combination with medicinal support (e.g. nicotine substitutes).

1. Psychoeducation: education, information and attitude change
2. Analysis of problem and behaviour: Analysis and documentation of smoking behaviour and the maintaining cognitive and situational or social conditions
3. Strengthening of motivation to change (motivational interview): Clear decision to quit smoking, determination of a deadline to stop smoking
4. Systematic preparation for abstinence, execution of smoke stop and modification of behaviour: Control of conditioning stimuli, development and training of alternative behaviour, contract management, self-reward, teaching of strategies of self-control
5. Activation of a supporting social network and teaching of health promotional behaviour
6. Relapse prevention: Dealing with risk situations, strategies against relapse risks (role play exercises)

Box 1. Components of complex behavioural therapy programmes for smoking cessation.

Primary goal in smoking cessation treatment is *total abstinence.* Controlled tobacco use leading to harm reduction is only aimed for in exceptional cases (in cases of severe disease or pregnancy with simultaneous inability to remain abstinent; Stead & Lancaster, 2007; Lumley et al., 2009). The medicinal treatment in smoking cessation primarily aims to soothe the somatic withdrawal symptoms and associated craving. The *pharmacological treatment* options are based on three different modes of action:

i. In *nicotine replacement therapy* a patient is given nicotine doses, which substitute the nicotine the patient does not take in anymore by smoking, by means of drugs containing nicotine (nicotine patch, gum, inhaler, lozenge, nasal spray, sublingual tablet). By means of retaining an equal level of nicotine withdrawal symptoms are soothed and the withdrawal is made easier by stepwise downdosing the pharmacological nicotine.
ii. The nicotine-free drug *bupropion (Zyban®)*, originally developed as *anti-depressant,* inhibits the synaptic absorption of catecholamines (adrenalin, dopamine) in the mesolimbic dopamine system, thereby compensating the dopamine lack caused by the nicotine withdrawal and, in this way, soothes the withdrawal symptoms without supplying nicotine. Due to serious contra-indications, side-effects and pharmaceutical risks, bupropion may only be applied under medical supervision.
iii. The *partial agonist varenicline (Chantix®)* binds to specific nicotine receptors of the subtype that is responsible for one of the addictive effects of the nicotine. The active agent stimulates the receptors and thereby eases withdrawal symptoms. At the same time, it inhibits the effect of externally supplied nicotine by blocking the receptors. Also due to the serious side-effects and risks (nausea, headache, insomnia, abnormal dreams, suicidal ideation and occasional suicidal behavior, erratic behavior and drowsiness) there are similarly strict regulations for varenicline in terms of prescription and medical supervision.

Multi-modal smoking cessation programmes can be divided into three stages: (i) reinforcement of the abstinence motivation and the patient's commitment to quit smoking, (ii) preparation and realisation of smoke stop, (iii) maintenance of abstinence and using new coping strategies to avoid a return to use.

i. Regular smokers generally are ambivalent towards quitting. Although almost every smoker is aware of the health risks and further disadvantages of smoking, most of them dread the burdens associated with smoke stop (fear of withdrawal symptoms and loss of positive reinforcement) and continually postpone their withdrawal, often for years. This is why it is necessary to make an explicit decision pro tobacco withdrawal at the beginning of the *withdrawal stage* (in case of smokers willing to stop) and/or to motivate in favor of a smoke stop (in case of smokers not yet willing to stop). For this purpose, *motivational interviewing* is a suitable approach (Miller & Rollnick, 2002 by which the motivation to quit smoking and the confidence to change can be analysed and systematically strengthened during the preparation stage. In smoking cessation practice, behavioural-therapeutic techniques (smoking diaries, behavioural analysis, CO-measurement, reinforcement plans, pros-cons lists, target hierarchies, aim in life analysis, short and long term benefits, strengthening of self-efficacy) as well as cognitive techniques (disputation of irrational ideas, worst case scenarios, development of rational alternatives) are applied for the preparation of the smoke stop. The explicit commitment of the smoker to his/her desire to quit smoking (importance) and his belief to being able to reach this goal (realisability) proves to be decisive in this stage.

ii. During the *quitting stage* the smoker is systematically prepared for the smoke stop and the time of abstinence. For this purpose, it is important, not only to create adequate commitment but also to enhance the optimism about one's ability to change and to strengthen self efficacy. Using the 'cold turkey method', a certain quit day is determined. In the sense of a stimulus control, all triggers (smoke utensils such as ashtray, cigarette boxes, lighter etc.) are removed from the immediate surrounding and/or typical smoke situations (e.g. local pub) are temporarily avoided for the time of the smoke stop preparation stage. The smoke stop can be supported by means of aversion therapy (excessive inhaling, retain smoke in lung, smelling of containers with cigarette butts and cold ash) or counter conditioning (presentation of unpleasant stimuli such as deterring photos of smoke-related diseases contingent to smoking).

iii. The treatment stage most important to keep long term abstinence is the *maintenance and relapse prevention*. The ex-smoker is supported in his/her self control management (response control) and self instruction in order for him/her to master craving and withdrawal symptoms and to successfully cope with high risky situation (refusal training). At the same time, positive alternatives to smoking (relaxation exercise, physical exercise, easy breathing, water drinking, pleasant activities and attentional distraction) are proposed and trained. Positive stimuli (e.g. appraisal, material rewards, amount of money saved, improvement of lung function, duration of abstinence) or contracting (written commitment, rewards vs punishment) are used to support abstinence and social resources are mobilised (workshop assistants, supporters). During abstinence a cognitive reframing shall be triggered in which the smokefree life comes to be seen as less unpleasant condition of withdrawal and loss but increasingly as an awarding situation in which a positive physical well-being and independence dominates. Finally, an individual emergency plan is drafted and structured relapse prevention management is trained (what to do when having a relapse).

2.5 Empirical evidence

Up to date, a large amount of professional and more or less *evidence-based smoking cessation treatments* have been developed, that range from minimal interventions (physician's advice to quit smoking) and medicinal withdrawal treatment (nicotine replacement therapy, psychotropic drugs such as bupropion or varenicline) to telephone counselling ('quit-line') and online quitting programmes as well as to multi-modal smoking cessation in behavioural group therapy described above. The efficacy of professional smoking cessation treatments is well determined. An impressive number of RCTs as well as several meta-analyses and *Systematic Cochrane Reviews* clearly proved the high efficacy of several cessation treatments towards the primary outcome of long-term abstinence.

In particular, *group behaviour therapy* programmes for smoking cessation yielded high effect sizes in many randomised controlled trials (RCT) and were found to be superior to self help, and other less intensive interventions (Stead & Lancaster, 2005). However, there is not enough evidence to evaluate whether groups are more effective, or cost-effective, than intensive individual counselling and only limited evidence that the addition of group therapy to other forms of treatment, such as advice from a health professional or nicotine replacement, produced extra benefit (Stead & Lancaster, 2005, p 2). *Individual behavioural counselling interventions* for smoking cessation have been well-proven, too (Lancaster & Stead, 2005). Individual counselling was more effective than control, but a greater effect of intensive counselling compared to brief counseling could not be found. *Aversion therapy*, which pairs the pleasurable stimulus of smoking a cigarette with some unpleasant stimulus in order to extinguish the urge to smoke, has been evaluated in a smaller number of RCT's that provide insufficient evidence to determine the efficacy of rapid smoking (Hajek & Stead, 2001).

Pharmaceutical treatment in smoking cessation is high efficient as well. All of the commercially available forms of *nicotine replacement therapy* (gum, transdermal patch, nasal spray, inhaler and sublingual tablets/lozenges) can help people who make a quit attempt to increase their chances of successfully stopping smoking by 50-70%, regardless of setting Stead et al., 2008). The empirical evidence show that the *antidepressants* bupropion and nortriptyline are equally effective and of similar efficacy to nicotine replacement therapy, but there is insufficient evidence that adding bupropion to nicotine replacement therapy provides an additional long-term benefit (Hughes et al., 2007, p 2). Also *varenicline* at standard dose increases the chances of successful long-term smoking cessation between two- and threefold compared with pharmacologically unassisted quit attempts (Cahill et al., 2011, p 2).

The trials to *internet-based interventions* for smoking cessation did not show consistent effects, but for some interventions there is evidence that online counselling can assist smoking cessation, especially if the information is appropriately tailored to the users and frequent automated contacts with the users are ensured (Civljak, Sheikh, Stead & Car, 2010, p 2). Similarly, proactive *telephone counselling* for smoking cessation can efficiently help smokers in quitting, but a minimum of three or more calls are required to increase the chances of quitting compared to a minimal intervention (providing standard self-help materials, brief advice), or compared to pharmacotherapy alone (Stead et al., 2006). *Motivational interviewing* for smoking cessation yielded a modest but significant increase in quitting compared to brief advice or usual care and was more effective, when delivered by primary care physicians and by counselors and when conducted in longer and multiple sessions (Lai et al., 2010).

In contrast, there is no consistent, bias-free evidence that *acupuncture, acupressure, laser therapy* or *electrostimulation* or *exercise interventions* for smoking cessation are effective for smoking cessation (White et al., 2011; Ussher et al., 2008). Also, the empirical evidence for *hypnotherapy* fails to show a greater effect on six-month quit rates than other interventions or no treatment (Barnes et al., 2010). *Standard self-help materials* may increase quit rates compared to no intervention, but the effect is likely to be small, and no additional benefit has been found alongside other interventions such as advice from a healthcare professional, or nicotine replacement therapy (Lancaster & Stead, 2005, p 2). Materials that are tailored for individual smokers are more effective than untailored materials, although the absolute size of effect is still small.

Smoking *reduction versus abrupt cessation* in smokers who want to quit makes no difference with regard to long-term abstinence (Lindson et al., 2010). According to the *transtheoretical model stage-based* self-help interventions (expert systems and/or tailored materials) and individual counselling were neither more nor less effective than their non-stage-based equivalents (Cahill et al., 2010, p 2).

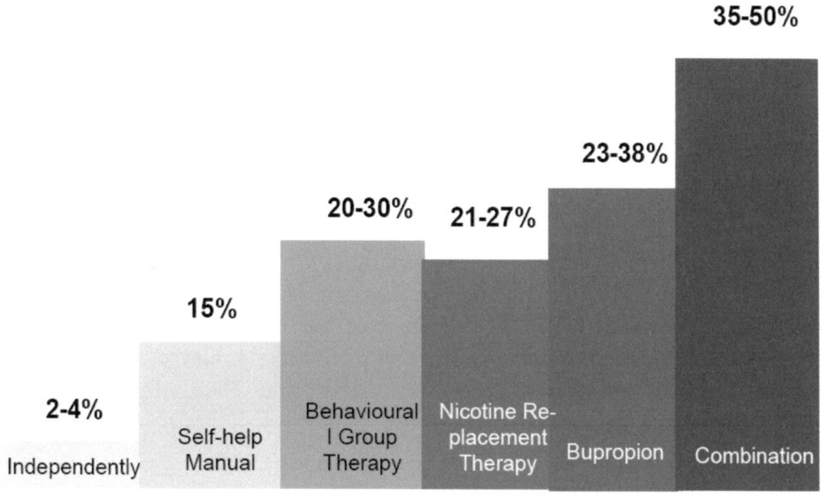

Fig. 4. Success rates (12-months abstinence) of measurements for tobacco withdrawal in clinical studies (efficacy) according to a meta-analysis of the US Department of Health and Human Services (Fiore et al., 2008)

In context of the *US Clinical Practice Guidelines*, sponsored by the U.S. Public Health Service, Guideline Panel conducted 2000 a large mega-metanalysis *'Treating Tobacco Use and Dependence'* which has been updated in 2008 (Fiore et al., 2008). The main results are shown in figure 7. In Detail, the effectiveness and abstinence rates of various interventions and medications in smoking cessation treatment are presented in table 6 and 7. In summary, the most effective smoking cessation treatment is a combination of group behavior therapy or individual counseling with pharmaceutical treatment, whereas a combination of more than one pharmaceutics has an extra benefit (e.g., NRT patch + NRT gum or NRT patch + oral medication).

Based on the empirical evidence of international trials in the field of smoking, tobacco dependence and smoking cessation in numerous countries specific clinical guidelines for treating tobacco addiction have been developed during the last decade, e.g. :

- The well-known *US 'Clinical Practice Guideline for Treating Tobacco Use and Dependence'* (Fiore et al., 2000, 2008) occurred as a result of an extraordinary partnership among Federal Government and nonprofit organizations;
- in UK the National Institute for Health and Clinical Excellence - NICE created a number of clinical guidelines:
  - Smoking cessation services in primary care, pharmacies, local authorities and workplaces, particularly for manual working groups, pregnant women and hard to reach communities (2008)
  - The Impact of Quitlines on Smoking Cessation (2007)
  - Economic Analysis of Interventions for Smoking Cessation Aimed at Pregnant Women (2007)
  - School-based interventions to prevent the uptake of smoking among children and young people: cost-effectiveness model (2010)
  - The effectiveness of smoking cessation interventions to reduce the rates of premature death in disadvantaged areas through proactive case finding, retention and access to services
  - Mass-media and point-of-sales measures to prevent the uptake of smoking by children and young people (2008)
  - Workplace health promotion: how to help employees to stop smoking (2007)
- *Association of the Scientific Medical Societies* in Germany co-ordinates the national programme of medical guidelines of its member organizations. In cooperation with numerous institutions and non-profit organizations (e.g. German Society of Addiction Research; German Association for Psychiatry and Psychotherapy) two smoking cessation guidelines have been developed:
  - Guidelines for Treating Substance Use Disorders (2004)
  - Smoking Cessation in COPD patients (2008)

These various national guidelines do explicitly consider the different conditions of the social, cultural or health care systems in each country and should be received by the health care professionals in the specific region they are developed for.

Various intensity levels of session length (n = 43 studies)[a]			
Level of contact	Number of arms	Estimated odds ratio (95% C.I.)	Estimated abstinence rate (95% C.I.)
No contact	30	1.0	10.9
Minimal counseling (< 3 minutes)	19	1.3 (1.01–1.6)	13.4 (10.9–16.1)
Low-intensity counseling (3–10 minutes)	16	1.6 (1.2–2.0)	16.0 (12.8–19.2)

Higher intensity counseling (> 10 minutes)	55	2.3 (2.0–2.7)	22.1 (19.4–24.7)
Total amount of contact time (n = 35 studies) [a]			
Total amount of contact time	Number of arms	Estimated odds ratio (95% C.I.)	Estimated abstinence rate (95% C.I.)
No minutes	16	1.0	11.0
1–3 minutes	12	1.4 (1.1–1.8)	14.4 (10.3–17.5)
4–30 minutes	20	1.9 (1.5–2.3)	18.8 (15.6–22.0)
31–90 minutes	16	3.0 (2.3–3.8)	26.5 (21.5–31.4)
91–300 minutes	16	3.2 (2.3–4.6)	28.4 (21.3–35.5)
> 300 minutes	15	2.8 (2.0–3.9)	25.5 (19.2–31.7)
Various types of formats (n = 58 studies) [a]			
Format Number	Number of arms	Estimated odds ratio (95% C.I.)	Estimated abstinence rate (95% C.I.)
No format	20	1.0	10.8
Self-help	93	1.2 (1.02–1.3)	12.3 (10.9–13.6)
Proactive tel. counseling	26	1.2 (1.1–1.4)	13.1 (11.4–14.8)
Group counseling	52	1.3 (1.1–1.6)	13.9 (11.6–16.1)
Individual counseling	67	1.7 (1.4–2.0)	16.8 (14.7–19.1)
Various types of counseling and behavioral therapies (n = 64 studies) [a]			
Type of counseling and behavioral therapy	Number of arms	Estimated odds ratio (95% C.I.)	Estimated abstinence rate (95% C.I.)
No counseling/ behavioral therapy	35	1.0	11.2
Relaxation/breathing	31	1.0 (0.7–1.3)	10.8 (7.9–13.8)
Contingency contracting	22	1.0 (0.7–1.4)	11.2 (7.8–14.6)
Weight/diet	19	1.0 (0.8–1.3)	11.2 (8.5–14.0)
Cigarette fading	25	1.1 (0.8–1.5)	11.8 (8.4–15.3)
Negative affect	8	1.2 (0.8–1.9)	13.6 (8.7–18.5)
social support	50	1.3 (1.1–1.6)	14.4 (12.3–16.5)
Extratreatment social support	19	1.5 (1.1–2.1)	16.2 (11.8–20.6)
Practical counseling (problem solving/skills)	104	1.5 (1.3–1.8)	16.2 (14.0–18.5)
Other aversive smoking	19	1.7 (1.04–2.8)	17.7 (11.2–24.9)
Rapid smoking	19	2.0 (1.1–3.5)	19.9 (11.2–29.0)

[a] Go to www.surgeongeneral.gov/tobacco/gdinrefs.htm for the articles used in this meta-analysis.

Table 6. Meta-analysis (2000): Effectiveness and abstinence rates of various interventions in smoking cessation treatment

Various medications and medication compared to placebo at 6-months post quit (n = 83 studies) [a]			
Medication	Number of arms	Estimated odds ratio (95% C.I.)	Estimated abstinence rate (95% C.I.)
Placebo	80	1.0	13.8
Monotherapies			
Varenicline (2mg/day)	5	3.1 (2.5–3.8)	33.2 (28.9–37.8)
Nicotine Nasal Spray	4	2.3 (1.7–3.0)	26.7 (21.5–32.7)
Hig-Dose Nicotine Patch (> 25mg) (These include both standard or ling-term-duration)	4	2.3 (1.7–3.0)	26.5 (21.3–32.5)
Long-Term Nicotine Gum (>14 weeks)	6	2.2 (1.5–3.2)	26.1 (19.7–33.6)
Varenicline (1mg/day)	3	2.1 (1.5–3.0)	25.4 (19.6–32.2)
Nicotine Inhaler	6	2.1 (1.5–2.9)	24.8 (19.1–31.6)
Clonidine	3	2.1 (1.2–3.7)	25.0 (15.7–37.3)
Bupropion SR	226	2.0 (1.8–2.2)	24.2 (22.2–26.4)
Nicotine Patch (6–14 weeks)	632	1.9 (1.7–2.2)	23.4 (21.3–25.8)
Long-Term Nicotine Patch (> 14 weeks)	3102	1.9 (1.7–2.3)	23.7 (21.0–26.6)
Nortriptyline	5	1.8 (1.3–2.6)	22.5 (16.8–29.4)
Nicotine Gum (6–14 weeks)	15	1.5 (1.2–1.7)	19.0 (16.5–21.9)
Combination therapies			
Patch (long-term; > 14 weeks) + ad llb NRT (gum or spray)	3	3.6 (2.5–5.2)	36.5 (28.6–45.3)
Patch + Bupropion SR	3	2.5 (1.9–3.4)	28.9 (23.5–35.1)
Patch + Nortriptyline	2	2.3 (1.3–4.2)	27.3 (17.2–40.4)
Patch + Inhaler	2	2.2 (1.3–3.6)	25.8 (17.4–36.5)
Patch + Second generation antidepressants (paroxetine, venlafaxine)	3	2.0 (1.2–3.4)	24.3 (16.1–35.0)
Medications not shown to be effective			
Selective Serotonin Re-uptake Inhibitors (SSRIs)	3	1.0 (0.7–1.4)	13.7 (10.2–18.0)
Naltrexone	2	0.5 (0.2–1.2)	7.3 (3.1–16.2)

[a] Go to www.surgeongeneral.gov/tobacco/gdinrefs.htm for the articles used in this meta-analysis.

Table 7. Meta-analysis (2000): Effectiveness and abstinence rates of various medications in smoking cessation treatment

3. Conclusion

The *smoking rates* in the population vary from country to country with a range between approximately 25-60% of adult population. Although only every third smoker meets the diagnostic criteria for *nicotine dependence*, tobacco addiction is the *most prevalent mental disorder* worldwide. Besides the well-known impact of tobacco smoking on physical health, there is a growing body of evidence that smoking increases the *vulnerability for mental disorders*, too. Point prevalence of tobacco smoking amongst persons with mental disorders (MD) is 40-50% and thus, on average, twice as high as amongst the general population. Smokers with psychiatric comorbidity do not only show increased somatic morbidity and mortality rates, but also a significantly worse prognosis in relation to their MD, up to a significant increase of lifetime *suicide risks*.
The *addiction potential of tobacco smoking* as well as the difficulty to quit and to permanently remain abstinent is often highly underestimated by smokers themselves, but by many health care professionals as well. The high failure and relapse rates in smoking cessation, even in patients with life threatening smoking-associated disorders (e.g. myocardial infarction, pulmonary emphysema or lung transplantation) demonstrates that nicotine dependence is a serious mental disorder and an addiction comparable harmful like in case of illicit drugs. Overcoming smoking as a serious 'substance use disorder' in many cases calls for *professional cessation treatment*. Although every second smoker succeeds to quit at some point in his/her life without professional help, however, this is only achieved after many years and after a number of failed trials. During this long lasting period since smokers are successful in quitting, in many cases serious harm to their physical or mental health has already been caused. Therefore, in *routine care*, smokers should be *encouraged to quit smoking* at an *early stage* and they should be tested on a routine basis for a *tobacco addiction* and, if necessary, be referred to a *smoking cessation specialist* or an outpatient cessation clinic.

4. Acknowledgment

I acknowledge Ph.D. Stefanie Fuchs and Ph.D. Anja Sehl for their helpful support in the systematic evidence search and Ms. Christina Bernd for editing this manuscript.

5. References

Balfour, D. J. K. & Ridley, D. L. (2000). The effects of nicotine on neural pathways implicated in depression: A factor in nicotine addiction? *Pharmacology, Biochemistry and Behavior*, Vol. 66, No. 1, pp. 79-85, ISSN 0091-3057

Barnes, J., Dong, C. Y., McRobbie, H., Walker, N., Mehta. M. & Stead, L. F. (2010). Hypnotherapy for smoking cessation. *Cochrane Database of Systematic Reviews*, Vol. 10, (October 2010), ISSN 13616137

Breslau, N., Johnson, E. O., Hiripi, E. & Kessler, R. (2001). Nicotine dependence in the United States - Prevalence, trends, and smoking persistence. *Archives of General Psychiatry*, Vol. 58, No. 9, (September 2011), pp. 810-816, ISSN 0003-990X

Breslau, N., Novak, S. P. & Kessler, R. C. (2004). Psychiatric disorders and stages of smoking. *Biological Psychiatry*, Vol. 55, No. 1, pp. 69-76, ISSN 0006-3223

Breslau, N., Schultz, L. R., Johnson, E. O., Peterson, E. L. & Davis, G. C. (2005). Smoking and the risk of suicidal behavior: a prospective study of a community sample. *Archives of General Psychiatry*, Vol. 62, No. 3, (March 2005), pp. 328-34, ISSN 0003-990X

Brown, S. L. & Owen, N. (1992). Self-help smoking cessation materials. *Australian Journal of Public Health*, Vol. 16, No. 2, (June 1992), pp. 188-191, ISSN 1035-7319

Brown, S., Inskip, H. & Barraclough, B. (2000). Causes of the excess mortality of schizophrenia. *British Journal of Psychiatry*, Vol. 177, (September 2000), pp. 212-217, ISSN 0007-1250

Brown, R., Kahler, C., Niaura, R. S., Abrams, D. B., Sales, S., Ramsey, S., Goldstein, M. G., Burgess, E. S. & Miller, I. W. (2001). Cognitive-behavioral treatment for depression in smoking cessation. *Journal of Consulting and Clinical Psychology*, Vol. 69, No. 3, (June 2001), pp. 471–480, ISSN 0022-006X

Buchkremer, G., Bents, H., Horstmann, M., Opitz, K. & Tölle, R. (1989). Combination of behavioral smoking cessation with transdermal nicotine substitutution. *Addictive Behaviors*, Vol. 14, No. 2, pp. 229-238, ISSN 0306-4603

Buchkremer, G., Minneker, E. & Block, M. (1991). Smoking-cessation treatment combining transdermal nicotine substitution with behavioral therapy. *Pharmacopsychiatry*, Vol. 24, No. 3, (May 1991), pp. 96-102, ISSN 0176-3679

Cahill, K., Lancaster, T. & Green, N. (2010). Stage-based interventions for smoking cessation. *Cochrane Database of Systematic Reviews*, Vol. 11, (November 2010), ISSN 13616137

Cahill, K., Stead, L. F. & Lancaster, T. (2011). Nicotine receptor partial agonists for smoking cessation. *Cochrane Database of Systematic Reviews*, Vol. 2, (February 2011), ISSN 13616137

Civljak, M., Sheikh, A., Stead, L. F. & Car, J. (2010). Internet-based interventions for smoking cessation. *Cochrane Database of Systematic Reviews*, Vol. 9, (September 2010). ISSN 13616137

Conklin, C. A., & Tiffany, St. (2002). Applying extinction research and theory to cue-exposure addiction treatment. *Addiction*, Vol. 97, No. 2, pp. 155-167, ISSN 09652140

De Leon, J. & Diaz, F. J., (2005). A meta-analysis of worldwide studies demonstrates an association between schizophrenia and tobacco smoking behaviors. *Schizophrenia Research*, Vol. 76, No. 2/3, (July 2005), pp. 135-157, ISSN 09209964

El-Guebaly, N., Cathcart, J., Currie, S., Brown, D. & Gloster, S. (2002). Public health and therapeutic aspects of smoking bans in mental health and addiction settings. *Psychiatric Services*, Vol. 53, No. 12, (December 2002), pp. 1617–1622, ISSN 10752730

Etter, J. F. & Sutton, S. (2002). Assessing stage of change in current and former smokers. *Addiction*, Vol. 97, No. 9, pp. 1171-1182, ISSN 09652140

ENSH. (2007). Tobacco Force United, 30. 03. 2010, Available from: http://www. ensh. eu/ensh/racine/

Fagerström, K. O., Schneider, N. G. & Lunell, E. (1993). Effectiveness of nicotine patch and nicotine gum as individual versus combined treatment for tobacco withdrawal symptoms. *Psychopharmacology*, Vol. 111, No. 3, (June 1993), pp. 271-277, ISSN 00333158

Fahrenkrug, H. & Gmel, G. (1996) Addictiveness: How Swiss experts rate alcohol and other drugs. *Alcologia*, Vol. 8, No. 3, pp. 225-229

Fiore, M. C. (2000). US Public Health Practice Guideline: Treating tobacco use and dependence. *Respiratory Care*, Vol. 45, No. 10, (October 2000), pp. 1200-1262, ISSN 0020-1324

Fowler, J. S., Logan, J., Wang, G. J. & Volkow, N. D. (2003). Monoamine oxidase and cigarette smoking. *Neurotoxicology*, Vol. 24, No. 1, (January 2003), pp. 75-82, ISSN 0161813X

Gallinat, J., Meisenzahl, E., Jacobsen, L. K., Kalus, P., Bierbrauer, J., Kienast, T., Witthaus, H., Leopold, K., Seifert, F., Schubert, F. & Staedtgen, M. (2006). Smoking and structural brain deficits: a volumetric MR investigation. *The European Journal of Neuroscience*, Vol. 24, No. 6, (September 2006), pp. 1744-1750; ISSN 0953816X

Grant, B. F., Hasin, D. S., Chou, S. P., Stinson, F. S. & Dawson, D. A. (2004). Nicotine dependence and psychiatric disorders in the United States - Results from the National Epidemiologic Survey on Alcohol and Related Conditions. *Archives of General Psychiatry*, Vol. 61, No. 11, (November 2004), pp. 1107-1115, ISSN 15383636

Gubbay, J. (1992). *Smoking and the Workplace*. Centre for Health Policy Research, University of East Anglia.

Gulliver, S. B., Rohsenow, D. J. & Colby, S. M. (1995). Interrelationship of smoking and alcohol dependence, use and urges to use. *Journal of Studies on Alcohol*, Vol. 56, No. 2, (March 1995), pp. 202-206, ISSN 0096-882X

Gulliver, S. B., Kalman, D. & Rohsenow, D. J. (2000). Smoking and drinking among alcoholics in treatment: cross-sectional and longitudinal relationships. *Journal of Studies on Alcohol*, Vol. 61, No. 1, (January 2000), pp. 157-163, ISSN0096-882X

Gulliver, S. B., Kamholz, B. W., & Helstrom, A. W. (2006). Smoking Cessation and Alcohol Abstinence: What Do the Data Tell Us?. *Alcohol Research & Health*, Vol. 29, No. 3, pp. 208-212, ISSN 15357414

Hajek, P. & Stead, L. F. (2001). Aversive smoking for smoking cessation. *Cochrane Database of Systematic Reviews*, Vol. 3, ISSN 13616137

Haug, N. A., Heinberg, L. J. & Guarda, A. S. (2001). Cigarette smoking and its relationship to other substance use among eating disordered inpatients. *Eating and weight disorders*, Vol. 6, No. 3, (September 2001), pp. 130-139, ISSN 1124-4909

Haustein, K. O. (2000). Pharmacotherapy of nicotine dependence. *Int J Clin Pharmacol Ther*, Vol. 38, No. 6, (June 2000), pp. 273-290, ISSN 0946-1965

Heatherton, T. F., Kozlowski, L. T., Frecker, R. C. & Fagerström, K. O. (1991). The Fragerström Test for Nicotine Dependence: a revision of the Fagerstrom Tolerance Questionaire. *British Journal of Addiction*, Vol. 86, No. 9, (September 1991), pp. 1119-1127, ISSN 0952-0481

Hughes, J. R., Oliveto, A. H., Riggs, R., Kenny, M., Liguori, A., Pillitteri, J. L. & MacLaughlin, M. A. (2004). Concordance of different measures of nicotine dependence: Two pilot studies. *Addictive Behaviors*, Vol. 29, No. 8, (November 2004), pp. 1527-1539, ISSN 03064603

Hughes, J. R., Stead, L. F. & Lancaster, T. (2007). Antidepressants for smoking cessation. *Cochrane Database of Systematic Reviews*, Vol. 1, (January 2007), ISSN 13616137

Hurt, R. D., Sachs, D. P., Glover, E. D., Offord, K. P., Johnston, J. A., Dale, L. C., Khayrallah, M. A.,Schroeder, D. R., Glover, P. N., Sullivan, C. R., Croghan, I. T. & Sullivan, P. M. (1997). A comparison of substained-release bupropion and placebo for smoking cessation. *New England Journal of Medicine,* Vol. 337, No. 17, (October 1999), pp. 1195-1202, ISSN 0028-4793

Jochelson, K. & Majrowski, W. (2006). *Clearing the Air: Debating Smoke-Free Policies in Psychiatric Units* (Vol. 1), King's Fund, ISBN 978 1 85717 550 9, London

John, U., Meyer, C., Rumpf, H-J. & Hapke, U. (2004). Smoking, nicotine dependence and psychiatric comorbidity - a population-based study including smoking cessation after three years. *Drug and Alcohol Dependence,* Vol. 76, No. 3, (December 2004), pp. 287-295, ISSN 03768716

Jorenby, D. E., Leischow, J. J., Nides, M. A., Rennard, S. I., Johnston, J. A., Hughes, A. R., Smith, S. S., Muramoto, M. L., Daughton, D. M., Doan, K., Fiore, M. C. & Baker, T. B. (1999). A controlled trial of substained-release Bupropion, a nicotine patch, or both for smoking cessation. *New England Journal of Medicine,* Vol. 340, No. 9, (March 1999), pp. 685-691, ISSN 0028-4793

Kalman, D., Baker Morissette, S. & George, T. P. (2005). Co-Morbidity of Smoking in Patients with Psychiatric and Substance Use Disorders. *The American Journal on Addictions,* Vol. 14, No. 2, (March-April 2005), pp. 106–123, ISSN 1055-0496

Keltner, N. L. & Grant, J. S. (2006). Smoke, smoke, smoke that cigarette. *Perspectives Psychiatric Care,* Vol. 42, No. 4, (November 2006), pp. 256-261, ISSN 00315990

Koenen, K. C., Hitsman, B., Lyons, M. J., Niaura, R., McCaffery, J., Goldberg, J., Eisen, S. A., True, W. & Tsuang, M. (2005). A twin registry study of the relationship between posttraumatic stress disorder and nicotine dependence in men. *Archives of General Psychiatry,* Vol. 62, No. 11, (November 2005), pp. 1258-1265, ISSN 15383636

Kunze, U., Schmeiser-Rieder, A. & Schoberberger, R. (1998). European Medical Association Smoking for Health (EMASH) - Consensus on smoking cessation: guidelines for physicians. *Sozial und Präventivmedizin,* Vol. 4, No. 3, pp. 167-172, ISSN 0303-8408

Lai, D. T. C., Cahill, K., Qin, Y. & Tang, J. L. (2010). Motivational interviewing for smoking cessation. *Cochrane Database of Systematic Reviews,* Vol. 1, (January 2010), ISSN 13616137

Lancaster, T. & Stead, L. F. (2005). Self-help interventions for smoking cessation. *Cochrane Database of Systematic Reviews,* Vol. 3, (July 2005), ISSN 13616137

Lasser, K., Boyd, J. W., Woolhandler, S., Himmelstein, D. U., McCormick, D. & Bor, D. H. (2000). Smoking and Mental Illness - A Population-Based Prevalence Study. *JAMA: Journal of the American Medical Association,* Vol. 284, No. 20, (November 2000), pp. 2606-2610, ISSN 15383598

Lawn, S., Pols, G. & Barber, J. (2002). Smoking and quitting: a qualitative study with community-living psychiatric clients. *Social Science and Medicine,* Vol. 54, No. 1, (January 2002), pp. 93- 104, ISSN 0277-9536

Lawn, S. & Condon, J. (2006). Psychiatric nurses' ethical stance on cigarette smoking by patients: Determinants and dilemmas in their role in supporting cessation. *International Journal of Mental Health Nursing,* Vol. 15, No. 2, (June 2006), pp. 111-118, ISSN 14458330

Levin, E. D., Wilson, W., Rose, J. E. & McEvoy, J. (1996). Nicotine-haloperidol interactions and cognitive performance in schizophrenics. *Neuropsychopharmacology,* Vol. 15, No. 5, (November 1996), pp. 429-436, ISSN 0893133X

Lindson, N., Aveyard, P. & Hughes, J. R. (2010). Reduction versus abrupt cessation in smokers who want to quit. *Cochrane Database of Systematic Reviews*, Vol. 3, (March 2010), ISSN13616137

Lumley, J., Chamberlain, C., Dowswell, T., Oliver, S., Oakley, L. & Watson, L. (2009). Interventions for promoting smoking cessation during pregnancy. *Cochrane Database of Systematic Reviews*, Vol. 3, (July 2009), ISSN 13616137

McChargue, D. E., Gulliver, S. B., & Hitsman, B. (2002a). A reply to the commentaries on schizophrenia and smoking treatment: more research is needed. *Addiction*, Vol. 97, No. 7, (July 2002), pp. 799-800, ISSN 09652140

McChargue, D. E., Gulliver, S. B., & Hitsman, B. (2002b). Would smokers with schizophrenia benefit from a more flexible approach to smoking treatment? *Addiction*, Vol. 97, No. 7, (July 2002), pp. 785-793, ISSN 09652140

McChargue, D. E., Collins, F. L., & Cohen, L. M. (2002). Effect of non-nicotinic moist snuff replacement and lobeline on withdrawal symptoms during 48-hour smokeless tobacco deprivation. *Nicotine and Tobacco Research*, Vol. 4, No. 2, (May 2002), pp. 195-200, ISSN 014622203

McCloughen, A. (2003). The association between schizophrenia and cigarette smoking: a review of the literature and implications for mental health nursing practice. *International Journal of Mental Health Nursing*, Vol. 12, No. 2, (June 2003), pp. 119-129, ISSN 14458330

Mester, R., Toren, P., Ben-Moshe, Y. & Weizman, A. (1993). Survey of smoking habits and attitudes of patients and staff in psychiatric hospitals. *Psychopathology*, Vol. 26, No. 2, (March-April 1993), pp. 69-75, ISSN 02544962

Meyer, C., Rumpf, H. -J., Hapke, U., & John, U. (2004). Impact of psychiatric disorders in the general population: satisfaction with life and the influence of comorbidity and disorder duration. *Social Psychiatry and Psychiatric Epidemiology*, Vol. 39, No. 6, pp. 435 - 441, ISSN 09337954

Miller, M., Hemenway, D., & Rimm, E. (2000). Cigarettes and suicide: a prospective study of 50,000 men. *American Journal of Public Health*, Vol. 90, No. 5, (May 2000), pp. 768-773, ISSN 00900036

Miller, W. R., & Rollnick, S. (2002). *Motivational interviewing: Preparing people for change (2nd ed.).* New York, NY US: Guilford Press

Morrell, H. E. R., & Cohen, L. M. (2006). Cigarette smoking, anxiety, and depression. *Journal of Psychopathology and Behavioral Assessment*, Vol. 28, No. 4, (December 2006), pp. 281-295, ISSN 08822689

Moxham, J. (2001). Mental health and smoking - an opening address. *Symposium report - smoking and mental health*, Royal Pharmaceutical Society, London, 9 November 2001

Mühlig, S. (2008). Smoking cessation in patients with COPD: the status of routine care in Germany. *Pneumologie, Vol.* 62, No. 10, (October 2008), pp. 616-622, ISSN 09348387

Nelson, C. B. & Wittchen, H. U. (1998). Smoking and nicotine dependence: Results from a sample of 14-24-years olds in Germany. *European Addiction Research*, Vol. 4, No. 1-2, (March 1998), pp. 42-49, ISSN 1022-6877

Nutt, D., King, L. A., Saulsbury, W. & Blakemore, C. (2007) Development of a rational scale to assess the harm of drugs of potential misuse. *The Lancet*, Vol. 369, No. 9566, (March 2007), pp. 1047-1053, ISSN 01406736

Oquendo, M. A., Lizardi, D., Greenwald, S., Weissman, M. M. & Mann, J. J. (2004). Rates of lifetime suicide attempt and rates of lifetime major depression in different ethnic groups in the United States. *Acta Psychiatrica Scandinavica*, Vol. 110, No. 6, (December 2004), pp. 446-451, ISSN 0001690X

Pabst, A., Piontek D., Kraus L. & Müller, S. (2010). Substance Use and Substance Use Disorders. Results of the 2009 Epidemiological Survey of Substance Abuse. *Sucht*, Vol. 56, No. 5, (October 2010), pp. 327–336, ISSN 0939-5911

Patkar, A. A., Gopalakrishnan, R., Lundy, A., Leone, F. T., Certa, K. M. & Weinstein, S. P. (2002). Relationship between tobacco smoking and positive and negative symptoms in schizophrenia. *Journal of Nervous and Mental Disease*, Vol. 190, No. 9, (September 2002), pp. 604-610, ISSN 00223018

Patten, C. A., Martin, J. E. & Owen, N. (1996). Can psychiatric and chemical dependency treatment units be smoke free? *Journal of Substance Abuse Treatment*, Vol. 13, No. 2, (March-April 1996), pp. 107-118, ISSN 07405472

Pelkonen, M. & Kankkunen, P. (2001). Nurses' competence in advising and supporting clients to cease smoking: a survey among Finnish nurses. *Journal of Clinical Nursing*, Vol. 23, No. 4, (July 2001), pp. 189-200, ISSN 09621067

Prochaska, J. O., DiClemente, C. C., Velicer, W. F. & Rossi, J. S. (1993). Standardized, individualized, interactive, and personalized self-help programs for smoking cessation. *Health Psychol*, Vol. 12, No. 5, (September 1993), pp. 399-405, ISSN 02786133

Prochaska, J., Butterworth, S., Redding, C. A., Burden, V., Perrin, N., Leo, M., Flaherty-Robb, M. & Prochaska, J. M. (2008). Initial efficacy of MI, TTM tailoring and HRI's with multiple behaviors for employee health promotion. *Preventive Medicine*, Vol. 46, No. 3, (March 2008), pp. 226-31, ISSN 00917435

Prochaska, J., Fromont, S. C. & Hall, S. M. (2005). How prepared are psychiatry residents for treating nicotine dependence? *Academic Psychiatry*, Vol. 29, No. 3, (August 2005), pp. 256-261, ISSN 10429670

Prochaska, J., Fletcher, L., Hall, S. E. & Hall, S. M. (2006). Return to smoking following a smoke-free psychiatric hospitalisation. *American Journal on Addictions*, Vol. 15, No. 1, (January 2006), pp. 15–22; ISSN 10550496

Prochaska, J., Fromont, S. C., Louie, A. K., Jacobs, M. H. & Hall, S. M. (2006). Training in Tobacco Treatments in Psychiatry: A National Survey of Psychiatry Residency Training Directors. *Academic Psychiatry*, Vol. 30, No. 5, (September 2006), pp. 372-379, ISSN 10429670

Prochaska, J., Gill, P. & Hall, S. M. (2004). Treatment of Tobacco Use in an Inpatient Psychiatric Setting. *Psychiatric Services*, Vol. 55, No. 11, (November 2004), pp. 1265-1270, ISSN 10752730

Rosen-Chase, C. & Dyson, V. (1999). Treatment of nicotine dependence in the chronically mentally ill. *Journal of Substance Abuse Treatment*, Vol. 16, No. 4, pp. 315-320, ISSN 07405472

Rowe, K. & Clark, J. M. (2000). The incidence of smoking amongst nurses: a review of the literature. *Journal of Advanced Nursing*, Vol. 31, No. 5, (May 2000), pp. 1046–1053, ISSN 03092402

Schmitz, N., Kruse, J. & Kugler, J. (2003). Disabilities, quality of life, and mental disorders associated with smoking and nicotine dependence. *The American Journal of Psychiatry*, Vol. 160, No. 9, (September 2003), pp. 1670-1676, ISSN 15357228

Schneider, B., Schnabel, A., Wetterling, T., Bartusch, B., Weber, B. & Georgi, K. (2008). How do personality disorders modify suicide risk?. *Journal of Personality Disorders*, Vol. 22, No. 3, (June 2008), pp. 233-245, ISSN 0885579X

Silagy, C., Mant, D., Fowler, G. & Lodge, M. (1994). Meta-analysis on efficacy of nicotine replacement therapies in smoking cessation. *The Lancet*, Vol. 343, (January 1994), pp. 139–142, ISSN 0140-6736

Stead, L. F. & Lancaster, T. (2005). Group behaviour therapy programmes for smoking cessation. *Cochrane Database of Systematic Reviews*, Vol. 2, (April 2005), ISSN 13616137

Stead, L. F., Perera, R. & Lancaster, T. (2006). Telephone counselling for smoking cessation. *Cochrane Database of Systematic Reviews*, Vol. 3, (July 2006), ISSN 13616137

Stead, L. F. & Lancaster, T. (2007). Interventions to reduce harm from continued tobacco use. *Cochrane Database of Systematic Reviews*, Vol. 3, (July 2008), ISSN 13616137

Stead, L. F., Perera, R., Bullen, C., Mant, D. & Lancaster, T. (2008). Nicotine replacement therapy for smoking cessation. *Cochrane Database of Systematic Reviews*, Vol. 1, (January 2008), ISSN 13616137

Sutton, S. (2001). Back to the drawing board? A review of applications of the transtheoretical model to substance use. *Addiction*. Vol. 96, No. 1, pp. 175-186, ISSN 09652140

Tiffany, S. T, & Conklin, S. A. (2000). A cognitive processing model of alcohol craving and compulsive alcohol use. *Addiction*, Vol. 95, No. 2, (August 200), pp. 145-154, ISSN 09652140

Tizabi, Y., Getachew, B., Rezvani, A., Hauser, S. R. & Overstreet, D. H. (2009). Antidepressant-like effects of nicotine and reduced nicotinic receptor binding in the Fawn-Hooded rat, an animal model of co-morbid depression and alcoholism. *Progress in Neuro-Psychopharmacology and Biological Psychiatry*, Vol. 33, No. 3, (April 2009), pp. 398-402, ISSN 02785846

Ussher, M. H., Taylor, A. & Faulkner, G. (2008). Exercise interventions for smoking cessation. *Cochrane Database of Systematic Reviews*, Vol. 4, (October 2008), ISSN 13616137

Vazquez-Palacios, G., Bonilla-Jaime, H. & Velazquez-Moctezuma, J. (2005). Antidepressant effects of nicotine and fluoxetine in an animal model of depression induced by neonatal treatment with clomipramine. *Progress in Neuro-Psychopharmacology and Biological Psychiatry*, Vol. 29, No. 1, (January 2005), pp. 39-46, ISSN 02785846

White, A. R., Rampes, H., Liu, J. P., Stead, L. F. & Campbell, J. (2011). Acupuncture and related interventions for smoking cessation. *Cochrane Database of Systematic Reviews*, Vol. 1, (January 2011), ISSN 13616137

WHO. (2001). Evidence based Recommendations on the treatment of tobacco dependence, In: *WHO-recommendations*, Available from: http://www. bvsde. paho. org/bvsacd/cd16/whoevidence. pdf

WHO. (2008). WHO Report on the Global Tobacco Epidemic, *The MPOWER package*. World Health Organization, ISBN 978 92 4 159628 2, Geneva

Wiesbeck, G. A., Kuhl, H. -C., Yaldizli, Ö. & Wurst, F. M. (2008). Tobacco smoking and depression - Results from the WHO/ISBRA study. *Neuropsychobiology*, Vol. 57, No. 2, (June 2008), pp. 26-31, ISSN 14230224

Wilhelm, K., Wedgwood, L., Niven, H. & Kay-Lambkin, F. (2006). Smoking cessation and depression: current knowledge and future directions. *Drug Alcohol Review*, Vol. 25, No. 1, (October 2005), pp. 97-107, ISSN 09595236

Williams, J. M. & Ziedonis, D. (2004). Addressing tobacco among individuals with a mental illness or an addiction. *Addictive Behaviors*, Vol. 29, No. 6, pp. 1067-1083, ISSN 03064603

Wye, P. M., Bowman, J. A., Wiggers, J. H., Baker, A., Knight, J., Carr, V. J., Terry, M. & Clancy, R. (2009). Smoking Restrictions and Treatment for Smoking: Policies and Procedures in Psychiatric Inpatient Units in Australia. *Psychiatric Services*, Vol. 60, No. 1, (January 2009), pp. 100-107, ISSN 10752730

Ziedonis, D. M. & George, T. P. (1997). Schizophrenia and nicotine use: report of a pilot smoking cessation programme and review of neurobiological and clinical issues. *Schizophrenia Bulletin*, Vol. 23, No. 2, pp. 247–254, ISSN 0586-7614

Ziedonis, D. M. & Williams, J. (2003). Management of smoking in people with psychiatric disorders. *Current Opinion in Psychiatry*, Vol. 16, No. 3, (May 2003), pp. 305-15, ISSN 0951-7367

17

Comorbidity of a Serious Mental Illness with an Addiction to Psychoactive Substances

Krzysztof Krysta, Irena Krupka-Matuszczyk,
Małgorzata Janas-Kozik and Małgorzata Stachowicz
Medical University of Silesia, Katowice
Poland

1. Introduction

Available data from literature show that among patients suffering from serious mental illnesses it was observed that about 50% of them abused psychoactive substances during their lives (Kessler et al., 1996). And the dependence on such substances like cannabis, amphetamine, or cocaine is more common in patients suffering from schizophrenia than in other psychiatric patients (May-Majewski, 2002). It was found that in the North American population every fourth person suffering from schizophrenia abused alcohol (Helzer & Pryzbeck, 1998). The objective of this study is to analyze data from literature concerning the reasons for psychoactive substance abuse by persons suffering from psychiatric disorders and to discuss the most effective treatment strategies for them. A very important part of this analysis is the so called self-treatment hypothesis formulated by Khantzian (1985). Its definition embraces two elements. Firstly ill persons use psychoactive substances, because they decrease their psychological discomfort. On the other hand there is a great degree in psychopharmacological specificity in choosing the abused substance.

2. Definition of dual diagnosis

In the diagnostic process in psychiatry it often happens to set two or more diagnoses in the same patient. "Dual diagnosis" is a concept that doesn't appear in the official nomenclature of mental health and is not included in the ICD-10 and DSM-IV classifications. In a very general sense it concerns a patient who presents a psychopathological picture, in which we find simultaneously fulfilled criteria for two different psychiatric disorders. However, in recent years, the term "dual diagnosis" has become synonymous with the coexistence of psychiatric disorders and psychoactive substance dependence (Solomon et al., 1993) and this coexistence can consist of the following options:

1. Mental illness and drug dependence.
2. Drug dependence and personality disorders.
3. Acute psychotic disorders resulting from substance use.
4. Drug dependence, mental illness and organic disorders in different combinations (Sciacca, 1987).

Patients with a dual diagnosis can cause many problems in the diagnostic process and therapy at different stages of treatment both in the psychiatric and in the addiction treatment systems. One of the most common examples of a dual diagnosis encountered in psychiatric clinical practice is comorbodity of schizophrenia or bipolar disorder and psychoactive substance dependence.

3. Epidemiology and demographics of dual diagnosis

In recent years, there has been a gradually growing awareness that the problems associated with abuse and addiction to psychoactive substances are very common in people with various mental disorders, including schizophrenia and bipolar disorder. But, although there is an increasing number of reports from the literature that these coexisting disorders are very common, as yet few therapeutic programs based on empirical data targeted specifically at this group of patients have been developed (Lewin & Hennesy, 1994). Based on available evidence, we can try to desribe the scale of the problem. The incidence of bipolar disorder and coexisting abuse of psychoactive substances has been described inter alia in the Epidemiological Catchment Area Study (Regier et al, 1990). This study was conducted among participants from five different municipalities in the U.S.. It showed that, in comparison with with patients with other psychiatric disorders, people with bipolar disorder had the highest comorbidity of disorders associated with alcohol use (46%) and drugs (41%). In addition, rates of disorders associated with the use of alcohol and drugs in people with bipolar disorder were much higher than the associated disorders in the general population (14% and 6%). It was also observed that in bipolar I there was a higher risk of co-existence of problems associated with substance abuse in comparison with bipolar II, wich were respectively 61% and 48% (Lewin & Hennesy, 1994). These results were confirmed by further epidemiological studies. In the National Comorbidity Study (NCS) focused on the respondents with a lifetime alcohol or drug use disorder, recruited for the evaluation, it was found that 51,4% of them also met criteria for at least one lifetime mental disorder. 50.9% of the NCS respondents with a lifetime mental disorder also had a history of alcohol or drug abuse or dependence (Kessler et al., 1996). As mentioned above, one of the most common example of dual diagnosic in the coexistence of schizophrenia and addiction to substances. In the studies of Helzer and Pryzbeck (1998) it was found out that four times more alcoholic than non-alcoholic subjects suffer from schizophrenia. The abuse of stimulants four times more common in schizophrenic than non-schizophrenic subjects (Leduc & Mittleman, 1995). In New York State among each 100 patients hospitalised for their first episode of schizophrenia, 35% of them were addicted to illicit drugs. During the relapses of schizophrenia 22% of the patients use psychoactive substances (DeLisi et al., 1991).

3.1 Young age of patients with dual diagnosis

Patients with dual diagnosis are often young people. De Millo (1989) observed the prevalence of various psychiatric disorders among adolescents addicted to drugs, which was much higher that a paralell incidence among adults, but he also emphasises the fact that there is a lack of standardisation of diagnostic tools for this population. According to Lysaker et al. (1994) among schizophrenic patients with concomitant use of cocaine, the age of first hospitalisation was earlier than in patients not biased. In turn, according to Menezes (1996) patients with dual diagnosis are mainly young men. These observations confirm the evaluations from the studies of Maynard and Cox (1998), who compared the demographic structure of patients hospitalised in psychiatric hospitals in the United States. They showed that among patients with dual diagnosis there was a larger number of younger ones (average age of 36-37 years), compared with those which had only a single psychiatric diagnosis (mean age of 42-43 years).

A study done in Swiss population, which was conducted in different groups of schizophrenic patients presented a higher average age of subjects without addiction, and also of those who were solely dependent on alcohol, in comparison with patients with a history of illicit drug abuse (Modestin et al., 2001).

Similarly, Kavanagh et al. (2004), examining patients with dual diagnosis in the population of Australia, found that the incidence of alcohol use in patients with dual diagnosis did not depend on the age group, whereas the use of other psychoactive substances was higher in younger groups. Epidemiological studies in England showed that the average age of patients with dual diagnosis is within the range of 34-38 years, but recent trends show a gradual decline of this age (Frisher et al., 2004).

3.2 Sex differences among dual diagnosis patients

When discussing issues related to the comorbidity of a seriuos maental disorder and addiction to psychoactive substances, an important factor to be considered is the sex. Lewine (1981) in his review of the literature devoted to the differences between men and women suffering from schizophrenia emphasises that men are characterized by poorer premorbid social functioning, earlier age of first hospitalisation, more severe negative symptoms, more severe disease. Better premorbid functioning of women with schizophrenia is an element often emphasised in the literature. Women at the time of onset have a better social contacts, higher education, more permanent job, most of them have already left home, got married, or have a regular partner (Kalisz et al., 2001). Girls more often than boys have a secondary education (Krupka-Matuszczyk, 1998). Research on gender differences in schizophrenia have shown that women experience a milder form of the disease than men, which is associated with better premorbid functioning. Gearon and Bellack (2000) draw attention to the gender difference in patients with dual diagnosis. In the group of outpatients with coexisting schizophrenia and psychoactive substance dependence found that women, despite a better premorbid functioning and later age of onset, experience a deterioration, when they begin to use drugs. This may indicate that women are particularly susceptible to the adverse effects of psychoactive substances. The use of these substances and related social deficits, and reduced ability to process information in them may impair the ability to recognise hazards, such as the threat of violence or rape and protect themselves against them (Bellack & Gearon, 1998). Prevalence of drug use also has a correlation with gender. As noted Sieroslawski, in studies conducted in Poland and Europe in the early 90's, the prevalence among boys was more than twice higher than in girls, though he stressed that in some other countries, like Britain or the USA differentiation based on gender was not so clear (Sierosławski, 1998). Since the age of onset of schizophrenia in men is lower than in women, and drug use among young men is more prevalent, perhaps it may result in a fact that the population of patients with dual diagnosis is dominated by young men. Numerous studies show a predominance of males among people with dual diagnosis. In 1994 DeQuardo et al. evaluated the frequency of substance use among schizophrenic patients. In a population of addicts analysed by them, there were 48% of men and 20% of women. Maynard and Cox (1998) analyzed cross-sectionally a population of patients hospitalized in the U.S. due to various psychiatric disorders, and they found that among those with a dual diagnosis, the majority were males. Swartz et al. (2000) conducted an epidemiological study including drug addicts in the U.S.. Among the people who developed a dual diagnosis, 70% were males, and most of them were in the age group of 30-40 years. Salyers and Mueser (2001), studying a group of 404 patients with schizophrenia and schizoaffective disorder, found that in the subgroup that had used alcohol or drugs, women constituted a minority. Other sources of demographic and social analyses of patients with dual diagnosis indicate that the population of such patients consists mostly of men, who often do not work and are poorly educated (Drake & Mueser, 2000). Hambrecht and Hafner (2000) conducted research among a population of a billion participants from Germany, noting that among patients with the first episode of schizophrenia, male gender is a greater risk factor when it comes to cannabis abuse. Similar observations were made by Cantor-Graae in studies conducted in Sweden (2001) in which it was found that among patients with schizophrenia who use substances were far fewer women. French researchers analysed the demographics of patients with schizophrenia and the use of psychoactive substances. It turned out that in that group only 16.7% were women (Dervaux et al., 2003). Kavanagh et al. (2004) examining the incidence of substance use psychoactive drugs in patients with psychoses of various aetiologies noted a prevalence of males in the evaluated group.

3.3 Level of education in the population of dual diagnosis patients

As stated by Chouinard et al. (2003), the first episode of a serious mental illness usually appears at the beginning of adult life, and this is the age when people take important life decisions on, inter alia, the occupation. Suffering from psychiatric disorders is often associated with failure to achieve an adequate education, which may be a consequence of reduced social and economic status. In a Polish follow-up study conducted by Krupka-Matuszczyk (1998) on a group of adolescents including 142 persons, it was observed that after the first hospitalisation 30% of young people did not continue education interrupted by illness. Patients with schizophrenia or bipolar disorder often appear to be poorer, positioned (economically and socially) in worse groups and regions. Achieving a lower educational level may be also the result of the use of psychoactive substances. Swaim et al. (1997) repeatedly observed a higher proportion of drug users in those who interrupted their education prematurely. In a study conducted in Australia it was found that weekly marijuana use in adolescents increases the risk of disruption of school before completing it (Lynskey et al., 2003). Oboth and Anthony (2000) found that among young Americans intravenous drug use causes frequent interruptions of education in high school. In further studies, Kavanagh et al., (2004) observed that having a lower educational attainment was correlated with the use of cannabis, but there was no such correlation with other drugs. In another study, devoted to patients with dual diagnosis, it was found that patients with schizophrenia addicted to alcohol or drugs achieve worse education in comparison to patients with schizophrenia without concomitant dependence (Potvin et al., 2003). Thus, the coexistence of addiction and a serious mental ilness may imply in a summation of the associated adverse factors affecting the level of education of the patients.

4. Diagnostic problems

Conducting epidemiological studies is complicated by the fact that the described problem is associated with a number of diagnostic questions. For example it is possible that some of the observed elevated rates of coexistence of bipolar disorder, or disorders of the bipolar spectrum, such as cyclothymia, and addiction may be caused by the effects of consumption of psychoactive substances. This diagnostic error is less likely in patients with chronic, severe bipolar disorder or in those patients who clearly developed symptoms of bipolar disorder before they began using substances (Lewin & Hennesy, 2004). It is also sometimes difficult to make a differential diagnosis between schizophrenia and a drug related psychosis. Some helpful observations from the patient's behaviour may suggest the clinician the possibility of substance abuse by persons treated for various mental disorders. For example, patients can often ask the nurse for painkillers, and pharmaceuticals to treat different symptoms. This behaviour often distinguishes them from patients without substance abuse problems who are reluctant to take medications because of unpleasant experiences with side effect and because of an association with a stigma of a mental illness. Another clue suggesting addiction is a behaviour of the patient in the community of patients. Patients with a co-dependency often show a better functioning in a group of mentally ill persons. They show higher social skills and they are more adequate in the field of sexual behaviour. Patients with a co-dependence more often have a tendency to intimidate others, causing fear and respect among the staff and other patients (Solomon et al., 1993).

5. Reasons for substance abuse among mentally ill people

Why are disorders related to substance use so common in patients with serious mental illnesses? One of the attempts to explain this phenomenon is the self-medication hypothesis formulated by Khantzian (1985). In defining the self-medication, he draws attention to its two aspects. 1) There is a considerable degree of specificity in the choice of a psychoactive substance. 2) People use, abuse and become addicted to psychoactive substances because they reduce the feeling of psychological discomfort. This suggests that people with psychiatric disorders use specific substances (e.g. use heroin during a manic episode or stimulants during a depressive episode) in an attempt to prevent or "self-medicate" unpleasant symptoms, which ultimately leads to the re-use of these substances. The motivation to do it is often a result of subjective profits that the patients using them experience. The patients with schizophrenia use those substances in order to handle depression, to experience more profoundly different emotions, and to reduce the side-effects of the medication they are prescribed. The data show that illicit drugs are used to reduce depression (72%), and tension (64%) to increase pleasant emotions (62%), to enhance the ability to work and to learn (17%), to decrease the side-effects of the medication.(15%), to reduce hallucinations (11%) , suspicion (4%) and other symptoms (Dixon et al., 1991). The analysis of the causes of abuse of psychoactive substances by subjects with schizphrenia was made by a Canadian team, which attempted to balance gains and losses incurred by the patients reaching for psychoactive substances. In the patients' opinion marijuana and alcohol improved their social functioning. However besides the positive outcomes, the respondents emphasised that the reduction of depressive symptoms was often only their wish, because except for achieving such effects as relaxation, pleasure, being more active etc., the psychoactive substances may happent to be an uncontrolled and unexpected reason for an increase of depressive symptoms. In addition, in spite of achieving a feeling of increased satisfaction, the patients might experience an exacerbation of existing, or develop new positive symptoms of schizophrenia (Addington & Duchak, 1997). When evaluating the attractiveness of different substances for the patients suffering from schizophrenia it is very important to distinguish between positive and negative symptoms of this disease. The positive symptoms usually implicate the abuse of tranquilisers, and the negative symptoms are most frequently a reason to develop a dependence than the positive symptoms. The incidence of negative symptoms is usually accompanied by increased suffering and the patient uses the substance to reduce it even if the relief is only transient. The study done in Australia (1995) was very important. 53 patients with comorbid diagnoses of schizophrenia and addiction to psychoactive substances were interviewed with the use of Brief Symptom Inventory and Schizophrenia/Substance Abuse Interview Schedule. Most of the patients reported that the use of substances was the reason for a development or exacerbation of their disease, 80% of them used drugs to handle their dysphoria and anxiety. The amphetamines caused their subjective improvement better than alcohol, however the choice of the substance depended mainly on what they could afford. Only cannabis exacerbated the positive symptoms and only amphetamines reduced negative symptoms (Baigent et al., 1995). In other studies it was proven that different substances have influence on different problems related to the disease. For example alcohol, cannabis and cocaine decrease depression, cannabis and alcohol decrease the level of anxiety and cocaine increases it (Coben & Levy, 1998). The analysis of subjective experiences of the patients shows that handling the positive symptoms is the most difficult for them as alcohol has here only a limited influence, cannabis increases these symptoms and the effect of cocaine may be diverse depending on the individual patients.

6. Impact of substance use on the course of psychiatric disorders

The observations of the clinicians treating the dual diagnosis patients concerning the influence of the substance abuse on the course of the mental illness are inconsistent. According to some of them the patients suffering from schizophrenia abusing substances present less positive and negative symptoms, according to others the substance abuse highly deteriorates the course of the disease. Especially the stimulants like cocaine have a negative impact on the intensity of psychiatric symptoms. According to data from literature the only result of substance abuse is the increase of frequency of hospitalizations (LeDuc & Mittleman, 1995), and according to some other studies the impact on different symptoms may be diverse, e.g. alcohol causes an increase of positive symptoms, and it is also responsible for a higher frequency of suicidal attempts (Soyka, 1994). We have available data from the literature on the relationship between substance use and severity of clinical symptoms. Lysaker et al., (1994), found that patients with schizophrenia who use cocaine have less intense negative symptoms than patients, who do not use cocaine. Serper et al. (1995) found in schizophrenic patients with a concomitant use of cocaine lower scores of negative symptoms and higher scores of depression and anxiety. Salyers and Mueser (2001) examining patients with schizophrenia who used alcohol and drugs, observed lower intensity of negative symptoms than in patients without concomitant dependence. However, Soyka et al., (2001) found that the coexistence of addiction, causes only minor differences in the scores of positive and negative symptoms. Clearer differentiation of severity was related only hallucinations among patients with dual diagnosis. Norwegian authors who analysed the relationship between substance use and severity of PANSS scores in psychotic patients who used and who did not use psychoactive substances, did not observe differences in positive negative and general symptoms (Moller & Linaker, 2004). In contrast, Canadian researchers found that patients with dual diagnosis had a higher score in

PANSS than patients with schizophrenia alone (Margolese et al., 2003). Buhler et al (2002) examined populations of nonabused patients with schizophrenia and those addicted to alcohol and drugs (mainly cannabis). They found that patients with dual diagnosis experienced more severe positive symptoms. Similar results have also resulted in a study conducted by Green et al. (2002). In the work of Addington and Addington (1997) there was no overall significant difference in symptoms measured by PANSS scale between the group using and not using psychoactive substances. The exception was the subgroup of people who used cocaine, in which a higher severity of positive symptoms was observed. In a study conducted by Pencer and Addington (2003) analysing the cognitive functions in patients with first episode of psychosis, using psychoactive substances, an assessment of PANSS at the start, after one year and two years of observation was done. There was no difference in negative symptoms between the two groups, while those who did not use drugs had less severe positive symptoms. It must be remembered that the subjects throughout the period of observation have used psychoactive substances. Substance abuse can also have a negative impact on the course of the bipolar disorder. For example, it may be associated with earlier age of onset of the disorder and cause more difficulties in the therapy of the subtypes of the disease, such as rapid cycling, dysphoria and mixed states. Salloum et al. (2002) conducted a study covering 256 patients with acute manic episode, done in a municipal psychiatric ward, in which it was found that patients with severe symptoms of disease, abusing alcohol presented a significantly higher lability of mood, impulsivity and increased incidence of aggressive behaviour than patients with an acute manic episode without accompanying alcohol abuse. Furthermore, the coexistence of bipolar disorder and substance abuse is associated with an increased number of psychiatric hospitalisations and it is more difficult to achieve remission of acute manic episodes.

7. Treatment strategies for patients with dual diagnosis

These observations lead to a conlusion that a specific approach for the treatment of comorbid mental ilness and disturbances associated with the use of psychoactive substances is necessary. Currently, clinicians must often rely on their own observations rather than on empirical data to determine which therapies are best for this group of patients.

7.1 Pharmacological treatment

In schizophrenic patients with comorbid substance abuse the treatment with second-generation antipsychotics may have beneficial effects on their symptoms. There are reports in the literature, which indicate the ability of these drugs to reduce other symptoms of the disease, as well as reducing the amount of drug used by patients treated with them.

In the studies of subjects with schizophrenia and schizoaffective disorder, previously diagnosed as drug resistant, a subgroup of patients with dual diagnosis was selected. When they were switch on clozapine from classical neuroleptics in within six months, the authors noted that patients with a coexistence and without a coexistence of drug dependence responsed equally to the treatment (Buckley et al., 1994). Similar observations were made Volavka (1999), who noted that during a 6-month treatment with clozapine it could not be determined whether the difference in the treatment response between patients with schizophrenia and schizoaffective disorder depends on the fact if they use or do not use psychoactive substances. In turn, Zimmet et al (2000) found that over 85% of patients who used psychoactive substances during their treatment with clozapine reduced the quanities of abused psychoactive substances. To similar conclusions also led the studies by Green et al., (2002) and also by Drake et al., (2000) in relation to patients who use alcohol, as well as research of Buckley et al. (1998) embracing patients with dual diagnosis abusing alcohol, cigarettes and cocaine. As it turned out, the classical neuroleptic treatment did not reduce the amount of abused substances. Probably the positive effects of clozapine treatment is due to the fact that it acts on mesocortical and mesolimbic dopaminergic neurons that are associated the reward system (Green et al., 1999). According to Noordsy et al., (2003) in patients with schizophrenia the reward system does not function properly, which increases the susceptibility to substance use. This may also underly the poorer tolerability of conventional antipsychotics in patients with dual diagnosis and the effectiveness of clozapine and, to a lesser extent, of other atypical antipsychotics in the treatment of this group of patients. According to Stip et al., (2003) and Weisman (2003) in the treatment of patients with dual diagnosis the most promising results were obtained with clozapine, and slightly worse results with olanzapine and quetiapine. Other studies have shown a reduction in the frequency of alcohol use after the change of treatment from classical neuroleptics to risperidone (Huang, 1996).

As for the effect of various drugs used to treat bipolar disorder, a summary is made here Maremmani et al (2010). According to them, for example, carbamazepine is beneficial in preventing relapse in abusers of cocaine and has a positive effect on discomfort associated with fluctuations in mood, but it has no effect on the behaviour directed to obtain the substance. Selective response to lithium is achieved in alcoholics with a coexisting depression. Oxcarbazepine has a good effect of aggressive patients, while valproic acid generally is considered the drug effective in patients with coexisting bipolar disorder and addiction, but also in people with anxiety disorders and the accompanying dependence on psychoactive substances. The authors of that study conclude that some of these medicines are safe and effective agents that can be used in the treatment of addicted persons with mood disorders.

7.2 Psychotherapy and rehabilitation

Due to the above-described specific problems associated with diagnosing and treatiment of patients with dual diagnosis, specific treatment programs should be developed for them, which combine elements of both psychiatric treatment and addiction therapy. Understanding the causes of the problems described above is necessary for an effective prevention of drug abuse by people with mental illnesses. An example of therapeutic program for dual diagnosis patients with comorbid addiction to substances, with which the authors have a possibility to co-operate, is the Therapeutic Community "Famila" in Gliwice, Poland, which was founded by May-Majewski in the 80-ties. A comprehensive model of treating patients with dual diagnosis, offered by the Center for Addiction Treatment "Familia" allows them to move freely between the settings of two therapeutic models. The program is stationary, conducted in three separate buildings. They have registered 100 beds. The whole program employs three psychiatrists, 6 psychologists and 8 specialists in addiction therapy and nurses. The therapy takes place in a therapeutic community in which the average age is 23 years and in various small groups depending on the current needs of the patient. The treatment of the patient in the psychiatric ward usually follows a complex diagnostic process. Depending on the patient's current condition, which for example may be acute or chronic, the patient may continue his or her treatment in a therapeutic community. The most important rules of the program are: 1) authority, 2) clear rules and principles. The fulfillment of these conditions is essential in building a therapeutic offer for the patients with an addiction to psychoactive substances and psychiatric disorders. These standards apply in therapeutic communities, where adherence to rules and principles is possible through the common responsibilty of all members of this community, both therapists and the patients. The most important factor in a succeful therapy are: receiving feedback from others, allowing to express emotions, a sense of belonging to a group, giving feedback to others, discovering that others have similar problems, receiving support from others, giving support to others, receiving tips and ideas from others. The participant of a therapeutic program is expected to make a gradual transition from the periphery of the therapeutic communitiy to a position, when he or she takes over certain responsibilities (May-Majewski, 2002). Training of social skills is also a very important part of rehabilitation of patients with dual diagnosis. It includes skills such as: communication, interpersonal problem solving, active participation in their pharmacotherapy, learning to take care of their own health (Sawicka, 2001). A very important element that should be included in these programs is also a cognitive skills training, because, according to the the literature, patients participating in cognitive skills training significantly improve their performance on neuropsychological tests, they increase their insight. Keshavan and Hogarty (1999) developed the concept of "social cognition", which is associated with the term "emotional intelligence". The so-called "social cognition" is the central element of pathophysiology of certainn mental disorders like schizophrenia. People predisposed to the development of schizophrenia may use immature (concrete as opposed to abstract) styles which are inadequate for the more complex and abstract cognitive requirements specific to adults. In this way, they do not understand the essence of the subtleties and nuances of social interaction (Lewis, 2004). It appears that cognitive impairment is associated with various aspects of social functioning and problems in vocational activities. Data from literature suggest that they are particularly important for social functioning, quality of life, social skills, ability to benefit from learning new skills (Tamminga, 1998).

8. Conclusion

Understanding the causes of the problem described above is necessary for effective prevention of substance abuse by people with mental health problems. The results of available studies suggest that these patients have an increased risk of a relapse of both the disease and the addiction to substances. In addition to the symptoms they experience, one of the very important problem in the lives of these patients is their difficulty in social functioning. Effective therapy for these individuals should include: making it possible to create a protective environment, assisting these people in makin important changes in their lives, such as finding a good job, friends abstaining from drugs and alcohol, a group of people who can help the patient to find sense their lives. Patients directed to a therapeutic program must be motivated to make changes in their current life. This decision must be conscious and and be a free choice of the patient. It is also necessary to apply specific, individualied forms of therapy of, mental disorders and those associated with subsatnce abuse.

9. References

Addington, J. & Addington, D. (1997). Substance Abuse And Cognitive Functioning in Schizophrenia, *Journal of Psychiatry and Neuroscience,* Vol.22, No.4, (March 1997), pp. 99-104, ISSN:1180-4882

Addington J.; & Duchak V. (1997). Reasons For Substance Use in Schizophrenia. *Acta Psychiatrica Scandinavica,* Vol.96, No.5 (December 1997), pp. 329-333, ISSN:0001 - 690X

Baigent, M.; Holme, G. & Hafner, R.J. (1995). Self Reports of the Interaction Between Substance Abuse and Schizophrenia, *Australian and New Zealand Journal of Psychiatry,* Vol.29, No.1 (March 1995), pp. 69-74, ISSN 0004-8674

Bellack, A.S. & Gearon, J.S. (1998). Substance Abuse Treatment for People with Schizophrenia. *Addictive Behaviors,* Vol.23, No.6 (November-December 1998), pp.749-766, ISSN 0306-4603

Buckley, P.F. (1998). Substance Abuse in Schizophrenia: a Review. *The Journal of Clinical Psychiatry,* Vol.59, Suppl.3, pp. 26-30, ISSN 0160-6689

Buckley, P.; Thompson, P.; Way, L. & Meltzer, H.Y. (1994). Substance Abuse Among Patients with Treatment-resistant Schizophrenia: Characteristics and Implications for Clozapine Therapy. *American Journal of Psychiatry,* Vol.151, No.3 (March 1994), pp. 385-389, ISSN 0002-953X

Bühler, B.; Hambrecht, M.; Löffler; W.; an der Heiden; W. & Häfner, H. (2002). Precipitation and Determination of the Onset and Course of Schizophrenia by Substance Abuse - a Retrospective and Prospective Study of 232 Population-based First Illness Episodes. *Schizophrenia Research,* Vol.54, No.3, (April 2002), pp. 243-251, ISSN 0920-9964

Cantor-Graae, E.; Nordström, L.G. & McNeil, T.F. (2001). Substance Abuse in Schizophrenia: a Review of the Literature and a Study of Correlates in Sweden. *Schizophrenia Research,* Vol.48, No.1, (March 2001), pp. 69-82, ISSN 0920-9964

Chouinard, S.; Stip, E.; Comtois, G.; Corbière, M.; Bolé, P.; Lamontagne, L.; Lecavalier, M. & Beauregard, F. (2003). Young Patients with Severe Mental Illness Returning to School: Results of a Pilot Project Conducted in Montreal. *Santé mentale au Québec,* Vol.28, No.2, (Autumn 2003), pp. 273-290, ISSN 0383-6320

DeLisi, L.E.; Boccio, A.M.; Riordan, H.; Hoff, A.L.; Dorfman, A.; McClelland, J.; Kushner, M.; Van Eyl, O. & Oden, N. (1991). Familial Thyroid Disease and Delayed Language Development in First Admission Patients with Schizophrenia. *Psychiatry Research,* Vol.38, No.1, (July, 1991), pp. 39-50, ISSN 0165-1781

DeMilio, L. (1989). Psychiatric Syndromes in Adolescent Substance Abusers. *American Journal of Psychiatry,* Vol.146, No.9, (September 1989), pp. 1212-1214, ISSN 0002-953X

DeQuardo, J. R.; Carpenter, C. F. & Tandon, R. (1994). Patterns of Substance Abuse in Schizophrenia: Nature and Significance. *Journal of Psychiatric Research,* 1994, Vol.28, No.3, (May-June 1994), pp. 267-275, ISSN 0022-3956

Dervaux, A.; Laqueille, X.; Bourdel, M.C.; Leborgne, M.H.; Olié, J.P.; Lôo, H. & Krebs, M.O. (2003) Cannabis and Schizophrenia: Demographic and Clinical Correlates. *L'Encéphale,* 2003, Vol.29, No.1, pp. 11-17, ISSN 0013-7006

Dixon, L.; Haas, G.; Weiden, P.J.; Sweeney, J. & Frances, A.J. (1991). Drug Abuse in Schizophrenic Patients: Clinical Correlates and Reasons for Use. *American Journal of Psychiatry,* Vol.148, No.2, pp. 224-230, ISSN 0002-953X

Drake, R.E. & Mueser, K.T. (2000). Psychosocial Approaches to Dual Diagnosis. *Schizophrenia Bulletin,* Vol.26, No.1, pp. 105-118, ISSN 0586-7614

Drake, R.E.; Xie, H.; McHugo, G.J. & Green, A.I. (2000). The Effects of Clozapine on Alcohol and drug use disorders among patients with schizophrenia. *Schizophrenia Bulletin,* Vol.26, No.2, pp. 441-449, ISSN 0586-7614

Frisher, M.; Collins, J.; Millson, D.; Crome, I. & Croft P. (2004). Prevalence of Comorbid Psychiatric Illness and Substance Misuse in Primary Care in England and Wales. *Journal of Epidemiology and Community Health,* Vol.58, No.12, (December 2004), pp. 1036-1041, ISSN 0143-005X

Gearon, J.S. & Bellack, A.S. (2000). Sex differences in illness presentation, course, and level of Functioning in Substance-abusing Schizophrenia Patients. *Schizophrenia Research,* Vol.43, No1, pp. 65-70, (May 2000), ISSN 0920-9964

Green, A.I., Salomon, M.S., Brenner, M.J., Rawlins, K. (2002). Treatment of schizophrenia and comorbid substance use disorder. *Current drug targets. CNS and neurological disorders,* Vol.1, No.2, (April 2002) pp.129-139, ISSN: 1568-007X

Green, A.I., Zimmet, S.V., Strous, R.D., Schildkraut, J.J. (1999). Clozapine for comorbid substance use disorder and schizophrenia: do patients with schizophrenia have a reward-deficiency syndrome that can be ameliorated by clozapine? *Harvard review of psychiatry,* Vol.6, No.6, (March-April 1999) pp.287-296, ISSN: 1067-3229

Hambrecht, M. & Häfner, H. (2000). Cannabis, Vulnerability, and the Onset of Schizophrenia: an Epidemiological Perspective. *Australian and New Zealand Journal of Psychiatry,* Vol.34, No.3 (June 2000), pp. 468-475, ISSN 0004-8674

Helzer, J.E. & Pryzbeck, T.R. (1988). The Co-occurrence of Alcoholism with Other Psychiatric Ddisorders in the General Population and its Impact on Treatment. *Journal of Studies on Alcohol and Drugs,* Vol.49, No.3, (May 1988), pp. 219 -224, ISSN 1937-1888

Kalisz, A. & Cechnicki, A. (2001). Różnice w Czynnikach Rokowniczych Między Mężczyznami, i Kobietami Hospitalizowanymi po raz Pierwszy z Rozpoznaniem Schizofrenii. *Psychiatria Polska,* Vol.35, No.6, (November-December 2001), pp. 951-963, ISSN 0033-2674

Kavanagh, D.J.; Waghorn, G.; Jenner, L.; Chant, D.C.; Carr, V.; Evans, M.; Hemnan, H.;

Jablensky, A. & McGrath, J.J. (2004). Demographic and Clinical Correlates of Comorbid Substance Use Disorders in Psychosis: Multivariate Analyses from an Epidemiological Sample. *Schizophrenia Research,* Vol.66, No.2-3, (February 2004), pp. 115-124., ISSN 0920-9964

Keshavan, M.S. & Hogarty, G.E. (1999). Brain Maturational Processes and Delayed Onset in Schizophrenia. *Development and Psychopathology,* Vol.11, No.3, (Summer 1999), pp. 525-543, ISSN 0954-5794

Kessler, R.C.; Nelson C.B.; McGonagle, K.A.; Edlund, M.J .; Frank, R.G.; & Leaf P.L. (1996). The Epidemiology of Co-occurring Addictive and Mental Disorders: Implications for Prevention and Service Utilization, *The American Journal of Orthopsychiatry,* Vol.66, No.1, (January 1996), pp. 17-3, ISSN 0002-9432

Khantzian, E.J. (1985). The Self-medication Hypothesis of Addictive Disorders: Focus on Heroin and Cocaine dependence. *The American Journal of Psychiatry*, (November 1985), Vo.142, No.11, pp. 1259-1264, ISSN 002-953X

Leduc, P. & G. Mittleman, G. (1995). Schizophrenia and Psychostimulant Abuse: a Review and Re-analysis of Clinical Evidence. *Psychopharmacology*, Vol.21, No.4, (October 1995), pp. 407–427, ISSN 0033-3158

Levin, F.R. & Hennessy, G. (2004). Bipolar Disorder and Substance Abuse. *Biological Psychiatry*, Vol.56, No.10, (November 2004), pp. 738–748, ISSN 0006-3223

Lewine, R.R. (1981). Sex Differences in Schizophrenia: Timing or Subtypes? *Psychological Bulletin*, Vo.90, No.3, (November 1981), pp. 432-434, ISSN 0033-2909

Lynskey, M.T., Coffey, C., Degenhardt, L., Carlin, J.B., Patton, G. (2003). A longitudinal study of the effects of adolescent cannabis use on high school completion. *Addiction*, Vol.98, No.5, (May 2003), pp. 685-692, ISSN: 0965-2140

Lysaker, P.; Bell, M.; Beam-Goulet, J. & Milstein, R. (1994). Relationship of Positive and Negative Symptoms to Cocaine Abuse in Schizophrenia. *The Journal of Nervous and Mental Disease*, Vol.182, No.2, (February 1994), pp. 109-112, ISSN 0022-3018

May-Majewski, A. (2002). Normy i Zasady Leczenia Pacjentów z Podwójną Diagnozą. *Wiadomości Psychiatryczne*, Vol.5, No.1, ISSN 1505-7429

Maynard, C. & Cox, G.B. (1998).Psychiatric hospitalization of persons with dual diagnoses: estimates from two national surveys. *Psychiatric Services*, No.49, (December 1998), pp. 1615-1617, ISSN 1075-2730

Margolese, H.C.; Malchy, L.; Negrete, J.C.; Tempier, R. & Gill, K. (2004). Drug and Alcohol Use Among Patients with Schizophrenia and Related Psychoses: Levels and Consequences. *Schizophrenia Research*, Vol.67, No.2-3, (April 2004), pp. 157-166, ISSN 0920-9964

Maremmani, I.; Pacini, M.; Lamanna, F.; Pani, P.P.; Perugi, G.; Deltito, J.; Salloum, I.M.& Akiskal, H. (2010). Mood Stabilizers in the Treatment of Substance Use Disorders. *CNS Spectrums*,Vol.15, No.2, pp. 95-109, ISSN 1092-8529

Modestin, J.; Gladen, C.J. & Christen, S. (2001). A Comparative Study on Schizophrenic Patients with Dual Diagnosis. *Journal of Addictive Diseases*, Vol.20, No.4, pp.41-51, ISSN 1055-0887

Møller, T. & Linaker, O.M. (2004). Symptoms and Lifetime Treatment Experiences in Psychotic Patients with and without Substance Abuse. *Nordic Journal of Psychiatry*, Vol.58, No.3, pp. 237-242, ISSN 0803-9488

Noordsy, D.L., & Green, A.I. (2003). Pharmacotherapy for Schizophrenia and Co-occurring substance use disorders. *Current Psychiatry Reports*,Vol.5, No.5, (October 2003), pp. 340-346, ISSN 1523-3812

Obot, I.S. & Anthony, J.C. (2000). School Dropout and Injecting Drug Use in a National Sample of White Non-Hispanic American adults. *Journal of Drug Education*, Vol.30, No.2, pp.145-155, ISSN 0047-2379

Pencer, A. & Addington, J. (2003). Substance Use and Cognition in Early Psychosis. *Journalof Psychiatry and Neuroscience*, Vol.28, No.1, (January 2003), pp. 48-54, ISSN 1180-4882

Potvin, S.; Stip, E. & Roy, J.Y. (2003). Schizophrenia and Addiction: An Evaluation of the Self-medication Hypothesis. *L'Encéphale*, Vo.29, No.3 Pt 1, (May-June 2003), pp.193-203, ISSN 0013-7006

Salloum, I .M.; Cornelius, J. R.; Mezzich, J. E. & Kirisci, L. (2002). Impact of Concurrent Alcohol Misuse on Symptom Presentation of Acute Mania at Initial Evaluation. *Bipolar Disorders,* Vol.4, No.6, (December 2002), pp. 418-21, ISSN 1398-5647

Salyers M.P., Mueser K.T. (2001). Social functioning, psychopathology, and medication sideeffects in relation to substance use and abuse in schizophrenia. *Schizophrenia Research,* Vol.48, No.1, (March 2001), pp.109-123, ISSN: 0920-9964

Sawicka, M. (2005). Podobieństwa i Różnice w Stylu Radzenia Sobie ze Stresem Pomiędzy Osobami Chorymi na Schizofrenię, Uzależnionymi a Osobami z Podwójnym Rozpoznaniem. *Psychiatria Polska,* Vol.29, No.6, pp. 1199-1210, ISSN 0033-2674

Serper; M.R., Alpert, M.; Richardson, N.A.; Dickson, S.; Allen, M.H. & Werner, A. (1995). Clinical effects of recent cocaine use on patients with acute schizophrenia. *The American Journal of Psychiatry,* Vol.152, No.10, (October 1995), pp. 1464-1469, ISSN 0002-953X

Sciacca, K. (1987). Alcohol and Substance Abuse Programs at New York State PsychiatricCenters Develop and Expand. *AID Bulletin Addiction Intervention with the Disabled,* Vol.9, No.2, (Winter 1987), pp. 1-3

Sierosławski, J. (1998). Używanie Narkotyków przez Młodzież Polską na Tle Wybranych Krajów Europy. Wyniki badań ESPAD 1995. *Serwis Informacyjny Narkomania,* No.2, pp. 25-40, ISSN 1233-9318

Solomon J.; Zimberg, S. & E. Shollar (1993). *Dual Diagnosis: Evaluation, Treatment, Trainingand Program Development,* Spinger, ISBN 978-0306445439, London, UK

Soyka, M. (1994). Addiction and Schizophrenia. Nosological, Clinical and Therapeutic Questions. 2. Substance Dependence and Schizophrenia. *Fortschritte der Neurologie-Psychiatrie,* Vol.62, No.6, (June 1994), pp. 186-196, ISSN 0720-4299

Soyka, M.; Albus, M.; Immler, B.; Kathmann, N. & Hippius, H. (2001). Psychopathology inDual Diagnosis and Non-addicted Schizophrenics - are There Differences? *European Archives of Psychiatry and Clinical Neuroscience,* Vol.,251, No.5, (October 2001) pp. 232-238, ISSN 0940-1334

Stip, E.; Remington, G.J.; Dursun, S.M.; Reiss, J.P.; Rotstein, E.; MacEwan, G.W.; Chokka, P.R.; Jones, B. & Dickson, R.A.; Canadian Switch Study Group. (2003). A Canadian Multicenter Trial Assessing Memory and Executive Functions in Patients with Schizophrenia Spectrum Disorders Treated with Olanzapine. *Journal of Clinical Psychopharmacology,*Vol.23, No.4, (August 2003), pp 400-404, ISSN 0271-0749

Swaim, R.C.; Beauvais, F.; Chavez, E.L. & Oetting, E.R. (1997). The Effect of School Dropout Rates on Estimates of Adolescent Substance Use among Three Racial/Ethnic Groups. *American Journal of Public Health,* Vol.87, (January 1997), No.1, pp. 51-55, ISSN 0090-0036

Regier, D.A.; Farmer, M.E.; Rae, D.S.; Locke, B.Z.; Keith, S.J.; Judd, L.L. & Goodwin, F.K. (1990). Comorbidity of Mental Disorders with Alcohol and Other Drug Abuse. *JAMA: The Journal of the American Medical Association,* Vol.264, No.19, (November 1990), pp. 2511–2518, ISSN 0098-7484

Swartz, J.A.; Lurigio, A.J. & Goldstein, P. (2000). Severe Mental Illness and Substance Use Disorders Among Former Supplemental Security Income Beneficiaries For Drug Addiction and Alcoholism. *Archives of General Psychiatry,* Vo.57, No., (July 2000), pp. 701-707, ISSN: 0003-990X

Tamminga, C.A.; Buchanan, R.W. & Gold, J.M. (1998). The Role of Negative Symptoms and Cognitive Dysfunction in Schizophrenia Outcome. *International Clinical Psychopharmacology,* Vo.13, Suppl.3, (March 1998), pp. 21-26, ISSN 0268-1315

Volavka, J. (1999). The Effects of Clozapine on Aggression and Substance Abuse inSchizophrenic Patients. *The Journal of Clinical Psychiatry,* Vol.60, Suppl.12, pp. 43-46, ISSN 0160-6689

Weisman, R.L. (2003). Quetiapine in the Successful Treatment of Schizophrenia with Comorbid Alcohol and Drug Dependence: a Case Report. *International Journal of Psychiatry and Medicine,* Vol.33, No.1, pp. 85-89, ISSN 0091-2174

Zimmet, S.V., Strous, R.D., Burgess, E.S., Kohnstamm, S. & Green, A.I. (2000). Effects of Clozapine on Substance Use in Patients with Schizophrenia and Schizoaffective Disorder: a Retrospective Survey. *Journal of Clinical Psychopharmacology,* Vol.20, No.1, (February 2000), pp.94-98, ISSN 0271-0749

Part 4

Biological Neuropsychiatry

18

Molecular Mechanism of the Involvement of the Susceptibility Genes, *DISC1, PACAP, TRAP1* and *Dysbindin* in Major Psychiatric Disorders Such as Schizophrenia, Depression and Bipolar Disease

Taiichi Katayama[1], Shinsuke Matsuzaki[1,2],
Tsuyosi Hattori[3] and Masaya Tohyama[1,2]
[1]*United Graduate School of Child Development, Osaka University, Kanazawa University and Hamamatsu University School of Medicine,*
[2]*Department of Anatomy and Neuroscience, Graduate school of Medicine, Osaka University*
[3]*Department of Molecular Neuropharmacology, Graduate School of Medicine, Osaka University,*
Japan

1. Introduction

No effective drugs are currently available for the treatment of mental diseases, primarily because the underlying mechanism of mental diseases have not been adequately explored at the molecular level. However, recent studies have examined several molecular cascades whose disturbances are associated with mental diseases such as schizophrenia, bipolar disease and major depression. The most common characteristics of these cascades us that they are all associated with neural circuit formation, suggesting that neurodevelopmental factors play a key role in the pathogenesis of mental diseases. The present review summarizes the available information on these molecular cascades and their association with mental disease.

2. Molecular mechanism of PACAP-stathmin1 dependent psychiatric disorders (Yamada et al., 2010)

Pituitary adenylate cyclase polypeptide (PACAP) is involved in multiple brain function such as neurotransmission and neural plasticity (Hashimoto et al., 2001; Vaudry et al., 2000). It also has a neurotrophic effect via three heptahekical G protein coupled receptors, one of which is specific for PACAP (PAC_1 receptor) and two others that are shared with vasoactive intestinal polypeptide ($VPAC_1$ and $VPAC_2$) (Hashimoto et al., 1993). Recently, mice that lack *Adcyap 1*, the gene encoding PACAP, (*Adcyap 1*$^{-/-}$ mice) were developed (Hashimoto et al., 2001, Shintani et al., 2002). *Adcyap 1*$^{-/-}$ mice display remarkable behavioral abnormalities providing evidence that PACAP plays a previously uncharacterized role in the regulation of psychomotor behavior. In addition, previous association study reported that several single nucleotide polymorphism (SNPs) in the vicinity of the PACAP gene locus were associated with schizophrenia (Hashimoto, R. et al., 2007). However, although nothing was known about the mechanism of PACAP deficiency-induced psychiatric illness, we have clarified these mechanisms.

2.1 Down-regulation of PACAP expression induces up-regulation of stathmin1 expression in the dentate gyrus both *in vivo* and *in vitro*

Real-time PCR showed that stathmin1 mRNA was markedly increased in the dentate gyrus of *Adcyap 1*$^{-/-}$ mice. An increased in stathmin1 protein levels in the dentate gyrus of *Adcyap 1*$^{-/-}$ mice was confirmed by western blot analysis. These findings were confirmed also *in vitro* using PC12 cells. PACAP stimulation of PC12 cells caused a decrease in stathmin1 mRNA levels after 3 h, and expression continued to decrease over the next 24 h (Fig. 1A). Stathmin1 protein levels also decreased in response to PACAP, which caused a dose-dependent decrease of stathmin1 mRNA levels. The decrease of stathmin1 expression caused by PACAP stimulation was slightly, but statistically significantly, inhibited by pretreatment with a $PAC_1/VPAC_2$ receptor antagonist (PACAP6-38). In addition, pretreatment with a p38 antagonist (SB202190) or an ERK antagonist (PD98059) also inhibited the PACAP-induced decrease of stathmin1 expression. Co-administration of SB202190 and PD98059 strongly inhibited the effect of PACAP, reflecting the key roles played by p38 and ERK in the PACAP signaling pathway. On the other hand, VIP did not decrease stathmin1 expression. These results indicate that PACAP regulates stathmin1 expression via the PAC_1 receptor in neurons of the dentate gyrus.

2.2 Up-regulation of stathmin1 induces abnormal axonal arborization in neurons of the dentate gyrus subgranular zone

In wild-type mice, cells expressing stathmin1 were preferentially located in the innermost part of the granular cell layer, the so-called subgranular zone (SGZ), where neurogenesis of granular cells occurs in adults. Two types of stathmin1 containing processes were found, namely; dendrites and axons. Immunoreactivity for stathmin1 was significantly increased in the SGZ neurons of *Adcyap 1*$^{-/-}$ mice, although the actual number of immunoreactive cells was similar in mutant and wild-type mice. . The number of dot-like immunoreactive fibers belonging to axons was significantly increased in the polymorphic layer of *Adcyap 1*$^{-/-}$ mice, compared with wild-type mice. In support of the *in vivo* datas, over-expression of stathmin1 in the hippocampal primary culture neurons caused dramatic changes of axon fibers. Arborization of axon fibers was markedly increased by stathmin1 over-expression compared with that in normal primary cultured neurons. The number of secondary neurites on axons was also increased following over-expression of stathmin1. These findings indicated that an increase in stathmin1 expression in SGZ neurons leads to abnormal axon arborization.

If PACAP directly regulates stathmin1 expression in vivo, SGZ neurons should express PAC_1. In fact, strong expression of PAC_1 mRNA was identified throughout the entire granular cell layer, including the SGZ. Furthermore, SGZ neurons expressed both stathmin1 protein and PAC_1 mRNA. These results show that PACAP inhibits stathmin1 expression via the PAC_1 receptor.

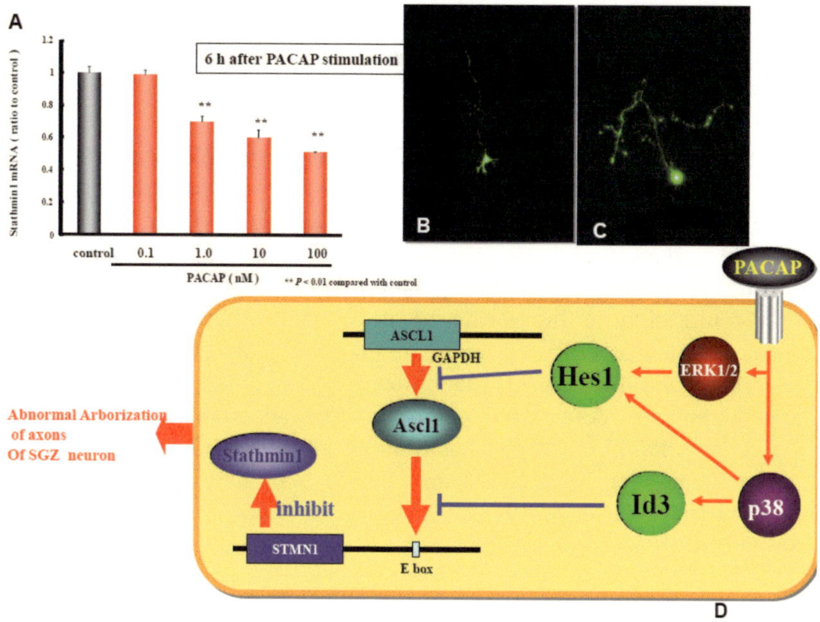

Fig. 1. PACAP-stathmin1 cascade
A: PACAP regulated stathmin1 expression via PAC1 in PC12 cells. Alteration of stathmin1 mRNA levels 24 h after PACAP treatment, at the indicated concentrations were quantified by real-time PRC. Data are expressed as mean ±SEM relative to control values (n=3, PACAP 1nM **P=0.0044, 10nM **P=0.0033, 100nM ***P=0.0003 compared with control. B,C; Stathmin1 over-expression in neurons caused abnormally pronounced arborization of axon fibers. Morphology of hippocampal primary neurons transfected with stathmin1. Over-expression of GFP (B) and GFP-stathmin1 (C). The neurons over-expressing stathmin1 have abnormally pronounced sprouting of axon fibers. D: Schematic drawing of the molecular pathway underlying PACAP regulation of stathmin1 expression. The schematic representation shows the pathway by which PACAP regulates the expression of stathmin1 by suppressing the function and expression of Ascl1 after increasing the expression of Hes1 and Id3 by activating ERK and p38.

2.2.1 Stathmin1 gene promoter activity is regulated by basic helix loop helix (bHLH) proteins via the E10 box

A BLAST search identified the genomic sequence of rat stathmin1 in a chromosome 5 contig. PCR amplification of a 1885bp genomic DNA fragment that consisted of 1561 nt upstream of the stathmin1 transcription start site (+1), exon1, and part of intron 1 (+325) was then performed. This fragment was sequenced and subcloned into a pGL3 luciferase reporter vector. This fragment was also analyzed for transcription factor-binding sites using the DNAsis program. The 1.8kbp rat stathmin1 5' genomic sequence contained 12 (E1-E12) putative E boxes (CANNTG), which are potential binding sites for bHLH proteins, including neuronal transcription activators. To investigate the promoter activity of stathmin1, we constructed several expression plasmids for the luciferase assay after transient transfection in PC12 cells. Constructs containing E10 (such as STMN1-1, STMN1-2 and STMN 1-3) showed a high level of luciferase activity compared with control cells, but constructs containing a stathmin promoter lacking the E10 box (such as STMN1-4) did not show luciferase activity. Therefore, the E10 box was found to be a key motif that regulates stathmin1 expression through bHLH factors.

2.2.2 An activating bHLH protein, Ascl1, activates the stathmin promoter

Among activating bHLH proteins, Ascl1was found to activate the stathmin1 promoter. Co-transfection of PC12 cells with the stathmin1-promoter plasmid and the Ascl1 expression plasmid induced a dose-dependent increase in luciferase activity compared with cells transfected with the stathmin1 promoter plasmid alone. To examine whether endogenous Ascl1 protein could bind to the stathmin1 promoter sequence in PC12 cells, sheared chromatin was immunoprecipitated with an anti-Ascl1 antibody or with control IgG, followed by PCR amplification of the corresponding DNA regions using stathmin1 promoter specific primers. Analysis of amplified DNA showed that more sequences were amplified by primers flanking the E10 box than by primers flanking the E10-E11 boxes. In addition, co-localization of Ascl1 and stathmin1 in SGZ neurons was demonstrated by immunohistochemistry. These results established that endogenous Ascl1 protein binds to stathmin1 promoter and act as a major regulator of stathmin1 promoter activity.

2.2.3 The inhibitory bHLH proteins, Hes1 and Id3, showed increased expression after PACAP stimulation

As described above, PACAP inhibits stathmin1 expression. In addition, PACAP stimulation of PC12 cells caused an increase in the expression of the inhibitory HLH proteins, Hes1 and Id3 expression which belong to inhibitory HLH proteins. Inhibition of the PACAP signaling pathway, as through the inhibition of p38 and ERK, suppresses the effect of PACAP on stathmin1 expression. Moreover, the increase of Id3 mRNA levels in response to PACAP stimulation was inhibited by a p38 inhibitor (SB202190), but not by an ERK inhibitor (PD98059), while induction of Hes1 mRNA by PACAP stimulation was inhibited by both an ERK inhibitor and a p38 inhibitor. Co-administration of p38 and ERK inhibitors strongly inhibited thePACAP-induced induction of Hes1 mRNA. These findings showed that Hes1 expression is regulated by both the PACAP-ERK and PACAP-p38 pathways, whereas Id3 expression is mainly controlled by the PACAP-p38 pathway.

2.2.4 Hes1 and Id3 suppress stathmin1 promoter activity via Ascl1 inhibition

PC12 cells were co-transfected with a stathmin1 promoter plasmid and a Hes1 expression plasmid or an Id3 expression plasmid with or without an Ascl1 expression plasmid. Even without exogenous Ascl1 expression, a high level of luciferase activity was detected, owing to the action of the stathmin1 promoter. Expression of Hes1 or Id3 in these cells inhibited luciferase activity related to the stathmin1 promoter activity through endogenous Ascl1. In PC12 cells transfected with the stathmin1 promoter plasmid and the Ascl1 expression plasmid, luciferase activity was higher than that in PC12 cells without the Ascl1 expression plasmid. Id3 expression in these cells inhibited the up-regulation of stathmin1 promoter luciferase activity, while Hes1 expression failed to reduce the luciferase activity induced by exogenous Ascl1.These findings suggested that Id3 inhibits activation of the stathmin1 promoter by both exogenous and endogenous Ascl1, while Hes1 only blocked the effect of endogenous Ascl1. Thus, it is likely that Id3 regulates Ascl1 at the protein level, while Hes1 regulates Ascl1 transcription. If so, inhibition of Hes1 expression should increase the transcription of Ascl1. In fact, the up-regulation of Hes1 in PC12 cells by PACAP stimulation led to inhibition of Ascl1 expression. In addition, a reduction of Hes1 expression also resulted in an elevation of Ascl1 expression to 1.2 fold the control level. These results indicate that Ascl1, which controls stathmin1 expression, was functionally regulated by Id3 and quantitatively regulated by Hes1, in response to PACAP signaling.

2.3 Role of the PACAP-stathmin1 cascade in psychiatric disorders

As described above, PACAP inhibits stathmin1 expression. In addition, over-expression of stathmin1 causes abnormal axonal arborization (Fig. 1B,C), indicating that stathmin1 regulates the maturation of neurons and neural circuit formation. Furtehrmore, *Adcyap 1*$^{-/-}$ mice are known to show behavioral abnormalities, some of which might have potential relevance to mental disorders such as schizophrenia (Hashimoto et al.,2001; Shintani et al., 2002), and several SNPs in the vicinity of the *PACAP* gene locus are associated with schizophrenia (Hashimoto et al., 2007). If so, stathmin1 expression should be altered in the brain of patients with schizophrenia. Our RT-PCR study showed that stathmin1 mRNA levels were significantly increased in schizophrenic patients compared with age-matched controls. In contrast, stathmin1 was not significantly increased in the brains of patients with bipolar disorder.

3. Mechanism of PACAP-DBZ/DISC1 dependent psychiatric disorders (Hattori et al.,2007; Katayama et al., 2009)

DBZ (DISC1-binding zinc finger protein) was found as a DISC1(disrupted-in schizophrenia 1)-interacting molecules by yeast-2-hybrid screening of a complementary DNA (cDNA) library. Subsequent co-immunoprecipitation studies and yeast-2 hybrid assays showed that amino acids 348-597 of DISC1 act as the DBZ binding region, which indicates that the regions of DISC1 near the translocation breakpoint (amino acid 598) participate in the interaction with DBZ. DISC1 and DBZ co-localize diffusely in the cytoplasm and centrosome, and are involved in neurite extension. PACAP regulates the association between DISC1 and DBZ (for details on DISC1, see the chapter 6).

3.1 DISC1-DBZ interaction inhibits the neurite outgrowth (Fig.2)

DBZ mRNA was expressed exclusively in the brain, but was not expressed in peripheral tissues. To examine the functional role of the DISC1-DBZ interaction, PC12 cells stably expressing DISC1-HA and mock-transfected cells were infected with Adv-DBZ-GFP or Adv-GFP for 24 h. Immunoprecipitation and western blot analysis confirmed the over-expression of DBZ-GFP and DISC1-HA as well as the association between these 2 molecules. Over-expression of both proteins in PC12 cells caused a significant reduction in the number of neurite bearing PC12 cells after PACAP stimulation. However, over-expression of either DBZ or DISC1 alone had no effect. The region of DBZ encompassing amino acids 152-301 interacts with DISC1. PC12 cells were transiently transfected with DBZ (152-301)-IRES-GFP or with GFP alone and treated with PACAP (100nM) for 48 h. The cells expressing DBZ (152-301) had a shorter neurite length than cells expressing GFP alone. Under these conditions, no significant change of apoptosis was detected and the number of transfected cells was similar. The effect of DBZ (152-301) on neurite growth was also confirmed in primary cultured hippocampal neurons.

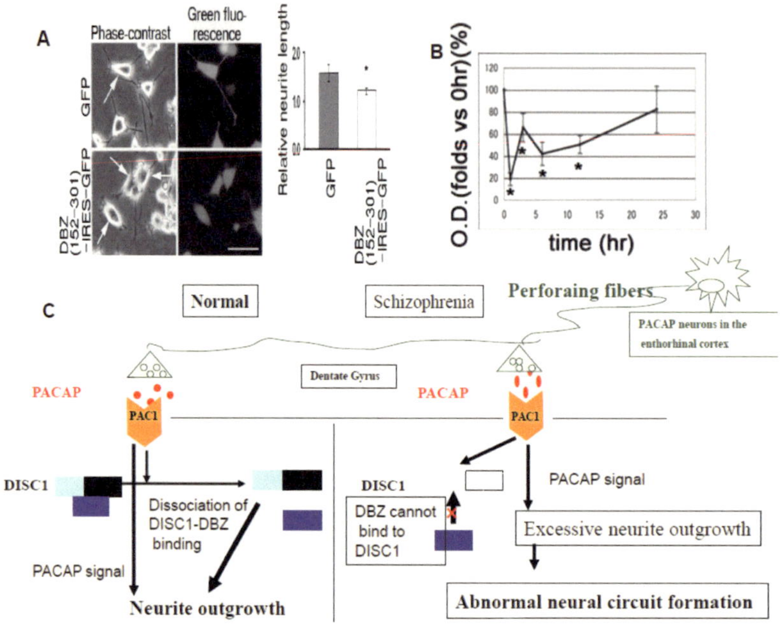

Fig. 2. A: Neurite outgrowth was inhibited by the DISC1-binding domain of DBZ [DBZ(152-301)-IRES-GFP]. PC12 cells were transfected with DBZ (152-301)-IRES-GFP or GFP alone at 2 days after plating. After 24 h , cells were starved of serum for 4h and treated with 100nM PACAP for 48h. Phase-contrast and fluorescence microscopy images are shown. Diagrams display neurite length relative to cell body diameter of transfected PC12 cells. B: PACAP-induced transient inhibition of the endogenous DISC1-DBZ interaction in PC12 cells. Immunoprecipitation and western blot analysis (with anti-DISC1 or anti-DBZ antibodies) of PC12 cells lysates collected at the indicated times after stimulation with 100nM PACAP. Immunoprecipitaes obtained with an anti-DBZ antibody incubated with 5% of each lysates (5% input), were subjected to western blot analysis with the same antibody. Quantitation of relative band densities for DISC1 co-immunoprecipitated with DBZ, as well as for total DISC1 or DBZ protein, was performed by scanning densitometry. Data were expressed as the mean ±SEM. of at least 3 independent experiments. *$P<0.05$ vs control (Student's t-test). C: A possible PACAP-DISC1/DBZ pathway . In the normal brain, PACAP leads to the temporal dissociation of the binding between DISC1 and DBZ , which in turn leads to normal neurite outgrowth. In the brain of schizophrenia patients, DBZ cannot bind to DISC1, and the PACAP pathway may proceed without inhibition, resulting in the formation of an abnormal neural circuit.

3.2 PACAP regulates DISC1-DBZ binding (Fig. 2)

Exposure to PACAP (100nM) increased the expression of endogenous DISC1 in PC12 cells by about 50% after 24 h, whereas it had no effect on DBZ expression. PACAP has a marked influence on the interaction between DBZ and DISC1. The co-immunoprecipitation of DISC1 and DBZ from PC12 cell lysates was reduced by approximately 80% 1h after treatment of cells with PACAP (100nM). However, this reduction was transient and there was a gradual return to control level by 24 h after treatment. Addition of an ERK inhibitor 24 h after PACAP treatment inhibited the rebinding of DBZ to DISC1, while an inhibitor of adenyl cyclase failed to influence the DISC1-DBZ interaction, showing that PACAP regulates DISC1-DBZ binding through the ERK cascade but not through the cAMP cascade.

3.3 Role of the PACAP-DBZ cascade with regard to PACAP-DBZ/DISC1 dependent psychiatric disorders (Fig.2)

The findings described above show that the DISC1-DBZ interaction inhibits neurite out growth, and PACAP dissociates this interaction, resulting in neurite outgrowth. The involvement of the DISC1-DBZ interaction and PACAP in neurite outgrowth suggests that these molecules should be expressed in the early ontogenetical stages. In fact, a marked elevation of both DBZ and PAC_1 (PACAP receptor) expression was observed during the perinatal stage (Hattori et al. in preparation). DISC1 shows a high level of expression in the developing cortex and hippocampus (Honda et al.,2004). In addition, down-regulation of DBZ caused a delay in the migration of cortical neurons (Sato et al., personal communication) and disturbance of cilia formation (Kumamoto et al., in preparation). The DISC1-DBZ interaction which is regulated by PACAP has therefore been shown to be involved in neurite out growth and the migration of neurons. In the brain of patients with PACAP-dependent psychiatric disorders, dissociation of the binding between DISC1 and DBZ does not occur and neurite extension may be inhibited. On the other hand, in brains in which translocation of DISC1 occurs, DBZ is unable bind to DISC1 and the dissociation of DISC1 from DBZ may not be induced, which results in an immature neural circuit.

4. Molecular mechanism of Dysbindin-MARCKS cascade dependent psychiatric disorders (Okuda et al., 2010)

Studies of postmortem brain tissue showed decreased Dysbindin (dystrobrevin binding protein 1; DTNBP1) protein and mRNA levels in patients with schizophrenia compared with controls (Bray et al., 2005; Talbot et al., 2004; Weickert et al., 2004). Chronic treatment of mice with antipsychotics did not affect the levels of Dysbindin protein and mRNA expression in their brains (Chiba et al., 2006; Talbot et al., 2004), suggesting the lower levels of Dysbindin protein and mRNA found in the postmortem brains of schizophrenia patients is not likely to be a simple artifact of antemortem drug treatment. In addition, several studies suggested that diverse high-risk SNPs and haplotypes could influence Dysbindin mRNA expression (Bray et al., 2005; Talbot et al., 2004; Weickert et al., 2004). These data indicate that the *Dysbindin* gene may confer susceptibility to schizophrenia through reduced Dysbindin expression. However, the molecular mechanisms underlying the effect of decreased Dysbindin expression on vulnerability to schizophrenia remain unknown.

4.1 Dysbindin- myristoylated alanin-rich protein kinase C substrate (MARCKS) cascade (Okuda et al., 2010)

4.1.1 Dysbindin exists within the nucleus in addition to the cytoplasm

Cell fractionation experiments using Dysbindin-FLAG-overexpressing HEK293 cells showed that Dysbindin exists mainly in the cytosol while a small amount is present in the nucleus. Immunohistochemical analysis also revealed that Dysbindin is localized mainly in the cytoplasm with a perinuclear high density region. However, a faint immunoreaction was seen within the nucleus. Furthermore, pretreatment with leptomycine-B(LPB), which inhibits the export of proteins from the nucleus to the cytoplasm, caused a slight increase of

Dysbindin and its nuclear localization. These findings show that the Dysbindin protein is shuttled between the nucleus and the cytoplasm.

4.1.2 Dysbindin binds to the transcription factor NF-YB

Using yeast 2-hybrid screening, several transcriptional factors including nuclear transcription factor Y beta (NF-YB), were identified as candidates for interaction with Dysbindin. NF-YB belong to a family of CCAAT-binding transcription factors that are important for the basal transcription of a class of regulatory genes and are involved in cellular reactions. HEK293T cells which express NF-YB endogenously were transfected with expression vectors for Dysbindin-V5 and subjected to immunoprecipitation to confirm the Dysbindin-NF-YB interaction. In addition, the Dysbindin-NF-YB interaction was shown in lysates from SH-SY5Y cells, which express both Dysbindin and NF-YB endogenously, as well as adult mouse brain lysates.

4.1.3 Downregulation of Dysbindin causes up-regulation of the expression level of MARCKS

The interaction between Dysbindin and NF-YB suggests that Dysbindin may be functionally involved in the transcription of genes regulated by NF-YB. We therefore screened for genes displaying altered expression by means of a DNA chip, using RNA extracts from the Dysbindin or NF-YB knockdown human neural cell line, SH-SY5Y. Among them identified, we focused on MARCKS, because protein kinase C has been involved in psychiatric diseases and because the promoter region of the *MARCKS* gene has the CCAAT binding motif specific for NF-YB.

The effect of Dysbindin on MARCKS *in vitro* was confirmed *in vivo* by examining the expression of the MARCKS protein product in the hippocampus of Dysbindin knockout mice with advanced age and comparing the levels with those of wild-type mice. In wild-type mice, a peak in MARCKS protein expression in the hippocampus was detected on postnatal days 15 and 20, and with a marked decrease in expression levels over time. However, this decrease was not observed in Dysbindin knockout mice, suggesting that down-regulation of Dysbindin may enhance the transcription of the MARCKS protein.

Chromatin immunoprecipitation analysis using SH-SY5Y cells over-expressing Dysbindin-Flag, was performed to explore the possibility that the Dysbindin-NF-YB complex could affect the transcription of *MARCKS via* interaction with the promoter region of *MARCKS*. PCR products from the chromatin immunoprecipitates suggested that Dysbindin and NF-YB simultaneously interact with the promoter region of *MARCKS*. These results indicate that the Dysbindin-NF-YB complex interacts with the promoter region of the *MARCKS* gene resulting in inhibition of MARCKS transcription.

4.1.4 The transcriptional level of the *MARCKS* gene is regulated by Dysbindin via the NF-YB binding motif, CCAAT-2

The 5'-UTR region of the *MARCKS* gene has 2 kinds of CCAAT sequences, namely; one CCAAT motif located between residues -1152 and -700 (CCAAT-1) and one located between UTR -700 and -614 (CCAAT-2). Because NF-YB binds to the CCAAT motif to regulate the transcription of target genes , the role of the CCAAT motifs in the regulation of *MARCKS* transcription was examined by luciferase assay with 5 vectors containing shorter RNA probes (Fig. 3A); These vectors were UTR(1152)-Luc, UTR (953)-Luc, UTR (700)-Luc, UTR

(614)-Luc, and UTR (462)-Luc. The luciferase activity detected in SH-SY5Y cells expressing the UTR (1152)-Luc after retinoic acid stimulation was used as a baseline. In the cells transfected with UTR (953)-Luc containing both CCAAT sequence and UTR (700)-Luc containing CCAAT-1 sequence but lacking the CCAAT-2 sequence, luciferase activity remained at baseline level after stimulation with retinoic acid. However luciferase activity was markedly increased in cells expressing UTR (614)-Luc after retinoic acid stimulation. These results suggest that the CCAAT-2 motif plays an important role in the inhibition of *MARCKS* transcription. Furthermore, SH-SY5Y cells transfected with UTR (462)-Luc lacking CCAAT-1, CCAAT-2 and SP1 region showed very low luciferase activity, indicating that the SP1 is indispensable for *MARCKS* transcription.

To confirm that the CCAAT-2 region is important for the regulation of MARCKS transcription, several probes were designed for the luciferase assay (Fig. 3B), namely; D1-UTR (1152)-Luc which lacks the CCAAT-2 motif and its downstream region including Sp1 from UTR (1152)-Luc, D2-UTR (1152)-Luc which lacks the SP1 region and the downstream sequence from UTR (1152)-Luc, D3-UTR (1152)-Luc which lacks only the sequence downstream of the SP1 region, D4-UTR (1152)-Luc which lacks only the CCAAT motif from UTR (1152)-Luc, and M-UTR(1152)-Luc, which has a point mutation in the CCAAT-2 motif. Luciferase activity was detected in SH-SY5Y cells transfected with each probe, using the activity in cells transfected with UTR (1152)-Luc as the baseline value. Cells transfected with M-UTR (1152)-Luc and those transfected with D4-UTR (1152)-Luc exhibited marked increases in luciferase activity, showing that the CCAAT-2 motif plays a key role in the inhibition of *MARCKS* transcription. Furthermore, cells expressing D1-UTR (1152)-Luc, D2-UTR (1152)-Luc or D3-UTR (1152)-Luc exhibited no luciferase activity. These findings suggest that the sequence downstream of the Sp1 region, and the Sp1 region itself, areindispensable for *MARCKS* transcription.

To confirm the involvement of Dysbindin in the altered MARCKS transcription levels via the CCAAT-2 motif, we compared the luciferase activity of UTR (1152)-Luc detected in Dysbindin knockdown cells with that of control cells. Knockdown of Dysbindin resulted in the up-regulation of luciferase activity in the UTR (1152)-Luc transfected cells. However, the effect of knockdown of Dysbindin knockdown on luciferase activity was not observed in D1-UTR (1152)-Luc transfected cells. These results suggest that Dysbindin regulates MARCKS transcription via the NF-YB binding motif CCAAT-2. On the other hand, the negligible levels of luciferase activity observed in cells transfected with probes lacking the sequence downstream of the Sp1 region, suggest that this this sequence is essential for *MARCKS* transcription. In fact, knockdown of Dysbindin caused the up-regulation of MARCKS expression (Fig. 3C).

4.2 Role of the Dysbindin-MARCKS cascade in psychiatric disorders (Fig. 3D)

SNPs in Dysbindin have been associated with intermediate cognitive phenotypes related to schizophrenia such as IQ and working and episodic memory, and a Dysbindin haplotype has been associated with higher educational attainment (Corvin et al., 2008; Donohoe et al., 2007). In addition, several papers show evidence of the involvement of Dysbindin in cognitive functions (Burdick et al., 2006; Zinkstok et al., 2007).

Furthermore, accumulating evidence suggests the involvement of Dysbindin in neurotransmission. At the cellular level, Dysbindin is located at both pre- and post-synaptic terminals., and is thought to be involved in postsynaptic density function and the

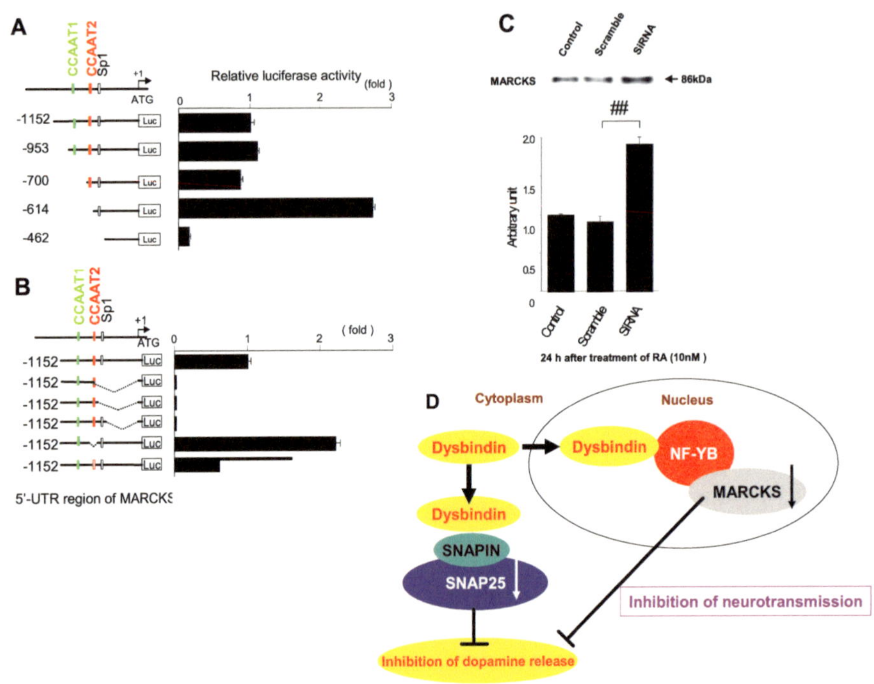

Fig. 3. A,B: Dysbindin regulates the transcription of MARCKSvia the CCAAT-2 sequence. A: The following 5 vectors containg shorter DNA probes were used for the luciferase assay; UTR(1152)-Luc, UTR (953)-Luc, UTR (700)-Luc, UTR (614)-Luc, and UTR (462)-Luc. Vectors were transfected into SH-SY5Y cells and luciferase activity was measured. The luciferase activity of UTR (1152) was used as the control. Columns and vertical bars denote the means ±SEM (triplicate independent experiments). B: The UTR (1152)-Luc vector and deletion or point mutations of the UTR (1152)-Luc vectors, [D10UTR(1152)-Luc], [D2-UTR (1152)-Luc], [D3-UTR (1152)-Luc], [D4-UTR(1152)-Luc] and [M-UTR (1152)-Luc], were transfected into SH-SY5Y cells and luciferase activity was measured. [D4-UTR(1152)-Luc], which lacks CCAAT-2, and [M-UTR (1152)-Luc], which has a point mutation in the CCAAT-2 sequence, showed increased luciferase activity. The luciferase activity of UTR (1152) was used as the control. Columns and vertical bars denote the means ±SEM(triplicate independent experiments). C: Dysbindin knockdown results in the up-regulation of MARCKS. SH-SY5Y cells were transfected with scrambled RNAi or siRNA for Dysbindin. Cell lysate of un-treated cells (cont.), scrambled RNAi-transfected cells (Scr.) and RNAi for Dysbindin-transfected cells (siRNA) were subjected to western blotting with an anti-MARCKS antibody. Columns and vertical bars denote the means ±SEM(triplicate independent experiments). Dysbindin knockdown cells exhibited significant up-regulation of MARCKS expression compared with control cells ($P<0.001$, Student's t-test). D: A possible Dysbindin pathway related to the regulation of dopamine release. In the cytoplasm of the nigrostriatal dopamine neurons, Dysbindin binds to Snapin. This binding inhibits the expression of SNAP25, which may suppress dopamine release. In the nuclei of these neurons, Dysbindin inhibits MARCKS expression via the binding to NF-YB. Reduction of MARCKS expression in dopaminergic neurons may causes the down-regulation of dopamine transport from the soma to the terminal. Thus Dysbindin inhibits dopamine release by 2 pathway.

trafficking of receptors (NMDA,GABAergic and nicotinic) (Sillitoe et al., 2003; Talbot et al., 2004). Over-expression of Dysbindin increases glutamate release from pyramidal neurons in cell culture, possibly because of its role in vesicular trafficking (Numakawa et al., 2004). Decreases in Dysbindin mRNA and protein levels have been reported in regions previously implicated in schizophrenia such as the prefrontal; cortex, midbrain and hippocampus (Talbot et al., 2004; Weickert et al., 2004). On the other hand, abnormal activation of nigrostriatal and mesolimbic dopaminergic systems is thought to be one of the most important etiologies for schizophrenia (Angrist & van Kammen, 1984; Creese et al., 1976; Lieberman et al., 1987; Seeman &Lee, 1975), suggesting a functional relationship between dopamine and Dysbindin. In support of this, midbrain dopamine neurons also contain Dysbindin (Kumamoto et al., 2006). Suppression of Dysbindin expression in PC12 cells resulted in an increase of the expression of SNAP25 which plays an important role in neurotransmitter release, and increased the release of dopamine. On the other hand, up-regulation of Dysbindin expression in PC12 cells showed a tendency to decrease the expression of SNAP25 and the release of dopamine. These findings show that Dysbindin inhibits dopamine release via down-regulation of SNAP25 expression (Kumamoto et al., 2006).

Thus, Dysbindin inhibits MARCKS expression and decreased expression of Dysbindin is characteristic of the schizophrenic brain. In addition, a decrease in Dysbindin levels up-regulates dopamine release. MARCKS influences neurotransmission *via* F-actin and vesicular transport *via* synaptic vesicles. The enhanced dopaminergic transmission produced by the lower expression level of Dysbindin may be partially attributed to activation of MARCKS. Thus, the impairment of neuronal transmission in the schizophrenic brain may be caused by alterations of MARCKS expression levels *via* changes in Dysbindin.

Sandy (*sdy*) mice that express no Dysbindin, showed behavioral abnormalities, which could be endophenotypes of schizophrenia (Feng et al., 2008). These mutant mice reportedly exhibit defective synaptic structure and function of CA_1 neurons (Chen et al., 2008), though the mechanism by which the loss of Dysbindin induces schizophrenia-like behaviors, remains unclear. Recently, we revealed that Dysbindin is involved in neural development through the regulation of the actin skeleton organization (Kubota et al., 2008). This study showed that knockdown of Dysbindin resulted in the aberrant organization of the actin cytoskeleton in SH-SY5Y cells. Furthermore, morphological abnormalities of the actin cytoskeleton were similarly observed in growth cones of cultured hippocampal neurons derived from sdy mice. In addition, a significant correlation was found between Dysbindin expression levels and the phosphorylation level of c-Jun N-terminal kinase (JNK), which is implicated in the regulation of cytoskeletal organization. These findings revealed that Dysbindin plays a key role in coordinating JNK signaling and actin cytoskeleton organization, which are required for neuronal development.

5. Mechanism of tumor necrosis factor receptor (TNFR) associated protein 1 (TRAP1)-N-cadherin alteration-induced psychiatric disorders

An increase in serum tumor necrosis factor-α (TNF-α) level is closely related to the pathogenesis of major depression (Irwin & Miller, 2007). The tumor necrosis factor receptor assoicated protein (TRAP1) was detected in whole brain lysates (Song et al., 1995). TRAP1 is a member of the heat shock protein 90 (HSP90) family and possesses ATPase activity, but lacks chaperone activity (Felts et al., 2000). However, the function and molecular mechanism of the TNF-TRAP system remain unclear. In the following section, we will describe the evidence that TRAP1 regulates the expression of adhesion molecule (Kubota et al., 2009).

5.1 TRAP1 is widely expressed in neurons through the brain, including in regions known to be affected in patients with major depression

In situ hybridization histochemistry and immunocytochemistry revealed that TRAP1 mRNA and protein are broadly expressed in neurons throughout the gray matter of the brain and the spinal cord, including in regions known to be affected in patients with major depression patients, such as the medial prefrontal cortex, hippocampus and nuclei producing monoamine: the substantia nigra pars compacta, dorsal raphe nucleus and locus ceruleus (Nestler et al., 2002; Berton and Nestler, 2006). However, glial cells such as astrocytes and oligodendrocytes are devoid of TRAP1. In addition, punctate immunostaining of TRAP1 was detected in the cytoplasm, which is consistent with previously reported mitochondrial localization of TRAP1 in a cell culture (Felts et al., 2000).

5.2 TRAP1 regulates cell adhesion

A striking cell-scattering phenotype was observed in TRAP1 knockdown SH-SY5Y cells. Cells transfected with siTRAP1 were dispersed throughout the dish, compared to cells transfected with control siRNA, which grew in aggregates resembling untransfected SH-SY5Y cells (Fig. 4A,B). This phenomenon was detectable as early as 24 h after transfection and became more prominent by 72 h after transfection. Immunostaining of actin filaments in siRNA-treated cells showed no difference in cytoskeletal structure. Quantification of the percentage of cells with no inter-cellular contacts after staining for actin detected a 6.2-fold increase in cells transfected with siTRAP1(36%) compared to cells transfected with control siRNA (5.8%). The cell aggregation assay revealed that TRAP1 knockdown cells were characterized by decreased efficacy of cell-cell adhesion compared with control cells, suggesting an alteration in calcium-dependent cell adhesion is affected. These results strongly indicate that TRAP1 regulates downstream molecules crucial for cell adhesion.

5.3 N-cadherin is transcriptionally down-regulated in TRAP1 knockdown cells

Expression levels of cell adhesion molecules, including N-cadherin, are directly related to the cell-scattering phenomenon (Hayashida et al., 2006; Yasuda et al., 2007) and N-cadherin mediates calcium-dependent cell adhesion in neuronal cells (Takeuchi and Nakagawa, 2007) Our findings showed that N-cadherin levels were remarkably decreased throughout the cytoplasm of TRAP1 knockdown cells, including around the membrane where cell-adhesion takes place, compared to control cells (Fig. 4C,D). Immunoblotting experiments confirmed this finding, showing a significant decrease in N-cadherin expression in TRAP1 knockdown cells from as early as 24 h until at least 2 h after transfection. However, the expression level of β-catenin, which is involved in the regulation of cell-adhesion, was unaffected. These results suggest that the cell scattering phenotype detected in TRAP1 knockdown cell is at least partially mediated by a reduction of N-cadherin expression in those cells.

To exclude the possibility that cell viability or migration may contributes to the cell-scattering phenotype in TRAP1 knockdown cells, we examined cell viability by the 3-(4,5-dimethylthiazol2-yl)-2,5-diphenyltetrazolium bromide (MTT) assay and migration by the wound-healing assay. Although a slight decrease in cell viability was observed in TRAP1 knockdown cells compared to control cells 48 h after transfection or later, no changes were

detected 24 h after transfection, when the cell-scattering phenotype of TRAP1 was already observed. No significant changes in the rate of cell migration were observed.
To determine if down-regulation of N-cadherin induced by siTRAP1 occurs at the transcriptional level, N-cadherin mRNA levels were measured by real-time RT-PCR analysis 48 h after siRNA transfection, which showed that N-cadherin mRNA levels in TRAP1 knockdown cells were approximately 45% lower than in control cells. These results indicate that TRAP1 knockdown induces transcriptional down-regulation of N-cadherin.

5.4 E2F1, a putative transcription factor of N-cadherin, is down-regulated in TRAP1 knockdown cells

To determine the possible involvement of a transcription factor in down-regulation of N-cadherin in TRAP1 knockdown cells, a search DBTSS (Database of Transcriptional Start Sites) and TRANSFAC (The Transcription Factor Database) database was conducted. This search revealed a putative binding site for E2F1 in the promoter region of the N-cadherin gene. Immunoblot analysis and real-time PCR showed that E2F1 mRNA and protein levels were significantly decreased in TRAP1 knockdown cells (Fig. 4E), although the mRNA level of c-Myc, another representative transcription factor, was not affected, In addition, SH-SY5Y cells transfected with the N-cadherin-luciferase plasmid showed strong activity of the reporter, and this activity was suppressed in TRAP1 knockdown cells, mimicking the signaling cascade detected *in vitro*. Furthermore, exogenously transfected E2F1 showed a 7.5-fold induction of luciferase reporter activity relative to the control vector. These results indicate that E2F1 plays a regulatory role upstream of N-cadherin in TRAP1 knockdown cells.

5.5 Reduced phosphorylation of STAT causes down-regulation of E2F1 in TRAP1 knockdown cells

A recognition sequence for STAT3 is located 89bp upstream of the transcription initiation site of the *E2F1* gene. Upon activation, STAT3 proteins are tyrosine-phosphorylated, dimerize and translocate to the nucleus where the nuclear phospho-STAT binds to STAT recognition sites located in the promoter region of downstream genes to promote the transcription of those genes. In TRAP1 knockdown cells, the amount of tyrosine-phosphorylated STAT3, but not the total amount of tyrosine-phosphorylated STAT3, was significantly reduced. In addition, the promoter activity of the *E2F*1 gene was significantly reduced if the STAT3 recognition site was deleted and if TRAP1 was knocked down. These data indicate that TRAP1 regulates the tyrosine phopsphorylation status of STAT3, which controls the expression of E2F1, and thus modulates the transcription of N-cadherin.

5.6 Role of the TRAP1-N-cadherin cascade in psychiatric disorders (Fig. 4G)

Because N-cadherin is involved in the morphogenesis of synapses (Okamura et al., 2004; Togashi et al., 2002), the regulation of the morphology of dendritic spines by TRAP1 via N-cadherin was analyzed in cultured hippocampal neurons. Spines are divided into 2 types based on morphology, namely: pedunculated and sessile with the former possessing a substantial stalk construction that is absent in the latter (Greg et al., 1999). In TRAP1 knockdown neurons, spines were predominantly sessile. Only 20.8% of spines displayed a pedunculate morphology compared with 66.7% in control neurons. Functionally, N-cadherin regulates synaptic plasticity; The activity dependent accumulation of N-cadherin

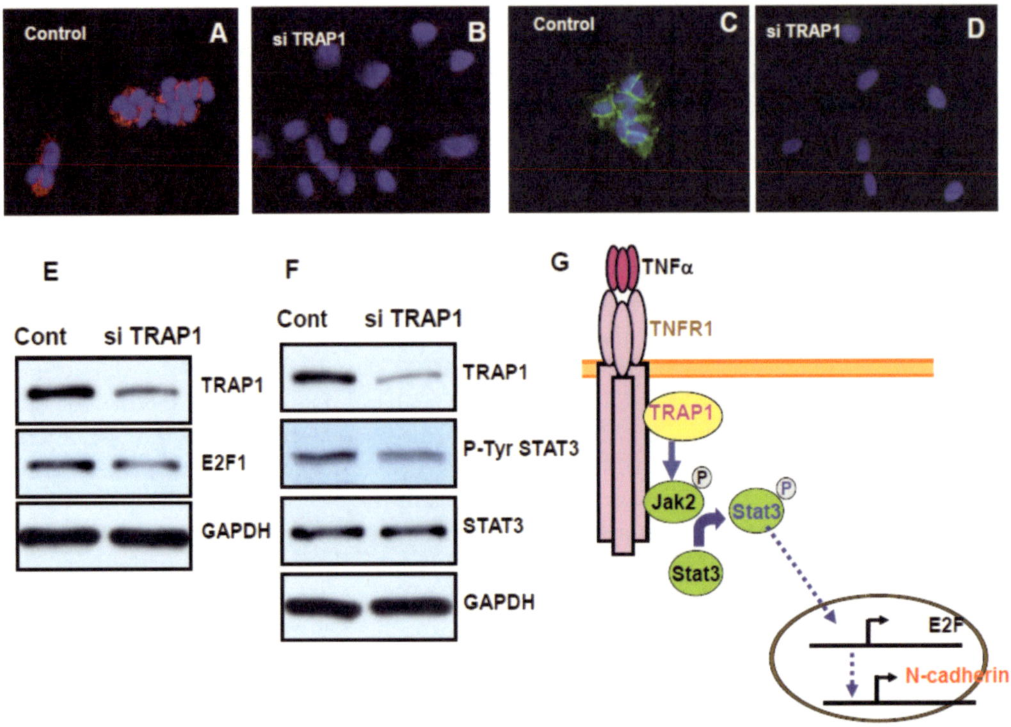

Fig. 4. TRAP1 is involved in cell-cell adhesion. A,B: Immunohistochemistry of TRAP1 knockdown and control cells stained with an anti-TRAP1 antibody (red) and DAPI(blue). TRAP1 protein levels are markedly reduced in B. In addition, cells transfected with siTRAP1 were dispersed throughout the dish (B), compared withcells transfected with control siRNAthat grew in aggregates resembling untransfected SH-SY5Y cells. C,D: TRAP1 knockdown results in the down-regulation of N-cadherin. Immunohistochemistry of TRAP1 knockdown cells (D) compared with that of control cells (C) stained with an anti-N-cadherin antibody (green) and DAPI (blue). In the TRAP1 knockdown cells (D), N-cadherin is remarkably decreased throughout the cytoplasm, including around the membrane where cell-adhesion takes place. C: Immunobloting of TRAP1 knockdown cells at 48 h after transfection with anti-TRAP1, E2F1 and GAPDH antibodies.E2F1 expression was significantly decreased in the TRAP1 knockdown cells, showing that TRAP1 knockdown decreases the transcription activity of the N-cadherin promoter. D: Immunoblotting of TRAP1 knockdown cells with anti-TRAP1, phosphorylated STAT3 (Tyr705) (p-Tyr STAT3), STAT3 and GAPDH antibodies 48h after transfection. The level of tyrosine-phosphorylated STAT was significantly reduced in the TRAP1 knockdown cells. D: Molecular pathway of the TRAP1-N-cadherin cascade. TRAP1 regulates the tyrosine phosphorylation of STAT3, which controls the expression of E2F, and thus, subsequently modulates the transcription of N-cadherin. As TRAP1 mutations are deeply involved in major depression, the disturbance of cell adhesion by the reduction of N-cadherin which causes abnormal neural circuit formation, may be important in the pathogenesis of major depression.

at synapse is essential for spine remodeling and long term potentiation, suggesting that N-cadherin plays important roles in higher brain function such as learning and memory. It is

therefore likely that altered expression of N-cadherin may be associated with the pathogenesis of mental disorders.
In support of this, we showed that 4 SNPs in the TRAP1 gene may be associated with the pathogenesis of mental disorders, particularly major depression, including 2 SNPs that cause an amino acid change in the TRAP1 protein:R07G (rs1 3926) and D395E (rs1 136948). Moreover, these 2 non-synonymous SNPs are located in the region critical for the binding of TRAP1 to TNFR1, suggesting that the binding affinity of TRAP1 to TNFR1 or the downstream signaling of TRAP1 might be altered in these disorders.

6. Involvement of DISC1 in psychiatric disorders (Fig. 5)

DISC1 has been identified as a potential susceptibility gene for major psychiatric disorders. Disruption of this gene by a balanced translocation (1:11,q42.1;q14.3) results in a predicted C-terminal truncation of the open reading frame. Furthermore, this anomaly is segregated with schizophrenia and affective disorders in a large Scottish family (Millar et al., 2000,2001). A frameshift mutation of DISC1 has been identified in an American family with schizophrenia and schizoaffective disorder (Sach et al., 2005), and the association of the SNPs of DISC1 with schizophrenia, schizoaffetive disorder and bipolar disorder has also been suggested (Hodgkinson et al., 2004).

6.1 Interacting partners bind to the area close to the translocation breakpoint of DISC1

DISC1 has been proposed to be a multifunctional protein that interacts with multifunctional protein that interact with multiple proteins of the centrosome and cytoskeletal system at a distinct domain (Morris et al., 2003; Ozaki et al., 2003). The function of DISC1 could therefore be regulated by DISC1 binding proteins. The DISC1 binding partners, fasciculation and elongation protein zeta-1 (Fez1), DBZ and kendrin were identified using yeast 2-hybrid analysis. The interaction between DISC1 and Fez1, DISC1 and DBZ, and DISC1 and Kendrin were confirmed by immunoprecipitation assays (Matsuzaki & Tohyama, 2007, Miyoshi et al., 2003, Hattori et al., 2007) .

6.2 Role of DISC1-Fez1 interaction in psychiatric disorders (Miyoshi et al.,2003)

The DISC1-Fez1 interaction identified *in vitro* was confirmed *in vivo* by showing the co-localization of DISC1 and Fez1 in neurons of the hippocampus, cerebral cortex and olfactory bulb. Analysis of the intracellular localization of DISC1 revealed that DISC1 and Fez1 co-localize in growth cones in cultured hippocampal neurons. The interactions of these proteins are associated with F-actin. The finding that a molecular complex composed of DISC1, Fez1 and actin is located in the growth cone of neurite suggests the involvement of the DISC1-Fez1 interaction in neurite extension. In support of this, both DISC1 and Fez1 were found to be expressed in the brain during an early ontogenetical stage Honda et al., 2004). The physiological role of the DISC1-Fez1 interaction in neuronal cells, especially at the stage of neurite outgrowth, was examined using PC12 cells. After stimulation with nerve growth factor (NGF), PC12 cells cease proliferation and begin to extend neuritis. The interaction between FLAG-tagged DISC1 and endogenous Fez1 was examined over the course of neuronal differentiation. The amount of Fez1 in immunoprecipitates obtained using an anti-FLAG antibody was drastically increased upon NGF stimulation, suggesting that the DISC1-

Fez1 interaction is up-regulated by NGF stimulation.. Furthermore, when treated with NGF, DISC1-stable lines exhibited enhanced neurite extension compared to mock-stable cells. These findings established that DISC1 participates in neurite outgrowth through its interaction with Fez1. In schizophrenia with DISC1 translocation carriers, in which Fez1 cannot bind to DISC1 owing to its translocation, neuronal circuit formation may remain immature. In addition, an association between the SNPs of the *Fez1* gene and schizophrenia has also been suggested in a Japanese population (Yamada et al., 2004).

6.3 Role of the DISC1-Kendrin interaction in psychiatric disorders (Miyoshi et al., 2004; Shimizu et al. 2008)

6.3.1 The carboxy-terminal region of DISC1 is essential for the DISC1-Kendrin interaction

Kendrin, also referred to as pericentrin-B, is a calmodulin-binding protein localized specifically on centrosomes. Through the presence of the PACT domain, Kendrin is targeted to the centrosome. Co-localization of DISC1 and Kendrin was demonstrated in SH-SY5Y neuroblastoma cells transfected. In addition, co-localization of DISC1 and Kendrin at the centrosome was confirmed by immunohisotchemistry. DISC1 lacking the putative Kendrin binding region (amino acid 446-553) (KBR) is unable to target to the centrosome and distributes diffusely throughout the cytoplasm, showing that interaction of DISC1 with Kendrinis essential for its centrosomal localization. A direct yeast 2-hybrid interaction assay suggested that a short fragment of amino acids 446-533 of DISC1 constituting the binding region (KBR) was essential for the interaction with Kendrin. A subsequent study using immunoprecipitation assays in HEK293 cells in which Kendrin was endogenously expressed confirmed that KBR is critical for the interaction with Kendrin as described below. Cells were transiently transfected with expression vectors for HA-tagged full-length DISC1 (DISC1-HA) and the HA-tagged DISC1 deletion muctant lacking the KBR (DSC1⊿KBR-HA). Endogenous Kendrin was coimmunoprecipitated with DISC1-HA, but not with DISC1⊿KBR-HA. These findings indicate that KBR is the binding region of DISC1 to Kendrin. To examine whether KBR itself could bind to Kendrin, several DISC1 deletion mutants were prepared: GDBP (amino acids 348-597—FLAG, BPC (amino acids 598-854)-FLAG, BR (amino acids 446-633)-FLAG, KBR-FLAG and KBRC (amino acids 446-854)-FLAG. Surprisingly, endogenous Kendrin was detected in immunoprecipitates from cells transfected with KBRC-FLAG, but it was barely detected in immunoprecipitates from cells transfected with GDBP-FLAG, BPC-FLAG, BR-FRAG or KBR-FLAG. These findings confirm KBR as the Kendrin binding region for DISC1 to Kendrin, but also show that the binding to Kendrin is enhanced remarkably in the presence of the carboxy-terminal region downstream of KBR. Thus, KBR is required but not sufficient for the interaction, and the carboxy-terminal region of DISC1 is also indispensable for the binding to Kendrin.

6.3.2 The carboxy-terminal region of DISC1 is required for the localization of DISC1 to the centrosome

Next, we determined which part of DISC1 is indispensable for co-localization of DISC1 with Kendrin at the centrosome. KBRC-FLAG showed a diffuse pattern in the cytoplasm but clearly revealed a strong 'dot' pattern in the perinuclear area. The merged image of KBRC-FLAG and Kendrin showed that they were colocalized at the centrosome. On the other hand, localization of KBR-FLAG showed a diffuse distribution pattern in the nucleus and cytoplasm without strong staining at the centrosome. Staining of BR-FLAG and GDBP-FLAG was characterized by a small punctate distribution pattern, while BPC-FLAG exhibited a diffuse distribution in the cytoplasm. However, BPC-FLAG was not detected at the centrosome. Taken together, these findings demonstrate that the carboxy-terminal half of the DISC1 protein containing KBR and the downstream region of KBR are necessary and sufficient to target the DISC1 protein to the centrosome.

6.3.4 Inhibition of the DISC1-Kendrin interaction perturbs the microtubule network formation

The interaction of DISC1 with Kendrin at the centrosome and the key role of Kendrin in microtubule nucleation at the centrosome suggest that the interaction between DISC1 and Kendrin may affect microtubule network formation. The DISC1-binding region of Kendrin (DBR) (amino acids 2918-305) was first identified. To inhibit the DISC1-Kendrin interaction specifically at the centrosome, a FLAG-tagged DRB-PACT (DBR-PACT-FLAG) construct was prepared including DBR and PACT (a conserved centrosomal targeting motif in CG-NAP and pericentrin). Microtubule aster formation was then observed in COS cells transfected with either the DBZ-PACT-FLAG or PACT-FLAG expression vector. Mock-transfected cells showed microtubule aster formation at the centrosome. However, over-expression of DBR-PACT-FLAG resulted in a significant decrease in the percentages of cells containing the microtubule aster compared with cells expressing PACT-FLAG. In addition, over-expression of DISC1 ⊿KBR-FLAG resulted in a significant decrease in the percentage of cells containing the microtubule aster compared with mock-transfected cells. These results show that the DISC1-Kendrin interaction is involved in brain maturation through the regulation of microtubule organization.

6.3.5 Role of the DISC1-Kendrin interaction in mental disorders

Over-expression of the DISC1-binding region of Kendrin perturbed the normal distribution of the stabilized microtubule network. The over-expression of DISC1 lacking the Kendrin binding site caused an impairment in microtubule aster formation. Carriers of the chromosomal translocation that segregates with mental diseases are expected to produce the truncated mutant DISC1 protein that lacks the carboxy-terminal region, or to have a reduced expression of the DISC1 protein. In the case of truncated mutant protein expression, this protein would not be able to target to the centrosome and interact with Kendrin, which might induce dysfunction of the microtubule network formation. Loss of DISC1 protein expression could lead to the dysfunction of microtubules by disrupting the DISC1-Kendrin interaction. In addition, involvement of Kendrin in olfactory cilia assembly was also reported (Miyoshi et al., 2009). Thus, the DISC1-Kendrin interaction plays a role in neuronal development by regulating microtubule organization, showing that mental diseases derived from DISC1 dysfunction are neurodevelopmental disease. In addition, our recent analysis showed an association between SNPs of the Kendrin gene and bipolar diseases (Anitha et al., 2005).

6.4 Role of DISC1 and its binding proteins with special reference to psychiatric disorders

The present review summarize results showing that DISC1 functions in neural network formation by interacting with several binding partners, including Fez1, DBZ, and

Kendrin, which binds to the area near the translocation site of DISC1. DISC1 interactions, including DISC1-Fez1, DISC1-DBZ and DISC1-Kendrin, all play a key role in neuronal development. Other groups have identified additional DISC1 interaction partner such as NudE-like (NUDEL) (Morris et al., 200; Ozeki et al., 2003), lissenchphaly-1 (LIS1) (Brandron et al., 2004), phosphodiesterase 4B (PDE4B) (Millar et al., 2005), glycogen synthase kinase 3 (GSK3) (Mao et al., 2009), the motor protein dynein and growth factor receptor bound protein 2 (Grb2) (Shinoda et al., 2007;Taya et al., 2007), and these binding partners suggested the functional involvement of DISC1 in neural development. DISC1 therefore plays crucial roles in brain development by affecting neuronal migration, neurite outgrowth and neural maturation through its interaction with several cytoskeletal proteins.

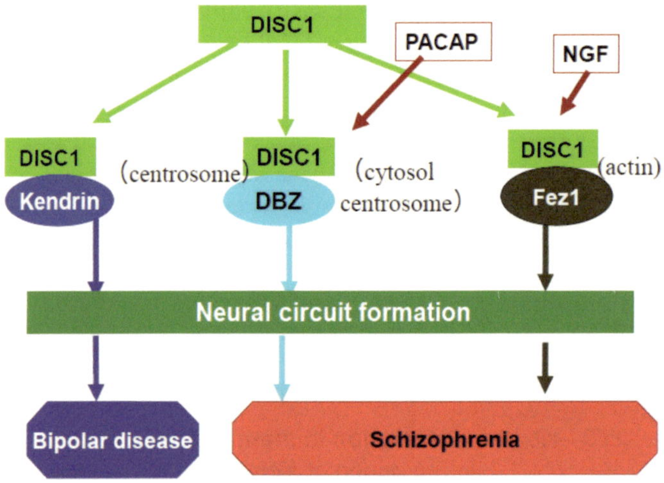

Fig. 5. DISC1 binding proteins that bind to an area near the translocation and their function. The binding between DISC1 and these molecules play a role in neurodevelopment. Accordingly mental disorders in which these molecules are implicated could be considered neurodevelopmental diseases.

7. Conclusion

The results summarized in this review indicate that the TRAP1 cascade, PACAP-stathmin1 cascade, PACAP-DBZ/DISC1 cascade, Dysbindin-MARCKS cascade, DISC1-Fez1 interaction and DISC1-Kendrin interaction are all involved in neural development. In addition, the molecules mentioned above are associated with schizophrenia or bipolar disease, showing that the neural development that is associated with these systems is disturbed in the brains of patients with either of these disease.

8. Acknowledgment

This research was partly supported by Ministry of Education, Culture, Sports, Science and Technology of Japan and by a grant from Dainippon Sumitomo Pharma Co. Ltd.
We thank Mrs. Etsuko Moriya for preparing this manuscript.

9. References

Angrist, B. & van Kammen, D.P., (1984). CNS stimulants as tools in the study of schizophrenia. *Trend Neurosci.* Vol.7, pp. 388-390

Anitha, A., Nakamura, K., Yamada, K. et al. (2008). Gene and expression analyses reveal enhanced expression of pericentrin2 (PCNT2) in bipolar disorder. *Biol. Psychiatry* Vol. 63, pp. 678-685

Berton, O. & Nestler, E.J. (2006). New approaches to antidepressant drug discovery: beyond monoamines. *Nat. Rev. Neurosci.* Vol. 7, pp. 372–377

Brandron, N.J., Handford, E.J., Schurov, I. et al. (2004). Disrupted in Schizophrenia 1 and Nudel form a neurodevelopmentally regulated protein complex: implication for schizophrenia and other major neurological disorders. *Mol. Cell Neurosci.* Vol. 25, pp. 42-55

Bray, N.J., Preece, A., Williams, N.M., et al. (2005). Haplotypes at the dystrobrevin binding protein 1 (DTNBP1) gene locus mediate risk for schizophrenia through reduced DTNBP1 expression. *Hum. Mol. Genet.* Vol. 14, pp. 1947-1954

Burdick, K.E., Lencz, T., Funke, B. et al. (2006). Genetic variation in DTNBP1 influences general cognitive ability. Hum. Mol. Genet. Vo. 15, No.10, pp.1563-1568

Chen, X.W., Feng, Y.Q., Hao,C.J. et al. (2008). DTNBP1, a schizophrenia susceptibility gene, affects kinetics of transmitter release. J. Cell Biol. Vol. 181, 791-801

Chiba, S., Hashimoto, R., Hattori, S. et al. (2006). Effect of antipsychotic drugs on DISC1 and dysbindin expression in mouse frontal cortex and hippocampus. J. Neural Transm. Vol.113, No.9, pp. 1337-1346

Corvin, A., Donohoe, G., Nangle, J.M. et al. (2008). A dysbindin risk haplotype associated with less severe mani-type symptoms in psychosis. *Neurosci. Lett.* Vol. 431, No.2, 146-149

Creese, I., Burt, D.R. & Snyder, S.H. (1976). Dopamine receptor binding predicts clinical and pharmacological potencies of antischizophrenic drugs. *Science* Vol. 192, pp. 481-483

Donohoe, G., Morris, D.W., Nangle, J.M. et al. (2007). Variance in neurocognitive performance is associated with dysbindin-1 in schizophrenia: a preliminary study. *Neuropsychologia* Vol. 45, No. 2, pp. 454-458

Felts, S.J., Owen, B.A., Nguyen, P. et al. (2000). The hsp90-related protein TRAP1 is a mitochondrial protein with distinct functional properties. *J. Biol. Chem.* Vol. 275, pp. 3305-3312

Feng, Y.Q., Zhou, Z.Y., He, X. et al. (2008). Dysbindin deficiency in sandy mice causes reduction of snapin and displays behabiors related to schizophrenia. *Schizophr. Res.* Vol. 106, pp. 218-227

Hashimoto, H., Ishiharas, T., Shigemoto, R. et al., (1993). Molecular cloning and tissue distribution of a receptor for pituitary adenylate cyclase activating polypeptide. *Neuron* Vol. 11. pp. 333-342

Greg, S., Nelson, S. &Michael, H. (1999). Dendrites. Oxford University Press, New York

Hashimoto, H., Shintani, N., Tanaka, K. et al. (2001). Altered psychomotor behaviors in mice lacking pituitary adenylate cyclase-activating polypeptide (PACAP). *Proc. Natl. Acad. Sci. USA* . Vol. 98, pp.13355-13360

Hashimoto, R., Hashimoto, H., Shintani, N. et al. (2007). Pituitary adenylate cyclase-activating polypeptide is asociated with schizophrenia. *Mol. Psychiatry* Vol. 12, pp. 1026-1032

Hattori, S., Murotani, T., Matsuzaki, S. et al., Behavioral abnormalities and dopamine reductions in sdy mice with a deletion in Dtnbp1, susceptibility gene for schizophrenia. *Biochem. Biophys. Res. Commun.* Vol. 373, pp. 298-302

Hattori, T., Baba, K., Matsuzaki, S., et al. (2007). A novel DISC1-interacting partner DISC1-binding Zinc finger protein: implication in the modulation of DISC1-dependent neurite outgroath. *Mol. Psychiatry* Vol. 12, pp. 398-407

Hayashida, Y., Urata, Y., Muroi, E. et al. (2006). Calreticulin represses E-cadherin gene expression in Madin-Darby canine kidney cells via Slug. *J. Biol. Chem.* Vol. 281, pp. 32469-32484

Hodgkinson, C..A., Goldman, D., Jaeger, J. et al. (2004). Disrupted in schizophrenia 1 (DISC1): association with schizophrenia, schizoaffective disorder,and bipolar disorder. *Am. J. Hum. Genet.* Vol. 75, pp. 862-872

Honda, A., Miyoshi, K., Baba, K., et al. (2004). Expression of fasciculation and elongation protein zeta-1 (Fesz1) in the developing rat brain. *Mol. Brain Res.* Vol. 122, pp. 89-92

Irwin, M.R. & Miller, A.H. (2007). Depressive disorders and immunity: 20 years of progress and discovery. *Brain Behav. Immun.* Vol. 21,pp. 374-383

Katayama,T., Hattori, T., Yamada,K. et al., Role of the PACAP-PAC1-DISC1 and PACAP-PAC1-stathmin1 systems in schizophrenia and bipolar disorder; novel treatment mechanisms? *Pharmacogenomics* Vol. 10, No. 12, pp. 1967-1978, ISSN1462-2416

Kubota, K., Inoue, K., Hashimoto, R. et al. (2009). Tumor necros i s factor receptor-associated protein 1 regulates cell adhesion and synaptic morphoogy via modulation of N-cadherin expression. *J. Neurochem.* Vol. 110, pp.496-508

Kubota, K., Kumamoto, N., Matsuzaki, S. et al. (2009). Dysbindin engages in c-Jun N-terminal kinase activity and cytoskeletal organization. *Biochem. Biophy. Res. Commun.* Vol. 73, pp. 191-195

Kumamoto N., Matsuzaki, S., Inoue, K. et al. (2006). Hyperactivation of midbrain dopaminergic system in schizophrenia could be attributed to the down-regulation of dysbindin. *Biochem. Biophy. Res. Comm.* Vol. 345, pp. 904-909.

Lieberman, J.A., Kane, J.M. & Alvir, J. (1987). Provocative tests with psychostimulant drugs in schizophrenia. *Psychopharmacol. (Berl)* Vol. 91, pp. 415-433

Mao, Y., Ge, X., Franki, C.L. et al. (2009). Disrupted in schizophrenia 1 regulates neuronal progenitor proliferation via modulation of GSK3β / β-catenin signaling. *Cell* Vol. 136, pp. 1017-1031

Matsuzaki, S. & Tohyama, M. (2007). Molecular mechanism of schizophrenia with reference to disrupted-in-schizophrenia 1 (DISC1). *Neurochem. Int.* Vol. 51, pp. 165-172

Millar, J.K., Wilson-Annan, J.C., Anderson, S. et al. (2000). Distribution of tw novel genes by a translocation co-segregating with schizophrenia. *Hum. Mol. Genet.* Vol. 9, pp. 1415-1423

Millar, J.K., Christie, A., Anderson, S. et al. (2001). Genomic structure and localization within a linkage hotspot of distrupted in schizophrenia 1, a gene disrupted by a translocation segregating withschizophrenia. *Mol. Psychaitry* Vol. 6, pp. 173-178

Millar, J.K., Pickard, B.S., Mackie, S. et al. (2005). DISC1 and PDE4B are interacting genetic factors in schizophrenia that regulate cAMP signaling. *Science* Vol. 310, pp. 1187-1191

Miyoshi, K., Asanuma, I., Miyazaki, F.J. et al. (2004). DISC1 localizes to the centrosome by binding to kendrin. *Biochem. Biophys. Res. Commun.* Vol. 317, pp. 1195-1199.

Miyoshi, K., Kasahara, K., Miyazaki, I. et al. (2009). Pericentrin, a centrosomal protein related to microcephalic primordial dwarfism, is required for olfactory cilia assembly in mice. *FASEB J*. Vol. 10, pp. 3289-3297

Miyoshi, K., Honda, A., Baba, K. et al. (2003). Disrupted-In-Schizophrenia 1, a candidate gene for schizophrenia, participates in neurite outgrowth. *Mol. Psychiatry* Vol. 8, pp. 685-684

Morris, J.A., Kandpal,G., Ma, L. et al. (2003). DISC1 (disrupted-in-schizophrenia 1) is a centrosome-associated protein that interacts with MAP1A, MIPT3,ATF4/5 and Nudel: regulation and loss of interaction with mutation. *Hum. Mol. Genet.* Vol. 12, 1591-1608

Nestler, E.J., Barrot, M., DiLeone, R.J. et al. (2002). Neurobiology of depression. *Neuron*, Vol. 34, pp. 13-25.

Numakawa, T., Yagasaki, Y., Ishimoto, T. et al. (2004). Evidence of novel neuronal functions of dysbindin, a susceptibility gene for schizophrenia. *Hum. Mol. Genet.* Vol. 13,2699-2708

Okuda, H., Kuwahara, R., Matsuzaki, S. et al. (2010). Dysbindin regulates the transcriptional level of myristoylated alanine-rich protein kinase C substrate via the interaction with NF-YBin mice brain. *PLoS one* Vol. 5, Issue1 pp.e8773

Okumura, K., Tanaka, H., Yagita, Y. et al. (2004). Cadherin activity is required for activity-induced spine remodeling. *J. Cell Biol.* Vol. 167, pp. 961-972

Ozeki, Y., Tomoda, T., Kleiderlein, J. et al. (2003). Disrupted-in-schizophrenia-1 (DISC-1): mutant truncation prevents binding to NudE-like (NUDEL) and inhibits neurite outgrowth. *Proc. Natl. Acad. Sc. USA.* Vol. 100, pp.289-294

Sachs, N.A., Sawa, A., Holmes, S.E. et al. (2005). A frameshift mutation in disrupted in schizophrenia 1 in an American family with schizophrenia, schizoaffective disorder. *Mol. Psychiatry* Vol. 10, pp. 758-764

Seeman, P. & Lee,T. (1975). Antipsychotic drugs; direct correlation between clinical potency and presynaptic action on dopamine neurons. *Science* Vol. 188, pp. 1217-1219

Shimizu, S., Matsuzaki, S., Hattori, T. et al. (2008). DISC1-kendrin interaction is involved in centrosomal microtubule network formation. *Biochem. Biophys. Res. Commun.* Vol. 377, pp. 1051-1056

Shintani, N., Mori, W., Hashimoto, H., et al. (2992). Defects in reproductive functions in PACAP-deficient femal mice. *Regul. Pep.* Vol. 109, pp. 45-48

Shinoda, T., Taya, S., Tsuboi, D et al. (2007). DISC1 regulates neurortophion-induced axon elongation via interaction with Grb2. *J. Neurosci.* Vol. 27, pp.4-14

Sillitoe, R.V., Benson, M.A., Blake, D.J. et al. (2003). Abnormal dysbindin expression in cerebellar mossy fiber synapses in the mdx mouse model of Duchenne muscular dystrophy. *J. Neurosci.* Vol. 23, No. 16, pp. 6576-6585

Song, H.Y., Dunbar, Y., Zhang, J.D. et al. (1995). Identification of a protein with homology to hsp90 that binds the type 1 tumor necrosis factor receptor. *J. Biol. Chem.* Vol. 270, pp. 3574-3581.

Takeuchi, M. & Nakagawa, S. (2001). Cadherin-dependent cell-cell adhesion. *Curr. Protoc. Cell Biol.* Chapter9, Unit 9.3

Talbot, K., Eidem, W.L., Tinsley, M.A. et al. (2004). Dysbindin-1 is reduced in intrinsic, glutamatergic terminals of the hippocampal formation in schizophrenia. *J. Clin. Invest.* Vol. 113, pp. 1353-1363

Taya, S., Shinoda, T., Tsuboi, D. et al. (2007). DISC1 regulates the transport of the NUDEL/LIS1/14silon complex through kinesin-1. *J. Neurosci.* Vol. 27, pp. 15-26

Togashi, H., Abe, K., Mizoguchi, A. et al. (2002). Cadhelin regulates dendritic spine morphogenesis. *Neuron*, Vol. 35, pp. 77-89

Vaudry, D., Gonzalez, BJ, Basille, M. et al. (2000). Pituitary adenylate cyclase-activating polypeptide and its receptors: from structure to function. *Pharmacol. Rev.* Vol. 52, pp. 269-234

Weicker, C.S., Straub, R.E., McClintock, B.W., Matsumoto, M. et al. (2004). Human dysbindin (DTNBP1) gene expression in normal brain and in schizophrenic prefrontal cortex and midbrain. *Arch. Gen. Psychiatry* Vol. 61, pp. 544-555

Yamada, K., Matsuzaki,S., Hattori, T. et al. (2010). Increased stathmin1 expression in the dentate gyrus of mice causes abnormal axonal arborizations. *PLoS one* Vol.5, Issue1, e8596

Yamada,K., Nakamura, K., Minabe, Y. et al. (2004). Association analysis of FEZ1 variants with schizophrenia in Japanese cohorts. *Biol.Psychiatry* Vol. 56, pp. 683-690

Yasuda, S., Tanaka, H., Sugiura, H. et al. (2007). Activity-induced procadherin arcadlin regulates dendritic spine number by triggering N-cadherin endocytosis via TAO2beta and p38 MAP kinases. *Neuron* Vol. 56, pp. 456-471

Zinkstok, J.R., de Wilde, O., van Amelsvoort, T.A. et al. (2007). Association between the DTNBP1 gene and intelligence: a case-control study in young patients with schizophrenia and related disorders and unaffected siblings. Behav, Brain Func. Vol., 3, pp.19

19

Neurotransmitter and Behaviour: Serotonin and Anxiety

André Rex and Heidrun Fink[1]
Department of Neurology, Center for Stroke Research,
Charité University Medicine, Berlin,
[1]Institute of Pharmacology and Toxicology, School of Veterinary Medicine,
Freie Universität Berlin, Berlin,
Germany

1. Introduction

There are many indications that mental disorders such as depression and anxiety disorders are directly related to mechanisms of central synaptic transmission of serotonin (5-HT).
5-HT is a peripherally and centrally occurring transmitter, which is involved in regulation of anxiety-related behaviour (Iversen 1984; Griebel 1995) and mood, but mediates also learning, appetite, food intake, sexual behaviour, sleep and influences body temperature as well as motor activity (Lucki 1998).

2. Central serotonergic system

In mammals 5-HT is distributed throughout the body. About 5% are located in the central nervous system (CNS). After 5-HT was found in the CNS (Twarog and Page 1953), detailed studies of the origin and projection areas of serotonergic neurons in the CNS began (Falck et al. 1962).
Only about 500 000 neurons in the CNS use 5-HT as a transmitter, but serotonergic neurons have connections to almost all structures of the brain and show a high degree of axonal branching. Dahlström and Fuxe (Dahlstrom and Fuxe 1964) demonstrated by histochemical methods that the raphe nuclei are the origin of almost all serotonergic neurons. Amin and colleagues (Amin et al. 1954) determined 5-HT levels in various brain areas and found the highest concentrations in hypothalamus, midbrain and area postrema.
5-HT receptors are distributed throughout the CNS, with different distribution patterns for the different receptor types. Most 5-HT postsynaptic receptors are located on the subsequent neurons. The release of 5-HT is regulated by presynaptic 5-HT receptors that are located either at the soma or at the nerve endings of the serotonergic neurons. Today, the "5-HT Receptor Nomenclature Committee of the International Union of Pharmacology (NC-IUPHAR) recognizes seven 5-HT receptor families with 16 receptor subtypes (Hoyer et al. 2002).
In the regulation of anxiety-related behaviour by serotonergic transmission, mainly 5-HT1A receptors, 5-HT2A/2C receptors and 5-HT3 receptors are involved (Griebel 1995; Rex et al. 2007). Involvement of 5-HT1B/1D receptors in the modulation of anxiety-related behaviour is discussed.

3. Anxiety and anxiety disorders

Fear or anxiety has protective functions to avoid situations that cause pain, injury or even death (Vaas 2000).

In man, fear is associated with arousal, characterized by symptoms such as restlessness, tremor, less α-waves and frequent β-waves in the electroencephalogram, tachypnea, and tachycardia, elevated systolic blood pressure, hyperemia of the skeletal muscles, decreased blood flow to the internal organs, hypermotility of the stomach, decreased salivation and mydriasis. Clinical studies however, found no uniform physiologic reaction pattern due to large individual differences (Kielholz and Battegay 1967). It was found that the decrease in the frequency of α-waves in the electroencephalogram and the increase in finger tremor and respiratory rate correlated best with the perceived anxiety of the subjects.

But what about anxiety and fear in animals? If one assumes that fear is ... "an emotional reaction to the recognition or the recognition of a perceived threat, regardless of whether that risk is also a given objective" is considered (Tembrock 2000) and that animals in an aversive environment or threatening situations show similar physiological symptoms as people, it can be expected that at least highly developed animals due to physiological and ethological homologies can feel anxiety or fear (Silverman 1978).

We are aware that anxiety and fear are human emotions. However, to ease reading also in relation to animals we speak of fear, anxious and less anxious behaviour.

A distinction between pathological and "normal" anxiety is difficult. If, however, continued intense fear without real danger and threat perception occurs, or the fear response is "unreasonable" compared to the sources of threats, they get disease value.

Anxiety disorders are among the most common mental disorders. Up to 15% of all people suffer during their life from an anxiety disorder (lifetime prevalence) (Kessler et al. 2010).

Treatment of anxiety disorders and consequences of the disease cause high costs and are connected with severe social problems (Wittchen and Jacobi 2005). One in four patients with generalized anxiety disorder is not in a position to meet its daily life requirements (Becker and Hoyer 2000). The course of anxiety disorders without adequate treatment is chronic recurrent and a spontaneous remission was found in only about 14% of the patients (Wittchen 1991).

4. Pharmacotherapy of anxiety disorders

A rational pharmacotherapy with anxiolytics is the basis for successful treatment of anxiety disorders, often combined with psychotherapy (Bandelow et al. 2005). In general, the drug therapy lasts for at least 12 months.

In the search for effective anxiolytic agents, chlordiazepoxide was synthesized in 1957 as the first benzodiazepine by Sternberg. The benzodiazepines, such as chlordiazepoxide and diazepam, were the first primary anti-anxiety agents. Until the mid-90s benzodiazepines were the most commonly prescribed anxiolytics. Despite known sedative effects and addictive potential, they are safe drugs for the short-term treatment of anxiety (Lader 2005).

During the last decade, a fundamental change has taken place in the pharmacotherapy of anxiety disorders.

Nowadays, benzodiazepines, which are still the primary acute intervention in panic disorder or drugs of second choice or for an interim treatment in generalized anxiety disorder and social phobias, are prescribed less often (Lohse et al. 2004). At present, mainly drugs that affect the serotonergic system, such as buspirone, SSRIs or NSMRI, are recommended as first choice (Bandelow, Zohar et al. 2005) (Table 1).

Anxiety Disorders	Recommended pharmacotherapy
Panic disorder	acute: benzodiazepines chronic: non-selective monoamine reuptake inhibitors (NSMRI), SSRI
Generalized anxiety disorder	SSRI, NSMRI, selective 5-HT-norepinephrine reuptake Inibitors (SSNRI), buspirone in treatment failure + start: benzodiazepines or opipramol
Social phobia	SSRI, moclobemide in treatment failure + to start: benzodiazepines
Obsessive compulsive disorder	NSMRI, SSRIs, in treatment failure: combination with neuroleptics

Table 1. Summary of drugs that are recommended for the treatment of anxiety and compulsive disorders by the Drug Commission of the German Medical Association and the German Society for Psychiatry, Psychotherapy and Neurology.

In Germany, phytotherapeutics, prescribed or self-prescribed by the patients, are used widely although there is no evidence-based proof of efficacy in anxiety disorders (Kinrys et al. 2009). A special role had preparations kava-kava herbal products (Piper methysticum). The use of kava-kava and similar "natural remedy" in the industrialized countries increased strongly. In some clinical studies, the substance proved to be similarly effective as benzodiazepines with very few adverse drug reactions (Witte et al. 2005). In higher doses, kava-kava has also sedative and hypnotic effects.

5. Neurotransmitter systems and anxiety

Since the discovery of the mode of action of benzodiazepines late 70s (Möhler and Okada 1977), γ-aminobutyric acid (GABA) is most frequently associated with anxiety disorders and their pharmacotherapy. Benzodiazepines augment the GABAergic inhibition via GABA-A receptors (Rudolph et al. 2001). Inverse agonists at the binding site for benzodiazepines, such as the beta-carboline-3-carboxylic acid N-methylamide, have anxiety-causing effects (Moriarty 1995).

In addition to GABA, 5-HT plays an important role in the development and the persistence of anxiety disorders (Griebel 1995). Studies show that patients with anxiety disorders may have genetic polymorphisms in the 5-HT transporter (Overview: (Lesch and Gutknecht 2005) or in the 5-HT2A receptor (Golimbet et al. 2004) and the 5-HT1A receptor (Gordon and Hen 2004). In patients with panic disorder the number of 5-HT1A receptors in the limbic system was shown to be reduced (Neumeister et al. 2004). Preclinical evidence also points towards an involvement of 5-HT3 receptors in the regulation of anxiety (Costall and Naylor 1992; Rex, Bert et al. 2007), but clinical efficacy is still uncertain (Adell 2010).

First indications of a link between 5-HT and anxiety-related behaviour resulted from the observation that methysergide and metergoline, later on known as 5-HT antagonists, had an anxiolytic effect in animal studies (Robichaud and Sledge 1969). The same anxiolytic effect was seen following inhibition of 5-HT synthesis by para-chlorophenylalanine in rats in the

Geller-Seifter test. This conflict-reducing effect was prevented by treatment with 5-hydxroxytryptophan (5-HTP), the precursor of 5-HT (Geller and Blum 1970). Therefore, it was expected that an increased activity of the central serotonergic system would be connected with anxiety and vice versa reduced activity with declined anxiety (Iversen 1984). Several studies have shown that an increase in 5-HT concentration in the brain increased anxiety and a reduction of 5-HT level reduces anxiety.

Other neurotransmitters that affect fear-related behaviour include the neuropeptide cholecystokinin (CCK), neuropeptide S, adenosine, excitatory amino acids and angiotensin.

While the fear-producing effect of cholecystokinin is firm, the role of other neurotransmitters/-modulators for the development of anxiety, however, is not sufficiently understood.

CCK,, one of the best characterized neuropeptides, was, like 5-HT, discovered originally in the digestive tract and found later in the CNS (Vanderhaeghen et al. 1975). Two major receptor types were discovered: CCK2 and CCK1 receptors in the brain, whereas in the periphery almost exclusively CCK1 receptors occur (Beinfeld et al. 1981).

The CCK2 receptor is involved in the regulation of fear-related behaviours in humans and animals (Fink et al. 1998). In patients with a history of panic disorder and in healthy volunteers panic attacks could be triggered by a CCK-4 injection (De Montigny 1989; Bradwejn and Koszycki 2001).

Adenosine is also involved in the regulation of anxiety-related behaviour. High doses of the nonselective adenosine receptor antagonist caffeine induce fear in healthy people (Nehlig et al. 1992) and trigger panic attacks in patients with known anxiety disorder (Charney et al. 1985). Rats treated with caffeine, were more anxious in the elevated plus-maze test (X-maze) (Kayir and Uzbay 2005) and a free exploratory paradigm (Bert et al. 2011), while an adenosine-1 agonist had an anxiolytic effect in the X-maze (Florio et al. 1998).

For long the renin-angiotensin system has been considered as a classical endocrine system, with main effects in the peripheral blood pressure regulation, before an independent renin-angiotensin system in the CNS was demonstrated (Fischer-Ferraro et al. 1971). In the CNS, angiotensinII (ATII) is acting as a neurotransmitter involved in the regulation of anxiety-related behaviour. In animal studies intraventricular administration of ATII caused anxiogenic (Braszko et al. 2003), but also anxiolytic (Holy and Wisniewski 2001) effects in the X-maze test. Both, angiotensin1-receptor (AT1) antagonists (Srinivasan et al. 2003) and AT2-receptor antagonists (Braszko, Kulakowska et al. 2003) and reduced ATII levels by ACE inhibitors reduce the fear in rats (Srinivasan, Suresh et al. 2003).

Although clinical reports point to an anxiety-reducing effects of ACE inhibitors and AT-receptor antagonists, there are no valid data in man available (Gard 2004).

6. Animal models of anxiety and animal anxiety tests

Anxiety tests in the clinic have the advantage that the volunteers may self-report their experiences. To trigger anxiety, the subjects receive either fear-inducing agents (caffeine, pentylenetetrazol, lactate infusions or CO2 inhalation), or they undergo psychological tests in an aversive environment (Graeff et al. 2003).

If animals can experience fear (Tembrock 2000), it would be possible to observe behaviour and neurochemical changes similar to changes in humans.

Animal anxiety tests are necessary for the development and characterization of novel anxiolytics. A disadvantage of animal studies is that only indirect conclusions about the emotions involved are possible by observing the behaviour and physiological side effects.

6.1 Historical developments

There are many animal tests for anxiety available (File 1985; Lister 1990). These tests may be divided roughly into three groups:
1. Tests in which anxiety is induced chemically, such as the drug discrimination test (Lal and Emmett-Oglesby 1983); 2. Tests based on conditioned fear / aversion, as the conditioned-emotional-response test (Davis 1990), the Geller-Seifter test, or the bird-punished-drinking test (Geller 1960) and last but not least 3. unconditioned tests, inducing anxiety by a new aversive environment, leading to behavioural inhibition. The unconditioned tests of anxiety include the X-maze (Handley and Mithani 1984), the black and white box test (Crawley and Goodwin 1980), the modified open field test (Rex et al. 1998), the social interaction test (Cappell and Latane 1969; File and Pope 1974) and the free exploratory paradigm (Griebel et al. 1993).
In unconditioned tests a conflict situation is created for the animals and changes in the innate behaviour in this aversive situation are observed. Examples for innate behaviour of animals and inhibiting factors used are: natural exploratory behaviour and avoidance of aversive open spaces without protection, co-existing curiosity and fear reactions to the appearance of a stranger of their own species, or vocalisations during sudden isolation.
The animal anxiety tests have to be validated pharmacologically with drugs whose anxiolytic or anxiety-inducing effects are known, and biologically by the variation of test conditions and their impact on the animals' behaviour (File 1985).
Since it is assumed that the different animal anxiety tests detect various forms of anxiety, for the determination of drug effects on behaviour also various anxiety tests should be used (Hagan et al. 2000).
In humans and animals two fundamentally different forms of anxiety can be distinguished: short-term changes in the emotional state (state anxiety) and a personality trait representing enduring anxiety (trait anxiety) (Cattell and Scheier 1958). In humans state anxiety and trait anxiety are differentiated with the "State Trait Anxiety Inventory"(Spielberger 1972).
To our knowledge only the free exploration test, in which home cage leaving behaviour in a real home environment is used to measure trait anxiety in rodents.

6.2 Recent developments and improvements

Despite the use of benzodiazepines, antidepressants and 5-HT1A agonists in the pharmacotherapy of anxiety disorders, only about 40-70% of the patients reach a symptom-free state (remission) or symptomatic improvement (response) (Kjernisted and Bleau 2004). Remission rates with SSRIs are even lower than under the conventional benzodiazepines (Pollack 2004). Therefore for the treatment of anxiety disorders, novel drugs with a rapid onset and with a constant therapeutic effect, and with fewer adverse effects are needed.
Consequently, there is still a need for improved animal tests for anxiety, which are capable to predict the anxiolytic efficacy of a drug and to mirror different facets of anxiety related disorders (Iversen 1984).
In the 80s and 90s of the last century, tests for anxiety were directed towards the discovery of drugs acting at the GABA receptors, because benzodiazepines were the gold-standard in the pharmacotherapy of anxiety disorders (Stephens and Andrews 1991). In contrast to the reliable detection of effects of GABAergic drugs on anxiety-related behaviour, it appeared that the anxiety tests available gained insufficient information regarding cholecystokininergic or serotonergic influences on anxiety-related behaviour (Griebel 1995; Rodgers and Johnson 1995). In order to assess fear-related behaviours more

comprehensively, new tests for anxiety were developed or established tests changed. Examples for this progress are the elevated zero maze test (Shepherd et al. 1994) and improvements of the open field test.

6.2.1 Modified open field test and its validation

The open field has been used since about 80 years to study the locomotor and exploratory activity in laboratory rodents (Hall 1934). It could be shown that the movement pattern of animals in the brightly lit open field depends on their anxiety. The duration and frequency of the stay of animals in the central region or the amount of thigmotaxis indicate the intensity of anxiety in the animals. In assessing the behaviour of animals in the open field it has to be taken into account that a complex behaviour, which is composed of anxiety-related behaviour, neophobia, exploration, motivation, habituation and spatial learning, is analyzed.

In pre-clinical testing easy and quick tests are needed, which in the ideal case, reduce the assessment of a complex behaviour to a "yes-no decision". We modified the open field test on the basis of existing tests (Britton and Britton 1981). In our test, hungry rats were placed in a brightly lit and unfamiliar open field, with a petri dish of the usual rat chow in the middle of the open field. The hungry animals had the conflict between food supply and the fear of an unknown and aversive environment that suppresses food intake. As a parameter of an anxiety- modifying effect, we determined the percentage of rats of a group, which began to feed in the open field and could simplify the test (Rex et al. 1996; Rex, Stephens et al. 1996).

The modified open field test has been validated behaviourally and pharmacologically (Rex, Voigt et al. 1998). A shorter fasting period results in a less frequent food intake in the open field, similar to the offer of unfamiliar food.

Variations in the illumination of the test arena also changed the incidence of feeding in the open field. Increased illumination prevented the food intake entirely, while a reduction of light intensity increased the proportion of rats that fed in the aversive open field (Rex et al. 1994). These findings are consistent with other studies of rat behaviour in an open, aversive environment, showing that rats in a dimly lit open field had more social interactions than in a brightly lit open field (File and Hyde 1978; Rex et al. 2004).

We were able to show in this simple animal test not only the known anxiolytic effects of GABA agonists, such as diazepam and the β-carboline abecarnil (Rex, Stephens et al. 1996), but also the dose-related anxiety-reducing effects of 5-HT1A agonists, 5-HT2A antagonists and 5-HT3A antagonists. Hypnotics, antipsychotics such as haloperidol and stimulants such as amphetamine, without fear-reducing effect, did not increase the incidence of feeding in the open field (Rex, Voigt et al. 1998). To exclude false positive or false negative results locomotor activity and substance-related effects on food intake were also determined (Rex, Voigt et al. 1998).

6.2.2 Risk assessment in the X-maze

Often, serotonergic drugs fail to change traditional parameters of anxiety-related behaviour (De Vry 1995; Griebel 1995). However, the risk assessment behaviour of animals treated with serotonergic drugs differed from the behaviour of the controls. Therefore, in addition to developing new anxiety tests, a more detailed analysis and precise description of the behaviour in the commonly used tests was suggested. The determination of the risk behaviour of rats and mice in the X-maze is now common in the assessment of anxiety-related behaviour (Rodgers et al. 1997). We observed that guinea pigs after placement on the X-maze remained motionless in the centre of the test apparatus ("freezing"). The duration of freezing was shortened by anxiolytics such as diazepam, the 5-HT1A agonist 8-OH-DPAT or the CCK2-receptor antagonist L365, 260 and significantly prolonged by fear-inducing substances, such as CCK-4 (Rex et al. 1994). Similar findings were observed in rats. Rats of a more anxious strain showed a longer freezing-period compared with a less anxious strain (Rex et al. 1999).

6.2.3 Variation of pre-test and test procedures

The widespread use of unconditioned tests (Lister 1990) also led to varying results across different laboratories, caused by various reasons.

Variations in the construction of the experimental apparatus, for example, can affect the explorative activity of the animals. These variations include the mechanical stability of the entire experimental apparatus (Jones et al. 2002), the use of different materials of the walls of the open fields (Ohl and Keck 2003) or the use of opaque or translucent wall materials for the closed arms of X-maze (Anseloni and Brandao 1997).

Similar effects have variations in the handling and husbandry of animals before and during the test, which can alter both the spontaneous behaviour and sensitivity to anxiety-modulating drugs. Examples include: repeated "handling" (Andrews and File 1993), stress factors in the environment (also in the animal unit) (Haller and Halasz 1999), light conditions in the animal unit and in the test arena, social stress or isolation (Rodgers and Cole 1993) or test-experience of the animals (Hagan, Harper et al. 2000).

We could show that the rearing conditions in rats have an impact on the fear-related behaviour of the animals. It appears that rats that were reared either single housed or in groups, differed in anxiety-related behaviour. Animals reared in social isolation, behaved much more fearless on the X-maze (Marsden et al. 1995).

For the above reasons, a pharmacological and a behavioural validation is needed to compare own results with those in the literature. As an example for our laboratory, we established and validated the social interaction test in rats.

6.2.4 Validation of the social interaction test

The social interaction test, based on the open field test, was developed by (Cappell and Latane 1969) and validated throughout (File, 1978). When two rats, unknown to each other, are placed in a test arena, there will be contacts between the two animals. The time and frequency of individual forms of active social interaction during the tests are measured. In the aversive environment of a brightly lit open field contacts between the two animals are less frequent than in a non aversive environment (File 1985). Benzodiazepines stimulate the interaction between the two rats under aversive conditions (File and Hyde 1978). The use of non-GABAergic drugs led to conflicting results (De Vry 1995; Griebel 1995).

To assess the influence of organismic test variations on the fear-related behaviour, we tested a generally more anxious rat strain (Wistar [Wist: Shoe] Dimed Schönwalde GmbH, Germany) and a less anxious rat strain (Sprague Dawley [SD: Shoe], Dimed Schönwalde GmbH, Germany). We found that the duration of individual housing before the test and the associated social deprivation, had a significant influence on the duration and frequency of

social contacts. Without a previous isolation we observed little interest in the other animal (Rex, Voigt et al. 2004).
Reduction of the aversive nature of the test arena by lower illumination or by a previous habituation to the test arena led to increased social interaction and confirmed the results of (File and Hyde 1978). Here, the change of behaviour of the more anxious Wistar rats was more pronounced. Diazepam increased social contacts only in the more anxious Wistar rats (Rex, Voigt et al. 2004). The well-known anxiogenic mCPP decreased the number and duration of mutual contacts in both rat strains (Rex, Voigt et al. 2004).

6.3 Impact of strain differences

Considering the widespread use of rodents in behavioural experiments, strain differences and their impact on the findings in the assessment and comparison of results with the available literature have to be considered. Genetic differences between individual strains or substrains in rodents may produce conflicting results and lead to misinterpretation of results (Jax 2003).
It is known that the fear-related behaviour differs between various strains of rats or mice (e.g. Trullas and Skolnick 1993; Rex, Sondern et al. 1996).
During the validation of the social interaction test, we observed that anxious Wistar rats and less anxious Sprague Dawley rats differed in the severity of behavioural changes after modifications of the test (Rex, Voigt et al. 2004). It was not known to what extend these behavioural differences were genetic determined or caused by environmental conditions during breeding and animal keeping. To determine the influence of breeding, husbandry and genetic conditions on the anxiety-related behaviour, we examined the anxiety-related behaviour of inbred and outbred rats under identical and different breeding and housing conditions.

6.3.1 Inbred laboratory rodents

We compared the fear-related behaviour of inbred Fischer 344 rats supplied by two national breeders (Charles River Laboratories Inc., Germany and Harlan-Winkelmann Ltd, Germany) and from a regional vendor (Dimed Schönwalde GmbH, Germany). Because of their extensive homocygosity inbred animals should show a small variation in behaviour. In the analysis of the anxiety-related behaviour in the X-maze, black and white box and the modified open field we found small but significant differences in anxiety-related behaviour between animals from different breeders (Bert et al. 2001).
In a second set of experiments we obtained pregnant Fischer 344 rats from the three above-mentioned vendors. The F1 generations were reared in our animal house. Interestingly, the F1 generation showed despite identical housing conditions behavioural differences between the stocks and strains (Bert, Fink et al. 2001).These differences in anxiety-related behaviour seem to be primarily innate. It is possible that a long term breeding of the rats with original genetic uniformity at different places led to the formation of substrains (Jax 2003).

6.3.2 Outbred laboratory rodents

In behavioural pharmacology experiments outbred rats, like Wistar rats or Sprague Dawley rats, are used more often. Outbred rats with their greater genetic diversity are thought to reflect the genetic diversity of the human population. We observed significant differences in anxiety-related behaviour between different outbred rat strains. These behavioural differences were detected in several unconditioned anxiety tests and are therefore not attributable to a specific test stimulus (Rex, Sondern et al. 1996). Interestingly, behavioural differences between different stocks of one strain and the behavioural differences between strains were similar (Rex, Sondern et al. 1996; Bert, Fink et al. 2001). Even when pregnant rats from different breeders were obtained and the F1 generation was raised under the same conditions, the F1 generation showed similar differences in anxiety-related behaviour.

This confirms again, that behavioural differences between the rat strains can be caused primarily by genetic differences (Rex, Sondern et al. 1996; Rex, Voigt et al. 1999; Rex et al. 2007).

In a second approach, we examined the fear-related behaviour of two lines of Sprague Dawley rats with common origin. 20 years ago the Institute of Cytology and Genetics in Novosibirsk (Russia) started breeding Sprague-Dawley (SD) rats obtained from Charles River Sulzfeld, Germany. To best knowledge, there were no further deliveries from Charles River to Novosibirsk (communication with Dr. J. Geller, CEO Charles River Germany). Examination of the anxiety-related behaviour and neurochemical experiments using both stocks revealed differences in their exploratory and anxiety-related behaviour, in habituation and learning, physical development, and serotonergic neurotransmission. Therefore, rats of the same stock but obtained from different breeders should be used with caution in research involving these measures (Rex, Kolbasenko et al. 2007).

Intentionally selectively bred sublines of rat strains have be used for more than 40 years. The selective breeding includes lines of rat strains, which differ significantly in anxiety-related behaviour, such as the HAB / LAB (high anxiety-related behaviour / low anxiety-related behaviour) rats (Liebsch et al. 1998) or the Maudsley (reactive / nonreactive) rat lines (Broadhurst 1975).

Since each of the selectively bred lines start from one common rat strain, there should be only minor genetic differences between the lines, causing the change in behaviour in anxiety tests (Landgraf 2003). Genetic and pharmacological investigations of these rat lines may contribute to the elucidation of the neurobiological basis of fear and anxiety disorders.

However, it has to be taken into account, that a complex emotion like fear has a polygenic base.

7. Combination of anxiety tests with neurochemical analysis

7.1 Brain microdialysis

The microdialysis as an in vivo sampling technique allows to gain a sterile and protein-free dialysate from one or more limited regions of the brain and subsequently to analyze changes in the levels of substances in the extracellular fluid in vivo in anesthetized and in awake animals over time.

Introduction of brain microdialysis in awake animals represented a major advance, since substance effects in anesthetized and in awake animals may differ dramatically (Boix et al. 1992; Boix et al. 1993).

Together with the group of C.A. Marsden at the University of Nottingham, U.K. we established the method of microdialysis in an awake animal during a behavioural experiment (Rex et al. 1991; Marsden, Beckett et al. 1995). This made it possible to detect changes in the release of neurotransmitters associated to drug administration and behavioural changes. Accompanying experiments in the open field (Cadogan et al. 1994)

and on the X-maze (Rex et al. 2003) ensured that the implanted microdialysis probe with the attached tubings does not change the natural behaviour of animals.
The microdialysis has been used in animal anxiety tests such as the X-maze (Rex, Marsden et al. 1991; Rex et al. 1993; Voigt et al. 1999), social interaction test (Cadogan, Kendall et al. 1994), and the Vogel-test (Matsuo et al. 1996). For our studies, the microdialysis probes were implanted into brain regions involved in the regulation of anxiety-related behaviour, such as the prefrontal cortex or the hippocampus (Rex et al. 2008).

7.2 Brain serotonin concentrations

Although the relationship between anxiety and the central serotonergic transmission system is not simple, it can be assumed that changes in the activity of the serotonergic transmission system may lead to a change in the anxiety-related behaviour as well as in brain 5-HT concentration. Therefore, we investigated the relationship between anxiety-related behaviour and 5-HT concentrations in brain regions, which are involved in the regulation of anxiety-related behaviour, such as the prefrontal cortex, the ventral hippocampus and the raphe nuclei. Both, intracellular stored 5-HT and the released, extracellular located, 5-HT are measured. In general, after release into the synaptic cleft 5-HT is transported back into the presynaptic terminal by the 5-HT transporter and metabolized mainly to 5-hydroxyindole aceticacid (5-HIAA), which also can be determined. Changes in the ratio of 5-HT and 5-HIAA in the tissue indicate functional changes in central serotonergic transmission system.

8. Anxiety and serotonin

8.1 Traditional concept of anxiety and serotonin

25 years ago, the role of the central serotonergic transmission system in the regulation of anxiety-related behaviour could be summarized as follows: An increased availability of 5-HT or stimulation of postsynaptic 5-HT receptors is associated with anxiety. A reduced availability or release of 5-HT or blockade of postsynaptic 5-HT receptors triggers an anxiolysis (Iversen 1984). Earlier studies in panic disorder patients with elevated 5-HT plasma levels supported the 5-HT hypothesis of anxiety disorders (Giannini et al. 1983).
Contrary to this paradigm, in animals a local application of 5-HT into the dorsal raphe nucleus had anxiety-reducing effects. In own studies, destruction of serotonergic neurons in the raphe nuclei by the neurotoxin 5.7-DHT reduced 5-HT tissue levels without changing the anxiety-related behaviour (Rex, Thomas et al. 2003).
These results indicate that the relationship between anxiety-related behaviour and central serotonergic transmission system is not as clear as originally described by Iversen (Iversen 1984).

8.2 Strain differences in anxiety and central serotonin

If there is a connection between anxiety-related behaviour and the 5-HT concentration in the CNS, it should be possible that rat strains that differ in their anxiety-related behaviour also differ in the 5-HT concentration in the brain, too. In rats of different strains (Rex, Sondern et al. 1996), the 5-HT levels in brain tissue were determined. It could be shown that rats with a more anxious behaviour had increased 5-HT levels in projection areas of the central serotonergic transmission system (Bert, Fink et al. 2001; Rex, Voigt et al. 1999 ; Rex, Voigt et al. 2004).

8.3 Anxiogenic drugs and serotonin release

8.3.1 SSRIs

The 5-HT-releasing drug fenfluramine increases 5-HT concentration in the rat cortex substantially (Thomas et al. 2000) and leads to a more anxious behaviour on the X-maze (File and Guardiola-Lemaitre 1988).

The acute administration of NSMRIs or SSRIs, which increase 5-HT levels in the synaptic cleft leads to a more fearful behaviour in rats on the X-maze (Bagdy et al. 2001). This fear-enhancing effect of SSRIs is also observed in humans (Stahl 1998). It is particularly pronounced at the beginning of therapy (Gunnell et al. 2005) and generally it declines within two to three weeks.

8.3.2 CCK-receptor agonists

As described, CCK2-receptor ligands are also involved in the regulation of anxiety-related behaviour (Crawley and Corwin 1994; Fink, Rex et al. 1998). We have shown that the CCK2-receptor agonist CCK-4 induced in rats and guinea pigs a clear anxious behaviour on the X-maze, in the modified open field, in the black and white box and ultrasonic vocalisation test (Rex, Barth et al. 1994; Fink, Rex et al. 1998). Since both, CCK and 5-HT, affect the anxiety-related behaviour, an interaction between the two neurotransmitter systems was suggested. In the modified open field test we could show that the 5-HT1A agonist 8-OH-DPAT reduced as an anxiolytic and consequently as a "functional antagonist" dose-dependently the anxiogenic effect of CCK-4 (Rex et al. 1996).

During exposure to the X-maze, CCK-4 increased the release of 5-HT up to threefold (but not in home cage), whereas administration of the CCK1-receptor agonist A71738 and the non-selective CCK1/2-receptor agonist CCK-8s, did not affect the fear-related behaviour nor did change the 5-HT release compared to control animals (Rex and Fink 1998). The anxiogenic effect of CCK-4 in tests for anxiety could be antagonized by the selective CCK2-receptor antagonist L365,260 (Rex et al. 1993; Rex and Fink 1998). We could show an anxiolytic-like effect of L365,260 that abolished not only the effects of CCK2-receptor agonists, but had even own anxiety-reducing effects in animal anxiety tests (Hughes et al. 1990; Fink, Rex et al. 1998).

Our results can be summarized as follows: CCK-4 affected the function of central serotonergic transmission system only slightly or not at rest, but stimulated during acute fear the release of 5-HT in the cortex and hippocampus.

8.4 Arousal and serotonin release

There is general agreement that aversion, based on animal models of anxiety in animals leads to activation in the limbic system and cortex (arousal reaction). So far, it is uncertain whether the increased release of 5-HT during the test for anxiety is caused by anxiety or by the arousal reaction.

Besides the results of various in vivo microdialysis experiments that confirm our hypothesis of an involvement of central serotonergic system in anxiety-related behaviour (Wright et al. 1992; Rex, Marsden et al. 1993; Matsuo, Kataoka et al. 1996; Rex, Voigt et al. 1999; Rex, Voigt et al. 2004), other studies suggested a link between stress-related hyperactivity of rats and the increased release of 5-HT in projection areas (Linthorst et al. 2002).

We could show that the mild stressor "white noise" (Buller et al. 2003), did not increase hippocampal 5-HT release in anxious rats, although the rats were highly active during exposure to white noise (Rex et al. 2005). Comparing our results with other findings in which increased 5-HT release was found during a forced stay in an inescapable stressful situation, like the forced swim test, we think that these situations most likely cause fear in this animals. This is supported by the results of Linthorst and colleagues who interpret an extremely increased 5-HT release in some animals as an anxiety / panic-stimulated release (Linthorst, Penalva et al. 2002).

It was also assumed by others that the increased release of 5-HT during the stay on the X-maze (Rex, Marsden et al. 1993), in the aversive open field (Cadogan, Kendall et al. 1994) or during the forced swim test (Linthorst, Penalva et al. 2002) is caused not by fear but just by exposure to a new unfamiliar environment per se. To check whether a new, but not aversive environment also causes an increased release of 5-HT, we performed microdialysis studies with anxious rats in a non-aversive version of the X-maze. By closing the open arms the remaining arms represented with their high walls rather a protective environment for the animals. The initial stay of the animals in the modified X-maze did not increase 5-HT release, although the animals actively explored the new environment (Rex, Voigt et al. 2005).

Another argument for an anxiety-related increased 5-HT release in hippocampus and cortex emerged from studies in which behavioural strain differences have been analyzed. In several microdialysis studies, we could measure an increased release of 5-HT during the stay on the X-maze only in anxious rat strains. In rats with a non-anxious behaviour, the release of 5-HT in the X-maze test under the same conditions was not increased as much (Rex, Voigt et al. 1999; Rex, Voigt et al. 2004).

Together, our results suggest that acute fear increases the extracellular 5-HT concentration in the serotonergic projection areas and there is a connection between the amount of released 5-HT and the anxiety of the animals.

9. Anxiolysis and serotonin

9.1 Role of 5-HT1A, 5-HT1B/1D receptors

The release of 5-HT is regulated by presynaptic somatodendritic 5-HT1A receptors and presynaptic 5-HT1B/1D receptors at the nerve endings of serotonergic neurons (De Vry 1995).

The functional significance of postsynaptic 5-HT1A receptors and 5-HT1B/1D receptors is still not completely clarified (Göthert and Schlicker 1997). Differentiation of effects mediated by pre-or postsynaptic receptors with the existing substances is difficult. While a stimulation of presynaptic 5-HT1A receptors and 5-HT1D receptors by agonists reduces 5-HT release in the projection areas (Rex, Fink et al. 1993; De Vry 1995; Rex et al. 1997) antagonists at the 5-HT1A and 5-HT1D receptors do not always induce an increase of 5-HT release (Roberts et al. 1999), as 5-HT is released tonically only to a small extent.

Also own microdialysis studies showed that blockade of autoreceptors without previous stimulation of 5-HT release had no measurable effect. If guinea pigs stayed in the familiar cage, neither the selective 5-HT1A antagonist WAY 100635 nor the 5-HT1B/1D-Antagonist GR 127 935, changed release of 5-HT in the ventral hippocampus and the prefrontal cortex (Rex et al. 1996; Rex, Voigt et al. 2008).

Whereas in the resting state the tonic 5-HT release and therefore the effects of antagonists on 5-HT1A and 5-HT1B/D receptors are small, in an aversive environment, such as the X-maze the release of 5-HT was stimulated. Treatment with the 5-HT1B/1D-antagonist GR 127935 led to a quicker but short-lasting increase in extracellular 5-HT concentration in the cortex, compared to treatment with saline (Rex, Fink et al. 1996).

In other studies in which a drug-induced increased extracellular 5-HT concentration was examined, the regulatory function of 5-HT1A and 5-HT1D receptors could be shown more clearly. If pre-treatment with a SSRI increased the 5-HT concentration in the synaptic cleft, both, 5-HT1A antagonists(Hughes et al. 2005), as well 5-HT1B/1D-antagonists had a potentiating effect on 5-HT release in the CNS. These results suggest that control of the firing rate of serotonergic neurons and thus of transmitter release by presynaptic 5-HT1A- and 5-HT1B/1D-receptors is pronounced when 5-HT release is stimulated.

5-HT1A agonists such as buspirone and tandospirone are used in the treatment of anxiety disorders. Their anxiety-reducing effect is explained by stimulation of presynaptic 5-HT1A receptors and the subsequent reduction in 5-HT release (Stahl 1998).

However, the role of postsynaptic 5-HT1A receptors for an anxiolytic effect is still not clear. So we used a neurobiochemical approach to try to discriminate the function of presynaptic and postsynaptic 5-HT1A receptors in vivo.

9.2 5-HT1A receptors and brain metabolic activity

It is known that the energy metabolism in the CNS is linked closely to the activity of the cells. Determination of the redox status of cells allows conclusions about the functional state of these cells (Ames 2000). Complementary to established methods, the laser-induced fluorescence spectroscopy offers the possibility of "on line" - measurements of the metabolic state of intact tissues.

After verification that in vivo laser-induced fluorescence spectroscopy detects changes in mitochondrial/metabolic activity in the CNS, we determined the mitochondrial activity in the ventral hippocampus after administration of the 5-HT1A agonist 8-OH-DPAT (Rex and Fink 2006).

Systemic administration of 8-OH-DPAT induced dose-dependent changes in mitochondrial activity of hippocampal neurons. In the highest dose 8-OH-DPAT significantly increased the NADH fluorescence, while the middle dose had no effect on NADH fluorescence and the lowest dose resulted in a slight but not significant increase in NADH fluorescence.

We interpret the results as follows: The highest dose of 8-OH-DPAT stimulates postsynaptic 5-HT1A receptors in the ventral hippocampus and thus inhibiting the activity of the following neurons, leading to an increase in NADH fluorescence. Our conclusions are sustained by electrophysiological studies, in which higher doses of 8-OH-DPAT lowered activity in the hippocampus and cortex (Tada et al. 1999).

Since 8-OH-DPAT has in behavioural tests an anxiety-reducing effect in doses that affect the postsynaptic 5-HT1A receptors it cannot be excluded that the postsynaptic 5-HT1A receptors play a role in the regulation of anxiety-related behaviour.

10. Anxiolytic drugs and serotonin

It was shown that aversive stimuli and substances with an anxiety-enhancing effect increase the 5-HT release in some serotonergic projection areas, such as the ventral hippocampus and the prefrontal cortex. Therefore, we investigated whether anxiolytics of different drug classes inhibit 5-HT release in general.

10.1 Different classes of anxiolytic drugs and serotonin release

Benzodiazepines and 5-HT1A agonists are therapeutically used anxiolytics. CCK2 antagonists were effective in various animal anxiety models, such as the X-maze (Rex, Barth et al. 1994), the modified open field (Rex, Voigt et al. 1998), social interaction and the elevated zero maze (Revel et al. 1998). Therefore, we investigated the effects of diazepam (Rex, Marsden et al. 1993; Rex et al. 1993a), 8-OH-DPAT (Rex et al. 1993) and the CCK2 antagonist L 365.260 (Rex, Fink et al. 1994) on 5-HT release in the prefrontal cortex using microdialysis during the X-maze test.

As shown before, exposure to the X-maze resulted always in a marked increased 5-HT release (Rex, Marsden et al. 1991; Marsden, Beckett et al. 1995). Pretreatment with diazepam or 8-OH-DPAT or L 365.260 reduced this aversion induced increase in 5-HT release in the prefrontal cortex and caused a less anxious behaviour of the animals on the X-maze.

Under non-aversive conditions, like before and after exposure to the X-maze, diazepam, 8-OH-DPAT and L 365.260 decreased basal 5-HT release in the prefrontal cortex.

Both the reduction in the aversion induced 5-HT release and the anxiolytic effects of diazepam, 8-OH-DPAT and L 365.260 were antagonized by pretreatment with the benzodiazepine antagonist flumazenil, the non-selective 5-HT1 antagonist methiothepine and the selective CCK2-receptor agonist CCK-4, respectively (Rex, Fink et al. 1993; Rex, Marsden et al. 1993; Rex, Marsden et al. 1993).

Our results indicate a receptor mediation of the observed effects and they are consistent with the hypothesis that an acute stay in an aversive environment is associated with increased 5-HT release and an anxiolytic effect with a decreased release of 5-HT. The results are supported by in vitro studies showing that both, diazepam and the 5-HT1A agonist buspirone as well as the CCK2 antagonist GV 150 013, decreased the electrically stimulated release of 5-HT from cortical slices significantly (Siniscalchi et al. 2001).

10.2 Benzodiazepines and serotonin concentrations

Already in the 70s it has been shown that benzodiazepines reduce 5-HT synthesis (Dominic et al. 1975) and the 5-HT turnover (Wise et al. 1972).

After systemic administration chlordiazepoxide inhibited the firing rate of serotonergic neurons in the dorsal raphe nucleus (Trulson et al. 1982) and after injection into the dorsal raphe chlordiazepoxide reduced anxious behaviour in the conditioned-emotional-response test (Thiebot et al. 1980).

The dorsal and median raphe nuclei have a high density of GABA receptors. Microinjections of GABA in the dorsal raphe nucleus and in serotonergic projection areas, such as the amygdala and the hippocampus, reduced the firing rate of serotonergic neurons. This reduced firing rate was reduced even further by administration of benzodiazepines (Gallager 1978). On the other hand, the anxiety-reducing effect of benzodiazepines in a conflict test was abolished by the intraventricular administration of 5-HT (Wise, Berger et al. 1972).

We have seen "antiserotonergic" effects of diazepam on both the tissue concentration as well as the 5-HT release (Rex, Marsden et al. 1993; Bert, Fink et al. 2001). In the rat brain diazepam reduced tissue concentrations of 5-HT in serotonergic projection areas, such as cortex and hippocampus which confirmed the results of Pei and colleagues (Pei et al. 1989).

Interestingly, diazepam had a greater effect in animals with high tissue concentrations of 5-HT, while the effect was smaller in animals with low 5-HT levels.

In a Wistar rat strain (HsdCpb: WU, Harlan, Germany), which showed a non-anxious behaviour in different anxiety tests, diazepam reduced the already low 5-HT levels in hippocampus and cortex only marginally and did not change the anxiety-related behaviour. In these non-anxious rats exposure to the X-maze did not increase 5-HT release in the hippocampus (Rex, Voigt et al. 1999).

In the more anxious Wistar rats (Han: Wist (SYN WI), Institute for Risk Assessment, Germany) and Fischer rats (F344/NHsd, Harlan, Germany) with higher 5-HT concentrations in the tissue and aversion-induced release of 5-HT on the X-maze (Rex, Voigt et al. 1999), diazepam induced an anxiolytic-like behaviour on the X-maze and reduced the concentration of 5-HT in the hippocampus and frontal cortex significantly (Bert, Fink et al. 2001).

Since similar doses of diazepam in rat strains with different 5-HT concentrations in the brain have different effects on anxiety-related behaviour (Bert, Fink et al. 2001), it can be assumed that the effect of benzodiazepines depends of the activity of the serotonergic neurotransmission system and the GABAergic system interacts with the central serotonergic transmission system.

To further test the hypothesis of a close link between anxiolytic effects and a decreased release of 5-HT, we examined an anxiolytic effective herbal product.

10.3 Herbal anxiolytic kava-kava

The herbal product kava-kava had been widely used as an anxiolytic. Although kava pyrones have been identified as the pharmacologically active ingredients of kava-kava (Singh and Blumenthal 1997), the mechanism of action has not been clarified (Smith et al. 2001). The kava-kava pyrones bind probably not to the GABA-A receptors (Garrett et al. 2003). We examined the effects of kava-kava in the X-maze and the social interaction test. In both tests a standardized kava-kava preparation caused dose-dependent anxiety-reducing effect in rats, similar to the effect of diazepam (Rex et al. 2002). Our results were later confirmed in mice (Garrett, Basmadjian et al. 2003).

In a second experiment we determined the concentration of 5-HT in a tissue sample (punch), containing the dorsal and the medial raphe nucleus and in tissue samples of the ventral hippocampus and the prefrontal cortex. Kava-kava led to a reduction in 5-HT concentration in the cortex and hippocampus.

Since the tissue concentration is not related strongly to the release of 5-HT, we investigated the release of 5-HT in the ventral hippocampus following administration of kava-kava. Using in vivo microdialysis we showed for the first time that kava-kava, like 8-OH-DPAT and diazepam, decreased the 5-HT release in the projection areas.

11. Long term reduction of serotonin and anxiolysis

Under the premise that a correlation between the amount of tissue concentration of 5-HT and the expression of anxiety-related behaviour exists, it could be assumed that a reduction of 5-HT concentration in the CNS would be associated with anxiolysis. The 5-HT concentration in the brain can be reduced by destruction of serotonergic neurons for a long time.

Systemic para-chloroamphetamine reduced the 5-HT content in the CNS of rats and these animals showed an anxiolytic-like behaviour in the Geller-Seifter test (Geller and Blum 1970).

Intracerebral administration of the neurotoxin 5.7-DHT, causing destruction of serotonergic neurons, reduced the 5-HT content in the CNS and induced anxiolytic-like effects in conditioned anxiety tests (Iversen 1984; Soderpalm and Engel 1992; Thiebot, Jobert et al. 1980). These studies confirmed seemingly a simple relation between 5-HT and anxiety.

However, studies in which unconditioned tests were used and/or individual nuclei in the raphe region were lesioned, showed contradictory results. While 5.7-DHT reduces anxiety after intraventricular application (Griebel 1995), administration of the neurotoxin into either the median or the dorsal raphe nucleus had no effect on behaviour in several anxiety tests (Griebel 1995, Thomas et al 2000). Only in the social interaction test (File et al. 1979) a lesion of the dorsal raphe nucleus caused a less anxious behaviour of the animals.

In our studies, neither the lesion of the median raphe nucleus (Thomas, Fink et al. 2000) nor of the dorsal raphe nucleus (Rex, Thomas et al. 2003) alone changed the fear-related behaviour of the rats. The 5-HT levels in the projection areas, such as cortex and hippocampus were decreased significantly (Thomas, Fink et al. 2000; Rex, Thomas et al. 2003) and comparable to the effects of 5.7-DHT lesion on 5-HT concentrations in the CNS described in the literature (Tabatabaie and Dryhurst 1998).

For the first time not only the 5-HT levels in the tissue, but also the release of 5-HT in lesioned and non-lesioned rats in the familiar cage and during exposure to the X-maze were determined. Rats in which either the dorsal or the median raphe nucleus was lesioned by 5.7-DHT, differed in the tissue concentrations of 5-HT, but not in anxiety-related behaviour and in the aversion induced 5-HT release, compared to untreated control animals (Rex, Thomas et al. 2003).A reason, that the lesion of only one of the two major raphe nuclei did not relate to the aversion induced 5-HT release and the behaviour of animals, could lie in the overlapping innervations' of the hippocampus and the cortex by the dorsal raphe nucleus and the median raphe nucleus. The lesion of one of the raphe nuclei can be compensated by the innervations' of the other raphe nuclei, at least in part.

A lesion of almost all serotonergic neurons by intraventricular administration of 5.7-DHT (Griebel 1995) or simultaneous lesions of the dorsal and of the median raphe nuclei (Thomas, Fink et al. 2000), however, interrupt all serotonergic projections to the hippocampus. The 5-HT concentrations were reduced much more and there was no increased release of 5-HT observed during the exposure to the X-maze and the rats behaved "anxiety-free" on the X-maze. The destruction of serotonergic neurons in the raphe nuclei prevents storage of 5-HT in the nerve endings in the projection areas. Consequently, 5-HT is not released due to aversion and thus no anxious behaviour was induced.

The findings presented so far support the hypothesis that there is a relationship between decreased release of 5-HT and less anxious behaviour of animals.

We could also show that reduced 5-HT release does not necessarily change the anxiety-related behaviour. The non-selective 5-HT1 agonist 5-carboxamidotryptamine (5-CT) reduced the basal release of 5-HT and prevented the increased 5-HT release on the X-maze, similar to the 5-HT1A agonist 8-OH-DPAT. Nevertheless, we observed no change in anxiety-related behaviour compared to control animals after treatment with 5-CT (Rex, Fink et al. 1996).

At the present it can be generalized that anxiolytics reduce the release of 5-HT in the brain. However, a reduced concentration of 5-HT and reduced 5-HT release under resting conditions does not automatically lead to an anxiety-free behaviour of animals.

12. Conclusions

Similar to humans, anxiety-related behaviour in animals appears to be influenced by genetic factors and environmental conditions. Changes in housing and breeding conditions and/or variations in experimental conditions and the experimental procedure may change the behaviour of the animals profoundly. Strain differences have a strong influence on the anxiety-related behaviour in the animals. Additionally, separate maintaining and breeding of rodents over several generations may lead to the development of sublines with different anxiety-related behaviour.

Further developments of animal anxiety tests, the knowledge of their limits and the evaluation of additional ethological behavioural parameters can be used to detect changes in anxiety-related behaviour more accurately.

A correlation between the level of 5-HT concentration in the CNS and the anxiety of rat strains, but not general activation, could be proved experimentally. Anxious rats have higher tissue levels of 5-HT in projection areas of neurons originating in the median and the dorsal raphe nuclei as rat strains with "fearless" behaviour. Anxiolytics decrease extracellular 5-HT levels in the projection areas of the serotonergic neurons in the CNS, especially in more anxious rat strains.

Studies using in vivo microdialysis while performing tests for anxiety in awake and freely moving animals with permanently reduced 5-HT concentrations in specific brain regions showed that not only the absolute level of 5-HT concentration in the CNS, but also the amount of 5-HT released during an aversive situation, can be related to the behaviour of the animals.

Anxiolytics of different drug classes reduce the serotonin release during an aversive situation, whereas anxiety-causing substances increase the serotonin release under the same conditions significantly. However, a reduced release of serotonin does not always lead to fearless behaviour in rodents.

The central serotonergic transmission is also influenced by other neurotransmission systems, e. g. GABA and CCK systems..

In summary our results demonstrate the major role of the serotonergic neurotransmission in the regulation of anxiety-related behaviour. Studies on the role of the serotonergic system under aversive and non-aversive conditions may lead to a better understanding of the mechanisms involved in the development of anxiety disorders and the possible development of novel therapeutic approaches in the treatment of anxiety disorders, too.

13. References

Adell, A. (2010). Lu-AA21004, a multimodal serotonergic agent, for the potential treatment of depression and anxiety. IDrugs 13(12): 900-10.

Ames, A., 3rd (2000). CNS energy metabolism as related to function. Brain Res Brain Res Rev 34(1-2): 42-68.

Amin, A. H., Crawford, T. B.&Gaddum, J. H. (1954). The distribution of substance P and 5-hydroxytryptamine in the central nervous system of the dog. J Physiol 126(3): 596-618.

Andreatini, R.&Bacellar, L. F. (1999). The relationship between anxiety and depression in animal models: a study using the forced swimming test and elevated plus-maze. Braz J Med Biol Res 32(9): 1121-6.

Andrews, N.&File, S. E. (1993). Handling history of rats modifies behavioural effects of drugs in the elevated plus-maze test of anxiety. Eur J Pharmacol 235(1): 109-12.

Anseloni, V. Z.&Brandao, M. L. (1997). Ethopharmacological analysis of behaviour of rats using variations of the elevated plus-maze. Behav Pharmacol 8(6-7): 533-40.

Bagdy, G., Graf, M., Anheuer, Z. E., Modos, E. A.&Kantor, S. (2001). Anxiety-like effects induced by acute fluoxetine, sertraline or m-CPP treatment are reversed by pretreatment with the 5-HT2C receptor antagonist SB-242084 but not the 5-HT1A receptor antagonist WAY-100635. Int J Neuropsychopharmacol 4(4): 399-408.

Bandelow, B., Zohar, J.&Hollander, E. (2005). Medikamentöse Behandlung von Angst- und Zwangs- und posttraumatischen Belastungsstörungen. Frankfurt, Wissenschaftliche Verlagsgesellschaft.

Becker, E.&Hoyer, E. J. (2000). Das Generalisierte Angstsyndrom - Häufig nicht erkannt. DNP: 36-39.

Beinfeld, M. C., Meyer, D. K.&Brownstein, M. J. (1981). Cholecystokinin in the central nervous system. Peptides 2 Suppl.2: 77-79.

Bert, B., Fink, H., Sohr, R.&Rex, A. (2001). Different effects of diazepam in Fischer rats and two stocks of Wistar rats in tests of anxiety. Pharmacol Biochem Behav 70(2-3): 411-20.

Bert, B., Schmidt, N., Voigt, J. P., Fink, H.&Rex, A. (2011). Evaluation of cage leaving behaviour as a free choice paradigm Journal of Pharmacological and Toxicological Methods under revision.

Boix, F., Huston, J. P.&Schwarting, R. K. (1992). The C-terminal fragment of substance P enhances dopamine release in nucleus accumbens but not in neostriatum in freely moving rats. Brain Res 592(1-2): 181-6.

Boix, F., Mattioli, R., Adams, F., Huston, J. P.&Schwarting, R. K. (1993). Peripherally administered substance P affects extracellular dopamine concentrations in the neostriatum but not in the nucleus accumbens under anesthesia. Brain Res Bull 31(6): 655-60.

Bradwejn, J.&Koszycki, D. (2001). Cholecystokinin and panic disorder: past and future clinical research strategies. Scand J Clin Lab Invest Suppl 234: 19-27.

Braszko, J. J., Kulakowska, A.&Winnicka, M. M. (2003). Effects of angiotensin II and its receptor antagonists on motor activity and anxiety in rats. J Physiol Pharmacol 54(2): 271-81.

Britton, D. R.&Thatcher Britton, K. (1981). A sensitive openfield measure of anxiolytic drug activity. Pharmacol.Biochem.Behav. 15: 577-582.

Broadhurst, P. L. (1975). The Maudsley reactive and nonreactive strains of rats: a survey. Behav Genet 5(4): 299-319.

Buller, K. M., Crane, J. W., Spencer, S. J.&Day, T. A. (2003). Systemic apomorphine alters HPA axis responses to interleukin-1 beta administration but not sound stress. Psychoneuroendocrinology 28(6): 715-32.

Cadogan, A. K., Kendall, D. A., Fink, H.&Marsden, C. A. (1994). Social interaction increases 5-HT release and cAMP efflux in the rat ventral hippocampus in vivo. Behav Pharmacol 5(3): 299-305.

Cappell, H.&Latane, B. (1969). Effects of alcohol and caffeine on the social and emotional behavior of the rat. Q J Stud Alcohol 30(2): 345-56.

Cattell, R. B.&Scheier, I. H. (1958). The nature of anxiety: a review of thirteen multi-variate analyses comprising 814 variables. Psychol Rep 4(4): 351-388.

Charney, D. S., Heninger, G. R.&Jatlow, P. I. (1985). Increased anxiogenic effects of caffeine in panic disorders. Arch Gen Psychiatry 42(3): 233-43.

Costall, B.&Naylor, R. J. (1992). Astra Award Lecture. The psychopharmacology of 5-HT3 receptors. Pharmacol Toxicol 71(6): 401-15.

Crawley, J.&Goodwin, F. K. (1980). Preliminary report of a simple animal behavior model for the anxiolytic effects of benzodiazepines. Pharmacol Biochem Behav 13(2): 167-70.

Crawley, J. N.&Corwin, R. L. (1994). Biological actions of cholecystokinin. 15: 731-755.

Cryan, J. F.&Kaupmann, K. (2005). Don't worry 'B' happy!: a role for GABA(B) receptors in anxiety and depression. Trends Pharmacol Sci 26(1): 36-43.

Dahlstrom, A.&Fuxe, K. (1964). Localization of monoamines in the lower brain stem. Experientia 20(7): 398-9.

Davis, M. (1990). Animal models of anxiety based on classical conditioning: the conditioned emotional response (CER) and the fear-potentiated startle effect. Pharmacol Ther 47(2): 147-65.

De Montigny, C. (1989). Cholecystokinin tetrapeptide induces panic-like attacks in healthy volunteers. Archives of General Psychiatry 46: 511-517.

De Vry, J. (1995). 5-HT1A receptor agonists: recent developments and controversial issues. Psychopharmacology (Berl) 121(1): 1-26.

Dominic, J. A., Sinha, A. K.&Barchas, J. D. (1975). Effect of benzodiazepine compounds on brain amine metabolism. European Journal of Pharmacology 32: 124-127.

Falck, B., Hillarp, N. A., Thieme, G.&Torp, A. (1962). Fluorescence of catechol amines and related compounds condensed with formaldehyde. J Histochem Cytochem 10: 348-354.

File, S. E. (1985). Models of anxiety. Br.J.Clin.Pract.Symp.Suppl. 38: 15-20.

File, S. E.&Guardiola-Lemaitre, B. J. (1988). l-fenfluramine in tests of dominance and anxiety in the rat. Neuropsychobiology 20(4): 205-11.

File, S. E.&Hyde, J. R. (1978). Can social interaction be used to measure anxiety? British Journal of Pharmacology 62: 19-24.

File, S. E.&Pope, J. H. (1974). The action of chlorpromazine on exploration in pairs of rats. Psychopharmacologia 37(3): 249-54.

Fink, H., Rex, A., Voits, M.&Voigt, J. P. (1998). Major biological actions of CCK--a critical evaluation of research findings. Exp Brain Res 123(1-2): 77-83.

Fischer-Ferraro, C., Nahmod, V. E., Goldstein, D. J.&Finkielman, S. (1971). Angiotensin and renin in rat and dog brain. J Exp Med 133(2): 353-61.

Florio, C., Prezioso, A., Papaioannou, A.&Vertua, R. (1998). Adenosine A1 receptors modulate anxiety in CD1 mice. Psychopharmacology (Berl) 136(4): 311-9.

Gallager, D. W. (1978). Benzodiazepines: potentiation of a GABA inhibitory response in the dorsal raphe nucleus. European Journal of Pharmacology 49: 133-143.

Gard, P. R. (2004). Angiotensin as a target for the treatment of Alzheimer's disease, anxiety and depression. Expert Opin Ther Targets 8(1): 7-14.

Garrett, K. M., Basmadjian, G., Khan, I. A., Schaneberg, B. T.&Seale, T. W. (2003). Extracts of kava (Piper methysticum) induce acute anxiolytic-like behavioral changes in mice. Psychopharmacology (Berl) 170(1): 33-41.

Geller, I. (1960). The acquisition and extinction of conditioned suppression as a function of the base-line reinforcer. J Exp Anal Behav 3: 235-40.

Geller, I.&Blum, K. (1970). The effects of 5-HTP on para-Chlorophenylalanine (p-CPA) attenuation of conflict behavior. Eur J Pharmacol 9(3): 319-24.

Giannini, A. J., Castellani, S.&Dvoredsky, A. E. (1983). Anxiety states: relationship to atmospheric cations and serotonin. J Clin Psychiatry 44(7): 262-4.

Golimbet, V. E., Alfimova, M. V.&Mitiushina, N. G. (2004). Polymorphism of the serotonin 2A receptor gene (5HTR2A) and personality traits. Mol Biol 38(3): 404-12.

Gordon, J. A.&Hen, R. (2004). Genetic approaches to the study of anxiety. Annu Rev Neurosci 27: 193-222.

Göthert, M.&Schlicker, E. (1997). Regulation of 5-HT release in the CNS by presynaptic 5-HT autoreceptors and by 5-HT heteroreceptors. Serotoninergic Neurons and 5-HT Receptors in the CNS. H. G. Baumgarten &M. Göthert. Berlin Heidelberg New York, Springer. 129: 307-350.

Graeff, F. G., Parente, A., Del-Ben, C. M.&Guimaraes, F. S. (2003). Pharmacology of human experimental anxiety. Braz J Med Biol Res 36(4): 421-32.

Green, E. (1981). Genetics and Probability in Animal Breeding Experiments. New York, Oxford University Press.

Griebel, G. (1995). 5-Hydroxytryptamine-interacting drugs in animal models of anxiety disorders: more than 30 years of research. Pharmacol Ther 65(3): 319-95.

Griebel, G., Belzung, C., Misslin, R.&Vogel, E. (1993). The free-exploratory paradigm: an effective method for measuring neophobic behaviour in mice and testing potential neophobia-reducing drugs. Behav Pharmacol 4(6): 637-644.

Gunnell, D., Saperia, J.&Ashby, D. (2005). Selective serotonin reuptake inhibitors (SSRIs) and suicide in adults: meta-analysis of drug company data from placebo controlled, randomised controlled trials submitted to the MHRA's safety review. BMJ 330(7488): 385.

Hagan, J. J., Harper, A. J., Elliott, H., Jones, D. N.&Rogers, D. C. (2000). Practical and theoretical issues in gene-targeting studies and their application to behaviour. Rev Neurosci 11(1): 3-13.

Hall, C. S. (1934). Emotional behavior in the rat. I. Defecation and urination as measures of individual differences in emotionality. J. Comp. Psychol. 18: 385- 403.

Haller, J.&Halasz, J. (1999). Mild social stress abolishes the effects of isolation on anxiety and chlordiazepoxide reactivity. Psychopharmacology (Berl) 144(4): 311-5.

Handley, S. L.&Mithani, S. (1984). Effects of alpha-adrenoceptor agonists and antagonists in a maze- exploration model of 'fear'-motivated behaviour. Naunyn Schmiedebergs Archive of Pharmacology 327: 1-5.

Holy, Z.&Wisniewski, K. (2001). Examination of the influence of 3,5-DHPG on behavioral activity of angiotensin II. Pol J Pharmacol 53(3): 235-43.

Hughes, J., Boden, P., Costall, B., Domeney, A., Kelly, E., Horwell, D. C., Hunter, J. C., Pinnock, R. D.&Woodruff, G. N. (1990). Development of a class of selective cholecystokinin type B receptor antagonists having potent anxiolytic activity. Proc.Natl.Acad.Sci.U.S A. 87: 6728-6732.

Hughes, Z. A., Starr, K. R., Langmead, C. J., Hill, M., Bartoszyk, G. D., Hagan, J. J., Middlemiss, D. N.&Dawson, L. A. (2005). Neurochemical evaluation of the novel 5-HT1A receptor partial agonist/serotonin reuptake inhibitor, vilazodone. Eur J Pharmacol 510(1-2): 49-57.

Iversen, S. D. (1984). 5-HT and anxiety. Neuropharmacology 23(12B): 1553-60.

Jax (2003). The importance of understanding substrains in the genomic age. JAX Notes(491): 1-3.

Jones, N., Duxon, M. S.&King, S. M. (2002). Ethopharmacological analysis of the unstable elevated exposed plus maze, a novel model of extreme anxiety: predictive validity and sensitivity to anxiogenic agents. Psychopharmacology (Berl) 161(3): 314-23.

Kayir, H.&Uzbay, I. T. (2005). Nicotine antagonizes caffeine- but not pentylenetetrazole-induced anxiogenic effect in mice. Psychopharmacology (Berl): 1-6.

Kessler, R. C., Ruscio, A. M., Shear, K.&Wittchen, H. U. (2010). Epidemiology of anxiety disorders. Curr Top Behav Neurosci 2: 21-35.

Kielholz, P.&Battegay, R. (1967). Angst: Psychische und somatische Aspekte. Bern, Hans Huber.

Kinrys, G., Coleman, E.&Rothstein, E. (2009). Natural remedies for anxiety disorders: potential use and clinical applications. Depress Anxiety 26(3): 259-65.

Kjernisted, K. D.&Bleau, P. (2004). Long-term goals in the management of acute and chronic anxiety disorders. Can J Psychiatry 49(3 Suppl 1): 51S-63S.

Lader, M. (2005). Management of panic disorder. Expert Rev Neurother 5(2): 259-66.

Lal, H.&Emmett-Oglesby, M. W. (1983). Behavioral analogues of anxiety. Animal models. Neuropharmacology 22: 1423-1441.

Landgraf, R. (2003). Neurobiologie und Genetik der Angst im Tiermodell. Nervenarzt 74(3): 274-8.

Lesch, K. P.&Gutknecht, L. (2005). Pharmacogenetics of the serotonin transporter. Prog Neuropsychopharmacol Biol Psychiatry 29(6): 1062-73.

Liebsch, G., Montkowski, A., Holsboer, F.&Landgraf, R. (1998). Behavioural profiles of two Wistar rat lines selectively bred for high or low anxiety-related behaviour. Behav Brain Res 94(2): 301-10.

Linthorst, A. C., Penalva, R. G., Flachskamm, C., Holsboer, F.&Reul, J. M. (2002). Forced swim stress activates rat hippocampal serotonergic neurotransmission involving a corticotropin-releasing hormone receptor-dependent mechanism. Eur J Neurosci 16(12): 2441-52.

Lister, R. G. (1990). Ethologically-based animal models of anxiety disorders. Pharmac.Ther. 46: 321-340.

Lohse, J. L., Lorenzen, A.&Mueller-Oerlinghausen, B. (2004). Psychopharmaka. Arzneiverordnungsreport 2004. U. Schwabe &D. Paffrath. Berlin, Heidelberg, New York, Springer Verlag: 769-810.

Lucki, I. (1998). The spectrum of behaviors influenced by serotonin. Biol Psychiatry 44(3): 151-62.

Marsden, C. A., Beckett, S. R. G., Wilson, W., Bickerdike, M., Fink, H., Rex, A.&Cadogan, A. K. (1995). Serotonin involvement in animal models of anxiety and panic. Serotonin in the central nervous system and periphery. E. Takada &G. Curzon. Amsterdam, Elsevier: 135-143.

Matsuo, M., Kataoka, Y., Mataki, S., Kato, Y.&Oi, K. (1996). Conflict situation increases serotonin release in rat dorsal hippocampus: in vivo study with microdialysis and Vogel test. Neurosci Lett 215(3): 197-200.

Möhler, H.&Okada, T. (1977). Benzodiazepine receptor: demonstration in the central nervous system. Science 198(4319): 849-51.

Moriarty, D. D. (1995). Anxiogenic effects of a beta-carboline on tonic immobility and open field behavior in chickens (Gallus gallus). Pharmacol Biochem Behav 51(4): 795-8.

Nehlig, A., Daval, J. L.&Debry, G. (1992). Caffeine and the central nervous system: mechanisms of action, biochemical, metabolic and psychostimulant effects. Brain Res Brain Res Rev 17(2): 139-70.

Neumeister, A., Young, T.&Stastny, J. (2004). Implications of genetic research on the role of the serotonin in depression: emphasis on the serotonin type 1A receptor and the serotonin transporter. Psychopharmacology (Berl) 174(4): 512-24.

Ohl, F.&Keck, M. E. (2003). Behavioural screening in mutagenised mice--in search for novel animal models of psychiatric disorders. Eur J Pharmacol 480(1-3): 219-28.

Pei, Q., Zetterstrom, T.&Fillenz, M. (1989). Both systemic and local administration of benzodiazepine agonists inhibit the in vivo release of 5-HT from ventral hippocampus. Neuropharmacology 28: 1061-1066.

Pollack, M. H. (2004). Unmet needs in the treatment of anxiety disorders. Psychopharmacol Bull 38(1): 31-7.

Rex, A. (1996). Verhaltenspharmakologische und neurochemische Untersuchungen zu Interaktionen zwischen dem Neuropeptid Cholezystokinin und dem Neurotransmitter Serotonin. Medizinische Fakultät. Berlin, Humboldt-Universität.

Rex, A., Barth, T., Voigt, J. P., Domeney, A. M.&Fink, H. (1994). Effects of cholecystokinin tetrapeptide and sulfated cholecystokinin octapeptide in rat models of anxiety. Neurosci Lett 172(1-2): 139-42.

Rex, A., Bert, B.&Fink, H. (2007). [History and new developments. The pharmacology of 5-ht3 antagonists]. Pharm Unserer Zeit 36(5): 342-53.

Rex, A.&Fink, H. (1998). Effects of cholecystokinin-receptor agonists on cortical 5-HT release in guinea pigs on the X-maze. Peptides 19(3): 519-26.

Rex, A.&Fink, H. (2006). Effects of 8-OH-DPAT on hippocampal NADH fluorescence in vivo in anaesthetized rats. J Neurosci Res 83(4): 551-6.

Rex, A., Fink, H.&Marsden, C. A. (1993). The effect of CCK-4 and L 365.260 on cortical extracellular 5-HT release on exposure to the elevated plus maze. Anxiety: Neurobiology, Clinic and Therapeutic Perspectives. M. Hamon, H. Ollat &M. H. Thiébot. London

Paris, Colloque INSERM/John Libbey Eurotext: 207-208.

Rex, A., Fink, H.&Marsden, C. A. (1994). Effects of BOC-CCK-4 and L 365.260 on cortical 5-HT release in guinea-pigs on exposure to the elevated plus maze. Neuropharmacology 33(3-4): 559-65.

Rex, A., Fink, H., Skingle, M.&Marsden, C. A. (1996). Involvement of 5-HT1D receptors in cortical extracellular 5-HT release in guinea-pigs on exposure to the elevated plus maze. J Psychopharmacol 10: 219-224.

Rex, A., Kolbasenko, A., Bert, B.&Fink, H. (2007). Choosing the right wild type: behavioral and neurochemical differences between 2 populations of Sprague-Dawley rats from the same source but maintained at different sites. J Am Assoc Lab Anim Sci 46(5): 13-20.

Rex, A., Marsden, C. A.&Fink, H. (1991). Increased 5-HT release in the guinea-pig frontal cortex on exposure to the X-Maze. Monitoring molecules in neuroscience. H. Rollema, B. Westerink &W. J. Drijfhout. Groningen, University Centre for Pharmacy. 5: 250-252.

Rex, A., Marsden, C. A.&Fink, H. (1993). 5-HT 1A receptors and changes in extracellular 5-HT in the guinea-pig prefrontal cortex: involvement in aversive behaviour. J Psychopharmacol 7: 338-345.

Rex, A., Marsden, C. A.&Fink, H. (1993). Effect of diazepam on cortical 5-HT release and behaviour in the guinea-pig on exposure to the elevated plus maze. Psychopharmacology (Berl) 110(4): 490-6.

Rex, A., Marsden, C. A.&Fink, H. (1997). Cortical 5-HT-CCK interactions and anxiety-related behaviour of guinea-pigs: a microdialysis study. Neurosci Lett 228(2): 79-82.

Rex, A., Morgenstern, E.&Fink, H. (2002). Anxiolytic-like effects of kava-kava in the elevated plus maze test--a comparison with diazepam. Prog Neuropsychopharmacol Biol Psychiatry 26(5): 855-60.

Rex, A., Sondern, U., Voigt, J. P., Franck, S.&Fink, H. (1996). Strain differences in fear-motivated behavior of rats. Pharmacol Biochem Behav 54(1): 107-11.

Rex, A., Stephens, D. N.&Fink, H. (1996). Anxiolytic action of diazepam and abecarnil in a modified open field test. Pharmacol Biochem Behav 53(4): 1005-11.

Rex, A., Thomas, H., Hortnagl, H., Voits, M.&Fink, H. (2003). Behavioural and microdialysis study after neurotoxic lesion of the dorsal raphe nucleus in rats. Pharmacol Biochem Behav 74(3): 587-93.

Rex, A., Voigt, J. P.&Fink, H. (1999). Behavioral and neurochemical differences between Fischer 344 and Harlan-Wistar rats raised identically. Behav Genet 29(3): 187-92.

Rex, A., Voigt, J. P.&Fink, H. (2005). Anxiety but not arousal increases 5-hydroxytryptamine release in the rat ventral hippocampus in vivo. Eur J Neurosci 22(5): 1185-9.

Rex, A., Voigt, J. P., Gustedt, C., Beckett, S.&Fink, H. (2004). Anxiolytic-like profile in Wistar, but not Sprague-Dawley rats in the social interaction test. Psychopharmacology (Berl) 177(1-2): 23-34.

Rex, A., Voigt, J. P., Voits, M.&Fink, H. (1998). Pharmacological evaluation of a modified open-field test sensitive to anxiolytic drugs. Pharmacol Biochem Behav 59(3): 677-83.

Rex, A., Voigt, J. P., Wicke, K. M.&Fink, H. (2008). In vivo/ex vivo and behavioural study on central effects of 5-HT1B/1D and 5-HT1A antagonists in guinea pigs. Pharmacol Biochem Behav 88(3): 196-204.

Roberts, C., Boyd, D. F., Middlemiss, D. N.&Routledge, C. (1999). Enhancement of 5-HT1B and 5-HT1D receptor antagonist effects on extracellular 5-HT levels in the guinea-pig brain following concurrent 5-HT1A or 5-HT re-uptake site blockade. Neuropharmacology 38(9): 1409-19.

Robichaud, R. C.&Sledge, K. L. (1969). The effects of p-chlorophenylalanine on experimentally induced conflict in the rat. Life Sci 8(17): 965-9.

Rodgers, R. J., Cao, B. J., Dalvi, A.&Holmes, A. (1997). Animal models of anxiety: an ethological perspective. Braz J Med Biol Res 30(3): 289-304.

Rodgers, R. J.&Cole, J. C. (1993). Anxiety enhancement in the murine elevated plus maze by immediate prior exposure to social stressors. Physiol Behav 53(2): 383-8.

Rodgers, R. J.&Johnson, N. J. (1995). Cholecystokinin and anxiety: promises and pitfalls. Crit Rev Neurobiol 9(4): 345-69.

Rudolph, U., Crestani, F.&Mohler, H. (2001). GABA(A) receptor subtypes: dissecting their pharmacological functions. Trends Pharmacol Sci 22(4): 188-94.

Shepherd, J. K., Grewal, S. S., Fletcher, A., Bill, D. J.&Dourish, C. T. (1994). Behavioural and pharmacological characterisation of the elevated zero-maze as an animal model of anxiety. Psychopharmacology 116: 56-64.

Silverman, P. (1978). Animal behaviour in the laboratory. London, Chapman and Hall.

Singh, Y. N.&Blumenthal, M. (1997). Kava: An Overview. Distribution, mythology, botany, culture, chemistry, and pharmacology of the South Pacific's most revered herb. HerbalGram 39: 33-55.

Siniscalchi, A., Rodi, D., Cavallini, S., Marino, S., Beani, L.&Bianchi, C. (2001). Effects of cholecystokinin tetrapeptide (CCK(4)) and anxiolytic drugs on the electrically evoked [(3)H]5-hydroxytryptamine outflow from rat cortical slices. Brain Res 922(1): 104-11.

Smith, K. K., Dharmaratne, H. R., Feltenstein, M. W., Broom, S. L., Roach, J. T., Nanayakkara, N. P., Khan, I. A.&Sufka, K. J. (2001). Anxiolytic effects of kava extract and kavalactones in the chick social separation-stress paradigm. Psychopharmacology (Berl) 155(1): 86-90.

Soderpalm, B.&Engel, J. A. (1992). The 5,7-DHT-induced anticonflict effect is dependent on intact adrenocortical function. Life Sci 51(5): 315-26.

Spielberger, C. D. (1972). Anxiety: current trends in theory and research. New York, Academic Press.

Srinivasan, J., Suresh, B.&Ramanathan, M. (2003). Differential anxiolytic effect of enalapril and losartan in normotensive and renal hypertensive rats. Physiol Behav 78(4-5): 585-91.

Stahl, S. M. (1998). Mechanism of action of serotonin selective reuptake inhibitors. Serotonin receptors and pathways mediate therapeutic effects and side effects. J Affect Disord 51(3): 215-35.

Stephens, D. N.&Andrews, J. S. (1991). Screening for anxiolytic drugs. Behavioural models in psychopharmacology: Theoretical, industrial and clinical perspectives. P. Willner. Cambridge, University Press: 50-75.

Tabatabaie, T.&Dryhurst, G. (1998). Molecular mechanisms of action of 5,6- and 5,7-dihydroxytryptamine. Highly Selective Neurotoxins: Basic and Clinical Applications. R. M. Kostrzewa. Totowa, Humana Press: 269 - 291.

Tada, K., Kasamo, K., Ueda, N., Suzuki, T., Kojima, T.&Ishikawa, K. (1999). Anxiolytic 5-hydroxytryptamine1A agonists suppress firing activity of dorsal hippocampus CA1 pyramidal neurons through a postsynaptic mechanism: single-unit study in unanesthetized, unrestrained rats. J Pharmacol Exp Ther 288(2): 843-8.

Tembrock, G. (2000). Angst. Darmstadt, Wissensch. Buchges.

Thiebot, M. H., Jobert, A.&Soubrie, P. (1980). Conditioned suppression of behavior: its reversal by intra raphe microinjection of chlordiazepoxide and GABA. Neurosci Lett 16(2): 213-7.

Thomas, H., Fink, H., Sohr, R.&Voits, M. (2000). Lesion of the median raphe nucleus: a combined behavioral and microdialysis study in rats. Pharmacol Biochem Behav 65(1): 15-21.

Trullas, R.&Skolnick, P. (1993). Differences in fear motivated behaviors among inbred mouse strains. Psychopharmacology (Berl) 111(3): 323-31.

Trulson, M. E., Preussler, D. W., Howell, G. A.&Frederickson, C. J. (1982). Raphe unit activity in freely moving cats: effects of benzodiazepines. Neuropharmacology 21(10): 1045-50.

Twarog, B. M.&Page, I. H. (1953). Serotonin content of some mammalian tissues and urine and a method for its determination. Am J Physiol 175(1): 157-61.

Ungerstedt, U.&Hallstrom, A. (1987). In vivo microdialysis--a new approach to the analysis of neurotransmitters in the brain. Life Sciences 41: 861-864.

Ungerstedt, U.&Rostami, E. (2004). Microdialysis in neurointensive care. Curr Pharm Des 10(18): 2145-52.

Vaas (2000). Emotionen. Lexikon der Neurowissenschaft. Heidelberg, Berlin, Spektrum Akademischer Verlag. 1: 386-397.

Vanderhaeghen, J. J., Signeau, J. C.&Gepts, W. (1975). New peptide in the vertebrate CNS reacting with antigastrin antibodies. Nature 257(5527): 604-5.

Voigt, J. P., Rex, A., Sohr, R.&Fink, H. (1999). Hippocampal 5-HT and NE release in the transgenic rat TGR(mREN2)27 related to behavior on the elevated plus maze. Eur Neuropsychopharmacol 9(4): 279-85.

Wise, C. D., Berger, B. D.&Stein, L. (1972). Benzodiazepines: anxiety-reducing activity by reduction of serotonin turnover in the brain. Science 177(44): 180-3.

Wittchen, H. U. (1991). Der Langzeitverlauf unbehandelter Angststörungen: Wie häufig sind Spontanremissionen? Verhaltenstherapie 1: 273-282.

Wittchen, H. U.&Jacobi, F. (2005). Size and burden of mental disorders in Europe--a critical review and appraisal of 27 studies. Eur Neuropsychopharmacol 15(4): 357-76.

Witte, S., Loew, D.&Gaus, W. (2005). Meta-analysis of the efficacy of the acetonic kava-kava extract WS1490 in patients with non-psychotic anxiety disorders. Phytother Res 19(3): 183-8.

Wright, I. K., Upton, N.&Marsden, C. A. (1992). Effect of established and putative anxiolytics on extracellular 5-HT and 5-HIAA in the ventral hippocampus of rats during behaviour on the elevated X-maze. Psychopharmacology (Berl) 109(3): 338-46.

Psychogenic Movement Disorders

Carlo Dallocchio
Department of Medical Specialities, Division of Neurology, Ospedale Civile
Voghera (Pavia)
Italy

1. Introduction

Abnormal movements and postures resulting from primary psychiatric disease are a diagnostic dilemma because all types of movement disorders may be mimicked by a psychogenic disease, including akinetic-rigid and hyperkinetic disorders, with the latter more frequent, particularly tremor, myoclonus, and dystonia (Williams et al., 2005; Reich, 2006).

Psychogenic movement disorders (PMDs), are a valuable model for all medically unexplained symptoms and raise arduous challenges for diagnosis and treatment indicating our restricted understanding of the true pathogenesis that causes them. A multiplicity of terms such as "hysterical conversion", "functional", "psychosomatic", "neuropsychiatric", "dissociative motor disorders",and so on, have been applied to describe neurological symptoms that cannot be attribute to any known organic disease (Mace & Trimble, 1991; Lang, 2006). The term "psychogenic" is the commonest in the movement disorder literature, but there is no unanimity whether it reflects the precise nature of a syndrome containing both neurologic and psychiatric components.

By the late-19th century, psychoanalytic theory ruled medical reasoning about these symptoms. Originally referring to these disorders as hysteria, neuropsychiatrists began illustrating the various clinical phenomenological aspects of such disorders. Paralysis, tremors, convulsions and sensory alterations were identified as sometimes being due to hysteria. Subsequently, different etiologies of dystonia, tremor, myoclonus and other movement disorders were recognized. Over the years, newer clinical criteria, laboratory investigations, particularly neurophysiological findings, and improved neuroimaging have provided significant insights about the psychogenicity of the diagnosis. However, a misdiagnosis is possible either on patients originally believed to have a conversion disorder or because PMD was never considered on differential diagnosis (Rosebush & Mazurek, 2006; Lang & Gupta, 2009).

The pathophysiology of PMDs are not yet well known, but functional brain imaging studies combined with other neurophysiologic techniques are starting to help understand them (Stone & Carson, 2011). These studies promise an understanding of these symptoms in parallel neurologic and psychiatric ways.

The diagnosis of a psychogenic movement disorder is often difficult and the level of diagnostics that the clinician has for PMD varies remarkably, depending on the clinical feature of the movement disorders and the accompanying signs and symptoms. PMDs are classified by the Diagnostic and Statistical Manual of Mental Disorders (DSM-IV) of the American Psychiatric Association as conversion disorder of motor subtype and must be differentiated from factitious disorder and malingering, in which the abnormal movements are purposefully forged. Since most patients with conversion symptoms are found to have "no psychiatric disease" by the psychiatric and "no neurologic disease" by the neurologist, a multidisciplinary treatment approach, including the movement disorders neurologist, the consulting psychiatrist, and frequently a physical therapist, is crucial in obtaining symptom remission in many subjects (Williams et al., 2005; Stone et al., 2010).

Although evidence for treatment of PMDs are lacking and is mainly based on case control, retrospective, or case report studies, the therapeutic process starts with the diagnosis and the explanation of the symptoms to the patient. To date, the treatment for each patient with PMDs is individualized and may include psychotherapeutic interventions, behavioral therapy, hypnosis, pharmachotherapy, physical therapy, and other approach.

Physicians should not underestimate the importance of distress and disability that subjects with these symptoms suffer. Failure to diagnose a PMDs inevitably delays treatment and may perpetuate a patient's situation of disability (Williams et al., 2005). In addiction, patients with somatisation had approximately twice the medical care utilisation and twice the annual medical care costs of non-somatizing patients and spend 1.3 to 3.9 days in bed per month compared to an average of one day or less for patients with major medical problems (Smith et al., 1986; Barsky et al., 2005). The current chapter reviews empirical evidence concerning clinical manifestations of PMDs and summarizes how PMDs are currently diagnosed, investigated and treated.

2. Epidemiology and risk factors

Although psychogenic neurological symptoms are common and account for 1-9% of neurological symptoms observed in the general population (Lempert et al., 1990; Factor et al., 1995), the following caveats should be borne in mind: (i) available reports result from tertiary movement disorders centers, and therefore it is difficult to valuate how common these disorders are in the general population or even what is the prevalence respect to all conversion disorders, (ii) the insufficiency of confirmatory diagnostic testing prejudices case definition even when clinical satisfactory criteria are applied and (iii) several clinical settings and situations (e.g., neurology or psychiatry in- or outpatient service, emergency room or general practitioner cases, chronic or refractory cases, etc.) may confound case ascertainment (Lang, 2006). In the only series dividing medically unexplained motor symptoms into "absence of motor function" and "presence of abnormal motor activity", 48% of the patients had index symptoms in the former category, while 52% had symptoms, such as tremor, dystonia or ataxia (Crimlisk et al., 1998).

PMDs also can occur over a wide range of ages from teenage to the mid seventies (Deuschl et al.,1998; Feinstein et al., 2001). The mean age at onset described in several case series on these disorders ranges between 37 years and 50 years and women are predominantly affected with a range of 61-87% (Hinson et al., 2005; Factor et al., 1995).

There are no data on racial distribution in the published research, however a trans-cultural comparison between patients with these disorders in the USA, in Spain, and in Brazil showed essentially similar demographic and clinical characteristics by ethnic origin (Cubo et al., 2005; Munhoz et al., 2010). Nearly 15% of patients with a psychogenic movement disorder have also an underlying organic movement disorder (Ranawaya el al., 1990).

Curiously, PMDs are frequently seen in subjects employed in health care professions or allied health care professionals possibly due to the exposure to disease and those who have witnessed the organic form of the movement disorder (e.g. Parkinson's disease) in other relatives (Miyasaki et al., 2003;)

More frequently, PMDs are encountered in the context of a second coexisting psychiatric illness. Feinstein and colleagues followed 88 patients suffering from psychogenic movement disorders, over an average of 3 years. 42 patients agreed to undergo a structured psychiatric interview. The most common life time prevalence rates were found for depression (42%), anxiety disorders (62%), a combination of depression and anxiety (29%) and conversion disorder (95%). Personality disorder (antisocial, borderline, dependent, avoidant or a mixture of those) was diagnosed in 42% of patients tested (Feinstein et al., 2001). Among the a series of 127 patients with psychogenic tremor, depression (51%) and anxiety (31%) were the most common psychiatric co-morbidities (Jankovic & Thomas, 2006).

Risk factors for these disorders include: history of sexual abuse or rape, physical trauma, previous surgery, major stressful life experiences (Williams et al., 2005; Feinstein et al., 2001). Many patients with functional neurologic symptoms report just as much physical disability and are more distressed than patients with neurologic disease. Furthermore, subjects with these symptoms are more likely to be out of work because of ill health than the general population (Stone et al., 2011).

3. Pathophysiology

In reviewing the history of psychogenic neurologic disorders, hysterical paralisis and sensory loss have been known presumably back in antiquity (Ng BY, 1999) and have been debated before the late 19th century, when Charcot, Janet, Breuer, and Freud gave a systematic psychological account of these phenomena. (Charcot, 1889; Janet, 1907; Freud, 1910). From then on, there has been a large body of literature regarding the possible psychogenic, psychoanalytical, cultural and biological mechanisms underlying PMDs.

According to Janet, traumatic events can cause a functional separation (dissociation) of structures of memory, identity, insight, and perception of the environment from conscious awareness. As a result, unexplained symptoms emerge from the activation of these dissociated structures (Janet, 1889). Patients suffering from non-organic motor symptoms are singularly susceptible to hypnosis, an inducible state of dissociation.

This theory was later developed by Breuer and Freud, who considered dissociation a psychological defence mechanism rather than a disorganizing phenomenon: the mental conflict is partially or completely resolved by the expression of physical symptoms, which is called primary gain. According to this psychodynamic model, dissociation preserves the subject from the invalidating affect associated with remembrances of trauma by its "conversion" in to somatic symptoms and once these latter have developed, may confer further advantages to the patient (attention, solicitude, social interaction, etc.) or "secondary gains"(Breuer & Freud, 1895).

In contemporary psychiatry, dissociative symptoms and dissociation as a mechanism are taken to point to a role traumatic events in pathogenesis. Various factors may provide to the pathway to conversion disorder, perhaps comprehending, concurrent somatic illness in adolescence or adulthood, parental illness in the subject childhood, and early illness. In particular physical or sexual abuse in childhood have considered key factors in the generation of vulnerability to unexplained somatic symptoms (Ovsiew, 2006).

The definite nature of emotional disorders responsible of psychogenic disorders, and their functional consequences on neural systems in the brain, still remain largely unknown.

In the closing decades of the 19th century, researchers have progressively been looking for organic correlates of PMDs and the neural mechanism perspective became more approved with the advent of novel functional neuroimaging methods. These new approaches have now allowed to detect in vivo regionally specific changes in cerebral blood flow and task-related changes in the attempt to identify specific neural correlates associated with conversion symptoms, that is the "dynamic lesion" that Charcot considered responsible for the neurological signs he observed in patients affected by "hysteric movement disorders".

PMDs evoke notable interest because, as protean disorders of willed action or intention, the underlying mechanism are supposed to be the result of unconscious processes, a sort of impairment to the volition system, once any demonstrative organic or feigning dysfunctions has been excluded (Fink, 2006). Psychogenic movements may be voluntary or involuntary. Factitious disorder and malingering describe when the disorder is voluntary, and the patients are lying. On the other hand, most patients with PMDs have a conversion aetiology and manifest movements that look voluntary, even if patients declare that the movements are involuntary. By a physiological point of view we can not tell the difference between voluntary and involuntary, but we know (most of time) that both are preceded by a normal "readiness potential" or so called Bereitschaftspotential, a manifestation of cortical contribution to the pre-motor planning of volitional movement (Shibasaki & Hallet, 2006) and share cortical structures that are involved in movement planning and execution.

In a go-nogo task, while a patient underwent functional magnetic resonance imaging (fMRI), Cojan et al. demonstrated that distinct inhibitory mechanism are implicated in simulation and conversion disorders and that conversion symptoms do not act through cognitive inhibitory circuits, but involve selective activations in midline brain regions associated with self-related representations and emotion regulation (Cojan, 2009). Other neuroimaging results have shown increase activation in limbic regions, such as orbitofrontal or cingulated cortex during conversion symptoms affecting different motor or sensory modalities (Vuilleumier, 2005, Nowak, 2009). A recent single photon emission computed tomography (SPECT) study by Czarnecki et al. suggested that the prominent hypoperfusion of the prefrontal and anterior cingulate cortex in patients with psychogenic tremor likely indicates deactivation of the anterior portion of the default mode network (the baseline state of the brain that deactivates during goal-directed activity), which could prove to be a peculiar marker of PMDs. Moreover, this study reported resting hyperperfusion in left insula and left inferior frontal gyrus in psychogenic tremor that may also prove to be a disease characteristic (Czarnecki et al. 2011).

Voon and colleagues used functional magnetic resonance imaging (fMRI) to study patients with psychogenic tremor who could voluntarily mimic their tremor and showed hypoperfusion of the right temporal parietal junction only during involuntary movements. The authors speculate that this hypoactivity may reflect the lack of an appropriate sensory prediction signal, being the right temporal parietal junction implicated as a general comparator of internal predictions with actual events. This suggests a loss of self-agency o awareness that made the movements feel involuntary (Voon et al., 2010).

There may be a pathologic unconscious influence on movement production associated with a disconnection between movement production and sense of volition (Hallet, 2010). Besides, earliest affective or stress-related factors, neuropsychological and psychosocial processes, perhaps involved primitive reflexive mechanisms of protection and alertness that are not fully independent of conscious control (Vuilleumier, 2005). This prominent evidence in favour of multi causes of PMDs requires a multifaceted approach integrating innovative neuroimaging and neurophysiological techniques with social, psychological and psychodynamic theories.

4. Clinical manifestations and diagnostic clues

The diagnosis of PMDs remains a fascinating and challenging dilemma in both clinical neurology and psychiatry. It should not be considered as a diagnosis of exclusion but should be established on positive clinical criteria to determine whether abnormal movements are produced by organic disease, psychiatric disorder, or both (Jankovic & Thomas, 2006). Taking into account that unnecessary investigations should be prevented, more notable evidence is required before a diagnosis of psychogenic disorder can be confirmed. Some studies, including exhaustive neurologic assessments and modern diagnostic techniques, have shown that a misdiagnosis is possible on long-term follow-up of patients initially diagnosed with a conversion disorder and later identified as having an organic disorder (Moene et al., 2000; Lang, 2006; Lang & Gupta, 2009). Otherwise, failure to make the diagnosis arises because PMDs were seldom contemplated in the differential diagnosis, especially in patients who have a coexistent neurologic disease, such as neurodegenerative or demyelinating disorder or epilepsy. Coexistent organic neurologic disease was present in 37% of patients with psychogenic tremor followed for over 3 years (Jankovic et al., 2004). Additionally, the problem is exacerbated by a tendency among physicians to be concerned about missing an "organic" diagnosis in order to relieve the patient from a "functional" one, even if the latter is treatable and the former is not (Rosebush & Mazurek, 2006). Another troubling side of these disorders is the reluctance of many physicians to put their judgments and conclusions into a transparent discussion with the patient. So an ambivalent communication wanes to deliver the presumed diagnosis in real terms and running the risk that patients continue to explore for months or years further opinion through "doctor shopping". (Friedman & LaFrance WC, 2010).

Because many patients or family members of patients with PMDs are strongly reluctant to the diagnosis not explained organically and may resistant to a psychiatric referral, a multidisciplinary approach, including the general or movement disorders neurologist and the consulting psychiatrist is essential. The role of the neurologist is primary in determining whether there is an underline neurologic disorder and whether it could explain the clinical picture. Hardly mental health professionals undertake a treatment of such patients without the neurologic diagnosis has been either established or dismissed (Feinstein et al., 2001; Williams et al., 2005).

Fahn and Williams developed four degrees of certainty for the diagnosis (Tab. 1) of psychogenic dystonia, which are commonly applied in clinical practice and research to all PMDs (Fahn & Williams, 1988). Shill and Gerber formulated further criteria with a denomination of "clinically proven PMDs" which requires remission when the patient is unobserved or with psychotherapy or when there is a Bereitschaftspotential on electroencephalography (for myoclonus only). Moreover, they added further criteria of PMDs to include excessive pain or fatigue and previous disease exposure (Shill & Gerber, 2006). Developing this idea, Hallett proposed that a new designation of "laboratory proven PMDs" could be considered (Peckham & Hallett, 2009). A recent study demonstrated that the finger tapping test may provide an objective tool to aid the clinical diagnostic criteria set by Fahn and Williams for identifying patients with PMDs (Criswell et al., 2010).

Documented psychogenic
Movements are persistently relieved by psychotherapy or psychological suggestion or with the administration of placebos. If the patient is observed to be symptom free when left alone, this may also be documented as psychogenic; however, this feature is usually indicative of malingering or factitious disorder.
Clinically Established Psychogenic
Inconsistent or incongruent with classical dystonia (on examination, the patient is unable to move the limbs but is able to dress herself in daily life). In addition, one or all of the following is highly suggestive: other neurologic signs present that are psychogenic (self-inflicted injuries, false weakness, false sensory findings), an obvious psychiatric disturbance is present, and multiple somatizations are present.
Probable Psychogenic
Movements are inconsistent or incongruent, but there are no other features (as above) to further support the diagnosis. Movements are consistent with organic dystonia, but there are other features on examination to suggest psychogenicity (self-inflicted injuries, false weakness, false sensory findings). Multiple somatizations are present, but movements are consistent with organic dystonia.
Possible Psychogenic
An obvious emotional disturbance is present, but movements are consistent with organic dystonia.

Table 1. The classification of psychogenic movement disorders (Williams & Fahn, 1995)

An additional support, that seems appropriate to capture the complexity of PMDs and that can be used to assess PMDs and test the efficacy of intervention strategies is the Psychogenic Movement Disorder Rating Scale (PMDRS). This clinimetric assessment describes and quantifies the complicated phenomenology of PMDs, and provides the following six types of information: movement phenomenology, anatomic distribution and severity of abnormal movements, duration of abnormal movements, assessment of two functions (gait and speech), impairment-based incapacitation by abnormal movement or function, and total severity score (Hinson et al., 2005).

It should be emphasized that observation and examination are the most important tools for the physician looking for inconsistency of movements. The first trace of psychogenicity in a patient presenting with such abnormal motor activity can be obtained by history (Table 2.A). This may comprise psychiatric history, childhood history, personality factors, drug experience, recent personal and family life events, stressful situations or work-related injury, litigation or compensation pending, personal encounter or knowledge of similar disorders serving as a "model" and possible secondary gain (Bhatia & Schneider, 2007; Nowak & Fink, 2009).

In general, the manner of onset characterizes the clinical presentation of PMDs (Table 2.B): symptoms appear abruptly, frequently in the context of precipitating factors and, the highest disability and severity are reached quickly (Feinstein et al., 2001). Important specifics of PMDs are an inconsistent character of movement (unusual presentation in amplitude, frequency, distribution), and they may increase with attention or decrease with distraction (Miyasaki, 2003). A deliberate slowness of movement is incongruent with an organic movement disorders, as well as simultaneous occurrence of variegated abnormal movements and disfunctions, and peculiarly, patients may seem to struggle and put in more effort than needed to complete the task (Hinson & Blacke Haren 2006; Bhatia & Schneider 2007). Often, this is manifest by sighing, grimacing, and using their whole body to do a movement. The movements themselves may appear bizarre and should be incongruous with a known movement disorder.

There are controversial points of view whether there is a place for placebo in management of PMDs, as it reflects ethical evaluations and can infringe the relationship between physician and patient. Although a response to placebo of a movement disorder is seriously supportive of a diagnosis of PMDs (Espay et al., 2009). Equally, spontaneous resolution and improvement of unexplained symptoms with psychiatric evaluation or psychotherapy are highly suggestive of psychogenic aetiology of them (Fahn, 1994).

Diagnostic testing should be used primarily to give further support to the underlying clinical suspicion that it is psychogenic. Routine blood test including haematology, thyroid function, renal and liver function, and evaluation for Wilson's disease may be helpful. Magnetic resonance imaging can be helpful for excluding an underlying structural, vascular or demyelinating lesion, particularly if the abnormal movement is unilateral or asymmetrical. Neurophysiology studies to evaluate tremor and myoclonus can aid in the diagnosis of PMDs. Dopamine transporter (DAT) SPECT and Fluorodopa (18F-dopa) PET scans have been proven quite helpful in distinguishing psychogenic parkinsonism from Parkinson's disease or essential tremor (Kagi et al., 2010; Czarnecki et al. 2011).

The role of the consulting psychiatrist is to interpret the psychopathology present, ascertain its relevance to the presenting PMDs symptoms and establish a positive rapport with the patient. If this appears feasible, the psychiatrist will then begin the treatment course, with adequate collaborative support from neurologist (Williams et al., 2005).

However, psychiatric aspects and categorical differentiations, which are discussed in detail elsewhere in this book, also apply to PMDs. In brief, the psychiatric examination includes research of individual psychodynamics and significant environmental events as well as a complete multiaxial delineation of specific psychopathology according to the official psychiatric classification system such as the Diagnostic and Statistical Manual of Mental Disorders, fourth Edition (DSM-IV). The primary psychopathology underlying PMDs can be divided into two categoric diagnostic subgroups: somatoform disorders on the one hand, and factitious disorders and malingering on the other. The first category includes conversion disorder and somatization disorder. Conversion disorder is likely the most common mechanism of PMDs and is defined by the DSM-IV criteria as a disorder including one or more symptoms, that are not the result of a neurological disorder, affecting voluntary motor or sensory function that suggest a medical condition and is associated with psychological factors.

The primary psychiatric diagnosis varies: most cases are considered to be conversion disorders, in which the problem is generated by an unconscious mechanism, but infrequently some are factitious disorders or malingering, in which the abnormal movements are purposefully forged. Factitious disorders include intentional production of physical or psychological symptoms, where the goal is to assume the role of a patient and external incentives, such as economic gain or avoiding legal responsibility, are absent. In malingering, the symptoms can also be physical or psychological, but the individual is consciously aware of external pragmatic incentives, such as gaining financial compensation, acquiring drugs, avoiding work or school, et cetera, and when the external incentives are removed, the symptoms resolve. Beyond a categorical diagnostic classification, it is often very intricate, especially initially, to face with a patient having PMDs and make a differential diagnosis among somatoform disorders, factious disorders, and malingering. Simplification may arise however, in the course further and exhaustive evaluation, by reinforcing the agreement between physician and patient and ensuring patient's confidence in the treatment plan (Williams et al.,2006). Moreover, most patients with PMDs have a coexisting variety of different psychiatric disturbances such as dysthymia, major depression, anxiety, adjustment disorders, obsessive-compulsive disorder, panic attacks, bipolar disorders and others (Williams et al., 2005; Bhatia & Schneider, 2007). Yet, it is important to add that many organic movement disorders have an important incidence of the above-named psychiatric diagnoses (Reich, 2006). Finally, the common occurrence of movement disorders complicating primary mental illness and their treatment makes it important for psychiatrists to be able to recognize the various movement disorders, some of which have singular phenomenology such as tardive akathisia, tardive dystonia, tourettism and some unusual form of parkinsonism or tremor (Factor et al., 2005).

A) Historical

1. **Abrupt onset**
2. **Static course**
3. **Spontaneous remission**
4. **Precipitated by minor trauma**
5. **Obvious psychiatric disturbance**
6. **Multiple somatization**
7. **Employed in health profession**
8. **Pending litigation or compensation**
9. **Presence of secondary gain**
10. **Young age (female>male) Inconsistent character of movement (amplitude, frequency, distribution, selective ability)**

B) Clinical

1. **Paroxysmal movement disorder**
2. **Movements increase with attention or decrease with distrction**
3. **Ability to trigger or relieve the abnormal movements with unusual or non physiological interventions (e.g.trigger points on the body, tuning fork)**
4. **False weakness**
5. **False sensory complaints**
6. **Self-inflected injuries**
7. **Deliberate slowness of movements**
8. **Functional disability out of proportion to exam findings**
9. **Movement abnormality that is bizarre, multiple or difficult to classifyUnresponsive to appropriate medications**

C) Therapeutic responses

1. **Response to placebos**
2. **Unresponsive to appropriate medication**
3. **Remission with psychotherapy**

Table 2. General clues suggesting that a movement disorder may be psychogenic (Miyasaki et al., 2003; Lang, 2006)

4.1 Types of psychogenic movement disorders

4.1.1 Psychogenic tremor

Although many patients has a mixture of different movement disorders, psychogenic tremor is the prevalent movement disorder, up to 55%, of all PMDs. Clinical sites affected include the hand (84%), the leg (28%), and generalized body tremor 20% (Thomas & Jankovic 2004). Clinically, absence of finger tremor can be a positive diagnostic sign for psychogenic tremor (Jankovic & Thomas, 2006; Bhatia & Schneider, 2007) and attempting to immobilize the affected limb often makes a functional tremor worse, as well as loading the limb with weights tends to make the tremor worse, whereas organic tremor usually improves with this operation.

The diagnosis may be supported by the "coactivation sign". As in the testing procedure for rigidity, the physician feels the increased muscle tone in the tremulous extremity in both directions and this cogwheel-like resistance is strictly related to tremor or if the patient can be made to relax completely (Deuschl et al. 1998). The technique of back-averaging electroencephalographic activity preceding the electromyographic ones, can be useful to detect premovement potential in subjects with psychogenic tremor, absent in organic involuntary movement (Brown & Thompson, 2001). Zeuner et al. using accelerometry to measure frequency changes during tapping showed that in contrast to parkinsonian and essential tremor, patients with psychogenic tremor revealed larger tremor frequency changes and marked variability in tapping (Zeuner et al., 2003). Entrainment of tremulous movements of different body parts into a single rhythm has been used clinically as a means of distinguishing these tremor forms. If functional tremor involves more than one limb, it usually has the same frequency. On the other hand, organic tremor usually has slightly different frequencies in different body parts. A quantified electrophysiological entrainment test performed on accelerometer or surface EMG tremor signals may provide supportive evidence of a functional tremor (McAuley & Rothwell 2004). Recently, Czarnecki and colleagues revealed distinct patterns of cerebral perfusion, during rest and motor task, as measured by SPECT that distinguish psychogenic tremor from essential tremor and controls (Czarnecki et al. 2011).

4.1.2 Psychogenic dystonia

Dystonia exemplifies one of the longest history of misdiagnosis: for many centuries it was considered a psychogenic condition, then, after torsion dystonia was accepted as an organic entity in the early-20th century and different aetiologies of this condition were recognized, it was thought that psychogenic dystonia rarely occurred (Fahn, 2006). In general, psychogenic dystonia represents only approximately 5% of subjects with dystonia, but in most centers, it is the second most commonly encountered among PMDs and accounts for 20% to 50% of cases (Miyasaki et al., 2003). Psychogenic dystonia, classified as a secondary dystonia, largely remains a clinical diagnosis and there are no physiologic tests available that distinguish a psychogenic aetiology from an organic form (Peckham & Hallett, 2009).

Psychogenic dystonia may not occur with the typical variability and distractibility of other PMDs and presents with fixed dystonic postures (Fig. 1) without return to the neutral position at rest from the beginning. Leg involvement is uncommon in adult-onset organic dystonia, as well as lack sensory tricks or relief by certain inexplicable trick action, and presence of severe pain suggest psychogenic dystonia, even if not in a specific way (Schrag, 2006).

Controversial patients are those with dystonia developing within ours or days after a minor injury, with a fixed distonic posture and severe pain. This kind of dystonia may be associated with features of complex regional pain syndrome type I. A study by Schrag and co-workers show that a substantial proportion of patients with fixed dystonia clearly fulfils criteria for a psychogenic dystonia (37%) or somatization disorder (29%). Although fixed dystonia sometimes developed in patients in whom a diagnosis of somatization disorder had already been made, a history of somatization was often unrecognized and, in many cases, only became evident after examination of primary care records (Schrag et al., 2004; Miyasaki et al., 2003). Various features of complex regional pain syndrome-related fixed dystonia suggest abnormal regulation of inhibitory interneuronal mechanisms at the brainstem or spinal cord level and impairment central synaptic reorganisation due to an interaction between neuroplastic activities and anomalous environmental necessities (Munts & Koehler, 2010).

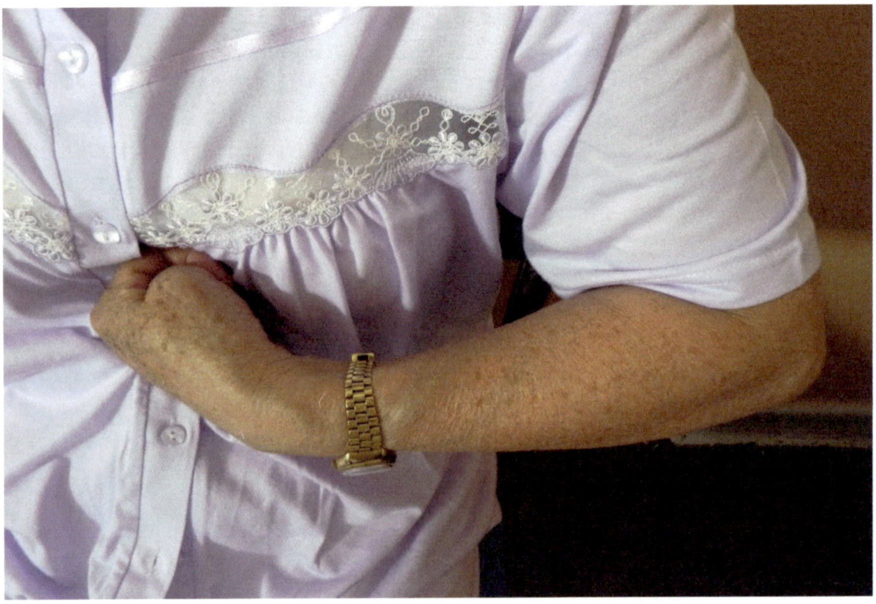

Fig. 1. A fixed dystonic posture of psychogenic origin

4.1.3 Psychogenic parkinsonism

Psychogenic parkinsonism is a rare syndrome accounting for 0.17–0.5% of all parkinsonism cases and representing nearly 10% of PMDs (Factor et al., 1995; Benaderette et al., 2006). In this disorder, atypical tremor occurs in conjunction with extremely slow movements that are often accompanied by grimacing, sighing, or whole-body movements when patients do a simple motor task. Common characteristics of organic parkinsonism, such as hypomimia, decreased blink rate, axial rigidity, and "cogwheel" phenomenon are usually absent in psychogenic parkinsonism. On postural stability testing, patients may have bizarre responses including flailing of the arms and reeling backward without falling (Thomas & Jankovic, 2004). Additionally, patients with psychogenic parkinsonism may also suffer from depression, which can cause psychomotor retardation, a clinical condition which may be difficult to distinguish from the bradyphrenia associated to Parkinson's disease (Morgan &

Sethi, 2006). It should be also remarked that parkinsonism or akinetic-rigid syndrome not uncommonly occur in the setting of major psychiatric disease and exposure to pharmacological agents.
Electrophysiology studies can be supportive in distinguishing a Parkinson's psychogenic tremor from other forms of tremor. Functional neuroimaging can be helpful in confirming a diagnosis of psychogenic parkinsonism. Loss of dopamine nerve function seen in organic parkinsonism can be measured by decreases in dopamine transporter density or presynaptic dopamine deficiency (I 123 B-CIT) on single positron emission computed tomography (SPECT) and Fluorodopa positron emission tomography (F-DOPA-PET). In psychogenic parkinsonism, these features are absent, but keeping in mind that other conditions, i.e. drug induced parkinsonism, dopa responsive dystonia-parkinsonism, have normal SPECT or F-DOPA-PET scans (Benaderette et al., 2006; Scherfler et al., 2006).
Table 3 summarizes the differences of clinical findings in Psychogenic parkinsonism, Drug-induced parkinsonism and Parkinson Disease.

	Psychogenic Parkinsonism	**Drug-Induced Parkinsonism**	**Parkinson Disease**
Onset	Abrupt, varied age of onset	Bilateral and symmetric, more common in the elderly	Gradual,unilateral or asymmetric, typically in the 6th or 7th decade
Cours	Usually static with maximum disability early, condition may abruptly or gradually remit	Acute or subacute	Insidious, slowly progressive
Tremor type	Unilateral or bilateral, rest, postural, action; usually involving the dominant hand, varying frequency and amplitude, spreads when immobilizing the affected limb	Not always present, bilateral, symmetric, postural or rest	Unilateral or asymmetric at rest, 4-6 Hz, worsens with distraction
Bradykinesia	Extremely slow movement often with fatigue, arrest or decrement; grimacing, sighing or whole body movements when performing simple task; normal speed of movements when not being examined	Often the earliest and commonest manifestation, facial hypomimia	Slowing of rapid repetitive movements without fatigue, arrest or decrement

Rigidity	Cogwheel absent, voluntary resistance which may decrease with distraction	Often uniform, inconstant cogwheel rigidity	Cogwheel rigidity
Postural instability	Impaired early, may have exaggerated or bizarre response to minimal backwards	Mild stooping, decreased arm swing	Impaired in moderate to advanced disease, retropulsion on pull test
Speech	Stuttering, bizarre dysarthria, distractible	Mild stuttering	Hypophonic, stuttering, tachyphemia
Motor fluctuation	Very rare complaint of "extra movements" on levodopa, no dyskinesias after long-term levodopa treatment	Absent	Dyskinesias in half of patients on levodopa after 5-7 years, on-off fluctuations
Psychiatric history	Previous conversion disorders, somatisation, factious disorder, anxiety, and depression	Relevant, particularly schizophrenia but also depression	Depression may precede diagnosis
Medication response	Usually unresponsive to multiple medical trials	Responds well to anticolinergic drugs, remittance within weeks or months when withdrawal of offending drug	Responds well to levodopa and dopamine agonist
Nonmotor problems	Sexual dysfunction and sleep disturbances occur	Possible swallowing less than normal, hallucination, rare costipation	Dysautonomia, constipation, sexual dysfunction, sleep problem, hallucination

Table 3. Clinical features of Psychogenic parkinsonism, Drug-induced parkinsonism and Parkinson Disease. Adapted from Morgan & Sethi, 2006.

4.1.4 Psychogenic gait

Abnormal gaits frequently occur in the setting of major psychiatric disease and represent 8% to 10% of all PMDs (Sudarsky, 2006). Psychogenic gate disorders are characterized by exaggerated effort or fatigue with grimaces, excessive slowness, convulsive shaking, often with knee buckling especially when the patient has unilateral functional weakness, astasia-abasia, arms are outstretched like a tightrope walker (Fig. 2), unusual uneconomic posture and bizarre movements (Bhatia, 2001; Baik & Lang, 2007). Patients with psychogenic require further strength and balance than an indifferent gait and they seem to be frightened of falling, and this gait allows them to be closer to the floor (Stone & Carson, 2010). The movement disorder is commonly accompanied by other psychogenic neurological symptoms, such as false weakness or sensory findings, or by excessive pain and tenderness (Thomas & Jankovic, 2004). Okun et al. described 9 consecutive patients who presented with a psychogenic gait disorder who underwent "chair testing." Each patient was asked to walk 20-30 feet forward and backward toward the examiner. Patients were then asked to sit in a swivel chair with wheels and to propel the chair forward and backward. Compared with their walking, 8 of the 9 patients in the psychogenic group performed well on the chair test, showing improved ability to propel a chair forward when seated. By contrast, all 9 control patients with nonpsychogenic gait problems, performed equally when walking or propelling utilizing the chair (Okun et al., 2007).

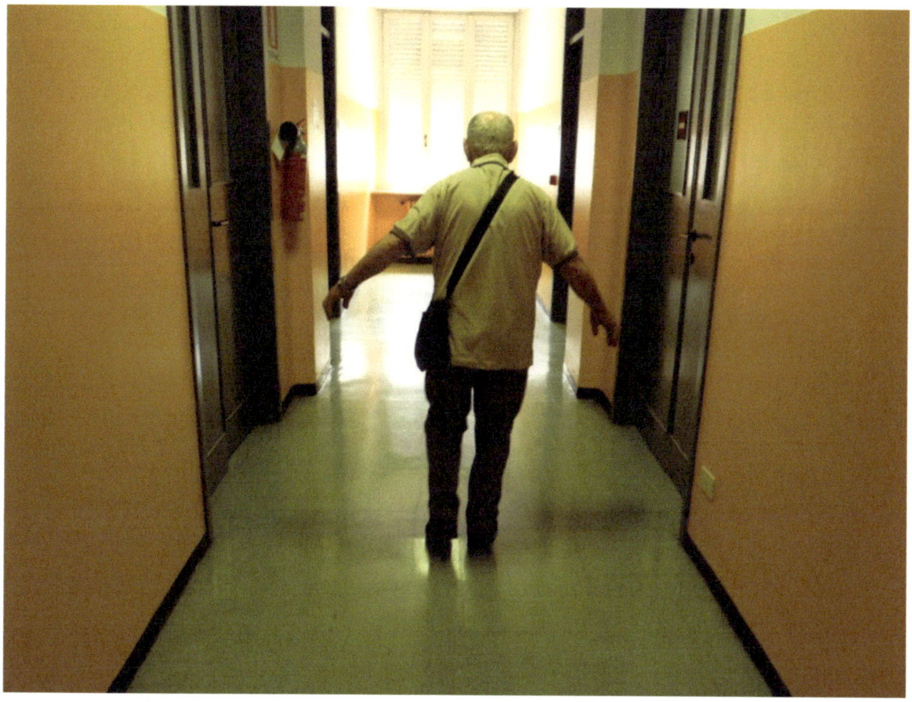

Fig. 2. Tightrope walking: the patient walks very slowly on a broad base with his arms extended.

4.1.5 Psychogenic myoclonus

Myoclonus account for 10% to 20% of PMDs. The clinical features of psychogenic myoclonus usually includes segmental or generalizes jerking, occurring at rest and during movement, commonly changing pattern, frequency, amplitude and anatomic distribution and may be stimulus sensitive (Monday & Jankovic 1993; Williams et al., 1995).

Neurophysiologic methods are particularly useful in distinguishing between voluntary jerking and cortical or brainstem myoclonus (Brown & Thomson, 2001). Organic myoclonus is characterized by burst length of less than 70 ms, and jerks lasting longer than that are suggestive of a psychogenic etiology. Functional myoclonus is often associated with a Bereitschaftpotential before the movement, which requires recording multiple events using an electroencephalogram and back averaging according to an electromyogram. In the absence of a Bereitschaftpotential, it is not possible to exclude a psychogenic etiology, as the Bereitschaftpotential can be absent in normal subjects (Brown & Thomson, 2001; Peckham & Hallett, 2009). Interestingly, in a recent case series of 35 consecutive patients with jerks of the trunk referred as possible proriospinal myoclonus, 34 patients showed features suggestive of a psychogenic origin even in the presence of a classic polymyography pattern or in the absence of a Bereitschaftpotential (van der Salm et al., 2010).

5. Treatment

There is no consensus even among the experts about the best treatment approach to patients with PMDs. Therefore, a common agreement is that treatment begins when the physician has made the diagnosis and mostly depending on the way of explaining PMDs to the patient, as well as a very close working relationship between neurologist, consulting psychiatrist, and frequently physical therapist, is crucial in obtaining symptom remission in many subjects. Table 4 emphasizes, by the acronym form THERAPIST, the essential basis for a treatment process.

Terminology must engage and not alienate the patient
Hear out the patient with interest, compassion, and empathy (and patience)
Explain the diagnosis and the mechanism of symptoms
Reassure that there is no evidence of neurologic damage
Address psychosocial and family issues
Prognosis is likely favorable, the patient has the potential to recovery fully
Individualize the therapy and customize it
Self-help is a crucial part of getting better
Treat concurrent psychiatric and medical illness (if present)

Table 4. Nine essential steps for an approach to management of patients with PMDs.

The objective of effective treatment is not only to provide symptoms remission in the short term, but to evaluate the causes that produced the heterogeneous symptomatology and to assess feasible strategies to remove them.

The issue about the terminology to use for the diagnosis is unresolved. Some authors find that "functional" disorder is an accurate term, which describe a disorder of the way the brain is working. Others find "psychogenic" an acceptable term with vagueness implication. Still others think that the latter arouses too much a "crazy" condition in the patient and family's mind and prefer the more broad word "neuropsychiatric" (Williams et al., 2005; Stone & Carson, 2010). In any case, whatever term is used it is important to find an explanatory language that engages the patient and gives a scenario within which to understand the disorder. In this regard, a self-rating approach reported that 49% of patients attributed a favorable outcome to a physician's described treatment (Jankovic & Thomas, 2006).

It is very important to reassure the patient early on, for example emphasizing that this is an "involuntary" condition and is most likely the result of an impairment of neural pathways. Another option is to explain that some of the symptoms are stress-related symptoms, pointing out that stress is a common cause of many physical afflictions. A sincere, supportive, hopeful and, professional manner of approach will allow to understand and, at the same time, have patients understand what the movement disorder means, what is its functions, why and when it evolved. Some experts and the authors also suggest an active physiotherapy program, from the beginning, in order to desensitized the stress-induced contraction that generate the anomalous muscle jerks. Overall, this aspect of the treatment may corroborate the "physical" dimension of the disorder and may allow decreasing the symptom without activating psychological defence mechanisms (Williams et al., 2006; Rosebush & Mazurek, 2006). Besides, the physiotherapist frequently recognizes the fears and unhelpful preconceptions which patients have, and can stimulate and compliment patients in their activity in a much more confidential mode than the allied psychotherapist.

Medication treatment can be initiated and the choice of a particular drug depends on the accompanying psychiatric or medical conditions. In authors experience these most frequently include anxiety, depression, insomnia and headache, and a low dose of tricyclic antidepressants or benzodiazepine can help with symptoms of pain and muscle tension.

Large randomized studies in patients with PMDs are lacking, and evidence for treatment is largely based on retrospective, case control, and case report studies. Several other clinical trials, not specifically designed for PMDs but for other forms of conversion or somatoform disorders, are treated more in detail elsewhere in this book.

In a study by Voon and co-workers, 23 patients were identified with PMDs, and 15 patients agreed to be treated with antidepressant drugs. Of the 15 patients, 10 were diagnosed with primary PMDs, and the remaining 5 were diagnosed with PMDs and another somatoform disorder. Patients were treated with either citalopram or paroxetine. Those who did not respond were switched to venlafaxine. Of the primary PMDs patients, 80% (8 patients) had marked improvement, and 7 patients had complete remission. None of the 5 patients with PMDs and other somatoform disorders improved. (Voon, & Lang, 2005).

An open-label trial of somatisation disorder studied the efficacy of nefazodone in patients with and without comorbid depression and showed improvement in clinical global impression and functioning in 73% of patients (Menza et al., 2001).

In a study by Rampello and colleagues, 18 patients were treated (6 with haloperidol and 12 with sulpiride). The latter group showed remarkable improvement in 8 patients, partial improvement in 2 patients, and no improvement in 1 patient. The haloperidol group showed 1 patient with remarkable improvement, 3 with partial improvement, and 2 with no improvement. This study showed a possible positive correlation between dopamine blockade, drug-induced plasma prolactine concentration, and improvement in a patient's conversion symptoms.

Hinson and colleagues recruited ten patients with PMDs for a single-blind clinical trial to receive 12 weeks of treatment with outpatient psychodynamic psychotherapy and use of antidepressants or anxiolytic drugs, depending on comorbid psychiatric diagnosis. The movement disorder was videotaped before and after treatment and rated in a random order by a rater unaware of treatment allocation using PMDRS. All patients were diagnosed with conversion disorder. Nine of ten recruited patients completed the study. Total mean PMDRS and total mean PMDRS function scores improved with psychotherapeutic intervention. There were significant treatment effects in Hamilton depression scores, Beck anxiety scores, and global assessment of function.

Shapiro and Teasell described a case series of 39 consecutive patients with conversion disorder who were told that they had a musculoskeletal problem that could resolve completely if they had an organic etiology. If the patients did not improve after 4 weeks, then they were told that it was a psychiatric condition, and the treatment would be modified to help them improve completely. If they did not improve, then they were given a final diagnosis of conversion disorder, and they were told that they could not improve because of an unconscious need to remain disabled. In 8 of 9 patients with acute conversion disorder (symptoms <2 months), the treatment was successful. In 1 of 28 chronic (>6 months duration) patients, behavioral treatment was successful (Shapiro & Teasell, 2004). In a randomised controlled clinical trial, Moene and colleagues assigned 48 patients to receive either hypnosis or a control intervention consisting of generic elements of psychotherapy. Outcome measures were a video rating scale for motor conversion symptoms, the symptom checklist-90, and elements of the international classification of impairments, disabilities, and handicaps. Independent of the treatment condition, 65% of patients showed substantial improvement at post-treatment assessment and 84% at 6-month follow-up, which suggests that both psychotherapy and hypnosis have a role in the treatment of conversion disorder.

A meta-analysis of studies of cognitive behavioral therapy for various somatisation syndromes showed a definite or possible treatment effect of cognitive behavioral therapy in 71 of patients (Kroenke et al., 2000). Randomized controlled studies support the efficacy of individual cognitive behavioral therapy for the treatment of hypochondriasis, body dysmorphic disorder, and undifferentiated somatoform disorders including medically unexplained symptoms, chronic fatigue syndrome, and noncardiac chest pain (Looper & Kirmayer, 2002; Allen et al., 2006).

In a single-blind study, 16 patients with PMDs completed a thrice-weekly, 12-weeks mild walking program. Assessments included DSM-IV interview, PMDRS, Beck Anxiety Inventory, Hamilton Depression Scale, V02 Max, and body mass index. A comparison of all measures taken at study onset and after completing the exercise program indicates statistically significant improvements. We observed a relevant improvement in 10 of 16 patients (62%). The mean difference for the primary outcome (PMDRS total) corresponded to about 70%. Compliance was good, and there were no adverse effects. This study provides preliminary evidence for regular low-medium intensity exercise as a safe, adequate, and pleasing intervention for PMD. (Dallocchio et al., 2010).

A retrospective study was performed in 10 patients with psychogenic gait. Patients were treated with physical therapy, occupational therapy, and recreational therapy, and psychological interventions were used in appropriate cases. All patients were able to ambulate normally before discharge (Speed, 1996).

A successful management of the three cases described in another report involved a combination of behavioral modification and physical therapy interventions Abnormal movement patterns were ignored, and correct movement patterns were reinforced using feedback and praise. All three patients showed complete resolution of their symptoms (Ness, 2007).

There is one published abstract report where EMG biofeedback as used as a treatment for psychogenic tremor; this open label study estimated the effectiveness of biofeedback therapy and found improvement in 60% of 15 subjects (Levy et al., 2006). One case report described a dramatic response to acupuncture in a patient with chronic, treatment-resistant PMD (Van Nuenen et al. 2007).

A preliminary experience with the application of transcranial magnetic stimulation to achieve symptom relief in psychogenic tremor showed its effectiveness in conversion disorder of motor subtype. In a group of 8 patients, 4 responded, 2 showed temporary improvement, and 2 did not respond. (Dafotakis et al., 2008). In a case report, a patient with psychogenic dysphonia was reported to have a dramatic improvement after 2 sessions of repetitive transcranial magnetic stimulation over the prefrontal cortex (Chastan et al., 2009).

6. Prognosis

The outcome of patients with PMDs is variable, and several elements that influence recovery have been described. These include the nature, chronicity, seriousness of the veiled psychopathology, the influence of external factors, the attitude of the patient, the capability of the patient's support system, as well as the modalities and the effectiveness of treatment. Predominantly, data are available on the outcome of conversion disorders in general.

Williams et al. found a permanent benefit in 52% of 131 patients, with complete, considerable and moderate relief in 25%, 21%, and 8% respectively, after a follow-up of an average of 1,8 years. They found that age, gender, intelligence, chronicity of illness, and types of symptoms had no influence on the outcome. In another longitudinal study of 228 patients with PMDs improvement symptoms was noticed in 56% of patients, 21% reported no change, and 22% were worse after an average duration of 3.4 years' follow-up. In this study, poor prognostic factors were inconsistent movements, dissatisfaction with the physician, long duration of illness, positive history of smoking, and suggestibility. Good prognostic factors were good physical health, positive social life, patients' perception of receiving effective treatment by the physician, elimination of a stressor, comorbid diagnosis of anxiety, and attribution of a specific medication (Thomas et al., 2006). A follow up report compared 66 patients with PMDs to 704 with Parkinson's disease and showed comparable levels of of disability and physical quality of life, increased psychiatric comorbidity and more severe mental health disorders, even if patients with PMDs were 20 years younger and had a shorter pathological condition (Anderson et al., 2007).

Feinstein et al. reported persistence of abnormal movements in 90% of 88 patients followed up for an average of 3,2 years. Poor outcome was associated with psychiatric, long duration of symptoms, and insidious onset of symptoms (Feinstein, (2001). Much higher rates of improvement was reported in another longitudinal study of 127 patients with psychogenic tremor followed for at least 3 years, 55% reported improvement in tremor. Dissatisfaction with the physician was identified as the stronger prognostic risk factor of poor long term outcome; good prognostic factors were physician's prescribed treatment, elimination of stressor, specific medication, stress management, biofeedback, and psychotherapy (Jankovic et al., (2004). Other authors described the presenting features and long-term outcomes of 33 patients with electrophysiologically-confirmed psychogenic tremor by a follow-up questionnaire. After a median follow-up of 3.2 years, 64% of patients valued their disability as moderate severe, 27% had complete resolution of symptoms, and 9% reported mild unchanged symptoms. Of the patients who had resolution of symptoms, in 15% the resolution occurred spontaneously and in 12% it occurred after an intervention (1 with an antidepressant, 1 with psychology/rehabilitation, 1 with hypnotherapy, 1 with behavioral therapy). (McKeon et al., (2008). In a follow study involving 64 patients affected by medically unexplained movement disorders, 28% showed complete resolution of symptoms, 20% improved, 14% remained unchanged, and 38% worsened after 6 years of follow-up (Crimlisk et al., 1998). Finally, other data showed that 83% of 42 patients with functional weakness or sensory symptoms, who have been investigated as inpatients, have symptoms and disability after a median of 12 years following initial assessment. In this study patients with only sensory symptoms and signs at presentation had significantly better outcome in terms of higher physical functioning, social functioning , and pain than patients with any symptoms or signs of weakness , a higher age of onset predicted lower physical functioning at follow up (Stone et al., 2003). If untreated, PMDs are inclined to become chronic, and follow-up data in several studies demonstrate 65-95% of patients are left with a high level of disability (Factor et al., 1995; Williams et al., 2005), undoubtedly asserting the necessity for un effective early intervention to convert the "sick role" of the patient and return to the suitable level of function as quickly as possible.

7. Conclusion

PMDs are important and underdiagnosed cause of major neurologic disability. Signs and symptoms must be interpreted in the overall clinical and psychological context. Neurophysiological and imaging findings may provide important understanding and confirmation of the diagnosis, but some cases pose a arduous challenge to both neurologists and psychiatrists. An adequate explanation of the symptoms to patients is a prerequisite to successful further treatment (Stone & Carson, 2010; Friedman & LaFrance, 2010). To date, the treatment for each patient with PMDs is individualized and may include psychotherapeutic interventions, behavioral therapy, pharmachotherapy, physical therapy, hypnosis and others. Recovery is sometimes delayed and can take place over the course of months and several patients are left with a high level of disability, but a supportive, nonjudgmental, and persistent multidisciplinary approach can divert the illness course to an excellent clinical outcome (Rosebush & Mazurek, 2006). Further researches are required, not only to improve the understanding and management of these heterogeneous diseases, but also for reconsidering conversion disorder terminology and positive rather than negative diagnostic criteria.

8. References

Allen, L.A., Woolfolk, R.L., Escobar JI, et al. (2006). Cognitive-behavioral therapy for somatization disorder: a randomized controlled trial. Arch Intern Med. 166(14):1512–8.

Anderson, K.E., GruberBaldini, A.L., Vaughan, C.G. et al. (2007). Impact of psychogenic movement disorders versus Parkinson's on disability, qualiy of life, and psychopathology. Movement Disord. 22:2204-2209.

Baik, J.S., Lang, A.E. (2007). Gait abnormalities in psychogenic movement disorders. Mov Disord. 22(3):395–9.

Barsky, A.J., Orav E.J., Bates D.W. (2005) Somatization increases medical utilization and costs independent of psychiatric and medical comorbidity. Arch Gen Psychiatry. 62(8):903-10.

Benaderette, S., Zanotti, F.P., Apartis, E. et al. (2006). Psychogenic parkinsonism: a combination of clinical, electrophysiological, and [(123)I]-FP-CIT SPECTscan explorations improves diagnostic accuracy. Mov Disord. 21(3):310–7.

Bhatia, K.P., (2001). Psychogenic gait disorders. Adv Neurol. 87: 251–54.
Bhatia, K.P., Schneider, S.A. (2007) Psychogenic tremor and related disorders. J Neurol. 254(5):569-74.
Breuer, J., Freud S., Studies on hysteria (1893-1895). In: Strachey J, Strachey A, eds. The standard edition of the complete psychological works of Sigmund Freud, (Vol. 2). London: Hogart Press & Institute of Psycho-Analysis, 1955.
Brown, P., Thomson, P.D. (2001). Electrophysiological aids to jerks, spasms and tremor. Mov Disord. 16:595.99.
Brown, R.J. Dissociation and conversion in psychogenic illness. In: Hallet M, Yudofsky SC, Lang AE, et al., editors. To psychogenic movement disorders. Philadelphia, USA: Lippincott Williams & Wilkins; 2006, pp. 131-143.
Carson, A., Stone, J., Hibberd C. et al. (2011). Disability, distress and unemployment in neurology outpatients with symptoms 'unexplained by disease'. J Neurol Neurosurg Psychiatry, in press.
Charcot, J.M. (1889). Clinical Lectures on Diseases of the Nervous System. In New Sydenham Society, London, pp. 220–259.
Chastan, N., Parain, D, Verin, E. et al. (2009). Psychogenic aphonia: spectacular recovery after motor cortex transcranial magnetic stimulation. J Neurol Neurosurg Psychiatr. 80(1):94.
Cojan, Y., Waber L., Carruzzo, A., Vuilleumier, P. (2009). Motor inhibition in histerical conversion paralisis; 47(3):1026-37.
Crimlisk, H.L., Bhatia, K., Cope, H., David, A., Marsden, C.D., Ron, M.A. (1998). Slater revisited: 6 year follow up study of patients with medically unexplained motor symptoms. Br. Med. J. 316, 582–586.
Criswell, S., Sterling, C., Swisher, L. et al. (2010). Sensitivity and specificity of the finger tapping task for the detection of psychogenic movement disorders. Parkinsonism Relat Disord. 16(3):197-201.
Cubo, E., Hinson, V.K., Goetz, C.G. et al. (2005). Transcultural comparison of psychogenic movement disorders. Mov Disord;20:1343-45.
Czarnecki, K., Jones, D.T., Burnett, M.S. et al. (2011). SPECT perfusion patterns distinguish psychogenic from essential tremor. Parkinsonism and related disorders (in press).
Deuschl, G., Koster, B., Lucking, C., Scheidt, C. (1998). Diagnostic and pathophysiological aspects of psychogenic tremors. Mov. Disord. 13, 294–302.
Espay, A.J., Goldenhar, L.M, Voon, V., et al. (2009). Opinion and clinical practices related to diagnosing and managing patients with psychogenic movement disorders: an international survey of Movement Disorder Society Members. Mov Disord. 24(9):1366-74.
Fahn, S. (1994). Psychogenic movement disorders. In: Marsden CD, Fahn S (eds) Movement Disorders 3. Buttenw Heinem, Oxford, pp. 359-72.
Fahn, S. The history of psychogenic movement disorders. In: Hallet M, Yudofsky SC, Lang AE, et al., editors. To psychogenic movement disorders. Philadelphia, USA: Lippincott Williams & Wilkins; 2006, pp. 24-31.
Factor, S.A., Podskalny,G.D., Molho, E.S. (1995). Psychogenicmovement disorders. Frequency, clinical profile and characteristics. J. Neurol. Neurosurg. Psychiatry 59, 406–412.
Factor, S, Lang, A.E, Weiner WJ. Drug Induced Movement Disorders. Mount Kisko, NY: Futura; 2005.

Feinstein A, Stergiopoulus V, Fine J, Lang AE. (2001). Psychiatric outcome in patients with a psychogenic movement disorder: a prospective study. Neuropsychiatry Neuropsychol Behav Neurol. 14:169-76.

Fink, G.R., Halligan, P.W., Marshall J.C. Neuroimaging og hysteria. In: Hallet M, Yudofsky SC, Lang AE, et al., editors. To psychogenic movement disorders. Philadelphia, USA: Lippincott Williams & Wilkins; 2006, pp. 230-237.

Friedman, J.H., LaFrance. W.C. Jr. (2010). Psychogenic disorders: the need to speak plainly. Arch Neurol. 67(6):753-5.

Freud, S., (1910). Psycho-analytic view of psychogenic disturbance of vision. The Standard Edition of the Complete Psychological Works of Sigmund Freud, 11. The Hogarth Press, London, pp. 209–218.

Gupta, A. Lang A.E. (2009). Psychogenic movement disorders. Current Opin Neurol. 22:430-436.

Hallet, M. (2010). Physiology of psychogenic movement disorders. J Clin Neuroscience. 17:959-65.

Hinson, V.K., Cubo, E., Comella, C., Leurgans, S., Goetz, C.G., (2005). Rating scale for psychogenic movement disorders: scale development and clinimetric testing. Mov Disord; 20: 1592–97.

Hinson, V.K., Cubo, E., Comella, C.L, Goetz, C.G., Leurgans, S. (2005) Rating scale for psychogenic movement disorders: scale development and clinimetric testing. Mov Disord;20:1592–1597.

Hinson, V.K., Weinstein, S., Bernard B., Leurgans, S.E, Goetz C.G., (2006) Single-blind clinical trial of pychotherapy for treatment of psychogenic movement disorders. Parkinsonism Relat Disord;12:177–180.

Hinson, V.K, Blacke Haren, W. (2006). Psychogenic movement disorders. Lancet Neurol;5:695-700.

Janet P., (1889). L'automatisme psychologique. Paris, NE: Felix Alcan.

Janet P., (1907) The major symptoms of hysteria. New York; Macmillan.

Jankovic, J., Thomas, M., Vuong, K.D. (2004). Long term outcome of psychogenic tremor. Neurology. 62(Suppl.5):A501.

Jankovic, J., Thomas, M., 2006. Psychogenic tremor and shaking. In: Hallett, M., Fahn, S., Jankovic, J., Lang, A.E., Cloninger, C.R., Yudofsky, C. (Eds.), Psychogenic Movement Disorders. InLippincott Williams and Wilkins, Philadelphia, pp. 42–47.

Jankovic, J., Cloninger, C.R., Fahn, S., Hallet, M., Lang, A.E,, Williams, D.T. Therapeutic approaches to psychogenic movement disorders. In: Hallet M, Yudofsky SC, Lang AE, et al., editors. To psychogenic movement disorders. Philadelphia, USA: Lippincott Williams & Wilkins; 2006, pp. 323–328.

Kagi, G., Bathia, K.P, Tolosa, E. (2010). The role of DAT-SPECT in movement disorders. J Neurol Neurosur Psychiatry. 81:5-12.

Kroenke, K., Swindle, R. (2000).Cognitive behavioral therapy for somatization and symptom syndromes: a critical review of controlled clinical trials. Psychother Psychosom. 69: 205–15.

Lang, A.E. General overview of psychogenic movement disorders: epidemiology, diagnosis, and prognosis. In: Hallet M, Yudofsky SC, Lang AE, et al., editors. To psychogenic movement disorders. Philadelphia, USA: Lippincott Williams & Wilkins; 2006, pp. 35-41

Lempert, T., Dieterich, M., Huppert, D., Brandt, T., (1990). Psychogenic disorders in neurology. Frequency and clinical spectrum. Acta Neurol. Scand. 82, 335–340.

Levy J.K., Thomas, M. Biofeedback therapy for psychogenic movement disorders. In: Hallet M, Yudofsky SC, Lang AE, et al., editors. To psychogenic movement disorders. Philadelphia, USA: Lippincott Williams & Wilkins; 2006. p 343-344.

Looper, K. J., Kirmayer, L. J. (2002). Behavioral medicine approaches to somatoform disorders. *J Consult Clin Psychol.* 70(3), pp. 810-827.

Mace, C.J., Trimble, M.,R. (1996). Ten year prognosis of conversion disorder. Br. J. Psychiatry 169, 282-288.

McAuley, J., Rothwell, J. (2004). Identification of psychogenic, distonic, and other organic tremors by a coherence entraiment test. Mov Disord. 19:253-67.

McKeon, A., Ahlskog, J.E., Bower, J.H. et al. (2008). Psychogenic tremor: long term prognosis in patients with electrophysiologically-confirmed disease.MovDisord. 24(1):72-6.

Menza, M., Lauritano, M., Allen, L. et al. (2001). Treatment of somatization disorder with nefazodone: a prospective, open-label study. Ann Clin Psychiatry. 13: 153-58.

Miyasaki, J.M., Sa, D.S., Galvez-Jmenez N. et al. (2003). Psychogenic movement disorders. Can J Neurol Sci; (30 Suppl 1):S94-100.

Moene, F.C., Landberg, E.H., Hoogduin, K.A. et al. (2000). Organic syndromes diagnosed as conversion disorder: identification and frequency in a study of 85 patients. J Psychosom Res. 49(1):7-12.

Monday, K., Jankovic, J. (1993). Psychogenic myoclonus. Neurology. 43(2):349-52.

Morgan. J.C., Sethi, K.D. (2006). Psychogenic parkinsonism. In: Hallet M, Yudofsky SC, Lang AE, et al., editors. To psychogenic movement disorders. Philadelphia, USA: Lippincott Williams & Wilkins. pp. 62-68.

Munhoz, R.P., Zavala, J.A., Becker. N., Teive H.A. (2010). Cross-cultural influences on psychogenic movement disorders - a comparative review with a Brazilian series of 83 cases. Clin Neurol Neurosurg. 113(2):115-8.

Munts, A.G., Koehler, P.J. (2010). How psychogenic is dystonia? Views from past to present. Brain. 133; pp. 1552-1564.

Ness, D. (2007). Physical therapy management for conversion disorder: case series. J Neurol Phys Ther. 31(1):30-9.

Ng, B.Y. (1999). Hysteria: a cross-cultural comparison of its origins and history. Hist Psychiatry. 10(39, pt 3):287-301.

Nowak, D., A., Fink, G.R. (2009). Psychogenic movement disorders: aetiology, phenomenology, neuroanatomical correlates and therapeutic approach. Neuroimage. 47:1015-25.

Okun, M.S., Rodriguez, R.L., Foote, K.D., et al. (2007). The "chair test" to aid in the diagnosis of psychogenic gait disorders. Neurologist. 13(2):87-91.

Ovsiew, F. An overview of the psychiatric approach to conversion disorder. In: Hallet M, Yudofsky SC, Lang AE, et al., editors. To psychogenic movement disorders. Philadelphia, USA: Lippincott Williams & Wilkins; 2006; pp. 115-121.

Peckham, E.L., Hallett, M. (2009). Psychogenic movement disorders. Neurol Clin. 27:801-819.

Rampello, L., Raffaele, R., Nicoletti. G. et al. (1996) Hysterical neurosis of the conversion type: therapeutic activity of neuroleptics with different hyperprolactinemic potency. Neuropsychobiology 1996; 33: 186-88.

Reich, S.G., (2006) Psychogenic movement disorders. Semin Neurol;26:289-206.

Rosebush, P., Mazurek, M.F. (2006). Treatment of conversion disorder. . In: Hallet M, Yudofsky SC, Lang AE, et al., editors. To psychogenic movement disorders. Philadelphia, USA: Lippincott Williams & Wilkins; 2006; pp. 289-301.

Scherfler, C., Schwarz, J., Antonini, A., et al. (2007). Role of DAT-SPECT in the diagnostic work up of parkinsonism. Mov Disord;22(9):1229–38.
Schrag, A., Trimble, M., Quinn, N., et al. (2004). The syndrome of fixed dystonia: an evaluation of 103 patients. Brain. 127:2360-72.
Schrag, A. Psychogenic dystonia and reflex sympathetic dystrophy. In: Hallett M, Yudofsky SC, Lang AE, et al, eds. Psychogenic movement disorders. Philadelphia, USA: Lippincott Williams & Wilkins, 2006: 53–61.
Shapiro, A.P., Teasell, R.W. (2004). Behavioural interventions in the rehabilitation of acute v. chronic non-organic (conversion/factitious) motor disorders. Br J Psychiatry. 185:140–6.
Shibasaky, H., Hallett, M. What is the Bereitschaftspotential? Clin Neurophysiol. 117:2341-56.
Shill, H., Gerber, P. (2006). Evaluation of clinical diagnostic criteria for psychogenic movement disorders. Mov Disord;21(8):1163–8.
Smith, G.R. Jr, Monson, R.A., Ray, D.C. (1986) Patients with multiple unexplained symptoms. Their characteristic, functonal health, and health care utilization. Arch Intern Med. 146(1):69-72.
Speed, J. (1996). Behavioral management of conversion disorder: retrospective study. Arch Phys Med Rehabil. 77(2):147–54.
Stone, J., Sharpe, M., Rothwell, P.M., et al. (2004). The 12 year prognosis of unilateral functional weakness and sensory disturbance. J Neurol Neurosurg Psychiatry. 74:591–6.
Stone, J., Carson, A. (2010). Functional neurologic symptoms: assessment and management. Neurol Clin. 29:1-18.
Stone, J., Vuilleumier, P., Friedman, J.H. (2010). Conversion disorders. Separating "how" from "why". Neurology; 74:190-91.
Sudarsky, L. Psychogenic gait disorders. (2006). Semin Neurol;26(3):351–6.
Thomas, M., Jankovic, J. (2004). Psychogenic movement disorders: diagnosis and management. CNS Drugs. 18(7):437–52.
Thomas, M., Vuong, K.D., Jankovic. J. (2006). Long-term prognosis of patients with psychogenic movement disorders. Parkinsonism Relat Disord. 12(6):382–7.
Van Nuenen, B.F., Wohlgemuth, M., Wong Chung, R.E. et al. (2007). Acupuncture for psychogenicmovement disorders: treatment or diagnostic tool? Mov Disord. 22(9):1353–5.
Voon, V., Lang, A.E. (2005) Antidepressant treatment outcomes of psychogenic movement disorder. J Clin Psychiatry;66:1529–1534.
Voon, V., Gallea, C., Hattori. et al. (2010). The involuntary nature of conversion disorder. Neurology. 19;74(3):223-8.
Vuilleumier, P., 2005. Hysterical conversion and brain function. Prog. Brain Res.150, 309–329.
Williams, D.T., Ford B, Fahn S. (1995). Phenomenology and psychopathology related to psychogenic movement disorders. Adv Neurol;65:233-57.
Williams D.T., Ford B., Fahn, S. (2005). Treatment issues in psychogenic-neuropsychiatric movement disorders. Adv Neurol. 96:350-63.
Williams, D.T., et al. Natural history of psychogenic movement disorder. In: Hallet M, Yudofsky SC, Lang AE, et al., editors. To psychogenic movement disorders. Philadelphia, USA: Lippincott Williams & Wilkins; 2006; pp. 274-286.
Zeuner K.E.,, Shoge, R.O., Goldstein, S.R. et al. (2003). Accelerometry to distinguish psychogenic from essential or parkinsonian tremor. Neurology. 61:548-550.